PENNINGTON CENTER NUTRITION SERIES

GEORGE A. BRAY, MD, *and* DONNA H. RYAN, MD, *Editors*

VOLUME 5

Molecular and Genetic Aspects of Obesity

PENNINGTON CENTER
NUTRITION SERIES

Sponsored by the Pennington Biomedical Research Center

VOLUME 5

Molecular and Genetic Aspects of Obesity

Edited by
GEORGE A. BRAY, MD
and
DONNA H. RYAN, MD

LOUISIANA STATE UNIVERSITY PRESS
BATON ROUGE AND LONDON

Designer: Laura Roubique Gleason
Typeface: Palatino
Typesetter: Impressions Book and Journal Services, Inc.
Printer and binder: Thomson-Shore, Inc.

Published with the assistance of the Pennington Biomedical Research Foundation.

LIBRARY OF CONGRESS CATALOGING-IN-PUBLICATION DATA

Molecular and genetic aspects of obesity / edited by George A. Bray and
  Donna H. Ryan.
     p.   cm. — (Pennington center nutrition series ; v. 5)
     "Published with the assistance of the Pennington Biomedical
  Research Foundation"—T.p. verso.
     Includes bibliographical references and index.
     ISBN 0-8071-2025-1 (cloth : alk. paper)
     1. Obesity—Molecular aspects—Congresses.   2. Obesity—Genetic
  aspects—Congresses.   I. Bray, George A.   II. Ryan, Donna H.
  III. Pennington Biomedical Research Foundation.   IV. Series.
     [DNLM: 1. Obesity—metabolism—congresses.   2. Obesity—genetics—
  congresses.   3. Adipose Tissue—metabolism—congresses.   4. Mice,
  Transgenic—congresses.   W1 PE289 v.5 1996 / WD 210 M718 1996]
  RC628.M59   1996
  616.3'98—dc20
  DNLM/DLC
  for Library of Congress   95-35680
                                                                         CIP

*To C. B. "Doc" Pennington, whose wisdom and generosity
make this series possible*

Contents

PART II

Biology of Animal Models

PART III

Regulation of Food Intake

PART VII
Transgenic Models of Obesity

Preface

Molecular biological techniques have permeated all fields of biology. The first conference to recognize this important dimension in the field of obesity was organized by the University of California at Los Angeles (UCLA) in 1989, and its proceedings subsequently were published in the Keystone Conference Series under the title *Obesity: Towards a Molecular Approach* (New York: Wiley-Liss, 1990). A second conference was held five years later at the Pennington Biomedical Research Center in Baton Rouge, Louisiana. The papers presented at the second conference build on the foundation of the first and document the rapid expansion in the field of molecular biology. In the five years between the two conferences, some major developments have occurred.

1. Three genes for models of obesity have been identified and cloned, and their molecular mechanisms are well on the way to being understood (see Klebig *et al.*).
2. Several genes have been introduced into transgenic mice that have produced or prevented obesity.

The first section of this volume deals with genetic models of obesity and the control of nutrient intake. An overview of animal models of obesity is presented in a review paper by Bray, which covers much of the literature published since the earlier conference was held. The primary mechanisms for the development of obesity include reduced thermogenesis often resulting from an imbalance in the autonomic nervous system, increased nutrient partitioning into fat because of hyperinsulinemia, low sympathetic activity, and high glucocorticoids. This review is followed by a series of papers dealing with specific aspects of genetic obesity.

In the first paper in this section, Friedman, whose group recently cloned the *ob* gene, reviews quantitative approaches to locating genetic abnormalities. Development of genetic maps by linkage has two pre-requisites. First, there must be defined genetic markers, and second, there must be a group of individuals in which variations among these markers can be scored. A landmark publication by Botstein (*Am J Hum Genet.* 1980;32:314–331) was the basis for the current widespread use of short simple sequence length polymorphisms (SSLP) to make detailed chromosomal maps of differences in linkage for genetic traits between groups of animals. These techniques have been supplemented by the use of yeast artificial chromosomes (YAC) as cloning vectors to further identify the potential genes located by the SSLP. Friedman discusses the information related to this technique as applied to the study of obesity with special reference to the *ob* and *db* genes, focusing primarily on the obese and diabetes mouse, with which his laboratory has been working. The next two papers in this section, by Fisler and Warden and by West and associates, respectively, look at the technique of SSLP for identification of genetic loci associated with the phenotypic expression of obesity in two particular strains of mice. Fisler and Warden have used the quantitative trait locus (QTL) system of SSLP to examine the polygenic obesity that develops by crossing two interfertile species of mice (*Mus spretus* × C57BL/6J). These animals develop obesity, hyperinsulinemia, insulin resistance, and hypertriglyceridemia. Two chromosomal locations, one on chromosome 7 and the other on chromosome 6, show significant associations with plasma cholesterol and carcass lipid. In the model used by Dr. West, QTL mapping has identified chromosomes 4, 9, and 15 as highly likely sites for genes that control total body fat and possibly regional fat distribution. The final presentation by Klebig *et al.* describes the recent advances following their identification of the genetic defect responsible for the obesity and yellow coat color in the obese yellow mouse. The defect in the yellow mouse is the result of ectopic expression of the agouti protein in many tissues in which this protein is normally not expressed. Whether the protein that is produced results in its myriad effects by interaction with the melanocyte-stimulating hormone receptor (MSH-R) or by interfering with the activity of other peptides such as melanocyte-stimulating hormone (α-MSH) corticotropin-releasing hormone (CRH), or corticotropin (ACTH) remains to be established.

Part II deals with some of the biological changes associated with genetic obesity. The first paper is by Smith and his colleagues and examines the control of meal size in the Zucker fatty rat. Two abnormalities that may account for the increased meal size of obese rats are suggested by these authors. First, there is increased positive oral-sensory feedback for corn oil in relation to sucrose. Second, there is a decreased negative feedback response to cholecystokinin, which has a sex-specific component present in male rats but not in female rats. That paper is followed by one from Rolland and her colleagues, who show the conjugate increase in enzymes involved in lipogenesis that occurs shortly after the development of hyperinsulinemia in the genetically obese rat. The primary mechanism for this increased activity is enhanced transcription of genetic messages. These authors provide data supporting earlier observations by Bray, York, Hainault, and Lavau that there may be an alteration in transacting transcription factors involved in the control of these lipogenic enzymes. In her paper, Bégin-Heick focuses on the mechanisms involved in the activation of adenylate cyclase in genetically obese mice. This work with adipose tissue has shown that the transduction of adenylyl cyclase messages for the production of cyclic adenosine monophosphate (cAMP) is abnormally low in several tissues of the obese (*ob/ob*) mouse. Bégin-Heick has shown that the β-3 adrenergic receptor is the major isoform in the mouse adipose tissue and that the levels of this receptor are severely decreased in the obese mouse. In contrast to most other defects, adrenalectomy does not restore the activity of this β-adrenergic receptor to normal in adipose tissue, although it does do so in liver. Of particular interest is the observation that the function of the β-3 adrenergic receptor in adipose tissue is extremely sensitive to small changes in the concentration of guanosine-triphosphate (GTP). The two remaining contributions in Part II deal with the critical role of glucocorticoids in the development of obesity. Braymer and his associates have demonstrated the presence of a nuclear factor that retards binding to the upstream regions of tyrosine aminotransferase (TAT), suggesting, along with the earlier paper of Rolland *et al.*, the importance of transacting genetic transcriptional factors in modulating the response to glucocorticoids. Finally, Hotamisligil and Spiegelman suggest that tumor necrosis factor alpha (TNF-α) released from adipose tissue may be involved in the development of insulin resistance in the genetically obese fatty rat.

Part III of this volume looks at the regulation of nutrient intake in the development of obesity. This process involves both central and peripheral mechanisms. Substantial new information has developed in this area in the years since the Keystone conference. One of these has been the understanding of the important role played by neuropeptide Y (NPY). Literature on this topic is reviewed by Kalra *et al.*, who suggest that the hyperphagia in both the genetic and hypothalamic models of obesity may be a result of enhanced NPY turnover. The role of galanin, a second peptide that stimulates food intake and may have specific stimulatory effects on fat intake, is reviewed by Leibowitz and Aka-bayashi. Also, the neural substrate for rewards in the nucleus ac-cumbens associated with food selection is discussed by Hoebel and his colleagues, who provide a global model for the monoaminergic mod-ulation of feeding.

A second series of papers in this section deals with the peripheral regulation of food intake. The pentapeptide enterostatin, described by York and Lin, suppresses fat intake whether injected peripherally or centrally. The peripheral inhibitory effects of this peptide appear to be modulated by afferent messages from the vagus nerve. The interface between the vagus nerve and the gastrointestinal tract and its anatomic connection to the brain forms a central theme in the presentation by Berthoud. The interface between hepatic messages and the vagus nerve is also a key part of the presentation by Friedman *et al.*, who argue that hepatic messages may be modulated by hepatic levels of adenosine triphosphate (ATP). The final paper in this section, by Brindley and Wang, examines the relationship between glucocorticoids and insulin as modulators of food intake.

The next section of the book begins with an overview by Brunzell on the relationship between low-density lipoproteins as a biochemical marker for visceral obesity and insulin resistance. It is now clear that the insulin resistance and other defects are associated with the small lipoprotein particle as opposed to the large, fluffy lipoproteins. Brunzell develops this theme and its implications for the onset of obesity. This is followed by a section dealing with the differentiation and metabolism of adipose tissue. Ailhaud *et al.* review the multistep phenomenon in the transformation of adipoblast to mature fat cell. The stages take fat cells from the adipoblast to the preadipocyte to the mature differenti-ated adipocyte. Ailhand identifies the markers that specify each of these phases and the critical hormonal factors involved in the transition from one phase to the next. One of these important factors is insulin-like growth factor-I (IGF-I). The relationship of IGF-I to the development of adipocytes is discussed in a paper by Ramsay. Both IGF-I and its binding protein (IGFBP) are paracrine factors. Growth hormone administration increases IGF-I, which may be counterbalanced by an increase in IGFBP. Defects in production of IGFBP to counteract the effects of IGF-I might be involved in the development of obesity. These two papers on development of adipocytes are followed by Strosberg's presentation on the molecular biology of the β-3 adrenergic receptor, which he and his colleagues have cloned. Its tissue localization and developmental control are dealt with in comparison to β-1 and β-2 adrenergic receptors. Lafontan and his colleagues discuss the α- and β-adrenergic receptors in fat cells and their control. These authors also discuss the important role of adenosine α-1 receptors, prostaglandin receptors, and the NPY/PYY (peptide YY) receptors as inhibitors of lipolysis. They point out that inhibitory regulation of lipolysis seems to involve two major systems. The first is a constitutive one using adenosine and prostaglandin receptors. The second is a regulatory system involving neuroendocrine messages provided by circulating norepinephrine, epinephrine NPY/PYY. Finally, Arner reviews the control of lipolysis in the human adipocyte and information being gleaned using microdialysis technology. Although defects have been demonstrated in the control of lipolysis in peripheral adipose tissue from human subjects, lipolytic defects in the more active visceral adipose tissue, if present, remain to be established in obese subjects.

Epidemiologic studies have contributed significantly to our understanding of the genetics of human obesity as described in Part V of this publication. Price reviews the population studies dealing with human obesity, and Sørensen reviews the adoption studies related to our understanding of this problem. In his review, Price suggests that on the basis of power calculations, African-American families may show particular promise for identifying obesity genes. Bouchard reviews the use of sib-pair linkage for understanding genetic epidemiology based on his work with the Quebec Family Study. The final two papers, by Burns *et al.* and Mitchell and Rao, respectively, review the data that has accumulated from the Muscatine Family Study and from the Quebec study in genetic epidemiologic terms.

Per Björntorp presents the final overview in this symposium. Björntorp and his colleagues have been leaders in understanding the effects of variation in regional fat distribution and its biology. In his presentation, Björntorp reviews his current concept of the central and peripheral control mechanisms involved in the development of visceral and subcutaneous fat patterns.

Molecular markers in human obesity have become more prevalent. Beales *et al.* review their experience with genetic markers, and this paper is followed by Weigle's presentation on potential candidate genes as a technique for approaching the problem of genetics in obesity. The work by Beales *et al.* suggests that the best hope of identifying the major gene believed to be associated with obesity will be through linkage studies in sib-pairs and by positional cloning. A complementary approach is to study candidate genes based on population association studies. With this method, this group has identified associations between either obesity, body fat distribution, or hyperinsulinemia, and the genes for insulin, apo-lipoprotein D, and the glucocorticoid receptor. The final paper in this section, by Nicholls *et al.,* reviews the advances in understanding the defect on chromosome 15 that is responsible for the development of the Prader-Willi syndrome. The Prader-Willi syndrome is transmitted by a defect on paternal chromosome 15. A similar genetic transmission by a defective maternal chromosome produces Angelman's syndrome, in which there is no obesity. The difference between these two syndromes is considered to result from intrauterine imprinting leading to expression of different genetic constellations in the conceptus.

Discussions of transgenic models make up the final section of this book. The relation of these models to energy expenditure is one of the new areas of molecular biology as applied to the study of obesity. The first paper is by Cassard-Doulcier *et al.,* who review information on uncoupling protein in brown adipose tissue and its regulation. Lowell and his colleagues have used a suicide transgene to abolish expression of the uncoupling protein in brown adipose tissue. In addition to being obese, the animals studied also develop hyperphagia as they mature. The relationship of the defect in expression of coupling protein in brown adipose tissue to the subsequent development of hyperphagia probably can be traced to the thermostatic hypothesis proposed by Brobeck more than forty years ago (Brobeck JR. Mechanism of the development of obesity in animals with hypothalamic lesions. *Physiol Rev.* 1946;26:541–559.). The introduction of transgenes that overexpress glucose 3-phosphate dehydrogenase has provided another model of thermogenic energy wasting. Kozak *et al.* observe that in lean animals overexpression of GPDH depresses UCP in brown adipose tissue. When this overexpression is bred into the *db/db* mouse, the obesity fails to develop, although the animals become markedly hyperphagic. This modification of the glycerophosphate cycle provides an important mechanism for modulation of energy expenditure. Gnudi *et al.* describe their work on the overexpression of the glucose transporter (GLUT4). In the affected animals, a mild degree of obesity is present. Finally, Barden describes his work on the incorporation of antisense RNA for glucocorticoid into the brain. His animals also developed obesity without hyperphagia. This may be a reflection of altered quantities of pro-opiomelanocortin processing with increased proportions of methylated and nonmethylated forms of melanocytes-stimulating hormone (MSH) and ACTH and endorphin in the hypothalamus.

The papers presented at this symposium open new doors to understanding the development of obesity using molecular biological tools. It is clear that before another five years have passed, a greater understanding will undoubtedly lead to new therapeutic approaches to the treatment of human obesity.

This fifth volume in the Pennington Center Nutrition Series, like its predecessors, is dedicated to C. B. "Doc" Pennington. His wisdom and philanthropic generosity made this important symposium possible. Through Mr. Pennington's encouragement, a planning committee consisting of Dr. David York, Dr. David West, Dr. Douglas Braymer, and Dr. Gary Truett worked to bring together the world's leading authorities in the field of molecular biology and genetics of obesity. This volume represents the proceedings of that meeting, which was held in Baton Rouge, Louisiana, on February 20–22, 1994.

In addition to the generous contributions of Doc Pennington, the work of other individuals was essential for the development and execution of this conference. They include Lloyd Moon and Mary Dawson of the Pennington Biomedical Research Foundation, Ben Phillips, Millie Cutrer, and the Pennington Center docents. Grateful appreciation goes to Mr. Phillips for his editorial work and to Louisiana State University Press for allowing us to publish this volume in the ongoing series.

PART I

Genetic Models of Obesity

GEORGE A. BRAY

Mechanisms for Development of Genetic, Hypothalamic, and Dietary Obesity

ABSTRACT

All animal models of obesity have three features in common; they have hyperinsulinemia; they show some degree of imbalance in the autonomic nervous system; and they are dependent for their expression on adrenal glucocorticoids. Several common final mechanisms appear to underlie the development of most types of obesity. Hyperphagia is a sufficient cause for most obesity, but most animal models become obese in the absence of hyperphagia. Animals with lesions in the paraventricular nucleus are an exception to this. A second common pathway is imbalance in the autonomic nervous system (the autonomic hypothesis). Obesity is associated with increased parasympathetic activity and decreased sympathetic activity. One consequence of this altered autonomic function is enhanced insulin secretion, which is a potent contributor to the channeling of nutrients into adipose tissue and to increasing fat-cell growth and development. A second consequence of reduced sympathetic function is reduced thermogenesis and hypothermia. Hypothermia is a necessary and sufficient cause for the increased storage of fat in the first two weeks in preweanling Zucker rats and probably obese (ob/ob) and diabetes (db/db) mice. Thereafter, hypothermia contributes to the nutrient partitioning into fat stimulated by hyperinsulinemia. A third common pathway is the endocrine system with adrenal glucocorticoids playing a critical role. In the absence of glucocorticoids, none of the obesities that have been examined will express itself completely, and if it does so at all it is only modestly. The fourth common mechanism involves hypothalamic disturbances associated with stunting, infertility, or reduced physical activity. These physiological mechanisms operate through one or more molecular mechanisms. Reduced activity of the stimulatory G-protein complex or increased activity of the inhibitory G-protein complex is one mechanism that could explain the reduced sympathetic activity, hypogonadism, and hyperphagia. The interaction of steroids with the gamma-aminobutyric-A receptor or other membrane receptors is a second possible general mechanism for the hyperphagia and other hypothalamic defects.

Introduction

The fifteen years since the proposal of an autonomic and endocrine hypothesis for obesity in 1979 (1) have seen rapid strides in molecular biology and genetics of obesity (2). It is thus fitting to review afresh the relationship between genetically transmitted forms of obesity and the kinds of obesity produced by diet or by manipulation of the hypothalamic or endocrine system. For this review, the models of obesity will be subdivided into three categories, shown in Table 1.

Most diseases are the result of an interaction between genetic susceptibility and environmental agents. This is the perspective I will use in looking at these models of obesity. The Zucker fatty rat (3), the obese (ob/ob) mouse, and the diabetes (db/db) mouse possess recessively inherited defects that lead unavoidably to obesity (4). At the other extreme are hypothalamic lesions and certain medications in which environment is predominant and genetics play only a minor role. That is, without an environmental disturbance these obesities would not have developed. A strong interaction between environment and genetics is seen in the dietary forms of obesity. Among the genetic types of obesity are those that are transmitted by single or recessive genes (4), those that are polygenic, and a recently described group of transgenic models (5–11) in which genetic manipulation is the basis for the observed obesity. In the second group, dietary obesities involve an interaction between environment and the genome. Exposing rodents to high-fat diets or diets with a variety of foods, commonly known as supermarket or cafeteria diets, will produce obesity in most but not all strains of rats (4). Some strains, such as the Osborne-Mendel rat (4) and the AKR mouse (12), readily develop obesity when eating high-fat diets. Other strains such as the S5B/Pl rat and the SWR mouse are resistant to developing obesity when eating high-fat diets. An example of dietary obesity that has little genetic involvement is the kind of obesity produced by forced feeding (13), either by conscious overeating or by chronic infusion of

Table 1. Models of Experimental Obesity

Genetic	Regulatory	Dietary
Dominant	Lesions	High-fat diet
Yellow mouse A^{vy} A^{iy} A^{sy} (chr 2)	Electrolytic or radio frequency in	Supermarket or cafeteria diet
Recessive	VMN	Meal feeding
Obese *ob/ob* (chr 6)	PVN	Tube feeding
Fatty Zucker (*fa/fa*) (chr 5)	Amygdala	Drink sucrose
[Koletsky (*fa*^{k})]	Chemical lesions	
[Corpulent (*fa*^{cp})]	6-hydroxydopamine lesion of ventral	
Diabetes (*db/db*) (chr 4)	noradrenergic bundle	
Adipose (*db*^{ad})	Monosodium glutamate	
Fat (chr 7)	Bipiperidyl mustard	
Tubby (chr 8)	Amphetamine (high dose)	
Polygenic	Chemical stimulation	
KK	Neuropeptide Y	
NZO	Norepinephrine	
C3H	5-Thioglucose	
Transgenic animals	Electrical stimulation	
Glucocorticoid receptor antisense		
Uncoupling protein knock-out		
GLUT4 (Overexpression)		
Glycerol 3-phosphate		
Dehydrogenase (overexpression)		

nutrients into the stomach of animals that would not otherwise become overweight.

In the third group, obesities are primarily the result of environmental manipulations. Hypothalamic lesions (1, 14), lesions in the amygdala (15), endocrine diseases, treatment with endocrine hormones, and several medications are all mechanisms by which body weight and body fat can be increased by "environmental agents" (4).

A number of features have been identified in most obesities, and these are summarized in Table 2, along with their relative level of importance in genetic, dietary and hypothalamic forms of obesity. Of these traits, hyperphagia, hyperinsulinemia, insulin resistance, and hyperglycemia are the most widely recognized. Other important traits include hypothermia, stunting, and infertility. Many of these abnormalities are much more severe in genetic forms of obesity than in dietary or hypothalamic obesity. In this paper I will discuss each of these characteristics with two questions in mind: first, what are the mechanisms that may be responsible for the characteristic, and second, is the characteristic sufficient and/or necessary for the development of obesity?

Hyperphagia

Hyperphagia is uniformly observed in animals with genetic obesity and in almost all forms of hypothalamic obesity (1, 16). The exceptions are weanling rats with hypothalamic lesions (17, 18) and animals with highly localized lesions in the ventromedial nucleus (19). In genetically obese animals, hyperphagia occurs after weaning, but by this time the

Table 2. Characteristics of Models for Experimental Obesity

	Necessary for Obesity	Sufficient for Obesity
Hyperphagia	No	Yes
Hyperinsulinemia	Yes	Yes
Insulin resistance	No	No
Stunting	No	No
Fat cell hyperplasia	No	No
Infertility	No	No
Hypothermia	Yes	Yes
Adrenal hyperfunction	Yes	Yes

animals are already obese (20). Although hyperphagia is sufficient to produce obesity, in only one instance is the hyperphagia necessary for its development, and that is in the animal with a lesion in the paraventricular nucleus (19). For the other forms of genetic and hypothalamic obesity it is clear that yoked feeding, tube feeding, or careful pair-feeding will not prevent the development of genetic or hypothalamic obesity (21, 22). The magnitude and duration of hyperphagia is greater when animals are eating a high-fat diet (4, 23). The Zucker fatty rat shows a delayed suppression of food intake following a carbohydrate preload (24). Collectively these findings suggest the presence, in one or more, of the mechanisms that integrate food intake with bodily needs. Figure 1 compares the weight gain and change in percent body fat of *ob/ob* mice fed identically to their lean littermates by yoked feeding. The lean animal pressed a bar to receive food. Each pellet received by the lean mouse led to a pellet appearing for the *ob/ob* mouse. The *ob/ob* mouse eating identical amounts of food gained more weight and more fat, indicating its increased efficiency. Several mechanisms including nutrients (25), monoamines, and peptides have been studied to understand the hyperphagia of obesity.

Monoamines and Amino Acids

Two major mechanisms have been proposed for the development of hyperphagia in genetically obese animals. The first is alterations in monoamine and amino acid neurotransmitters, and the second is alterations in neuropeptides. The feeding response to centrally administered norepinephrine (NE) appears to be similar in genetically obese (Zucker) and lean rats (26). However, intracerebroventricular (ICV) injection of clonidine, an α-2 agonist, increased food intake more in lean rats than in genetically obese rats (27). In contrast to the response to ICV clonidine, a β-3 agonist (BRL-37344) injected into the cerebral ventricles had little effect on food intake of lean animals, but it significantly reduced food intake in a dose-dependent way in Zucker fatty rats (27). When Pesonen *et al.* (28) gave clonidine peripherally to Zucker rats there were no differences in food intake compared to lean rats. In *ob/ob* mice NE and clonidine both stimulated food intake more than in lean mice (29). Using amphetamine as a probe for the noradrenergic feeding system in Zucker rats showed similar suppression in ad-lib fed animals but a loss of the anorexic response in "dieted" fatty rats (30). In *ob/ob*

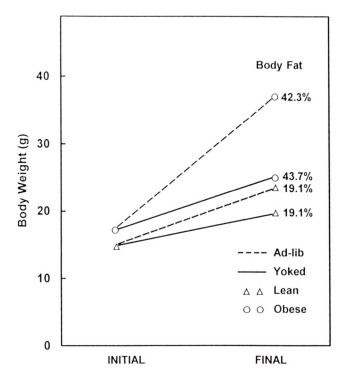

Figure 1. Effect of yoked feeding on change in body-fat content of *ob/ob* and lean mice. Food was provided in pellets to one group of lean mice ad lib (triangle and dashed line) and a second group that bar-pressed for it (triangle and solid line). The yoked *ob/ob* littermates received the same amount of food and at the same time as the lean bar-pressed mice (circle and solid line), and a second group of *ob/ob* mice received food ad lib (circle and dashed line). Initial body composition was 12% in the lean mice and 19% in the *ob/ob* mice. During feeding, the *ob/ob* mice gained more weight than their lean littermates, regardless of the feeding regime. In addition, their body fat increased proportionally, indicating their enhanced efficiency of food storage.

mice anorexia was less than in lean mice at comparable brain amphetamine levels, even though hypothalamic NE content was higher (31). In the yellow mouse, Shimizu *et al.* (32) have reported decreased turnover of norepinephrine and dopamine. Collectively these data appear to implicate an altered response of the noradrenergic system in the overall control of food intake in genetic obesity.

Measurements of adrenergic receptor binding in lean and genetically obese animals show discrepant results (33). Whereas Pesonen *et al.* (28) and Levin *et al.* (34) found no differences in α-2 adrenergic receptors in many regions of the brain of Zucker fatty rats compared to lean animals, Jhanwar-Uniyal *et al.* (35) reported a significant increase in α-1 and α-2 receptor binding in the paraventricular nucleus, but not elsewhere in 14-month-old fatty rats. Two proposals have been formulated from these observations. First, Levin *et al.* (36, 37) suggested that the increased ratio of α-2/α-1 adrenergic receptors in the ventromedial nucleus of Zucker rats may be important in their feeding deficit. Alternatively, Tsujii and Bray (27) have proposed that Zucker rats have increased tonic activity of α-2 adrenergic receptors and reduced tonic activity of β-2 adrenergic receptors to account for the hyperphagia in the fatty rats.

In contrast to the confusing data on adrenergic receptors, the data on the serotonin and serotonin receptors are more congruent (38). A reduction in the concentration of brain tryptophan (39, 40) and a reduction in 5-hydroxy-3-indole acetic acid (5-HIAA), the principal serotonin metabolite (33, 41), support a reduction in a serotonergic tone in the Zucker fatty rat. Indolepyruvic acid (IPA), a keto-analogue of tryptophan, reduced food intake and body weight for a longer period in fatty rats than in lean controls. The anorexia of IPA was blocked by meteorgoline, a drug that blocks serotonin receptors (42). Altered blood levels of tryptophan to long chain neutral amino acids in the Zucker fatty rat may be related to these changes (43, 44). Currie (29) has also reported a reduced response to serotonin in the obese (*ob/ob*) mouse, and Shimizu *et al.* (45) have made similar observations in the yellow obese mouse. Reducing brain serotonin by lesioning the raphe nucleus does not prevent obesity in ventromedial hypothalamus (VMH)–lesioned rats or ovariectomized rats (46).

Histamine is a third possible monoaminergic mechanism for hyperphagia in the Zucker fatty rat. Histamine, acting through histamine receptors, is known to decrease food intake (47). When chlorpheniramine, an H-1 receptor–blocking drug is injected into normal rats, food intake increases, but similar treatment of Zucker fatty rats does not increase food intake (48). Thioperamide, an H-3 receptor antagonist, will enhance hypothalamic neuronal histamine and decrease food intake in lean rats. However, this drug had no significant effect on food intake in the Zucker fatty rat, a result that is consistent with the finding of a lower histamine concentration in the hypothalamus and cortex of Zucker fatty rats. Collectively these data suggest a defect in a histamine inhibitory system that may play a role in the hyperphagia of the Zucker fatty rat (49).

The Zucker fatty rat also shows an impaired response to glucoprivic feeding. Injections of 2-deoxyglucose, which impairs glucose metabolism, failed to increase food intake in Zucker fatty rats in contrast to the brisk stimulation in lean animals (26, 50, 51). Tsujii and Bray also observed that the hyperphagic response to phlorizin of normal rats was absent in the obese rat (51). The disturbed glucoprivic feeding may be related to defective gamma-aminobutyric acid-A (GABA-A) receptor function. Stimulation of food intake by 2-deoxy-D-glucose can be blocked by picrotoxin, an antagonist of GABA-A receptors (52). Injections of muscimol, a GABA agonist, into the paraventricular nucleus, dorsomedial nucleus, or lateral hypothalamus had essentially identical effects in both the lean and the Zucker fatty rat (53). In contrast, injections of muscimol into the ventromedial hypothalamus produced a much greater hyperphagia in lean rats than in Zucker fatty rats. Injection of picrotoxin, the GABA-A antagonist, actually decreased food intake in the fatty rat but was without effect in lean animals, suggesting that there might be a tonic stimulatory GABA system operating in the ventromedial nucleus of the Zucker rat producing hyperphagia. These observations give added weight to the suggestion by Levin et al. (38) that the altered ratio of $\alpha2/\alpha1$ adrenergic receptors in the ventromedial nucleus of fatty Zucker rats may be important in the hyperphagia of these animals. Of interest, picrotoxin, which decreased food intake when injected into the ventromedial nucleus of the fatty rat, had a strong stimulatory effect of comparable magnitude in lean and fatty rats when injected into the lateral hypothalamus, showing the importance of the reciprocal effects of GABA feeding systems in these two regions. Coscina et al. (54) extended these observations on GABA neurotransmission by showing that the Zucker fatty rat is refractory to the anorexia produced by ethanol-0-sulphate, an inhibitor of GABA-transaminase, the enzyme that produces GABA. They also showed that the GABA level in brain tissue from lean and obese rats was comparable, indicating that a reduced response to GABA, not a reduced production of GABA, is responsible for the altered feeding patterns.

PEPTIDES

Because a variety of peptides stimulate (55, 56) or suppress (57, 58) food intake, peptidergic mechanisms have been used as an explanation for the hyperphagia of genetically obese animals. This was supported by studies demonstrating that the response to cholecystokinin (CCK) may be reduced (30), that β-endorphin in the pituitary is increased (59), and that neuropeptide Y (NPY) was increased in the brain of Zucker fatty rats (60–62). In contrast with the consistent increase in NPY, the level of bombesin, calcitonin gene-related peptide (CGRP), galanin (63), neurotensin (64), substance-P, somatostatin (SRIF), vasoactive intestinal peptide (VIP), and CCK are not altered in the Zucker fatty rat (62, 65–67). The neuropeptide pattern differs between *ob/ob* and *db/db* mice (68, 69). This contrasts with the yellow obese mouse in which an increase in brain CCK has been reported (70). An increase in NPY and in the mRNA for preproNPY in the Zucker rat occurs as early as 5 weeks of age, the time at which hyperphagia appears. Changes in mRNA for NPY are specific to the arcuate nucleus, where NPY is produced (71, 72). Hypothalamic NPY is increased by starvation and reduced by injections of insulin (73). The finding of lower levels of NPY in the paraventricular nucleus (PVN) may reflect the hyperinsulinemia of the Zucker fatty rats (see Kalra *et al.* in this volume). In contrast to the lower NPY levels, release of NPY is increased (74). In lean animals, injection of insulin decreased the mRNA for preproNPY in the arcuate nucleus, but this does not occur under similar conditions in the fatty rat (75). Beck *et al.* (60) observed that acute intraventricular injection of NPY increased food intake in Zucker fatty rats. However, Brief *et al.* (76) did not find a response to NPY in the fatty rat at any dose tested. Data on the response to NPY after adrenalectomy of Zucker rats have not been published.

Neuropeptide Y stimulates food intake in the *ob/ob* mouse and the lean mouse to a similar degree (77). In addition, when both *ob/ob* and lean mice had been adrenalectomized, NPY reduced sympathetic activity, as assessed by guanosine diphosphate binding to brown adipose tissue (BAT) mitochondria, and reduced oxygen consumption to a similar degree. Thus, these effects of NPY clearly do not require the presence of adrenal steroids.

Chronic infusion of NPY into the cerebral ventricular system has been carried out in two laboratories to test the hypothesis that elevated release of NPY might account for the syndrome. Both studies have shown chronic increases in food intake and weight gain (78, 79). The possibility that NPY is a major contributor to the hyperphagia in obesity comes from studies with VMH-lesioned rats. Infusion of antibodies to NPY into the third ventricle reduced food intake by more than 90% (see Kalra in this volume). Neuropeptide Y release from the PVN was increased, suggesting enhanced turnover in these animals. It is interesting that the chronic infusion of NPY does not appear to down-regulate NPY receptors.

Insulin may also be an important feedback signal for satiety (80, 81). Insulin uptake through endocytosis into the neuropil and thus into the cerebrospinal fluid (CSF) is decreased in Zucker fatty rats (82) possibly because of the reduced insulin binding to brain capillaries (83), and this may account for the reduced uptake of inositol in *fa/fa* rats (84). This reduced entry of insulin into the brain CSF of fatty Zucker rats might reduce the feedback inhibition of NPY and thus account for the increased NPY turnover and hyperphagia.

Several observations also suggest that opioid systems may be involved in genetic forms of obesity. Naloxone decreases body weight gain in *ob/ob* mice (85, 86). Dynorphin is increased in brain tissue from Zucker fatty rats (87). This finding would be consistent with the potent effects of phenylpiperidine opioid antagonists that act on kappa 2-B receptors and promote weight loss in Zucker fatty rats (88–90). Dynorphin and endorphin levels have been reported to be increased in the hypothalamus (91) and in the posterior pituitary of *ob/ob* mice (92), but in another report there were no differences in dynorphin in seven brain regions (93). Thus, changes in dynorphin levels in the brain of the *ob/ob* mouse may be an epiphenomenon. In one report, food intake in *ob/ob* mice was more sensitive to a kappa agonist and was suppressed more after a kappa antagonist than were lean littermates (92). In another report (93) *ob/ob* mice were more resistant to the effects of three kappa agonists than lean mice. This was surprising, since dynorphin acts primarily through kappa receptors. The differences may lie in the specificity of kappa receptors that are stimulated, since there are several subtypes of kappa receptors.

Corticotropin-releasing hormone (CRH) reduces food intake of lean and Zucker fatty rats (94–96). Chronic infusions of CRH into the third ventricle will reduce body weight or slow weight gain. Nakaishi and coworkers (97) found a significant decrease in immunoreactive-CRH in the median eminence but not in the PVN of obese Zucker fatty rats and suggested that "CRH tonus" may play a role in expression of obesity in these animals (97). The decrease in food intake by CRH is partially attenuated by an antagonist to CRH and by alpha-melanocyte-stimulating hormone (α-MSH) (98).

An increase in desacetyl-melanocyte-stimulating hormone (d-MSH) or a blockade of α-MSH might account for hyperphagia in some animal models of obesity. Desacetyl-melanocyte-stimulating hormone is produced by posttranslational processing of pro-opiomelanocortin (POMC) in the middle lobe of the anterior pituitary and in the hypothalamus. The final step in this processing is N-acetylation of d-MSH to produce α-MSH. The pituitary content of d-MSH is increased in the yellow obese mouse (99). Peripheral injections of d-MSH stimulate food intake but have very little effect on pigmentation of the skin in the yellow obese mouse. On the other hand, α-MSH, the N-acetylated form of melanocyte-stimulating hormone (MSH) stimulates pigmentation of the skin but has only a small effect on food intake (100). When injected into the brain, α-MSH reduces food intake (101), possibly by interfering with the effects of CRH on feeding (98). Recent data by Klebig *et al.* (in this volume) show that in the yellow obese mouse the defect is over-expression in many tissues of a peptide. This peptide might compete with binding of α-MSH to the melanocyte-stimulating hormone receptor. Such a model would explain the reduced pigmentation (yellow coat color), the hyperphagia, and the altered balance of the autonomic nervous system through competition with CRH. This is shown in Figure 2 (102). An alternative mechanism for the slow increase in body weight and food intake in the yellow obese mouse could be the augmented production of d-MSH and reduced production of α-MSH.

Desacetyl-melanocyte–stimulating hormone or competition with α-MSH may also be important in models of obesity. When the Furth corticotropin (ACTH) producing tumor was reported to produce obesity (103), the mechanism was attributed to the increased production of ACTH by this tumor (104), since ACTH stimulates corticosteroid secretion by the adrenal gland. However, neither ACTH injections nor treatment with corticosteroids produces a significant obesity either in lean rats or mice. Like d-MSH, ACTH is an acetylated peptide produced by post-translational processing of POMC. In a tumor, the possibility of cleavage of POMC without acetylation of the ACTH or MSH

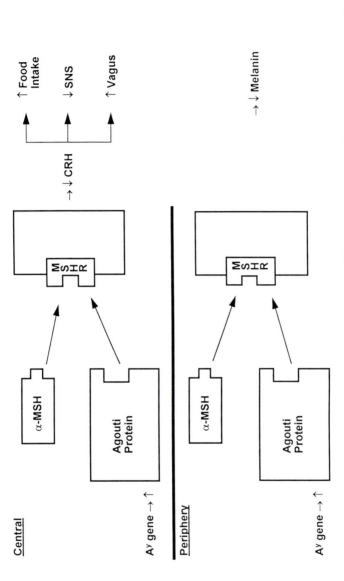

Figure 2. A model for the phenotypic expression in the yellow mouse. The agouti protein, which is widely expressed in tissues from the yellow mouse, is restricted in its expression in the black mouse. If this agouti protein were a competitive inhibitor of the MSH-receptor (MSHR), then the effects of α-MSH would be reduced at the sites at which this protein was produced. At the melanocyte this would decrease melanin production. In the hypothalamus, this would inhibit effects of CRH, leading to some increase in food intake and a shift in the balance of the autonomic nervous system to increased parasympathetic and decreased sympathetic activity. SNS = sympathetic nervous system; CRH = corticotropin-releasing hormone.

fragment would produce d-MSH and d-ACTH, a product which is known to increase food intake of mice when administered peripherally.

A third model in which production of d-MSH may be a component in the hyperphagia is the glucocorticoid antisense transgenic mouse, reported by Pepin *et al.* (105). In these animals, an antisense message decreases glucocorticoid receptor levels in the hypothalamus. Such animals fail to receive the negative inhibitory message from circulating corticosteroids and overproduce ACTH. Overproduction of ACTH, however, may well result in overproduction of d-MSH, which could increase food intake and body weight.

Apoprotein A-IV (Apo A-IV) is a constituent of the high density lipoproteins (HDL). Fujimoto *et al.* (106) have shown that Apo A-IV can inhibit food intake whether given systemically or into the ventricular system of the brain. Moreover, they found that the Zucker fatty rat was less responsive to Apo IV. Relative to other peptides, however, high doses of Apo A-IV are required to inhibit food intake, making it an unlikely physiological agent.

Neurotensin is a tridecapeptide that decreases food intake. Levels of neurotensin are unchanged in the obese (*ob/ob*) mouse (66, 107). One study on neurotensin levels in hypothalamic tissue from the fatty Zucker rat reported no differences but a second reported that neurotensin is decreased in the PVN and lateral hypothalamus of rats eating a high-fat diet (108). The final verdict on neurotensin in obesity is still out.

Hyperglycemia, Hyperinsulinemia, and Insulin Resistance

The Zucker fatty rat is normoglycemic, whereas a second strain carrying the fatty gene, the Wistar diabetic fatty (WDF) rat, is hyperglycemic. This hyperglycemia in WDF rats occurs in males but not in females and is not corrected by gonadectomy (109). Most mouse models with obesity are hyperglycemic. This is not prevented by Brewer's yeast containing glucose-tolerance factor (110). The mechanism by which normoglycemia is maintained in the fatty rat has been evaluated in studies using glucose kinetics and glucose utilization (111). In the suckling preweaning period, glucose turnover rates in the basal state, as well as glucose production and utilization during glucose infusion, were identical in lean and obese pups. Moreover, the utilization by individual tissues was similar between the two groups, except for brown adipose tissue. After weaning, the glucose turnover rates and rates of glucose utilization were identical in the two genotypes in the basal state. However, alanine uptake by liver is increased twofold and may provide the substrate for additional glucose production or for lipogenesis (112). During glucose infusion production of glucose by the liver was suppressed less in the Zucker obese rats than in the lean ones. Glucose utilization was significantly lower in muscles from the fatty rat and higher in white adipose tissues from these animals. Increased glycogen synthase phosphatase has been described in Zucker fatty rats (113) and may account for the highly activated glycogen synthase in hepatocytes from these animals, which could play a role in controlling glucose levels. Glucose tolerance can be improved by injecting CRH intravenously (114), probably because of its effects on insulin secretion (115).

Differences in the activity of hepatic steroid sulfotransferences may account for the hyperglycemia in some strains of the obese mice. Leiter *et al.* (116, 117) have shown that androgenization of the liver is associated with hyperglycemia. Androgenization can be produced by either inactivating estrogen through sulfation, or activating androgens such as dehydroepiandrosterone (DHEA) by sulfation. In the hyperglycemic *db/db* mouse, the level of estrogen sulfotransferase is high, which reduces the effect of estrogen by sulfating them. Treatment of yellow (A^{vy}/a) mice with dexamethasone increases hyperglycemia by inducing estrogen sulfotransferase, which increases the level of sulfated estrogen and thus androgenizes the liver. Hepatic androgenization may also explain the hyperglycemia in the male WDF rat.

Hyperinsulinemia characterizes both genetic and hypothalamic obesity, but is present to a lesser degree in dietary obesity (4). In animals with dietary obesity, the changes in insulin concentration are a function of diet and food intake. In all three models, however, insulin resistance occurs in part as a consequence of hyperinsulinemia.

Hyperinsulinemia is among the earliest defects detected in the genetically obese Zucker rat and the *ob/ob* mouse (101, 118–120). At 5 days of age, insulin secretion from perfused pieces of pancreas showed a significantly greater response to acetyl choline but not to glucose either with or without theophylline or arginine. The ability to block these effects by atropine or by vagotomy in the fatty rat suggests enhanced vagal activity. This scenario fits well with the proposals by Jeanrenaud (121) of increased vagal activity in the Zucker fatty rat. Altered function of glucokinase may play a role in this hypersecretion of insulin from islets of Zucker *fa/fa* rats (122). Similarly altered sensitivity of voltage-dependent events at the islet surface may play a role in hyperinsulinemia (123). Glucose homeostasis is improved in *ob/ob* mice and *fa/fa* rats by the transition metal vanadate (124, 125).

Increased vagal activity is also present in rats with hypothalamic obesity. Hyperinsulinemia is observed within minutes following VMH lesions and can be reversed by vagotomy (126–128). Similarly, isolated islets from VMH-lesioned rats show enhanced sensitivity to neurotransmitters in the early postlesion period that gradually shifts as the islets mature in a rat that is rapidly increasing in weight (129–131).

Reduced sympathetic activity is a second mechanism that may enhance insulin secretion. In the studies with 5-day-old pancreatic tissue from Zucker fatty rats, Atef *et al.* (132) found a suggestive, but not quite statistically significant, reduction in insulin secretion in response to added norepinephrine, which would be consistent with receptor hypersensitivity. Convincing evidence shows reduced sympathetic activity in animals with VMH lesions (133) and genetic obesity (134, 135). This decreased sympathetic activity would remove the inhibitory effects that sympathetic neurotransmitters could have on activation of α-adrenergic receptors that inhibit insulin secretion from the pancreas. This is consistent with the in vitro studies of islet function by Campfield and his colleagues (130). Disturbances in GABA in the medulla and pons may be the integrating mechanism for these neural effects. The GABA levels are lower in these brainstem areas of fatty rats than in lean controls (136).

Changes in blood flow to the pancreas may be another feature of altered autonomic function and might account for enhanced glucose cycling (137). Using radioactive microspheres, Atef *et al.* (138) showed a significantly higher blood flow to pancreatic islets of animals with VMH lesions and in the Zucker fatty rat. Vagotomy significantly reduced the blood flow to the islets of obese Zucker rats. Treatment with an α-2 adrenergic agonist, clonidine, induced a greater decrease in blood flow in the obese Zucker rat, which is consistent with the observations of greater stimulation of food intake in lean rats using peripheral injections of clonidine (33). The alterations in blood flow in response to manipulations of the sympathetic and parasympathetic nervous system add strength to the argument that this is a major mod-

ulator of insulin secretion in genetic and hypothalamic forms of experimental obesity.

Peptides may also play a role in modulating insulin secretion. Gastric inhibitory peptide (GIP) released from the gastrointestinal tract of
the *ob/ob* mouse (139), the Zucker fatty rats (140), or the JCR:LA-cor-
pulent (*cp/cp*) obese rat (140) is one peptide that might be involved in
insulin hypersecretion. Using isolated pancreas tissue from *cp/cp, fa/fa,*
and lean rats, Pederson *et al.* (140) observed that GIP increased the
integrated insulin response by twofold in the Zucker fatty rats and by
fivefold in the *cp/cp* strain. The anatomic size of the islet of Langerhans
was significantly greater in the *cp/cp* rats than in the fatty rats, which
were in turn greater than the lean animals, as would be expected in
response to chronic hypersecretion of insulin. β-Endorphin is a second
peptidergic mechanism for hyperinsulinemia. However, in the fatty rat
base-line levels of β-endorphin are similar to control, and treatment
with naloxone does not change base-line insulin, making this mechanism unlikely (141).

Using 8- to 12-week-old Zucker rats, Cawthorn and Chan (142)
found that in isolated pancreatic islets of Langerhans, both epinephrine
and somatostatin inhibited insulin secretion by approximately 75% in
both groups of animals. In islets cultured overnight, more insulin was
released from islets of lean animals than from islets of obese animals.
Pertussis toxin completely reversed the inhibition by somatostatin, but
galanin had no effect on insulin secretion in either group. Although the
islets of obese and lean rats responded normally to inhibitors of insulin
release, the authors noted a subtle difference in sensitivity to pertussis
toxin, an inhibitor of G_i proteins, between the islets of obese and lean
animals. These changes in function of G proteins may have the same
mechanisms as the changes in G-protein function in fat cells (see below)
and may be a part of the general mechanism underlying genetic obesity
(143, 144).

In summary, hyperinsulinemia appears to be a necessary component
of all forms of experimental obesity (Table 2). It is also clear that hyperinsulinemia is a sufficient cause of obesity, since chronic treatment
with exogenous insulin will produce hyperphagia and weight gain in
experimental animals and in human beings alike.

Many of the consequences of obesity can be directly traced to hyperinsulinemia. The increase in lipoprotein lipase, an enzyme whose
levels can be modified by treatment with insulin, is one example. In-

creased triglyceride production and secretion from the liver is a second manifestation of hyperinsulinemia. The development of insulin resistance may also be a consequence, in part, of hyperinsulinemia and the associated down regulation of insulin receptors. Finally, the alterations in many adipose tissue and hepatic enzymes may be related to continuing exposure to insulin and its anabolic role in lipogenesis (121).

Insulin resistance is also a characteristic feature of experimental forms of obesity, but it does not appear to be a necessary or sufficient cause for the obesity. The mechanism for induction of insulin resistance is unclear (145). Muscle is among the earliest tissues to become insulin resistant. This occurs by 28 days of age in the obese (*ob/ob*) mouse (146), the diabetes mouse (*mdb/mdb*) (147), and at a similar age in the Zucker fatty rat (148). Immediately following a hypothalamic lesion in weanling animals, there is an increase in insulin, a decrease in glucose concentration, and increased glucose clearance, indicating a normal insulin response (17, 149). It takes approximately three to six weeks for insulin resistance to appear in this model. In a longitudinal study of mice with hypothalamic obesity (121, 150), the syndrome of insulin resistance was observed to be complete within six weeks following an initial transient period of hypersensitivity to insulin. In rats fed high-fat diets, insulin resistance develops rapidly, regardless of whether they become obese (151, 152).

To establish the sequential development of insulin resistance in the Zucker fatty rat, Zarjevski *et al.* (79, 153) examined the uptake of 2-deoxy-D-glucose by diaphragm from 21-, 31-, and 70-day-old Zucker fatty rats and lean controls. At the youngest age (21 days), there was an enhanced response to insulin in the diaphragm from fatty rats. By 31 days of age, the insulin-stimulated glucose uptake by the diaphragm was similar in the two groups of animals, and by day 70 the syndrome of insulin resistance in the diaphragm muscle was clearly evident by the reduced uptake of 2-deoxy-D-glucose in response to insulin. In spite of these changes in insulin responsiveness, there were no changes in the mRNA for GLUT4 nor in the quantity of GLUT4 protein in these muscles (154). This contrasts with the obesity in mice treated with monosodium glutamate or gold thioglucose where GLUT4 protein was decreased in brown adipose tissue, skeletal, and cardiac muscle of obese insulin-resistant mice (155). GLUT1, on the other hand, showed no changes. Thus, the syndrome of insulin resistance in muscles appears after the development of the syndrome rather than playing an etiologic role. The development of insulin resistance in the fatty rat does not occur equally in all tissues. Insulin resistance develops readily in muscles from fatty rats but sensitivity of white fat cells remains, accounting for the enhanced lipogenesis in this tissue (41).

Amylin, an amyloid polypeptide from pancreatic islet cells (islet amyloid polypeptide [IAPP]), has been suggested to play a role in the development of insulin resistance (156–158). In a study by Tokuyama *et al.* (159), the amylin (IAPP) content measured by radioimmunoassay was increased in the islets of VMH-lesioned rats compared to sham-operated controls. The isolated islets from VMH-lesioned rats secreted larger quantities of amylin than did islets from lean animals. A similar study in 14-week-old Zucker fatty rats also showed an elevation of IAPP in pancreatic islets and a greater stimulation of IAPP release from isolated islets in response to hyperglycemia (159).

Tumor necrosis factor (TNF-α) may play a role in the insulin resistance of the fatty rat (160, 161). Tumor necrosis factor-α was increased in adipose tissue of Zucker fatty rats and secreted into the circulation. Infusion of TNF-α into rats produces profound insulin resistance (162). Conversely, infusion of a soluble fusion protein of TNF-α and immunoglobulin G greatly improves insulin resistance in the fatty rat (160). Whether these changes in TNF-α are the result of the enlarged fat cell or may be an early causal mechanism in insulin resistance in these animals remains to be determined.

The liver may be involved in the development of insulin resistance. Hepatic glycogen levels are higher in the *fa/fa* rat (163) and gold thioglucose obese mice (164) than in lean controls. The level of particulate N-myristoyl transferase is reduced in fatty rats and appears to be inversely related to the level of insulin concentration (165). Finally, an abnormality in regulation of fructose-1, 6-1 bisphosphates, in the New Zealand obese mouse may contribute to their hepatic overproduction of glucose (166).

Regardless of its etiology, the insulin resistance in genetic and hypothalamic obesity is reversed by adrenalectomy. Transplantation of islets of Langerhans from lean animals into the spleens of *ob/ob* mice, however, has no effect on the hyperinsulinemia or obesity (167). Attenuation by adrenalectomy was first convincingly demonstrated in the studies of Ohshima *et al.* (168), using perfused hindquarter preparations from the genetically obese (*ob/ob*) mouse. There was a shift to the right and a reduction in maximal response to infused insulin by muscle from the untreated *ob/ob* mouse. Within seven days after adrenalectomy, however, the responsiveness of muscle measured by uptake of 2-deoxy-D-glucose had returned to normal. To assess whether the effects of steroids were directly on muscle or required a secondary intermediary, Ohshima and colleagues (169) perfused isolated hind limbs from adrenalectomized animals with dexamethasone for five hours before examining the response to insulin. The perfusion with glucocorticoid increased insulin resistance and altered the basal uptake of 2-deoxy-D-glucose. This effect on muscle involves primarily the synthesis of muscle protein that is impaired in comparison with the normal rates of turnover. In addition to removing the barriers to insulin resistance, adrenalectomy also increases the mass of muscle tissue in obese (*ob/ob*) mice (170). However, the pattern of muscle fibers does not return to normal (171).

Muscle plays an important role in the development of insulin resistance in animals with experimental obesity. One potential explanation for this insulin resistance may be a decrease in number or a defect in translocation of glucose transporters in muscle (172). This hypothesis has been examined in genetic obesity (173–175) and hypothalamic obesity (176) and found wanting. The high level of insulin resistance was not associated with changes in GLUT4 protein or its messenger RNA.

Exercise training may improve insulin resistance in obese animals (177, 178, 180, 298). During low intensity training, only the fast twitch red fibers demonstrate improved insulin-stimulated glucose transport, whereas with high intensity training there are improvements in both fast twitch red and white fibers. 3-O-methyl glucose (3-O-MG) uptake by perfused hind limbs was increased in rats during both high and low intensity exercise, and compared with sedentary rats (180), there was no difference in GLUT4 and 3-O-MG transport in the red quadriceps muscle between rats trained at high and low intensity. Of interest, there were no differences at all in the rates of 3-O-MG uptake in the white quadriceps from exercised rats, regardless of their intensity of exercise when compared with sedentary rats. The concentration of GLUT4 protein and the activity of citrate synthase were increased in the muscles from rats trained at high intensity as compared with sedentary rats. GLUT4 content and citrate synthase activity were significantly correlated as were GLUT4 content and 3-O-MG transport. These authors (177, 178, 180, 298) conclude that the improvement in insulin resistance after exercise in Zucker obese rats is partly due to an increased GLUT4 concentration.

Electrical stimulation of muscle glucose uptake is unimpaired in the Zucker fatty rat (181, 182), in contrast to the marked impairment of glucose uptake after exposure to insulin. To evaluate the effect of exercise training, Brozinick *et al.* (181, 182) examined the effect of glucose uptake in the absence and presence of maximally stimulating concentrations of insulin with muscle contraction elicited by electrical stimulation of the sciatic nerve. Exercise training increased the insulin-stimulated uptake of glucose in several muscles (plantaris, red gastrocnemius, and white gastrocnemius) but not in others (soleus and extensor digitorum longus). Perfusion with insulin and electrically stimulated contraction resulted in significant increases in plasma membrane GLUT4 protein only in the untrained rats. The GLUT4 protein concentration in the insulin and the electrically stimulated muscle from trained rats remained, respectively, 53% and 30% higher than in the corresponding muscles from untrained rats. Thus, the increase in glucose uptake after aerobic training in response to insulin or electrical stimulation was due in part to an increase in plasma membrane GLUT4 protein and not to altered rates of GLUT4 protein translocation or in its functional activity.

Defects in activation of protein kinase-C (PKC) have been reported in the heart and liver from obese rats. A defect in PKC might account for the altered muscle response to insulin (183–184). Cooper *et al.* (185) found that the levels of diacylglycerol (DAG) were significantly increased in soleus muscles from 15- to 19-week-old obese Zucker rats. Yet the levels of PKC were diminished in soleus muscles from Zucker fatty rats. Both the common PKC and the novel isoforms of PKC were decreased by 70% to 90%. Thus, the levels of the common PKC isozyme, mRNA, protein, and enzyme activity in the soleus muscle of the obese Zucker rats are decreased, even though the endogenous PKC activator, DAG, is elevated. These decreased levels of PKC may well relate to the insulin resistance in the muscle of the fatty rats.

Growth and Development

Most animal models with the recessively transmitted forms of obesity are stunted, meaning their body length and muscle mass are reduced relative to their lean littermates. Weanling rats with hypothalamic lesions are also stunted, and a similar trend is observed in adult animals with hypothalamic lesions. The obese yellow mouse, which inherits obesity as an autosomal dominant, appears to be an exception to this generalization.

The relative reduction in muscle mass in the face of increased fat tissue in many forms of obesity is often associated with mild hypothermia. It may well be that this combination of altered nutrient channeling or altered nutrient partitioning to fat, rather than protein and the associated hypothermia, is a fundamental reflection of the basic disturbance in these animals.

The defect in growth reflected by the stunting in recessively inherited forms of obesity and hypothalamic obesity is reversed by adrenalectomy. This suggests that the presence of glucocorticoids form part of a critical system modulating nutrient channeling or nutrient partitioning. A more detailed discussion of the role of adrenal steroids in these models is presented in a later section of this paper.

A number of other mechanisms have also been suggested for the disturbance in growth in these animals. The first and most obvious would be an impairment in growth hormone. Growth hormone levels are low in most forms of obesity (186). The release of growth hormone in response to growth hormone–releasing hormone (GHRH) (187) added to isolated pituitaries in vitro or injected in vivo was significantly lower in the Zucker fatty rats (188) as was the expression of the GHRH gene (189). When GHRH and a hexapeptide called growth hormone–releasing peptide (GHRP-6), an orally active growth hormone–releasing peptide, were combined they significantly increased growth hormone release in Zucker fatty rats, but the levels were still far below those observed in lean animals (190). Although growth hormone levels are reduced, plasma insulin-like growth factor-I (IGF-I) is higher in obese Zucker rats than in lean controls (187, 190–192). The fact that IGF-I, the major peripheral mediator for the effects of growth hormone, is elevated in the Zucker fatty rat suggests that the relative stunting in this animal model results from resistance to the effects of the growth hormone/IGF-I rather than the result of impaired growth hormone secretion alone.

It is possible that diet and diet selection may play a role in impaired growth of these animals. Zucker fatty rats have a disturbance in their circadian rhythm that becomes worse with aging (193). The fatty rat also selects increased quantities of high-fat foods, which may be a reflection of the altered adrenal steroid system in these animals (194). Clearly, however, the most important component of the stunting must be the presence of adrenal glucocorticoids and their interaction with other systems, which lead to decreased protein synthesis and increased channeling or partitioning of nutrients into fat. As noted above, muscle mass is increased to normal following adrenalectomy, and the alterations in muscle response to insulin, which are improved following adrenalectomy, will revert toward the resistant state when adrenal steroids are perfused through muscle tissue from adrenalectomized animals (169).

The Fat Cell and Fat Metabolism in Experimental Forms of Obesity

The obesity in genetic, hypothalamic, and dietary models has led to a vast literature on adipose tissue, physiology, and development (195). An increase in fat cell size can be detected experimentally as early as 10 to 14 days of age (16). Other phenotypic markers, such as hypothermia, can also be detected in animals with recessively inherited obesity at a very early age. The recent introduction of a probe, which is specific for the gene on chromosome 5 in the fatty rat, will make it possible to explore the sequence of developments prior to day 10 of life (196).

Most studies on the development of these animals have been done in animals older than 14 days of age, when it is possible to make early phenotypic differentiation. By 16 days of age, the Zucker fatty rat and the *ob/ob* mouse are already more obese than their lean littermates because of increased lipogenesis (197, 198). The fat cells from these animals are increased in size. Adipocytes from preweaning 16-day-old animals show enhanced lipogenesis. The structure of fatty acid synthase (FAS) is identical in lean and fatty rats, but FAS and its mRNA are both overproduced in Zucker rats as young as 16 days of age (199). To explore this problem in more detail, Dugail and her colleagues (200) have examined the temporal sequence for the development of lipogenic enzymes in the fatty Zucker rat and have observed a coordinate increase in lipoprotein lipase (LPL), glyceraldehyde-3-phosphate dehydrogenase (GAPDH), malic enzyme, and FAS. All of these enzymes are elevated in the early preweaning days, with a much further elevation after weaning, at a time when hyperinsulinemia is present. In 16-day-old Zucker fatty rats, when insulin is not yet significantly elevated, the mRNA for malic enzyme is increased twofold, for LPL fivefold, and for GAPDH threefold, but there was no increase in glucose 6-phosphate dehydrogenase (G6PDH). By 30 days of age, the level of mRNA increased further for all of these enzymes with values ranging between six- and tenfold above the levels found in lean littermates. Adipocytes from young fatty rats show a marked increase in insulin-stimulated glucose uptake. These same cells also show an increase in glucose transporters as measured by cytochalasin-B binding (201). In both 16- and 30-day-old rats, that is, normoinsulinemic and hyperinsulinemic ages, there is an increase in the level of mRNA from 2.3- to 6.2-fold for GLUT4, but no difference in the noninsulin responsive GLUT1 protein or its mRNA.

The report by Flier et al. (202) that adipsin, a serine protease secreted into the circulation by fat cells, was reduced in ob/ob and db/db mice suggested that adipsin or other substances regulated by the adipocyte genome (203) may be involved as a feedback signal. Adipsin was found to be identical with complement factor D, which is involved in the alternate pathway for coagulation. Subsequent reports showed that adipsin was normal in 10-day-old db/db mice, which are already fat, and that it only fell to low levels after weaning (204). Likewise, adipsin mRNA in the fatty rat is normal in the preweaning period and only declines after weaning (205). The decline in adipsin after weaning suggests that the change may be secondary to the low level of sympathetic activity and/or marked hyperinsulinemia in these animals.

Fat cell size is increased in all forms of obesity. Genetically obese animals also have a marked increase in the number of their adipocytes. In hypothalamic obesity, an increased number of fat cells are present in animals eating high-fat diets, but this increase is absent or limited in animals eating low-fat diets, implying that the obesity occurs by enlargement of fat cells to nearly their maximal size before new fat cells are recruited. In an elegant series of experiments, Ashwell, Mead, and their colleagues (195, 206) showed that the size of the adipocytes was primarily a function of the environment in which the cells resided (Fig. 3). They transplanted segments of adipose tissue from obese to lean animals and vice versa, and examined the subsequent histology of the transplanted tissue. It is clear that the fat cells adopt the size of fat cells in the recipient rather than retaining the characteristics of the donor.

Lipolysis is controlled by stimulatory and inhibitory processes. Neu-

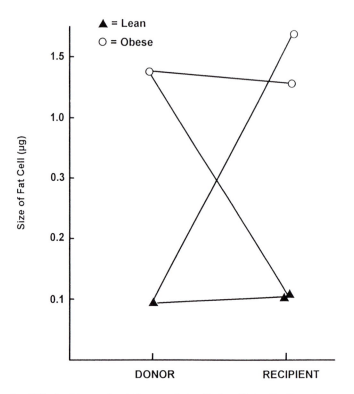

Figure 3. Effect of transplantation on fat cell size. Fat cells from lean or *ob/ob* mice (donors) were transplanted beneath the renal capsule of recipients that were either lean or *ob/ob*. It is clear that the fat cells adapted the size of the recipient, regardless of the genotype of the animal.

rotransmitters, hormones, and drugs that modulate lipolysis act through specific receptors that are coupled to G proteins. The G proteins are either stimulatory (G_s) or inhibitory (G_i) and each is composed of three subunits (α, β, γ). Two bacterial toxins, pertussis and cholera toxin, respectively, activate or inhibit lipolysis by ribosylation of the corresponding α-subunit of the G protein. The *ob/ob* mouse, the *db/db* mouse, and the fatty rat are resistant to activation of adenylyl cyclase. In the *ob/ob* mouse the α-subunits of the G_s and G_i proteins ($G_{s\alpha}$ and $G_{i\alpha}$) are lower than in adipose tissue and liver of lean mice. The fatty rat also shows a decrease in $G_{s\alpha}$ and $G_{i\alpha}$ ($\alpha 1$, $\alpha 2$, and $\alpha 3$). The diabetes mouse (*db/db*), on the other hand, shows similar levels of the $G_{s\alpha}$ and $G_{i\alpha}$. This suggests that alterations in the control of G proteins may be involved in the resistance to lipolysis in the *ob/ob* mouse and fatty rat. In the diabetes mouse a different explanation possibly involving adenylyl cyclase itself may be the explanation (143, 207, 208).

In addition to the alterations in G proteins, there are decreased levels of β-adrenoceptors in 20- to 25-week-old animals (209, 210). One explanation for reduced responsiveness could be reduced rates of dephosphorylation. The resistance of phosphorylation by PKC in hepatocyte membranes from Zucker rats could be overcome by treating the membranes with alkaline phosphates (211).

The changes in LPL in fat cells from obese rats have been examined in relation to the total number of cells and on a per cell basis. Fried and her colleagues (212) have found that the rates of LPL turnover are increased in the larger fat cells from Zucker rats, but that there is no specific abnormality in the cellular regulation of LPL. The increased level of LPL activity in the fat cell from the obese Zucker rat appears to be related to an overall hyperresponsiveness rather than to the effects of insulin on protein synthesis. One of the peculiarities in regulation of LPL metabolism is that it increases further with weight reduction in the Zucker rat, rather than returning toward normal as is observed with most of the other defects in these animals (213).

Several efforts have been made to identify protein abnormalities in genetic obesity. Lynch and his colleagues (214, 215) used two-dimensional isoelectric focusing on sodium dodecyl-sulfate polyacrylamide gel electrophoresis (SDS Page) to separate adipose tissue proteins in the fatty rat. With this technique, they demonstrated an increased expression of the lipogenic enzymes, fatty acid synthetase, ATP-citrate lyase and acetyl-CoA carboxylase. A 116-kDa particulate protein from these animals was found to be identical with pyruvate carboxylase. Maeda and Kasahara have used a similar technique to identify a 120 kd cytosolic fraction from liver that is related to lipogenesis (216). Differential expression of several peptides from adipose tissue were reported in 7-day-old *fa/fa* rats, but these differences were not present in 3-day-old animals (217).

In addition to the increase in several enzymes, Lynch *et al.* (214) have reported that other enzymes are decreased. One of these proteins is carbonic anhydrase-III. This 28 kd cytosolic adipocyte protein is the most abundant protein in adipocytes from lean Zucker rats. Its increase appears to be due to hyperinsulinemia. This insulin responsiveness is consistent with the altered activities of LPL and the coordinate changes in lipogenesis and the gluconeogenesis observed as a response of the hyperinsulinemic state (121).

One of the difficulties in evaluating functional changes in the adipocyte of lean and obese animals is the difference in adipocyte size (104, 126). This is clearly illustrated in the work of Pederson *et al.* (218). They examined the relationship between glucose uptake and the levels of protein and mRNA for GLUT1 and GLUT4 in lean and obese Zucker rats at 5, 10, and 20 weeks of age. The insulin responsiveness of fat cells from 5-week-old animals was high. In contrast it was markedly reduced by 20 weeks of age, showing the age relationship to the development of insulin resistance. When the levels of mRNA for GLUT1 and GLUT4 were compared in relation to total RNA and total membrane protein, respectively, they were lower in the adipocytes from obese rats. At all ages, however, the fat cells from obese rats were larger than those from lean rats with a several-fold increase in total RNA and in the total membrane protein per cell. Thus, on a cellular basis, mRNA and protein levels of GLUT4 increased in young obese rats and gradually declined as a function of age. Induction of diabetes with streptozocin at 20 weeks of age caused a profound decrease in glucose uptake and a concomitant reduction in both GLUT1 and GLUT4 protein levels.

In contrast with the difficulty of interpreting data on glucose transport from fat cells, studies in muscle are more straightforward because the size of muscle cells does not show the same variation. The Zucker fatty rat, the diabetes mouse (*db/db*) (174), and the gold thioglucose–treated mouse (176) show little, if any, change in glucose transporter levels in spite of the marked degree of insulin resistance in these obese animals (175). Alterations in the translocation process, in the transporter itself, or in the intrinsic signaling pathways may provide alternative explanations for reduced glucose transport by muscle from these obese animals. The WDF rat, an animal that carries the fatty (Zucker) (*fa*) gene and is hyperglycemic, showed reductions in GLUT4 relative to lean controls and a return to normal levels when hyperglycemia was corrected by adding acarbose to the animal's diet. The decrease in GLUT4 was 40% to 45% in red fibers from the quadriceps muscle. The correction of the defect by correction of the hyperglycemia points up the importance of hyperglycemia in the change in GLUT4 gene expression in muscle (219).

A reduction in fatty acid oxidation by perfused livers from Zucker fatty rats (220, 221) is well known. Isolated hepatocytes from fatty rats also show reduced fatty acid oxidation (222–225). In contrast, oxidation of fatty acids by isolated mitochondria from obese Zucker rats is equal to that in the lean animal (77, 226–228). This suggested that the cytosol might differ between the groups. To test this, Azain and Ontko (229) examined the cytosol from the fatty rat and showed that it decreased fatty acid oxidation when added to mitochondria from either group of animals. Malonyl CoA and glycerol 3-phosphate also decreased fatty acid oxidation, suggesting that the increased concentrations of malonyl CoA and glycerol 3-phosphate in the cytosol from fatty rats may account for the decreased fatty acid oxidation and ketogenesis.

Altered metabolism of ketones may be one mechanism for the efficiency of obese animals. Coleman (230) showed that the obese (ob/ob) mouse could carboxylate acetone and thus produce pyruvic acid, leading to the return of ketone bodies to the glucose-producing pathway. Such a mechanism could allow maximal oxidation of fatty acids.

Abnormalities in lipoproteins and cholesterol have been noted in the Zucker fatty rat since its earliest description (231). These changes are related to diet and hyperinsulinemia. When fatty rats are fed a chow diet, there is increased gene expression for Apo A-IV, but normal gene expression for Apo A-I and Apo C-III. In contrast, a diet high in fish oil decreases the Apo A-IV expression in lean rats, but not in the obese Zucker rats. Strobl et al. (232) reported alterations in hepatic Apo A-IV gene expression to lipid-lowering fish oil diets by a mechanism affecting regulation of transcription. The level of arachidonic acid is reduced in phospholipids from genetically obese Zucker rats when compared to their controls (233, 234). To test the possibility that correcting this difference might influence weight gain, Phinney and his colleagues (235) fed black currant oil, which is rich in arachidonic acid precursors, to Zucker and lean fatty rats to compare it with soybean oil, which is lower in arachidonic acid. The black currant oil reduced spontaneous food intake, weight gain, and adiposity in the Zucker obese rats, but not in the lean rats. Other studies using fish oils have also shown that they reduce body fat deposition in obese rodents (236–238).

Infertility

Infertility is a variable component of most experimental and human forms of genetically transmitted obesity. In some animals, such as the ob/ob mouse and humans with Prader-Willi syndrome, there is nearly complete infertility. In other experimental animals, such as the yellow obese mouse, there is a relative infertility (1). The infertility associated with hypothalamic lesions is a function of lesion size and location. In animals with dietary obesity, and in most forms of human obesity, infertility is a minimal or absent feature. Thus, it is clear that infertility is not necessary for the development of obesity, nor is infertility a sufficient cause of obesity (Table 2).

Understanding the existence of infertility in genetically obese (*ob/ob*; *db/db*) mice and in the Zucker fatty rat must eventually be part of the overall explanation for the syndrome. Since modulation of fertility is not associated with hyperphagia, with alterations in glucose metabolism, with the presence of insulin resistance, or with disturbances of fat cell size and number, the mechanism that leads to the development of recessively transmitted forms of obesity cannot simply be due to a primary disturbance in one of these other areas, but must encompass a mechanism that is altered in all of them.

Studies of the gonadal axis in the obese mouse have produced several important observations. First, the genetic defect is not a primary cause of the infertility. Ovarian transplants between obese and lean animals show that with the proper hormonal milieu, the ovary from the obese mouse can function normally (104). Moreover, appropriate hormonal support allows fertilization, pregnancy, and delivery in the obese (*ob/ob*) mouse. The gonadal system in both the obese mouse and the female Zucker fatty rat appears to be prepubertal in their functional characteristics. That is, the concentrations of luteinizing hormone (LH), follicle-stimulating hormone (FSH), testosterone, and estradiol are low. The gonadotropins can be released by treatment with gonadotropin-releasing hormone (GnRH). Following castration in lean male *ob/ob* mice, the suppression of gonadotropins with testosterone is shifted to the left, showing increased sensitivity of the pituitary-gonadal axis, similar to what is observed in the prepubertal state.

Two mechanisms may be involved in the infertility and in the other manifestations of the genetically obese syndromes. The first of these is the disturbance in the central regulation of sympathetic activity. The secretion of gonadotropins is pulsatile. The overall pattern differs significantly between males and females because of the cyclic pattern of estrogen release and ovulation. The signal for gonadotropin hormone release involves adrenergic receptors in the central nervous system. It is possible that a disturbance in hypothalamic α-1, α-2, and β-2 adrenoceptors could account for the disturbance in GnRH secretion. A disturbance in adrenoceptor function may also be influenced by steroids. In contrast to most of the defects in the *ob/ob* mouse and the fatty rat, which are reversed by adrenalectomy, the pituitary-gonadal axis is not (239). Shimizu *et al.* (239) have proposed that alterations in androgen receptor mechanisms similar to those proposed by Bray *et al.* (240) for glucocorticoid receptors may be involved in the disturbed feedback mechanisms producing infertility and altered sympathetic activity in the *ob/ob* mouse and fatty rat. This is consistent with the identification of decreased androgen receptors by Bannister and Whittiker (241).

Hypothermia and Thermogenesis

Evidence for hypothermia is clear cut in the genetically obese mice (*ob/ob; db/db*), in the Zucker fatty rat (1), and in the tube-fed hypothalamic obese rat (18). There is also suggestive data for hypothermia in the Prader-Willi syndrome in human beings (242). The hypothermia in the fatty rat and obese mouse is among the earliest demonstrated defects. Desautels and Himms-Hagen (243) in their studies of the obese mouse observed that impaired thermogenesis is primarily due to enhanced torpor. Torpor refers to the periods of spontaneous hypothermia observed primarily in mice.

One approach to examining thermoregulation in genetically obese animals is to use operant systems. This has been done for the obese (*ob/ob*) mouse and the fatty rat. When the obese (*ob/ob*) mouse is allowed to bar press for infrared heat, it shows a similar but displaced dose-response curve when compared with lean mice (244, 245). Wilson *et al.* (246) using a warming board with a gradient found that *ob/ob* mice at 6, 12, and 18 days preferred warmer locations than homozygous lean mice. Studies in the Zucker fatty rat using epinephrine as a mechanism for disrupting thermoregulatory behavior led Carlisle and Stock (247) to conclude that alterations in α-adrenergic receptors may be involved in the thermoregulatory effects of epinephrine.

Energy turnover and energy exchange of adult Zucker fatty rats is similar to that in lean rats. Demes and his colleagues (248) measured energy expenditure and heat loss by direct and indirect calorimetry at three separate ambient temperatures throughout a 24-hour period during both the light and dark cycles. Energy turnover, that is, heat production and heat loss in the lean and Zucker obese animals, increased as ambient temperature fell. The obese animals had a relatively greater rate of heat production and a greater rate of heat loss, expressed as kilocalories per day (kcal/d) or as kilocalories per kilogram of fat-free mass per day (kcal/kgFFM/d), than did the lean animals at each of the three temperatures that were studied. These animals were nine months old and had little change in weight or growth to complicate these measurements. These authors conclude that there is no difference in energy turnover between Zucker fatty and lean rats.

In contrast to the studies of thermogenesis in the whole animal, studies of heat production in response to norepinephrine in brown adipose tissue of the Zucker fatty rat and obese (*ob/ob*) mouse suggest that the capacity of this tissue as a "heat furnace" is impaired (249). The observations supporting these conclusions are the following.

1. Although the mass of interscapular brown adipose tissue (BAT) is increased, this increase is due primarily to fat, since the mitochondrial content is reduced.
2. The binding of guanosine 5'-diphosphate to mitochondrial membranes from BAT, as an index of thermogenic capacity in this tissue, is impaired in genetic obesity.
3. The quantity of uncoupling protein (UCP) and its messenger (mRNA) is reduced.
4. The activity of sympathetic nerves supplying BAT is reduced.
5. Physiologic signals related to food, which normally stimulate BAT, are impaired.

Brown adipose tissue thermogenesis is particularly important in the early postnatal life as a mechanism for heat production in mammals (249). For this reason, the function of this tissue in the fetal and early neonatal period has been particularly relevant in explaining the early pathogenesis of the Zucker fatty rat, the corpulent (*cp/cp*) mouse (250), and the obese (*ob/ob*) mouse. The hypothermia, which characterizes the suckling fatty rat pups, vanishes at the time of weaning, suggesting that this preweaning postnatal period is particularly important (251–253). During this suckling period, disturbances in fat metabolism are evident as early as the first week, and by the end of the second week in excess of one gram of adipose tissue has been deposited in fatty rats compared with lean littermates (254–256). Using techniques by which the core temperature can be continuously monitored and oxygen consumption continuously measured, lean and fatty rat pups were fed the same amount of milk at the same ambient temperature. Under these conditions, the lean pups at weaning were fatter than the lean pups reared in litters. When core temperatures were allowed to vary as a function of exposure to the mother, the Zucker fatty pups deposited even more fat than their lean littermates by 21 days of age, indicating that a disturbance in thermoregulation and thermogenesis could not be the primary cause of the lipid deposition throughout the entire pre-weaning period (251). The major increase in fat occurred between day 16 and day 21. In pups reared at the thermoneutrality for 16 days with low feeding rates there was a small but significant increase in fat content between the lean and the Zucker fatty pups, which could not be accounted for by differences in oxygen consumption or lean body mass. Markewicz *et al.* (257) suggested that this difference might be accounted for by a slightly, but significantly, lower fecal energy loss by the fatty pups. When the ambient temperature of pups was varied to simulate that of pups that were left alone by their mothers for up to 60% of the day, the differences in oxygen consumption between the lean and fatty animals could account for 100% of the extra fat deposition, suggesting that reduced energy expenditure provided the energy for the excess fat deposition in the fatty genotype during the first 16 days of life.

Reduced activity of BAT also occurs in hypothalamic obesity (4, 249), probably due to decreased activity of the sympathetic nervous system (23, 133, 258). The glucose transporter, GLUT4, is significantly reduced in BAT from mice that become obese after treatment with gold thioglucose (176). Treatment of these mice with a β-3 agonist (BRL-26830-A), which may mimic sympathetic activity, increased GLUT4 in BAT to normal.

Activity of the sympathetic nervous system is reduced in the Zucker fatty rat. Spontaneous electrical activity of nerves supplying BAT was reduced in fatty rats compared with lean animals. In both genotypes there was an inverse linear relationship between core temperature and electrical firing rate of these sympathetic nerves (134). Electrical stimulation of the ventromedial hypothalamus resulted in similar increments in BAT temperature for both lean and obese rats, but this was associated with a smaller increase in firing rate in the fatty rat. Intracerebroventricular administration of glucose enhanced nerve activity, whereas 2-deoxy-D-glucose reduced nerve activity in both rats. Although sympathetic tone was suppressed, the genetically obese Zucker rat was responsive to alterations in temperature and metabolic stimuli (134).

Sympathetic stimulation of BAT increases the level of thyroxin-5'-deiodinase, the enzyme that converts thyroxin to 3,5,3'-triiodothyronine (T_3) in BAT. In the *ob/ob* mouse (259) and the fatty rat this is impaired and thyroid function is altered (260). Thyroxine 5'-monodeiodinase is significantly reduced in BAT from obese mice (261) and from fatty rats at 2, 7, 14, and 16 days of age compared with age-matched lean rats (262). Since this conversion process in BAT can be an important source of serum triiodothyronine, it was not surprising that the circulating levels of T_3 were significantly lower in the fatty rats (1.1 to 0.73 pmol/L). Exposure of 14-day-old lean and fatty pups to cold or injection with a thermogenic drug (BRL-35135) significantly increased the activity of thyroxine 5'-monodeiodinase in both fatty and lean pups, but the genotype difference was still readily detectable. After weaning on day 21, the level of thyroxine 5'-deiodinase in BAT of Zucker fatty rats increased to levels significantly higher than those in the lean littermates. However, serum T_3 concentrations remained significantly lower because the postweanling rats had a reduction in the hepatic concentration of thyroxine 5'-deiodinase. Thermogenic drugs also increase GLUT4 in white adipose tissue but not in muscle of obese mice (176).

Mitochondrial oxidation is coupled to the generation of ATP with an efficiency approaching 50%. There is a mitochondrial proton leak in BAT, which is not coupled to the generation of ATP. In addition there are two other thermogenic mechanisms that may enhance oxidation by reducing ATP generation. The first of these is the glycerophosphate shunt, in which the oxidation and reduction of glycerol 3-phosphate through the mitochondrial-coupled glycerol phosphate cycle reduces the number of ATP molecules generated per mole of substrate oxidized, as compared with the usual oxidation throughout the citrate cycle and the cytochrome oxidase system. Lardy has suggested that activation of the glycerophosphate cycle may be involved in the responses to thyroid hormone and to dehydroepiandrosterone (263).

A variant of this futile cycle may be involved in thermogenic control. Overexpression of the glycerol 3-phosphate dehydrogenase in white and brown fat of transgenic mice reduced the uncoupling protein activity of BAT. When mated with misty *db/db* mice the cycling of glycerol to glycerol-3-D and back reduced the body fat of these *db/db* mice to normal, in spite of the continuing hyperphagia. Thus, the glycerophosphate cycle may be a functionally important one (Kozak *et al.*, in this volume).

A second oxidative pathway involving oxidation of fatty acids is through proliferation of peroxisomes. Peroxisome proliferation occurs in response to hypolipidemic drugs such as clofibrate and nafenopin. Assimacopoulos-Jeannet *et al.* (264) have examined the effect on fatty rats of a peroxisome-proliferating drug called nafenopin. As a control they pair-fed fatty rats at the reduced food intake noted during nafenopin treatment. Using nine-week-old animals, food intake was decreased in fatty rats from 33 to 26 grams per day with nafenopin treatment. This was associated with a reduction in body-fat content. The pair-fed animals had similar food intakes to the nafenopin-treated animals, but their body-fat content was not reduced. The difference may well be accounted for by the stimulation of energy expenditure observed comparing the food-restricted animals whose metabolic rate (watts/[kg]$^{0.66}$) fell by 13% compared with no change in the drug-treated animals.

In summary, the relative hypothermia in the first 16 days of life appears to be a necessary and sufficient basis for the increased fat storage in genetically obese rodents. This is shown in Figure 4. After day 14–16, a time at which a number of physiologic systems have reached maturity, increased fat accretion no longer depends solely on hypothermia. The most likely explanation for the change is a shift in "nutrient partitioning" leading to enhanced fat storage at the expense of linear growth. Both hyperinsulinemia and altered responsiveness to adrenal steroids may be involved in this shift (Fig. 4).

Nutrient Partitioning and Adrenal Steroids

The channeling of nutrients into growth, milk production, muscle formation, or fat is controlled by a variety of hormonal mechanisms. Growth hormone, gonadal steroids, adrenal steroids, and sympathomimetic drugs all fall in this category. From the whole animal perspective the *fa/fa* rat absorbs less dietary nitrogen than lean controls (265). Nitrogen excretion is almost entirely urea, which accounts for only 75% of urinary nitrogen in lean rats. The percentage of nitrogen retention was lower in the fatty rat, consistent with an increased nutrient partitioning of carbon from protein into fat and excretion of the nitrogen.

Adrenal glucocorticoids play a critical role in the development of all

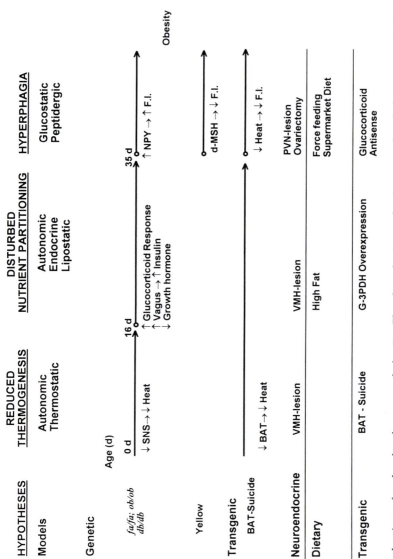

Figure 4. Mechanisms for the development of obesity. The three basic mechanisms—reduced thermogenesis due to impaired function of the autonomic nervous system; disturbed nutrient partitioning due to an imbalance in the autonomic nervous system, the endocrine system, and the lipostatic system; and finally, the hyperphagic model due to glucostatic or peptidergic means—are listed. For the genetic obesity, reduced thermogenesis is necessary and sufficient for early obesity. After 16 days of age, nutrient partitioning mechanisms become important and later hyperphagia. The time course or major mechanisms for the transgenic, neuroendocrine, and dietary forms of obesity.

forms of experimental obesity (266) after weaning, but may not be essential before that (267). Both Type I and Type II (glucocorticoid) receptors may be involved in modulating food intake and food choices (268, 269). Early studies by Naeser (270) and Solomon *et al.* (271) showed that adrenalectomy improved glucose tolerance. Studies on the fatty rat and the obese mouse, by Bray and his colleagues, clearly pointed to an essential role of glucocorticoids in a wide variety of phenotypic responses in both of these genetically obese animals (1, 272–277). King and his colleagues (278) subsequently showed the essential role of glucocorticoids for the expression of obesity following ventromedial hypothalamic lesions and the work of Hausberger (103) on the yellow mouse was complemented by the work of Shimizu *et al.* (279), which showed that adrenal steroids played a critical role in this species as well. Finally, the work of Okada *et al.* (280) showed that glucocorticoid receptor expression was critical in the development of obesity following exposure to a high-fat diet in the Osborne-Mendel rat, and Langley and York (281) made similar observations in the fatty rat.

A number of studies have examined the hypothalamic-pituitary control of adrenal corticoid secretion in relation to the expression of obesity (282, 283). The Zucker fatty rat appears to lack the normal circadian rhythm of serum corticosterone, with somewhat higher values in the morning when they are usually low in these animals (284–286). The *ob/ob* mice also show higher levels (287). The metabolic clearance rate of corticosterone is greater in the fatty rat, suggesting an increased rate of corticosterone production. This is consistent with the increased concentration of ACTH and the larger size of the adrenals in these animals (276, 288–290). If differences in the concentration of corticosterone were sufficient to explain the development of these syndromes, then treatment of lean animals with glucocorticoids would produce obesity. This is not the case. Treatment of lean animals with corticosterone will shift the percentage of fat and lean tissue (269, 291) but will not produce hyperphagia or significant weight gain. However, a disturbance in the glucocorticoid axis may provide important clues to the basis of the defect.

One hypothesis for the marked reduction in phenotypic expression of genetic obesity after adrenalectomy has been the possibility that elevated levels of corticotropin-releasing hormone (CRH) produced by adrenalectomy might serve to: 1) reduce food intake; 2) to stimulate the sympathetic nervous system; and 3) to inhibit the parasympathetic nervous system (94, 292, 293). This hypothesis has been supported by studies showing that the infusion of CRH into the ventricular system of experimentally obese animals reduces food intake, increases the activity of the sympathetic nervous system, and decreases body weight (94, 95, 115). It is also supported by the observation that a CRH antagonist can block the anorectic effect of estradiol (294). Hypothalamic CRH and pituitary ACTH are both elevated in the structurally abnormal hypothalamic nuclei (295). The CRH hypothesis has been explored in detail by measurements of CRH and arginine vasopressin (AVP) in the hypothalamus and pituitary of Zucker fatty rats (296). Neither the median eminence content of CRH or AVP nor the hypothalamic levels of CRH or AVP mRNA differed between obese and lean phenotypes. Moreover, there were no phenotypic differences in either basal or stimulated CRH release from isolated hypothalamic tissues nor were there any differences in the pituitary adrenal response to stressors. However, the release of CRH and AVP into the hypophyseal-portal circulation of obese fatty rats was significantly reduced, compared with lean animals. The output of CRH in the pituitary-portal circulation following adrenalectomy was threefold higher in fatty rats than in lean controls. Moreover, corticosterone infusion suppressed CRH levels more effectively in adrenalectomized fatty rats than in adrenalectomized lean animals. These data suggest that there is a reduced tone to the CRH regulatory system because of a dysfunction of the hypothalamic-pituitary axis at a site proximal to the point at which the CRH system affects glucocorticoid feedback regulation.

The altered responsiveness of the hypothalamic-pituitary axis to corticosterone is consistent with a variety of data, suggesting that adrenalectomized genetically obese animals and adrenalectomized hypothalamic obese animals have an enhanced sensitivity to corticosteroids. Early studies by Shimomura et al. (86) showed a dose-response stimulation of food intake in the genetically obese (ob/ob) mouse and the genetically diabetes (db/db) mouse compared with its lean littermates. Enhanced responsiveness to corticosterone was also shown by Freedman et al. (297) in replacement studies of adrenalectomized fatty rats (285). One possible site for these differential responses to corticosterone on the hypothalamic pituitary axis and in other areas is in the binding characteristics of the glucocorticoid receptors. White and Martin (179) reported a decrease in the affinity of receptors in the pituitary and liver from fatty rats, but not in the hypothalamus or hippocampus. Langley and York (299) also reported an increase in the Kd for corticosterone binding to type II receptors in the brain, but in contrast to the observations of White and Martin, they also observed these differences in the hippocampus and in the hypothalamus. Langley and York (299) concluded that glucocorticoid binding to both type I (mineralocorticoid) and type II (glucocorticoid) receptors is abnormally regulated in the Zucker fatty rat. In *ob/ob* mice glucocorticoid receptor numbers were lower in the liver, brain, and BAT of 8-week-old mice but were the same as lean mice at 8 weeks of age, suggesting that these changes were the result rather than the cause of the sensitivity to glucocorticoids (300). The sensitivity to glucocorticoids cannot be explained by a change in transport of steroids across the blood brain barrier (301). In studies on mRNA in adrenalectomized lean and fatty rats, Bray and colleagues (240) have shown that the induction of mRNA for male enzyme and GAPDH after treatment with corticosterone is abnormally controlled in adipose tissue and in the liver from these animals.

The phenotypic effects of adrenalectomy in the *ob/ob* mouse (170) are dependent in part on prior diet (244). After adrenalectomy *ob/ob* mice showed reduced energetic efficiency resulting from a decrease in food intake and an increase in energy expenditure (32) that persists even with ambient temperature of 35°C (302). High-glucose diets (303) and high-fat diets (304) increase food intake and fat storage. These dietary responses after adrenalectomy do not, however, modify the increased brain weight, do not increase protein content, nor improve thyroid hormone status (304). Additional support for the involvement of adrenal steroids in obesity comes from the work with DHEA. In the yellow mouse (305), in the obese and diabetes mouse (306, 307), and the fatty rat (308–310) dehydroepiandrosterone added to the diet reduces weight gain and percent body fat. One mechanism for this effect of DHEA may be by inhibiting the effects of glucocorticoids to stimulate the genome to transcribe new messages (175, 311, 312). A second possibility is that DHEA might act as a neurosteroid to modulate neuronal responses to glucocorticoids.

Summary and Conclusions

Glucocorticoids play a permissive role for the expression of most phenotypic features in genetically obese mice and rats and are necessary for obesity and hyperphagia in animals with hypothalamic injury and in animals eating a high-fat diet. Steroids can produce their effect by one of two mechanisms. First, they can bind to cytoplasmic receptors, enter the nucleus, bind to steroid receptor elements on the regulatory part of genes, and initiate or inhibit transcription of steroid-dependent messenger RNA. Alternatively they can bind to membrane elements to alter neuronal transmission. The fact that steroid replacement enhances food intake in response to norepinephrine almost immediately suggests that the latter may be the more important. This possibility is strengthened by the observation that the injection of dexamethasone into the ventricular system of adrenalectomized *ob/ob* mice will measurably decrease sympathetic activity and increase insulin within 30 minutes of injection (331, 314). This appears to be very rapid for a change resulting from transcriptional-translational processes.

A growing literature deals with neuronal action of steroids (315–318). The chloride channel of the GABA-A receptor appears to be one site at which some steroids act. Abnormalities in steroid action are not the primary defect in the genetically obese animals, though their interaction with neuronal elements and/or transacting genetic factors may be critical.

Where then does the defect in genetic obesity lie? (Fig. 4). One clue comes from the mechanism for early development in the Zucker fatty rat (257). In the first two weeks hypothermia appears to be necessary and sufficient. At this age activation of the BAT to maintain body temperature is essential. Activity of BAT in turn depends on effective modulation by the sympathetic nervous system. Abnormalities in the adenylyl cyclase and/or G protein coupled protein kinase could be a sufficient explanation. Since kinase-phosphatase cascades seem to be a critical part of many membrane events, I would suggest that these are highly viable candidates for the defect in recessively transmitted obesity. Kinase-phosphatase abnormalities could easily explain the similarity between the *db* and *ob* gene when they are on the same genetic background. One gene could affect one phosphatase and the other a second phosphatase in the same sequence. There are clearly other potential candidates, but these would be at the top of my list.

REFERENCES

1. Bray GA, York DA. Hypothalamic and genetic obesity in experimental animals: an autonomic and endocrine hypothesis. *Physiol Rev.* 1979;59:719–809.

2. Bray GA, Ricquier D, Spiegelman B. Obesity: Towards a Molecular Approach. Proceedings of a UCLA Symposium, held at Keystone, Colorado, April 17–23, 1989. New York, NY, Wiley-Liss, 1990; 1.

3. Zucker LM, Zucker FT. Fatty, a new mutation in the rat. *J Hered.* 1961;52:275–278.

4. Bray GA, Fisler JS, York DA. Neuroendocrine control of the development of obesity: understanding gained from studies of experimental animal models. *Front Neuroendocrinol.* 1990;11:128–181.

5. Kozak LP, Kozak UC, Clarke GT. Abnormal brown and white fat development in transgenic mice overexpressing glycerol 3-phosphate dehydrogenase. *Genes Dev.* 1991;5:2256–2264.

6. Kozak UC, Held W, Kreutter D, Kozak LP. Adrenergic regulation of the mitochondrial uncoupling protein gene in brown fat tumorcells. *Mol Endocrinol.* 1992;6:763–772.

7. Kahn BB, Pedersen O. Tissue-specific regulation of glucose transporter in different forms of obesity. *Proc Soc Exp Biol Med.* 1992;200:214–217.

8. Lowell BB, S-Susulic V, Hamann A, *et al.* Development of obesity in transgenic mice after genetic ablation of brown adipose tissue. *Nature.* 1993;366:740–742.

9. Olson AL, Liu M, Moye-Rowley WS, Buse JB, Bell GI, Pessin JE. Hormonal/metabolic regulation of the human GLUT4/muscle-fat facilitative glucose transporter gene in transgenic mice. *J Biol Chem.* 1993;269:9839–9846.

10. Ross SR, Graves RA, Spiegelman BM. Targeted expression of a toxin gene to adipose tissue: transgenic mice resistant to obesity. *Genes Dev.* 1993;7:1318–1324.

11. Shepherd PR, Gnudi L, Tozzo E, Yang HM, Leach F, Kahn BB. Adipose cell hyperplasia and enhanced glucose disposal in transgenic mice overexpressing GLUT4 selectively in adipose-tissue. *J Biol Chem.* 1993;268:2243–2246. Technical Note.

12. Warwick B, Suzuki H, Romsos DR. Corticosterone and tri-iodothyronine transport into brain of obese (*ob/ob*) mice. *Int J Obes.* 1992;16:377–382.

13. Hiremagalur BK, Vadlamudi S, Johanning GL, Patel MS. Long-term effects of feeding high-carbohydrate diet in preweaning period by gastrostomy: a new rat model for obesity. *Int J Obes.* 1993;17:495–502.

14. Oku J, Bray GA, Fisler JS, Schemmel R. Ventromedial hypotha-
    lamic knife-cut lesions in rats resistant to dietary obesity. *Am J
    Physiol.* 1984;246:R943–R948.
15. King BM, Kass JM, Cadieux NL, Sam H, Neville KL, Arceneaux
    ER. Hyperphagia and obesity in female rats with temporal-lobe
    lesions. *Physiol Behav.* 1993;54:759–765. Technical Note.
16. Bray GA, York DA. Studies on food intake of genetically obese
    rats. *Am J Physiol.* 1972;223:176–179.
17. Frohman LA, Bernardis LL, Schnatz JD, Burek L. Plasma insulin
    and triglyceride levels after hypothalamic lesions in weanling rats.
    Am J Physiol. 1969;216:1496–1501.
18. Han PW. Hypothalamic obesity in rats without hyperphagia. *Trans
    NY Acad Sci.* 1967;30:229–242.
19. Parkinson WL, Weingarten HP. Dissociative analysis of ventro-
    medial hypothalamic obesity syndrome. *Am J Physiol.* 1990;259:
    R829–R835.
20. Wilson LM, Currie PJ, Gilson TL. Thermal preference behavior in
    preweaning genetically obese (*ob/ob*) and lean (+ /?, + / +) mice.
    Physiol Behav. 1991;50:155–160.
21. Coleman DL. Obese and diabetes: two mutant genes causing di-
    abetes-obesity syndromes in mice. *Diabetalogia.* 1978;14:141–148.
    Review.
22. Cox JE, Powley TL. Development of obesity in diabetic mice pair-
    fed with lean siblings. *J Comp Physiol Psychol.* 1977;91:347–358.
23. Vander Tuig TG, Knehans AW, Romsos DR. Reduced sympathetic
    nervous activity in rats with ventromedial hypothalamic lesions.
    Life Sci. 1982;30:913–920.
24. Van de Werve G, Zaninetti D, Lang U, Vallotton MB, Jeanrenaud
    B. Identification of a major defect in insulin-resistant tissues of
    genetically obese (*fa/fa*) rats: impaired protein kinase C. *Diabetes.*
    1987;36:310–314.
25. Arase K, Fisler JS, Shargill NS, York DA, Bray GA. Intracerebro-
    ventricular infusions of 3-OH-butyrate and insulin in a rat model
    of dietary obesity. *Am J Physiol.* 1988;255:R974–R982.
26. Ikeda H, Nishikawa K, Matsuo T. Feeding responses of Zucker
    fatty rat to 2-deoxy-D-glucose, norepinephrine, and insulin. *Am J
    Physiol.* 1980;239:E379–E384.
27. Tsujii S, Bray GA. Food intake of lean and obese Zucker rats fol-

lowing ventricular infusions of adrenergic agonists. *Brain Res.* 1992;587:226–232.

28. Pesonen U, Miettinen T, Scheinin M, Koulu M. α2-adrenoceptor density in forebrain areas of Zucker rats: no effect of genetic obesity or antiglucocorticoid treatment. *Brain Res.* 1992;574:353–356.

29. Currie PJ. Differential effects of NE, CLON, and 5-HT on feeding and macronutrient selection in genetically obese (*ob/ob*) and lean mice. *Brain Res Bull.* 1993;32:133–142.

30. McLaughlin CL, Baile CA. Cholecystokinin, amphetamine and diazepam and feeding in lean and obese Zucker rats. *Pharmacol Biochem Behav.* 1979;10:87–93.

31. Kuprys R, Oltmans GA. Amphetamine anorexia and hypothalamic catecholamines in genetically obese mice ob/ob. *Pharmacol Biochem Behav.* 1982;17:271–282.

32. Smith CK, Romsos DR. Effects of adrenalectomy on energy balance obese mice are diet dependent. *Am J Physiol.* 1985;249:R13–R22.

33. Koulu M, Huuppone R, Hanninen H, Pesonen U, Rouru J, Seppala T. Hypothalamic neurochemistry and feeding behavioral responses to clonidine, an alpha-2 agonist, and to trifluoromethyl-phenylpiperazine, a putative 5-hydroxytryptamine-1B agonist, in genetically obese Zucker rats. *Neuroendocrinology.* 1990;52:503–510.

34. Levin BE, Planas B, Routh VH, Hamilton J, Stern JS, Horwitz BA. Altered α1-adrenoceptor binding in intact and adrenalectomized obese Zucker rats (*fa/fa*). *Brain Res.* 1993;614:146–154.

35. Jhanwar-Uniyal M, Awad IR, Gearhart GM, Finkelstein JA, Leibowitz SF. Higher alpha-noradrenergic receptors in paraventricular nucleus of obese Zucker rats: decline after food deprivation. *Pharmacol Biochem Behav.* 1991;40:853–859.

36. Levin BE. Defective cerebral glucose utilization in diet-induced obese rats. *Am J Physiol.* 1991;261:R787–R792.

37. Levin BE, Planas B. Defective glucoregulation of brain a2-adrenoceptors in obesity-prone rats. *Am J Physiol.* 1993;264:R305–R311.

38. Duhault J, Lacour F, Espinal J, Rolland Y. Effect of activation of the serotonergic system during prolonged starvation on subsequent caloric intake and macronutrient selection in the Zucker rat. *Appetite.* 1993;20:135–144.

39. Chaouloff F, Laude D, Serrurier B, Merino D, Elghozi JL. Periph-

eral and central consequences of immobilization stress in genetically obese Zucker rats. *Am J Physiol.* 1989;256:R435–R442.

40. Finkelstein JA, Chance WT, Fischer JE. Brain serotonergic activity
    and plasma amino acid levels in genetically obese Zucker rats.
    Pharmacol Biochem Behav. 1982;17:939–944.

41. Routh VH, Murakami DN, Stern JS, Fuller CA, Horwitz BA. Neu-
    ronal activity in hypothalamic nuclei of obese and lean Zucker
    rats. *Int J Obes.* 1990;14:879–891.

42. Squadrito F, Calapai G, Campo M, *et al.* Indolpyruvic acid, a tryp-
    tophan keto analogue, reduces food intake in obese Zucker rats.
    Neurosci Res Commun. 1991;9:27–36.

43. Serra F, Johnston J, Carnie J, Palou A. Altered blood amino acid
    distribution in genetically obese mice. *Biochim Biophys Acta.* 1991;
    1079:289–292.

44. Serra F, Pico C, Johnston J, Carnie J, Palou A. Opposite response
    to starvation of TRP/LNAA ratio in lean and obese Zucker rats.
    Biochem Mol Biol Int. 1993;29:483–491.

45. Shimizu H, Uehara Y, Negishi M, *et al.* Altered monoamine me-
    tabolism in the hypothalamus of the genetically-obese yellow (A-
    Y/A) mouse. *Exp Clin Endocrinol.* 1992;99:45–48.

46. Coscina DV, Chambers JW. Serotonin depleting midbrain lesions
    do not prevent ovariectomy induced weight gain. *Physiol Behav.*
    1991;50:1051–1056.

47. Sakata T, Ookuma K, Fukagawa K, *et al.* Blockade of the histamine
    H1-receptor in the rat ventromedial hypothalamus and feeding
    elicitation. *Brain Res.* 1988;441:403–407.

48. Sakata T, Fukagawa K, Ookuma K. Hypothalamic neuronal his-
    tamine modulates ad libitum feeding by rats. *Brain Res.* 1990;537:
    303–306.

49. Machidori H, Sakata T, Yoshimatsu H, *et al.* Zucker obese rats:
    defect in brain histamine control of feeding. *Brain Res.* 1992;590:
    180–186.

50. Allars J, York DA. The effects of 2-deoxy-D-glucose on brown ad-
    ipose tissue of lean and obese Zucker rats. *Int J Obes.* 1986;10:147–
    158.

51. Tsujii S, Bray GA. Effects of glucose, 2-deoxyglucose, phlorizin,
    and insulin on food intake of lean and fatty rats. *Am J Physiol.*
    1990;258:E476–E481.

52. Kamtachi GL, Veeraragavan K, Chandra D, Bapna JS. Antagonism

of acute feeding response to 2-deoxyglucose and 5-thioglucose by GABA antagonists: the relative role of ventromedial and lateral hypothalamus. *Pharmacol Biochem Behav.* 1986;25:59–62.

53. Tsujii S, Bray GA. GABA-related feeding control in genetically obese rats. *Brain Res.* 1991;540:48–54.

54. Coscina DV, Castonguay TW, Stern JS. Effect of increasing brain GABA on the meal patterns of genetically-obese vs lean Zucker rats. *Int J Obes.* 1992;16:425–433.

55. Morley JE, Levine AS. Appetite regulation: modern concepts offering food for thought. *Postgrad Med.* 1985;77:42–48. Review.

56. Morley JE, Levine AS, Gosnell BA, Kneip J, Grace M. Effect of neuropeptide Y on ingestive behaviors in the rat. *Am J Physiol.* 1987;252:R599–R609.

57. Arase K, Sakaguchi T, Takahashi M, Bray GA, Ling N. Effects on feeding behavior of rats of a cryptic peptide from the c-terminal end of prepro-growth hormone-releasing factor. *Endocrinology.* 1987;121:1960–1965.

58. Morley JE. Neuropeptide regulation of appetite and weight. *Endocr Rev.* 1987;8:256–287.

59. Margules DL, Boisset B, Lewis MJ, Shibuya H, Pert CB. β-endorphin is associated with overeating in genetically obese mice (*ob/ob*) and rats (*fa/fa*). *Science.* 1978;202:988–991.

60. Beck B, Burlet A, Nicolas JP, Burlet C. Hyperphagia in obesity is associated with a central peptidergic dysregulation in rats. *J Nutr.* 1990;120:806–811.

61. Tannenbaum GS, Lapointe M, Gurd W, Finkelstein JA. Mechanisms of impaired growth hormone secretion in genetically obese Zucker rats: roles of growth hormone releasing factor and somatostatin. *Endocrinology.* 1990;127:3087–3095.

62. Williams G, Cardoso H, Lee YC, *et al.* Reduced hypothalamic neurotensin concentrations in the genetically obese diabetic (*ob/ob*) mouse: possible relationship to obesity. *Metabolism.* 1991;40:1112–1116.

63. Beck BB, Nicolas JP, Burlet C. Galanin in the hypothalamus of fed and fasted lean and obese Zucker rats. *Brain Res.* 1993;623:124–130.

64. Beck B, Burlet A, Bazin R, Nicolas JP, Burlet C. Early modification of neuropeptide Y but not of neurotensin in the suprachiasmatic nucleus of the obese Zucker rat. *Neurosci Lett.* 1992;136:185–188.

65. Finkelstein JA, Steggles AW. Levels of gastrin-cholecystokinin-like immunoreactivity in the brains of genetically obese and non-obese rats. *Peptides*. 1981;2:19–21.

66. Oku J, Inoue S, Glick Z, Bray GA, Walsh JH. Cholecystokinin, bombesin and neurotensin in brain tissue from obese animals. *Int J Obes*. 1984;8:171–182.

67. Schneider BS, Monahan JW, Hirsch J. Brain cholecystokinin and nutritional status in rats and mice. *J Clin Invest*. 1979;64:1348–1356.

68. Timmers K, Coleman DL, Voyles NR, Powell AM, Rokaeus A, Recant L. Neuropeptide content in pancreas and pituitary of obese and diabetes mutant mice: strain and sex differences. *Metabolism*. 1990;39:378–383.

69. Timmers KI, Palkovits M, Coleman DL. Unique alterations of neuropeptide content in median eminence, amygdala, and dorsal vagal complex of 3-week-old and 6-week-old diabetes mutant mice. *Metabolism*. 1990;39:1158–1166.

70. Shimizu H, Shimomura Y, Uehara Y, Fukatsu A, Kobayashi I. Increased brain cholecystokinin concentrations in the genetically obese yellow (Ay/a) mouse. *Neuroendocrinol Lett*. 1990;12:465–470.

71. Pesonen U, Rouru J, Huuppone R, Koulu M. Effects of repeated administration of mifepristone and 8-oh-dpat on expression preproneuropeptide-y messenger-RNA in the arcuate nucleus of obese Zucker rats. *Mol Brain Res*. 1991;10:267–272.

72. Sanacora G, Finkelstein JA, White JD. Developmental aspect of differences in hypothalamic preproneuropeptide Y messenger ribonucleic acid content in lean and genetically obese Zucker rats. *J Neuroendocrinol*. 1992;4:353–357.

73. Chua SC, Brown AW, Kim JH, Hennessey KL, Leibel RL, Hirsch J. Food deprivation and hypothalamic neuropeptide gene expression: effects of strain background and the diabetes mutation. *Brain Res Mol Brain Res*. 1991;11:291–299.

74. Beck B, Burlet A, Nicolas JP, Burlet C. Unexpected regulation of hypothalamic neuropeptide Y by food deprivation and refeeding in the Zucker rat. *Life Sci*. 1992;50:923–930.

75. Schwartz MW, Marks JL, Sipols AJ, *et al*. Central insulin administration reduces neuropeptide Y mRNA expression in the arcuate nucleus of food-deprived lean (Fa/Fa) but not obese (*fa/fa*) Zucker rats. *Endocrinology*. 1991;128:2645–2647.

76. Brief DJ, Sipols AJ, Woods SC. Intraventricular neuropeptide Y

injections stimulate food intake in lean, but not obese Zucker rats. *Physiol Behav.* 1992;51:1105–1110.

77. Walker HC, Romsos DR. Similar effects of NPY on energy-metabolism and on plasma-insulin in adrenalectomized *ob/ob* and lean mice. *Am J Physiol.* 1993;264:E226–E230.

78. Beck B, Stricker-Krongrad A, Nicolase JP, Burlet C. Chronic and continuous intracerebroventricular infusion of neuropeptide Y in Long-Evans rats mimics the feeding behavior of obese Zucker rats. *Int J Obes.* 1992;16:295–302.

79. Zarjevski N, Cusin I, Vettor R, Rohner-Jeanrenaud F, Jeanrenaud B. Chronic intracerebroventricular neuropeptide-Y-administration to normal rats mimics hormonal and metabolic changes of obesity. *Endocrinology.* 1993;133:1753–1758.

80. Israel PA, Park CR, Schwartz MW, *et al.* Effect of diet-induced obesity and experimental hyperinsulinemia on insulin uptake into CSF of the rat. *Brain Res Bull.* 1993;30:571–575.

81. Schwartz MW, Figlewicz DP, Baskin DG, Woods SC, Porte D Jr. Insulin in the brain: a hormonal regulator of energy balance. *Endocr Rev.* 1992;13:387–414.

82. Stein LJ, Dorsa DM, Baskin DG, Figlewicz DP, Porte D Jr, Woods SC. Reduced effect of experimental peripheral hyperinsulinemia to elevate cerebrospinal fluid insulin concentrations of obese Zucker rats. *Endocrinology.* 1987;121:1611–1615.

83. Schwartz MW, Figlewicz DF, Kahn SE, Baskin DG, Greenwood MR, Porte DJ. Insulin binding to brain capillaries is reduced in genetically obese, hyperinsulinemic Zucker rats. *Peptides.* 1990;11:467–472.

84. Figlewicz DP, Szot P, Greenwood MRC. Insulin stimulates inositol incorporation in hippocampus of lean but not obese Zucker rats. *Physiol Behav.* 1990;47:325–330.

85. Recant L, Voyles NR, Luciano M, Pert CB. Naltrexone reduces weight gain, alters "beta-endorphin," and reduces insulin output from pancreatic islets of genetically obese mice. *Peptides.* 1980;1:309–313.

86. Shimomura Y, Bray GA, Lee M. Adrenalectomy and steroid treatment in obese (*ob/ob*) and diabetic (*db/db*) mice. *Horm Metab Res.* 1987;19:295–299.

87. Roane DS, Iadarola MJ, Porter JR. Decreased [3H]-naloxone bind-

ing and elevated dynorphin-A (1-8) content in Zucker rat brain. *Physiol Behav.* 1988;43:371–374.

88. Rothman RB, Xu H, Char GU, *et al.* Phenylpiperidine opioid antagonists that promote weight loss in rats have high affinity for the K2B (enkephalin-sensitive) binding site. *Peptides.* 1993;14: 17–20.

89. Shaw WN, Mitch CH, Leander JD, Mendelsohn LG, Zimmerman DM. The effect of the opioid antagonist-LY255582 on body-weight of the obese Zucker rat. *Int J Obes.* 1991;15:387–395.

90. Shaw WN, Mitch CH, Leander JD, Zimmerman DM. Effect of phenylpiperdine opioid antagonists on food consumption and weight gain of the obese Zucker rat. *J Pharm Exp.* 1990;253:85–89.

91. Khawaja XZ, Chattopadhyay AK, Green IC. Increased beta-endorphin and dynorphin concentrations in discrete hypothalamic regions of genetically-obese (*ob/ob*) mice. *Brain Res.* 1991;555: 164–168. Technical Note.

92. Ferguson-Segall M, Flynn JJ, Walker J, Margules DL. Increased immunoreactive dynorphin and leu-enkephalin in posterior pituitary of obese mice (*ob/ob*) and super-sensitivity to drugs that act as kappa receptors. *Life Sci.* 1982;31:2233–2236.

93. Morley JE, Levine AS, Gosnell BA, Kneip J, Grace M. The kappa opioid receptor, ingestive behaviors and the obese mouse *ob/ob.* *Physiol Behav.* 1983;31:603–606.

94. Arase K, Shargill NS, Bray GA. Effect of corticotropin releasing factor on genetically obese (fatty) rats. *Physiol Behav.* 1989;45:565–570.

95. Holt SJ, York DA. Studies on the sympathetic efferents of brown adipose tissue of lean and obese Zucker rats. *Brain Res.* 1989;491: 106–112.

96. Rohner-Jeanrenaud F, Walker CD, Greco-Perotto R, Jeanrenaud B. Central corticotropin-releasing factor administration prevents the excessive body weight gain of genetically obese (*fa/fa*) rats. *Endocrinology.* 1989;124:733–739.

97. Nakaishi S, Nakai Y, Fukata J, *et al.* Immunoreactive corticotropin-releasing hormone levels in discrete hypothalamic nuclei of genetically obese Zucker rats. *Neurosci Lett.* 1993;159:29–31.

98. Oohara M, Negishi M, Shimizu H, Sato N, Mori M. α-melanocyte stimulating hormone (MSH) antagonizes the anorexia by corticotropin releasing factor (CRF). *Life Sci.* 1993;53:1473–1477.

99. Shimizu H, Shargill NS, Bray GA, Yen T, Gesellchen P. Effects of MSH on food intake, body weight and coat color of the yellow obese mouse. *Life Sci.* 1989;45:543–552.

100. Shimizu H, Shimomura Y, Uekara Y, Kobayashi I. Reduced pituitary acetylation and possible role of hypothalamic monoamines in the yellow obese mouse. *Neuroendocrinol Lett.* 1990;12:31–42.

101. Tsujii S, Bray GA. Acetylation alters the feeding response to MSH and beta-endorphin. *Brain Res Bull.* 1989;23:165–169.

102. Yen T, Gill A, Frigeri L, Barsh G, Wolff G. Obesity, diabetes, and neoplasia in yellow A^{vy}/-mice: ectopic expression of the agouti gene. *FASEB J.* 1994;8:479–488.

103. Hausberger FX, Ramsay AJ. Islet hypertrophy in obesity of mice bearing ACTH-secreting tumors. *Endocrinology.* 1959;65:165–171.

104. Bray GA, York DA. Genetically transmitted obesity in rodents. *Physiol Rev.* 1971;51:598–646.

105. Pepin MC, Pothier F, Barden N. Impaired type II glucocorticoid-receptor function in mice bearing antisense RNA transgene. *Nature.* 1992;355:725–728.

106. Fujimoto K, Fukagawa K, Sakata T, Tso P. Suppression of food intake by apolipoprotein A-IV is mediated through the central nervous system in rats. *J Clin Invest.* 1993;91:1830–1833.

107. Willems MET, Brozinic JT, Torgan CE, Cortez MY, Ivy JL. Muscle glucose uptake of obese Zucker rats trained at two different intensities. *J Appl Physiol.* 1991;70:36–42.

108. Beck B, Stricker-Krongrad A, Burlet A, Nicolas JP, Burlet C. Changes in hypothalamic neurotensin concentrations and food intake in rats fed a high fat diet. *Int J Obes.* 1992;16:361–366.

109. Kava RA, West DB, Lukasik VA, *et al.* The effects of gonadectomy on glucose tolerance of genetically obese (*fa/fa*) rats: influence of sex and genetic background. *Int J Obes.* 1992;16:103–111.

110. Flatt PR, Juntti-Berggren L, Berggren P, Gould BJ, Swanston-Flatt SK. Failure of glucose tolerance factor-containing brewer's yeast to ameliorate spontaneous diabetes in C57BL/KsJ db/db mice. *Diabetes Res.* 1990;10:147–151.

111. Pujol A, Berthault MF, Picon L, Penicaud L. Regulation of glucose homeostasis in pre-obese Zucker rats before and after weaning. *Int J Obes.* 1991;15:505–511.

112. Ruiz B, Felipe A, Casado J, Pastoranglada M. Amino-acids uptake

by liver of genetically-obese Zucker rats. *Biochem J.* 1991;280:367–372.

113. Lavoie L, Bollen M, Stalmans W, Van de Werve G. Increased synthase phosphatase activity is responsible for the super-activation of glycogen synthase in hepatocytes from fasted obese Zucker rats. *Endocrinology.* 1991;129:2674–2678.

114. Rohner-Jeanrenaud F, Jeanrenaud B. Beneficial effect of intravenous bolus of corticotropin-releasing factor on glucose intolerance of genetically obese (*fa/fa*) rats. *Diabetes.* 1992;41:493–498.

115. Rohner-Jeanrenaud F, Jeanrenaud B. Acute intravenous corticotropin-releasing factor administration: effects on insulin secretion in lean and genetically obese *fa/fa* rats. *Endocrinology.* 1992;130:1903–1908.

116. Leiter EH, Beamer WG, Coleman DL, Longcope C. Androgenic and estrogenic metabolites in serum of mice fed dehydroepiandrosterone: relationship to antihyperglycemic effects. *Metabolism.* 1987;36:863–869.

117. Leiter EH, Chapman HD, Falany CN. Synergism of obesity genes with hepatic steroid sulfotransferases to mediate diabetes in mice. *Diabetes.* 1991;40:1360–1363.

118. Blonz ER, Stern JS, Curry DL. Dynamics of pancreatic insulin release in young Zucker rats: a heterozygote effect. *Am J Physiol.* 1985;248:E188–E193.

119. Khawaja XZ, Green IC, Thorpe JR, Bailey CJ. Increased sensitivity to insulin-releasing and glucoregulatory effects of dynorphin A1-13 and U 50488H in *ob/ob* versus lean mice. *Diabetes.* 1990;39:1289–1297.

120. Lee HC, Curry DL, Stern JS. Selective muscarinic sensitivity in perfused pancreases of obese Zucker rats. *Int J Obes.* 1993;17:569–577.

121. Jeanrenaud B, Halimi S, Van de Werve G. Neuro-endocrine disorders seen as triggers of the triad: obesity—insulin resistance—abnormal glucose tolerance. *Diabetes Metab Rev.* 1985;1:261–291.

122. Chan CB. Glucokinase activity in isolated islets from obese *fa/fa* Zucker rats. *Biochem J.* 1993;295:673–677.

123. Fournier LA, Heick HMC, Begin-Heick N. The influence of K+-induced membrane depolarization on insulin secretion in islets of lean and obese (*ob/ob*) mice. *Biochem Cell Biol.* 1989;68:243–248.

124. Brichard SM, Bailey CJ, Henquin JC. Marked improvement of glu-

cose homeostasis in diabetic *ob/ob* mice given oral vanadate. *Diabetes.* 1990;39:1326–1332.

125. Brichard SM, Ongemba LN, Kolanowski J, Henquin JC. The influence of vanadate on insulin counter-regulatory hormones in obese *fa/fa* rats. *J Endocrinol.* 1991;131:185–191.

126. Berthoud HR, Jeanrenaud B. Changes of insulinemia, glycemia and feeding behavior induced by VMH-procainization in the rat. *Brain Res Bull.* 1979;174:184–187.

127. Rohner-Jeanrenaud F, Jeanrenaud B. Vagal mediation of corticotropin-releasing-factor-induced increase in insulinemia in lean and genetically-obese *fa/fa* rats. *Neuroendocrinology.* 1990;52:52–56.

128. Tokunaga K, Fukushima M, Kemnitz JW, Bray GA. Effect of vagotomy on serum insulin in rats with paraventricular or ventromedial hypothalamic lesions. *Endocrinology.* 1986;119:1708–1711.

129. Campfield LA, Smith FJ. Alteration of islet neurotransmitter sensitivity following ventromedial hypothalamic lesion. *Am J Physiol.* 1983;244:R635–R640.

130. Campfield LA, Smith FJ, Larue-Achagiotis C. Temporal evolution of altered islet neurotransmitter sensitivity after VMH lesion. *Am J Physiol.* 1986;251:R63–R69.

131. Smith FJ, Campfield LA. Pancreatic adaptation in VMH obesity: in vivo compensatory response to altered neural input. *Am J Physiol.* 1986;251:R70–R76.

132. Atef N, Brule C, Bihoreau MT, Ktorza A, Picon L, Penicaud L. Enhanced insulin secretory response to acetylcholine by perfused pancreas of 5-day-old preobese Zucker rats. *Endocrinology.* 1991; 129:2219–2224.

133. Sakaguchi T, Arase K, Bray GA. Sympathetic activity and food intake of rats with ventromedial hypothalamic lesions. *Int J Obes.* 1988;12:43–49.

134. Holt SJ, York DA. The effects of adrenalectomy, corticotropin releasing factor and vasopressin on the sympathetic firing rate of nerves to interscapular brown adipose tissue in the Zucker rat. *Physiol Behav.* 1989;45:1123–1129.

135. Van Zeggeren A, Li ETS. Food intake and choice in lean and obese Zucker rats after intragastric carbohydrate preloads. *J Nutr.* 1990; 120:309–316.

136. Squadrito F, Cucinott D, Arcoraci V, *et al.* A decreased brain stem

content of GABA mediates hyperinsulinemia in obese Zucker rats. *Neurosci Res Commun.* 1991;8:1–10.

137. Khan A, Chandram V, Ostenson CG, *et al.* Glucose cycling is markedly enhanced in pancreatic-islets of obese hyperglycemic mice. *Endocrinology.* 1990;126:2413–2416.

138. Atef N, Ktorza A, Picon L, Penicaud L. Increased islet blood-flow in obese rats: role of the autonomic nervous-system. *Am J Physiol.* 1992;262:E736–E740.

139. Flatt PR, Kwasowsk P, Howland RJ, Bailey CJ. Gastric-inhibitory polypeptide and insulin responses to orally-administered amino-acids in genetically-obese hyperglycemic (*ob/ob*) mice. *J Nutr.* 1991; 121:1123–1128.

140. Pederson RA, Campos RV, Buchan AMJ, Chisholm CB, Russell JC, Brown JC. Comparison of the enteroinsular axis in two strains of obese rat, the fatty Zucker and the JCR:LA-corpulent. *Int J Obes.* 1991;15:461–470.

141. Elias AN, Vaziri ND, Pandian MR, Ansari MA. Relationship between β-endorphin/β-lipotropin, hyperglycemia, and hyperinsulinemia in obese male Zucker rats. *Proc Soc Exp Biol Med.* 1989;192: 157–160.

142. Cawthorn EG, Chan CB. Effect of pertussis toxin on islet insulin secretion in obese (*fa/fa*) Zucker rats. *Mol Cell Endocrinol.* 1991;75: 197–204.

143. Begin-Heick N. αSubunits of Gs and Gi in adipocyte plasma membranes of genetically diabetic (*db/db*) mice. *Am J Physiol.* 1992;263: C121–C129.

144. Chan CB, MacPhail RM. Functional characterization of alpha-adrenoceptors on pancreatic islets of *fa/fa* Zucker rats. *Mol Cell Endocrinol.* 1992;84:33–37.

145. Pujol A, Cousin B, Burnol AF, *et al.* Insulin receptor kinase activity in muscles and white adipose tissue during course of VHM obesity. *Am J Physiol.* 1992;262:E161–E166.

146. Grundleger ML, Godbole VY, Thenen SW. Age-dependent development of insulin resistance of soleus muscle in genetically obese (*ob/ob*) mice. *Am J Physiol.* 1980;239:E363–E371.

147. Le Marchand-Brustel Y, Jeanrenaud B. Pre- and postweaning studies on development of obesity in *mdb/mdb* mice. *Am J Physiol.* 1978; 234:E568–E574.

148. Penicaud L, Ferre P, Terretaz J, *et al.* Development of obesity in

Zucker rats: early insulin resistance in muscles but normal sensitivity in white adipose tissue. *Diabetes.* 1987;36:626–631.

149. Frohman LA, Goldman JK, Bernardis LL. Metabolism of intravenously injected 14 C-glucose in weanling rats with hypothalamic obesity. *Metabolism.* 1972;21:799–805.

150. Penicaud L, Rohner-Jeanrenaud F, Jeanrenaud B. In vivo metabolic changes as studied longitudinally after ventromedial hypothalamic lesions. *Am J Physiol.* 1986;250:E662–E668.

151. Buchanan TA, Fisler JS, Underberger S, Sipos GF, Bray GA. Whole body insulin sensitivity in Osborne Mendel and S5B/Pl rats eating a low- or high-fat diet. *Am J Physiol.* 1992;263:R785–R789.

152. Pedersen O, Kahn CR, Flier JS, Kahn BB. High fat feeding causes insulin resistance and a marked decrease in the expression of glucose transporters (GLUT-4) in fat cells of rats. *Endocrinology.* 1991; 129:771–777.

153. Zarjevski N, Doyle P, Jeanrenaud B. Muscle insulin resistance may not be a primary etiological factor in the genetically obese *fa/fa* rat. *Endocrinology.* 1992;130:1564–1570.

154. Kahn BB, Cushman SW. Subcellular translocation of glucose transporters: role in insulin action and its perturbation in altered metabolic states. *Diabetes Metab Rev.* 1985;1:203–227.

155. Machado UF, Shimizu Y, Saito M. Decreased glucose-transporter (GLUT-4) content in insulin-sensitive tissues of obese aurothioglucose-treated and monosodium glutamate-treated mice. *Horm Metab Res.* 1993;25:462–465.

156. Gill AM, Yen TT. Effects of ciglitazone on endogenous plasma islet amyloid polypeptide and insulin sensitivity in obese diabetic viable yellow mice. *Life Sci.* 1991;48:703–710.

157. Koranyi L, Tanizawa Y, Penicaud L, Atef N, Girard J, Permutt MA. Developmental regulation of amylin and insulin-gene expression in lean (*Fa/Fa*) and obese (*fa/fa*) Zucker rats. *Diabetes.* 1992;41:685–690.

158. Tokuyama Y, Kanatsuk A, Ohsawa H, *et al.* Hypersecretion of IAPP from the islets of VMH-lesioned rats and obese Zucker rats. *Diabetes Res Clin Pract.* 1992;15:23–30.

159. Tokuyama Y, Kanatsuk A, Ohsawa H, *et al.* Hypersecretion of islet amyloid polypeptide from pancreatic-islets of ventromedial hypothalamic-lesioned rats and obese Zucker rats. *Endocrinology.* 1991;128:2739–2744.

160. Hotamisligil GS, Shargill NS, Spiegelman BM. Adipose expression of tumor necrosis factor-α: direct role of obesity-linked insulin resistance. *Science.* 1993;259:87–91.

161. Spiegelman BM. Through thick and thin: wasting, obesity, and TNF. *Cell.* 1993;73:625–627.

162. Lang CH, Dobrescu C, Bagby GJ. Tumor necrosis factor impairs insulin action on peripheral glucose disposal and hepatic glucose output. *Endocrinology.* 1992;130:43–52.

163. Koubi H, Duchamp C, Geloen A, Freminet A, Minaire Y. Resistance of hepatic glycogen to depletion in obese Zucker rats. *Can J Physiol Pharmacol.* 1991;69:841–845.

164. Chen C, Williams PF, Caterson ID. Liver and peripheral tissue glycogen metabolism in obese mice: effect of a mixed meal. *Am J Physiol.* 1993;265:E743–E751.

165. King MJ, Pugazhenthi S, Khandelwal RL, Sharma RK. Membrane-associated N-myristoyltransferase activity is reduced in obese (*fa/fa*) Zucker rat liver. *Biochem Biophys Res Commun.* 1993;196:665–670.

166. Andrikopoulos S, Rosella G, Gaskin E, Thorburn A, Kaczmarczyk S, Proietto J. Impaired regulation of hepatic fructose-1,6-bisphosphatase in the New Zealand obese mouse model of NIDDM. *Diabetes.* 1993;42:1731–1736.

167. Andersson A, Korsgren O, Naeser P. DNA replication in transplanted and endogenous pancreatic islets of obese-hyperglycemic mice at different stages of the syndrome. *Metabolism.* 1989;38:974–978.

168. Ohshima K, Shargill NS, Chan TM, Bray GA. Adrenalectomy reverses insulin resistance in muscle from obese (*ob/ob*) mice. *Am J Physiol.* 1984;246:E193–E207.

169. Ohshima K, Shargill NS, Chan TM, Bray GA. Effects of dexamethasone on glucose transport by skeletal muscles of obese (*ob/ob*) mice. *Int J Obes.* 1989;13:155–163.

170. Saito M, Bray GA. Adrenalectomy and food restriction in the genetically obese (*ob/ob*) mouse. *Am J Physiol.* 1984;246:R20–R25.

171. Almond RE, Enser M. Effects of adrenalectomy on muscle fibre growth and fibre-type composition in obese hyperglycemic *ob/ob* and lean mice. *Int J Obes.* 1989;13:791–800.

172. King PA, Horton ED, Hirshman MF, Horton ES. Insulin resistance in obese Zucker rat (*fa/fa*) skeletal muscle is associated with a fail-

ure of glucose transporter translocation. *J Clin Invest.* 1992;90: 1568–1575.

173. Hainault I, Guerre-Millo M, Guichard C, Lavau M. Differential regulation of adipose tissue glucose transporters in genetic obesity (fatty rat): selective increase in the adipose cell/muscle glucose transporter (GLUT 4) expression. *J Clin Invest.* 1991;87:1127–1131.

174. Koranyi L, James D, Mueckler M, Permutt MA. Glucose transporter levels in spontaneously obese (*db/db*) insulin-resistant mice. *J Clin Invest.* 1990;85:962–967. Technical Note.

175. Wright BE, Porter JR, Browne ES, Svec F. Antiglucocorticoid action of dehydroepiandrosterone in young obese Zucker rats. *Int J Obes.* 1992;16:579–583.

176. Le Marchand-Brustel Y, Olichonb C, Gremeaux T, Tanti JF, Rochet N, Vanobber E. Glucose transporter in insulin sensitive tissues of lean and obese mice: effect of the thermogenic agent BRL-26830A. *Endocrinology.* 1990;127:2687–2695.

177. Becker-Zimmerman K, Berger M, Berchtold P, Gries FA, Herberg L, Schwenen M. Treadmill training improves intravenous glucose tolerance and insulin sensitivity in fatty Zucker rats. *Diabetologia.* 1982;22:468–474.

178. Cortez MY, Torgan CE, Brozinick JT, Ivy JL. Insulin resistance of obese Zucker rats exercise trained at two different intensities. *Am J Physiol.* 1991;261:E613–E619.

179. Zaninetti D, Greco-Perotto R, Assimacopoulos-Jeanner F, Jeanrenaud B. Dysregulation of glucose transport and transporters in perfused hearts of genetically obese (*fa/fa*) rats. *Diabetologia.* 1989;32:56–60.

180. Banks EA, Brozinic JT, Yaspelki BB, Kang HY, Ivy JL. Muscle glucose-transport, GLUT-4 content, and degree of exercise training in obese Zucker rats. *Am J Physiol.* 1992;263:E1015–E1020. Technical Note.

181. Brozinick JT, Etgen GJ, Yaspelkis BB, Ivy JL. Contraction-activated glucose-uptake is normal in insulin-resistant muscle of the obese Zucker rat. *J Appl Physiol.* 1992;73:382–387.

182. Brozinick JT, Etgen GJ, Yaspelkis BB, Kang HY, Ivy JL. Effects of exercise training on muscle GLUT-4 protein-content and translocation in obese Zucker rats. *Am J Physiol.* 1993;265:E419–E427.

183. Garcia-Sainz JA, Alcantar R, Roblesfl M, *et al.* Modulation by protein kinase C of the hormonal responsiveness of hepatocytes from

lean (*Fa/?*) and obese (*fa/fa*) Zucker rats. *Biochim Biophys Acta.* 1992; A1135:221–225.

184. Turkenkopf IJ, Kava RA, Feldweg A, Horowitz C, Greenwood MR, Johnson PR. Zucker and Wistar diabetic fatty rats show different response to adrenalectomy. *Am J Physiol.* 1991;261:R912–R919.

185. Cooper DR, Watson JE, Dao ML. Decreased expression of protein-kinase-C alpha, beta, and epsilon in soleus muscle of Zucker obese (*fa/fa*) rats. *Endocrinology.* 1993;133:2241–2247.

186. Finkelstein JA, Jervois P, Menadue M, Willoughby JO. Growth hormone and prolactin secretion in genetically obese Zucker rats. *Endocrinology.* 1986;118:1233–1236.

187. Renier G, Gaudreau P, Deslauriers N, Brazeau P. In vitro and in vivo growth hormone responsiveness to growth hormone releasing factor in male and female Zucker rats. *Neuroendocrinology.* 1989;50:454–459.

188. Renier G, Gaudreau P, Deslauriers N, Petitcle D, Brazeau P. Dynamic of the GRF-induced GH response in genetically obese Zucker rats: influence of central and peripheral factors. *Regul Pept.* 1990;28:95–106.

189. Ahmad I, Finkelstein JA, Downs TR, Frohman LA. Obesity-associated decrease in growth hormone–releasing hormone gene-expression: a mechanism for reduced growth-hormone messenger-RNA levels in genetically-obese Zucker rats. *Neuroendocrinology.* 1993;58:332–337.

190. Bercu BB, Yang SW, Masuda R, Hu CS, Walker RF. Effects of coadministered growth hormone (GH) releasing hormone and GH-releasing hexapeptide on maladaptive aspects of obesity in Zucker rats. *Endocrinology.* 1992;131:2800–2804.

191. Davies RR, Turner SJ, Cook D, Alberti KG, Johnston DG. The response of obese subjects to continuous infusion of human pancreatic growth hormone–releasing factor 1–44. *Clin Endocrinol (Oxf).* 1985;23:521–525.

192. Jacob RJ, Sherwin RS, Greenawalt K, Shulman GI. Simultaneous insulin-like growth factor-I and insulin resistance in obese Zucker rats. *Diabetes.* 1992;41:691–697.

193. Fukagawa K, Sakata T, Yoshimatsu H, Fujimoto K, Uchimura K, Asano C. Advance shift of feeding circadian rhythm induced by obesity progression in Zucker rats. *Am J Physiol.* 1992;263:R1169–R1175.

194. Castonguay TW. Glucocorticoids as modulators in the control of feeding. *Brain Res Bull.* 1993;27:423–428.

195. Ashwell M. Symposium on the manipulation of adiposity: why do people get fat: is adipose tissue guilty? *Proc Nutr Soc.* 1992;51: 353–365.

196. Truett GE, Bahary N, Friedman JM, Leibel RL. Rat obesity gene fatty (*fa*) maps to chromosome 5: evidence for homology with the mouse gene diabetes (*db*). *Proc Natl Acad Sci USA.* 1991;88:7806–7809.

197. Penicaud L, Ferre P, Assimacopoulos-Jeannet F, *et al.* Increased gene expression of lipogenic enzymes and glucose transporter in white adipose tissue of suckling and weaned obese Zucker rats. *Biochem J.* 1991;279:303–308.

198. Trayhurn P, Wusteman MC. Lipogenesis in genetically diabetic (*db/db*) mice: developmental changes in brown adipose tissue, white adipose tissue and the liver. *Biochim Biophys Acta.* 1990;1047: 168–174.

199. Guichard C, Dugail I, Le Liepvre X, Lavau M. Genetic-regulation of fatty-acid synthetase expression in adipose-tissue: overtranscription of the gene in genetically-obese rats. *J Lipid Res.* 1992;33: 679–687.

200. Dugail I, Quignard-Boulange A, Le Liepvre X, Ardouin B, Lavau M. Gene expression of lipid storage-related enzymes in adipose tissue of the genetically obese Zucker rat: co-ordinated increase in transcriptional activity and potentiation by hyperinsulinemia. *Biochem J.* 1992;281:607–611.

201. Guerre-Millo M, Lavau M, Horne JS, Wardzala LJ. Proposed mechanism for increased insulin-mediated glucose transport in adipose cells from young, obese Zucker rats: large intracellular pool of glucose transporters. *J Biol Chem.* 1985;260:2197–2201.

202. Flier JS, Cook KS, Usher P, Spiegelman BM. Severely impaired adipsin expression in genetic and acquired obesity. *Science.* 1987; 237:405–408.

203. Spiegelman BM, Choy L, Hotamisligil GS, Graves RA, Tontonoz P. Regulation of adipocyte gene expression in differentiation and syndromes of obesity/diabetes. *J Biol Chem.* 1993;268:6823–6826.

204. Dugail I, Quignard-Boulange A, Le Liepvre X, Lavau M. Impairment of adipsin expression is secondary to the onset of obesity in *db/db* mice. *J Biol Chem.* 1990;265:1831–1833. Technical Note.

205. Dugail I, Le Liepvre X, Quignard-Boulange A, Pairault J, Lavau M. Adipsin mRNA amounts are not decreased in the genetically obese Zucker rat. *Biochem J.* 1989;257:917–919.

206. Meade CJ, Ashwell M, Sowter C. Is genetically transmitted obesity due to an adipose tissue defect? *Proc R Soc Lond (Biol).* 1979;205: 395–410.

207. Gettys TW, Ramkumar V, Uhing RJ, Seger L, Taylor IL. Alterations in mRNA levels, expression, and function of GTP-binding regulatory proteins in adipocytes from obese mice (C57BL/6J-ob/ob). *J Biol Chem.* 1991;266:15949–15955.

208. McFarlane-Anderson N, Bailly J, Begin-Heick N. Levels of G-proteins in liver and brain of lean and obese (*ob/ob*) mice. *Biochem J.* 1992;282:15–23.

209. Naim M, Katz Y, Brand JG, Kare MR. Nonreceptor-mediated responses of adenylate cyclase in membranes from liver, muscle, and white and brown adipose tissue of obese (*fa/fa*) and lean (*Fa/?*) Zucker rats. *PSEBM* 1990;195:369–374.

210. Strassheim D, Palmer T, Milligan G, Houslay MD. Alterations in G-protein expression and the hormonal regulation of adenylate cyclase in the adipocytes of obese (*fa/fa*) Zucker rats. *Biochem J.* 1991;276:197–202.

211. Bushfield M, Pyne NJ, Houslay MD. Changes in the phosphorylation state of the inhibitory guanine nucleotide binding protein Gi-2 in hepatocytes from lean Fa/Fa and obese *fa/fa* Zucker rats. *Eur J Biochem.* 1990;192:537–542.

212. Fried SK, Turkenkopf IJ, Goldberg IJ, *et al.* Mechanisms of increased lipoprotein lipase in fat cells of obese Zucker rats. *Am J Physiol.* 1991;261:E653–E660.

213. Bessesen DH, Robertson AD, Eckel RH. Weight-reduction increases adipose but decreases cardiac LPL in reduced-obese Zucker rats. *Am J Physiol.* 1991;261:E246–E251.

214. Lynch CJ, Brennan WA, Vary TC, Carter N, Dodgson SJ. Carbonic anhydrase III in obese Zucker rats. *Am J Physiol.* 1993;264:E621–E630.

215. Lynch CJ, McCall KM, Billings ML, *et al.* Pyruvate carboxylase in genetic obesity. *Am J Physiol.* 1992;262:E608–E616.

216. Maeda H, Kasahara K. Increased 120-KDA protein in liver cytosol of genetically-obese Zucker rats. *J Nutr Sci Vitaminol (Tokyo).* 1993; 39:365–372.

217. Laurent-Winter C, Dugail I, Quignard-Boulange A, Le Liepvre X, Lavau M. Differential polypeptide expression in adipose tissue of lean and obese Zucker rats: evidence of specifically repressed peptides in 7-day-old pre-obese rats. *Biochem J.* 1992;284:813–817.
218. Pedersen O, Kahn CR, Kahn BB. Divergent regulation of the GLUT-1 and GLUT-4 glucose transporters in isolated adipocytes from Zucker rats. *J Clin Invest.* 1992;89:1964–1973.
219. Friedman JE, De Vente JE, Peterson RG, Dohm GL. Altered expression of muscle glucose transporter GLUT-4 in diabetic fatty Zucker rats (ZDF/Drt-fa). *Am J Physiol.* 1991;261:E782–E788.
220. Azain MJ, Fukuda N, Chao FF, Yamamoto M, Ontko JA. Contributions of fatty acid and sterol synthesis to triglyceride and cholesterol secretion by the perfused rat liver in genetic hyperlipemia and obesity. *J Biol Chem.* 1985;260:175–181.
221. Fukuda N, Azain MJ, Ontko JA. Altered hepatic metabolism of free fatty acids underlying hypersecretion of very low density lipoproteins in the genetically obese Zucker rats. *J Biol Chem.* 1982; 257:14066–14072.
222. Azain MJ, Martin RJ. Effect of genetic obesity on the regulation of hepatic fatty acid metabolism. *Am J Physiol.* 1983;244:R400–R406.
223. Azain MJ, Ontko JA. Ketone body utilization for lipogenesis in the perfused liver of the obese Zucker rat. *Hormone Met.* 1990;22:561– 565.
224. Malewiak MI, Griglio S, Le Liepvre X. Relationship between lipogenesis, ketogenesis, and malonyl-CoA content in isolated hepatocytes from the obese Zucker rat adapted to a high-fat diet. *Metabolism.* 1985;34:604–611.
225. Triscari J, Greenwood MR, Sullivan AC. Oxidation and ketogenesis in hepatocytes of lean and obese Zucker rats. *Metabolism.* 1982; 31:223–228.
226. Brady LJ, Hoppel CL. Hepatic mitochondrial function in lean and obese Zucker rats. *Am J Physiol.* 1983;245:E239–E245.
227. Clouet P, Henninger C, Bezard J. Study of some factors controlling fatty acid oxidation in liver mitochondria of obese Zucker rats. *Biochem J.* 1986;239:103–108.
228. Clouet P, Henninger C, Pascal M, Bezard J. High sensitivity of carnitine acyltransferase I to malonyl-CoA inhibition in liver of obese Zucker rats. *FEBS Lett.* 1985;182:331–334.
229. Azain MJ, Ontko JA. An explanation for decreased ketogenesis in

the liver of the obese Zucker rat. *Am J Physiol.* 1989;257:R822–R828.

230. Coleman DL. Acetone metabolism in mice: increased activity in mice heterozygous for obesity genes. *Proc Natl Acad Sci USA.* 1980; 77:290–293.

231. Barry W, Bray GA. Plasma triglycerides in genetically obese rats. *Metabolism.* 1969;18:833–839.

232. Strobl W, Knerer B, Gratzl R, Arbeiter K, Lin-Lee YC, Patsch W. Altered regulation of apolipoprotein A-IV gene expression in the liver of the genetically obese Zucker rat. *J Clin Invest.* 1993;92: 1766–1773.

233. Blond JP, Henchiri C, Bezard J. Delta 6 and delta 5 desaturase activities in liver from obese Zucker rats at different ages. *Lipids.* 1989;24:389–395.

234. Guesnet P, Bourre JM, Guerre-Millo M, Pascal G, Durand G. Tissue phospholipid fatty-acid composition in genetically lean (*Fa/-*) or obese (*fa/fa*) Zucker female rats on the same diet. *Lipids.* 1990;25: 517–522.

235. Phinney SD, Tang AB, Thurmond DC, Nakamura MT, Stern JS. Abnormal polyunsaturated lipid-metabolism in the obese Zucker rat, with partial metabolic correction by gamma-linolenic acid administration. *Metabolism.* 1993;42:1127–1140.

236. Hill JO, Lin D, Yakubu F, Peters JC. Development of dietary obesity in rats: influence of amount and composition of dietary fat. *Int J Obes.* 1992;16:321–333.

237. Jen KLC. Lipid lowering effect of omega-3 fatty acids in genetically obese Zucker rats. *Nutr Res.* 1989;9:1217–1228.

238. Parrish CC, Pathy DA, Angel A. Dietary fish oils limit adipose tissue hypertrophy in rats. *Metabolism.* 1990;39:217–219.

239. Shimizu H, Ohshima K, Bray GA, Peterson M, Swerdloff RS. Adrenalectomy and castration in the genetically obese (*ob/ob*) mouse. *Obesity Res.* 1993;1:377–383.

240. Bray GA, York DA, Lavau M, Hainault I. Adrenalectomy in the Zucker fatty rat: effect on m-RNA for malic enzyme and glyceraldehyde 3-phosphate dehydrogenase. *Int J Obes.* 1991;15:703–709.

241. Bannister P, Whitaker EM. Reduced tissue androgen receptors in the congenitally obese male Zucker rat. *J Endocrinol.* 1985;107:R13–R15.

242. Bray GA, Dahms WT, Swerdloff RS, Fiser RH, Atkinson RL, Carrel RE. The Prader-Willi syndrome: a study of 40 patients and a review of the literature. *Medicine (Baltimore)*. 1983;62:59–80.

243. Himms-Hagen J, Desautels M. A mitochondrial defect in brown adipose tissue of the obese (*ob/ob*) mouse: reduced binding of purine nucleotides and a failure to respond to cold by an increase in binding. *Biochem Biophys Res Commun*. 1978;83:628–634.

244. Dubuc PU, Carlisle HJ. Food restriction normalizes somatic growth and diabetes in adrenalectomized *ob/ob* mice. *Am J Physiol*. 1988;255:R787–R793.

245. Dubuc PU, Wilden NJ, Carlisle HJ. Fed and fasting thermoregulation in *ob/ob* mice. *Ann Nutr Metab*. 1985;29:358–365.

246. Williams G, Cardoso HM, Lee YC, *et al*. Hypothalamic regulatory peptides in obese and lean Zucker rats. *Clin Sci*. 1991;80:419–426.

247. Carlisle HJ, Stock MJ. Effect of conventional (mixed b1/b2) and novel (b3) adrenergic agonists on thermoregulatory behavior. *Pharmacol Biochem Behav*. 1991;40:249–254.

248. Demes GL, Buskirk ER, Alpert SS, Loomis JL. Energy turnover and heat exchange in mature lean and obese Zucker rats acutely exposed to three environmental temperatures for 24 hours. *Int J Obes*. 1991;15:375–385.

249. Himms-Hagen J. Neural control of brown adipose tissue thermogenesis, hypertrophy and atrophy. *Front Neuroendocrinol*. 1991; 12:38–93.

250. Marette A, Mauriège P, Deprés JP, Tulp OL, Bukowiecki LJ. Norepinephrine- and insulin-resistant glucose transport in brown adipocytes from diabetic SHR/N-cp rats. *Am J Physiol*. 1993;265: R577–R583.

251. Kaul R, Heldmaie G, Schmidt I. Defective thermoregulatory thermogenesis does not cause onset of obesity in Zucker rats. *Am J Physiol*. 1990;259:E11–E18.

252. Kaul R, Schmidt I, Carlisle H. Maturation of thermoregulation in Zucker rats. *Int J Obes*. 1985;9:401–409.

253. Schmidt I, Kaul R, Carlisle HJ. Body temperature of huddling newborn Zucker rats. *Pflugers Arch*. 1984;401:418–420.

254. Bazin R, Eteve D, Lavau M. Evidence for decreased GDP binding to brown-adipose-tissue mitochondria of obese Zucker (*fa/fa*) rats in the very first days of life. *Biochem J*. 1984;221:241–245.

255. Bell GE, Stern JS. Evaluation of body composition of young and obese and lean Zucker rats. *Growth.* 1977;41:63–80.

256. Planche E, Joliff M, Bazin R. Energy expenditure and adipose tissue development in 2- to 8-day-old Zucker rats. *Int J Obes.* 1988; 12:353–360.

257. Markewicz B, Kuhmichel G, Schmidt I. Onset of excess fat deposition in Zucker rats with and without decreased thermogenesis. *Am J Physiol.* 1993;265:E478–E486.

258. Niijima A, Rohner-Jeanrenaud F, Jeanrenaud B. Role of ventromedial hypothalamus on sympathetic efferents of brown adipose tissue. *Am J Physiol.* 1984;247:R650–R654.

259. Kates AL, Himms-Hagen J. Defective regulation of thyroxine 5'-deiodinase in brown adipose tissue of *ob/ob* mice. *Am J Physiol.* 1990;258:E7–E15.

260. Bray GA, York DA. Thyroid function of genetically obese rats. *Endocrinology.* 1971;88:1095–1099.

261. Kates A, Zaror-Behrens Z, Himms-Hagen J. Adrenergic effects on thyroxine 5'-deiodinase in brown adipose tissue of lean and *ob/ob* mice. *Am J Physiol.* 1990;258:R430–R435.

262. Marie V, Dupuy F, Bazin R. Decreased T(4)-to-T(3) conversions on brown adipose-tissue of Zucker *fa/fa* pups before the onset of obesity. *Am J Physiol.* 1992;263:E115–E120.

263. Lardy H, Stratman F. *Hormones, Thermogenesis, and Obesity.* New York: Elsevier; 1989.

264. Assimacopoulos-Jeannet F, Moinat M, Muzzin P, et al. Effects of a peroxisome proliferator on beta oxidation and overall energy balance in obese *(fa/fa)* rats. *Am J Physiol.* 1991;260:R278–R283.

265. Esteve M, Rafecas I, Remesar X, Alemany M. Nitrogen balances of lean and obese Zucker rats subjected to a cafeteria diet. *Int J Obes.* 1992;16:237–244.

266. Bray GA, Stern J, Castonguay T. Effect of adrenalectomy and high-fat diet on the fatty Zucker rat. *Am J Physiol.* 1992;262:E32–E39.

267. Bazin R, Planche E, Dupuy F, Krief S, Lavau M. Deprivation of corticosterone does not prevent onset of obesity in Zucker *fa/fa* pups. *Am J Physiol.* 1987;252:E461–E466.

268. Devenport L, Knehans A, Thomas T, Sundstrom A. Macronutrient intake and utilization by rats: interactions with type I adrenocorticoid receptor stimulation. *Am J Physiol.* 1991;260:R73–R81.

269. Devenport L, Stith R. Mimicking corticosterone's daily rhythm

with specific receptor agonists: effects on food, water, and sodium intake. *Physiol Behav.* 1992;51:1247–1255.

270. Naeser P. Effects of adrenalectomy on the obese-hyperglycemic syndrome in mice (gene symbol *ob*). *Diabetologia.* 1973;9:376–379.

271. Solomon J, Bradwin G, Cocchia H, *et al.* Effects of adrenalectomy on body weight and hyperglycemia in 5-month-old *ob/ob* mice. *Horm Metab Res.* 1977;9:152–156.

272. Bray GA. Regulation of energy balances: studies on genetic, hypothalamic and dietary obesity. *Proc Nutr Soc.* 1982;41:95–108.

273. Turkenkopf IJ, Johnson PR, Greenwood MR. Development of pancreatic and plasma insulin in prenatal and suckling Zucker rats. *Am J Physiol.* 1982;242:E220–E225.

274. Vander Tuig JG, Ohshima K, Yoshida T, Romsos D, Bray G. Adrenalectomy increases norepinephrine turnover in brown adipose tissue of obese (*ob/ob*) mice. *Life Sci.* 1984;34:1423–1432.

275. Yukimura Y, Bray GA. Effects of adrenalectomy on body weight and the size and number of fat cells in the Zucker (fatty) rat. *Endocr Res Commun.* 1978;5:189–198.

276. Yukimura Y, Bray GA. Effect of adrenalectomy of thyroid function and insulin levels in obese (*ob/ob*) mice. *Proc Soc Exp Biol Med.* 1978;159:364–367.

277. Yukimura Y, Bray GA, Wolfsen AR. Some effects of adrenalectomy in the fatty rat. *Endocrinology.* 1978;103:1924–1928.

278. King BM, Banta AR, Tharel GN, Bruce BK, Frohman LA. Hypothalamic hyperinsulinemia and obesity: role of adrenal glucocorticoids. *Am J Physiol.* 1983;245:E194–E199.

279. Shimizu H, Shargill NS, Bray GA. Adrenalectomy and response to corticosterone and MSH in the genetically obese yellow mouse. *Am J Physiol.* 1989;256:R494–R500.

280. Okada S, York DA, Bray GA. Mifeprostone (RU-486), a blocker of type-II glucocorticoid and progestin receptors, reverses a dietary form of obesity. *Am J Physiol.* 1992;262:1106–1110.

281. Langley SC, York DA. Effects of antiglucocorticoid RU 486 on development of obesity in obese *fa/fa* Zucker rats. *Am J Physiol.* 1990;259:R539–R544.

282. Guillaume-Gentil C, Rohner-Jeanrenaud F, Abramo F, Bestetti GE, Rossi GL, Jeanrenaud B. Abnormal regulation of the hypothalamo-pituitary-adrenal axis in the genetically obese *fa/fa* rat. *Endocrinology.* 1990;126:1873–1879.

283. Pesonen U, Koulu M, Heikinheimo O, Huupponen R. The gluco-corticoid antagonist mifepristone reveals abnormal regulation of the adrenocortical system in obese Zucker rats. *J Endocrinol.* 1992; 132:425–431.

284. Fletcher JM. Effects of adrenalectomy before weaning and short or long term glucocorticoid administration on genetically obese Zucker rat. *Biochem J.* 1986;238:459–463.

285. Fletcher JM, McKenzie N. The effects of dietary fat content on the growth and body composition of lean and genetically obese Zucker rats adrenalectomized before weaning. *Br J Nutr.* 1988;60: 563–569.

286. Martin RJ, Wangsness PJ, Gahagan JH. Diurnal changes in serum metabolites and hormones in lean and obese Zucker rats. *Horm Metab Res.* 1978;10:187–192.

287. Saito M, Bray GA. Diurnal rhythm for corticosterone in obese (*ob/ob*), diabetes (*db/db*) and gold thioglucose induced obesity in mice. *Endocrinology.* 1983;113:2181–2185.

288. West DB, Boozer CN, Moody DL, Atkinson RL. Dietary obesity in nine inbred mouse strains. *Am J Physiol.* 1992;262:1025–1032.

289. White BD, Corll CB, Porter JR. The metabolic clearance rate of corticosterone in lean and obese male Zucker rats. *Metabolism.* 1989;38:530–536.

290. Yen TT, Allan JA, Pearson DV, Acton JM, Greenberg MM. Prevention of obesity in Avy/a mice by dehydroepiandrosterone. *Lipids.* 1977;12:409–413.

291. Devenport L, Thomas T, Knehans A, Sundstrom A. Acute, chronic, and interactive effects of type-I and type-II corticosteroid receptor stimulation on feeding and weight-gain. *Physiol Behav.* 1990;47: 1221–1228.

292. Arase K, Shargill NS, Bray GA. Effects of intraventricular infusion of corticotropin-releasing factor on VMH-lesioned obese rats. *Am J Physiol.* 1989;256:R751–R756.

293. Arase K, York DA, Shimizu H, Shargill N, Bray GA. Effects of corticotropin releasing factor on food intake and brown adipose tissue. *Am J Physiol.* 1988;255:E255–E259.

294. Dagnault A, Ouerghi D, Richard D. Treatment with alpha-helical-CRF-(9-41) prevents the anorectic effect of 17-beta-estradiol. *Brain Res Bull.* 1993;32:689–692.

295. Bestetti G, Abramo F, Guillaume-Gentil C, Rohner-Jeanrenaud F,

Jeanrenaud B, Rossi G. Changes in the hypothalamo-pituitary-adrenal axis of genetically obese *fa/fa* rats: a structural, immuno-cytochemical, and morphometrical study. *Endocrinology.* 1990;126:1880–1887.

296. Plotsky PM, Thrivikraman KV, Watts AG, Hauger RL. Hypothalamic-pituitary-adrenal axis function in the Zucker obese rat. *Endocrinology.* 1992;130:1931–1941.

297. Freedman MR, Stern JS, Reaven GM, Mondon CE. Effect of adrenalectomy on in vivo glucose metabolism in insulin resistant Zucker obese rats. *Horm Metab Res.* 1986;18:296–298.

298. White BD, Davenport WD, Porter JR. Responsiveness of isolated adrenocortical cells from lean and obese Zucker rats to ACTH. *Am J Physiol.* 1988;255:E229–E235.

299. Langley SC, York DA. Glucocorticoid receptor numbers in the brain and liver of the obese Zucker rat. *Int J Obes.* 1992;16:135–143.

300. Tsai HJ, Romsos DR. Glucocorticoid and mineralocorticoid receptor-binding characteristics in obese (*ob/ob*) mice. *Am J Physiol.* 1991;261:E495–E499.

301. Wardlaw GM, Kaplan ML. Oxygen consumption and oxidative capacity of hepatocytes from young male obese and nonobese Zucker rats. *PSEMB.* 1986;183:199–206.

302. Kim HK, Romsos DR. Adrenalectomy increases brown adipose tissue metabolism in *ob/ob* mice housed at 35C. *Endocrinol Metab.* 1990;22:E362–E369.

303. Nei YM, Romsos DR. Dietary glucose increases plasma insulin and decreases brown adipose tissue thermogenic activity in adrenalectomized *ob/ob* mice. *J Nutr.* 1991;121:1407–1413.

304. Kang JS, Pilkington JD, Ferguson D, Kim HK, Romsos DR: Dietary glucose and fat attenuate effects of adrenalectomy on energy balance in *ob/ob* mice. *J Nutr.* 1992;122:895–905.

305. Yamamoto T, Fukumoto H, Koh G, *et al.* Liver and muscle fat type glucose transporter gene expression in obese and diabetic rats. *Biochem Biophys Res Commun.* 1991;175:995–1002.

306. Coleman DL, Leiter EH, Applezweig N. Therapeutic effects of dehydroepiandrosterone metabolites in diabetes mutant mice (C57BL/KsJ-db/db). *Endocrinology.* 1984;115:239–243.

307. Coleman DL, Schwizer RW, Leiter EH. Effect of genetic background on the therapeutic effects of dehydroepiandrosterone

(DHEA) in diabetes-obesity mutants and in aged normal mice. *Diabetes.* 1984;33:26–32.

308. Berdanier CD, Parente JA, McIntosh MK. Is dehydroepiandroc-terone an antiobesity agent? *FASEB J.* 1993;7:414–419.

309. Brady LJ, Ramsay RR, Brady PS. Regulation of carnitine acyltrans-ferase synthesis in lean and obese Zucker rats by dehydroepian-drosterone and clofibrate. *J Nutr.* 1991;121:525–531.

310. Cleary MP, Shepherd A, Jenks B. Effect of dehydroepiandrosterone on growth in lean and obese Zucker rats. *J Nutr.* 1984;114:1242–1251.

311. Browne ES, Porter JR, Correa G, Abadie J, Svec F. Dehydroepian-drosterone regulation of the hepatic glucocorticoid receptor in the Zucker rat: the obesity research program. *J Steroid Biochem Mol Biol.* 1993;45:517–524.

312. Browne ES, Wright BE, Porter JR, Svec F. Dehydroepiandroster-one: antiglucocorticoid action in mice. *Am J Med Sci.* 1992;303:366–371.

313. Vasselli JR. Diet composition determines course of hyperphagia in developing Zucker obese rats. *Physiol Behav.* 1990;48:805–811.

314. Walker HC, Romsos DR. Glucocorticoids in the CNS regulate BAT metabolism and plasma-insulin in *ob/ob* mice. *Am J Physiol.* 1992; 262:E110–E117.

315. Baulieu EE. Neurosteroids: an overview. *Adv Biochem Psychophar-macol.* 1992;47:1–16.

316. Majewska MD. Neurosteroids: endogenous dimodal modulators of the GABAa receptor: mechanism of action and physiological significance. *Prog Neurobiol.* 1992;38:379–395.

317. Nemere I, Norman AW. Steroid hormone actions at the plasma membrane: induced calcium uptake and exocytotic events. *Mol Cell Endocrinol.* 1991;80:C165–C169.

318. Paul SM, Pudy RH. Neuroactive steroids. *FASEB J.* 1992;6:2311–2322.

JEFFREY M. FRIEDMAN

Molecular Genetic Approaches to Complex Traits

ABSTRACT

The tools necessary for the genetic analysis of human variation are at hand and will have a profound impact on our understanding of the molecular basis of human disease. This paper will serve to discuss these newly developed genetic approaches and review the molecular and analytic methods that can be applied to study genetically complex traits, such as obesity. The initial discussion focuses on the steps in the process by which one can positionally clone a single Mendelian locus (*i.e.,* a single gene trait). This is followed by a discussion of the analytical approaches to genetically complex traits.

The Tools of Mammalian Genetics

Discussed below are the steps in the process of positional cloning: genetic mapping, physical mapping, gene isolation, and mutation detection.

GENETIC MAPS

The elemental principle of genetics is based on the premise that when two or more variable traits (polymorphisms) are inherited together at a higher than expected frequency the genes encoding those traits are in proximity to one another along the chromosome. Such traits are said to be linked to one another (1). The precise rates with which such traits are associated with one another can be used to predict the order of each trait relative to one another along the chromosome (2). Moreover, once linkage is demonstrated, the rate of recombination between two loci can be used to calculate genetic distance, the unit of which is the centimorgan, which equals a rate of recombination of 1%. Genetic distance

67

is a crude indicator of physical distance, which is measured in base pairs of DNA.

Two requirements must be satisfied to begin a comprehensive genetic analysis to localize traits relative to one another: genetic markers and a group of individuals among whom variations can be scored. These components have long been available in a number of invertebrate organisms in which a rapid generation time and an ability to select for variants led to the identification of a sufficient number of genetic loci to compile dense genetic maps.

Until recently, genetic analysis of mammalian organisms, including man, has been limited by a paucity of genetic markers. With the publication of a landmark paper by Botstein *et al.* thirteen years ago, this limitation was addressed by the suggestion that the technologies of recombinant DNA could be used to define an arbitrarily large number of polymorphic loci (3). This largely theoretical paper suggested that DNA probes could be used to identify polymorphisms in the DNA sequences of different individuals by their ability to detect differences in the size of particular restriction fragments resolved on southern blots. The polymorphisms defined by the use of these probes were called RFLPs (restriction fragment length polymorphisms). It was first proposed in this paper that the RFLPs could be assembled by themselves into genetic maps that could be applied to further studies of the inheritance of phenotypic traits in human pedigrees. The predictions made in this prescient paper have been borne out in part because of organized worldwide efforts to establish dense genetic maps in a variety of organisms using DNA-based polymorphisms. In retrospect, it is rather remarkable that the development of recombinant DNA in the late 1970s was followed so closely by an appreciation of the ways in which cloned DNA could be applied to genetics.

Progress in mammalian genetics was further accelerated by the introduction of polymerase chain reaction (PCR) based genetic markers. The direct application of PCR for the detection of genetic differences was first suggested by Weber and Mays, who noted that $(GT)^n$ microsatellite sequences were widely distributed throughout the mammalian genome (4). It was further shown that the length of the microsatellite repeats was highly variable and that length differences could be demonstrated by synthesizing PCR primers flanking the repeat and resolving the PCR products on an acrylamide gel. An example of a simple sequence length polymorphism (SSLP) is shown in Figure 1. The mu-

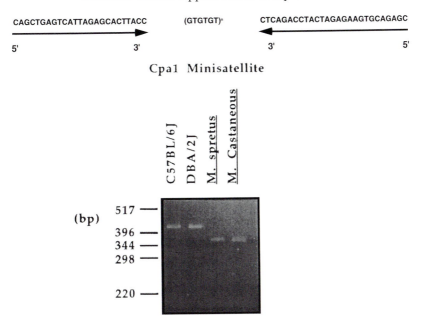

Cpa1 Minisatellite

Figure 1.   An example of an SSLP. Genomic clones encoding the mouse *cpa* (carboxypeptidase A) gene were isolated. Subclones containing GT repeats were isolated by probing with a 32P-(GT)[15] oligonucleotide. The PCR primers, shown on the upper panel, flanking the repeat were synthesized. These primers were used to PCR amplify genomic DNA from various mouse strains. Electrophoresis of the PCR products on agarose or acrylamide gels revealed length differences among *Mus spretus, Mus castaneous,* and the two *Mus domesticus* strains, DBA/2J and C57BL/6J. This SSLP can be used as a genetic marker in genetic crosses.

tation rate of microsatellite sequences is estimated as $\approx 10^{-4}$, a hundredfold higher rate than the base changes that are detected as RFLPs (5). Thus, SSLPs are highly polymorphic, a crucial attribute for genetic markers. The PCR-based markers are also suitable for use in genetics owing to the ease with which the process of scoring genetic differences can be automated and the simplicity of transferring primer sequences electronically as opposed to having to manually distribute DNA probes (6). The high polymorphism rates and suitability for automated genotyping has led to the development of very dense genetic maps in the human, mouse, and other species (7, 8). Several thousand genetic markers have thus been localized to discrete positions along each of the human and mouse chromosomes. The ways in which these powerful reagents can be applied to the study of human disease rests in the relationship between genetic and physical maps as discussed below.

Physical Maps

The ability to clone mutant genes from mammals depends on the fact that the recombination-based genetic map mirrors the physical map (double helix) of DNA along the chromosome. In most cases recombination events in proximity to the disease gene are used to delineate the minimal segment in which the gene must reside: the nonrecombinant region (9). To the extent that the rate of recombination is proportional to the physical distance (in base pairs of DNA), one can use a genetic map to predict the physical locations of individual traits. Estimates of the relationship between the physical and genetic maps have been given as 1% recombination equals one million base pairs in man and two million base pairs in mice. This is based on the facts that both genomes are three billion base pairs in length and the aggregate length of the genetic map is 3200 centimorgans in man and 1600 centimorgans in mouse. This estimate is highly variable at different regions of the genome, 1 centimorgan having been shown to range between approximately 100 kilobases and 2 megabases (10, 11, 12). This variability reflects the fact that the frequency of recombination is also a function of the DNA sequences in a given region. Thus, sequences that tend to suppress recombination (cold spots) tend to expand the physical distance per centimorgan and sequences that promote recombination (hot spots) tend to contract the physical maps. Although the precise relationship between the rate of recombination and physical distance is variable, the order of the traits relative to one another is uniformly identical in both genetic and physical maps. It is this feature that is the basis of positional cloning; once RFLPs or SSLPs are demonstrated to flank a phenotypic trait (such as a disease gene), one can clone the DNA between those markers and begin searching for the disease gene in that interval.

The principal difficulty in correlating the genetic and physical maps is that in mammals even subcentimorgan genetic distances often correspond to several hundred kilobases of DNA. This fact makes the use of conventional cloning methods impractical. This difficulty has been circumvented by the development of new yeast artificial chromosome

(YAC) cloning methods that make possible the cloning of contiguous stretches of DNA in excess of one megabase (13, 14). Yeast artificial chromosome cloning depends on the initial observation that if one ligates yeast telomeres, centromeres, and selectable markers together with random DNA fragments greater than 50 kilobases in length, the resulting product can be carried as an extra chromosome in suitable yeast stains (15). Although YACs with inserted fragments less than 50 kilobases are unstable, there is no strict upper size limit. Thus, random fragments up to 2 megabases in length have been stably inserted in these vectors to constitute complete genetic libraries with large inserts. Yeast artificial chromosome libraries are generally screened using PCR of library pools, and mouse and human libraries are currently available (13, 14, 16).

Alternative cloning vectors have recently been developed including recombinant P1 phage and bacterial artificial chromosomes (BACs). These vectors accommodate less DNA than YACs (up to 100 kilobases for P1 clones, and 250 kilobases for BAC clones) but offer an advantage in that cloned DNA can be more easily purified than can YACs (17, 18, 19).

With the use of these new cloning vectors, and available tightly linked genetic markers, the genetic and physical maps across a particular subgenomic interval can be cloned as a prelude to the identification of mutant disease genes. Indeed, physical maps in the region of a large number of disease loci have been built, although, as expected, substantial variability in the relationship between genetic physical distances has been observed.

At present, the process of physical mapping involves substantial efforts on the part of individual laboratories in which YACs are isolated, characterized, and used in turn to isolate new YACs. However, the rapid progress of the genome project will soon make much of this work superfluous, particularly when physical maps of the entire genome of mouse, human, and other organisms become available. Indeed, physical maps in YACs of several human chromosomes are already available, and a complete physical map of the human genome is forthcoming (20, 21, 22). In the case of the mouse physical map, it can be anticipated that the availability of 6000 microsatellite markers will rapidly lead to a complete physical map in this organism as well (8). Once these efforts are completed the principal bottleneck in the process of identifying disease genes will be in the development of a high resolu-

tion genetic map and the subsequent identification of genes in a defined
subchromosomal region.

GENE IDENTIFICATION

The objective of the efforts to build a dense genetic and physical map
is to narrow the search for the contributing gene to a subgenomic segment of DNA. Inside that region each gene is, by definition, a candidate
for the contributing gene. In attempts to isolate genes that contribute
to the development of obesity, this caveat is especially relevant, since
a number of sites of synthesis can be considered as potentially important in determining body weight (fat, liver, brain, pancreas, etc.). In this
context the most complete method for obtaining a comprehensive gene
inventory across a genomic region is large-scale DNA sequencing. The
use of modern computer programs such as GRAIL to analyze DNA
sequences from a segment of the genome offers a high likelihood that
almost all genes in a specific region will be identified (23). However,
even in the most favorable of cases, the implementation of this approach would require that several hundred thousand base pairs of
DNA be sequenced. Although current technology enables sequencing
of up to one million base pairs of DNA per year, only a small number
of labs are capable of this output (24). It can be anticipated that improved sequencing technologies will result in the more frequent use of
large-scale sequencing followed by computer analysis of DNA sequences to identify genes. This approach has the added advantage of
providing DNA sequences from introns. Primers derived from intron
sequences can be used to directly amplify genomic DNA as a first step
toward identifying mutations. (For human disease genes, in particular,
this is often simpler than analyzing RT PCR products derived from
tissue RNA.)

The standard methods for gene isolation now in common usage are
either hybridization based (analogous to library screening) or dependence on the presence of functional DNA elements that encode splice
donor and acceptor sites or polyadenylation signals. To date, the most
successful method based on hybridization is known as cDNA selection
(25, 26). In this method linkers capable of initiating a PCR reaction are
linked to random cDNA fragments. These cDNA fragments, derived
from an RNA source thought to express the mutant gene, are hybridized to genomic DNA, that is, YACs, P1s, etc., from the relevant sub-

genomic region. In one variation of this method the genomic DNA is bound to a membrane (25). The hybridized cDNA is subsequently eluted, PCR amplified using the ligated linker, and rehybridized to the genomic DNA. This procedure is repeated two to three times at which point the eluted material is often enriched several hundred times for gene sequences from the YAC (or P1s) of interest. A modification to this method that has produced useful hybrids makes use of genomic DNA that has been biotinylated (27). Hybrids between the cDNA and genomic DNA are captured using streptavidin beads; the DNA is then eluted, reamplified, and processed as above. This later method has an advantage in that it depends on a solution hybridization, thus enhancing the efficiency of hybridization. Gene sequences isolated are further characterized and sequenced as part of efforts to identify mutations.

The methods of exon trapping or poly A site trapping are alternatives to cDNA selection (27, 28). These methods make use of plasmid constructs containing a test gene with a highly active promoter, two exons, and a polyadenylation signal. Thus, the wild type construct has a single intron. Random genomic fragments from a subgenomic region are inserted into the intron of the test gene. These plasmids, when introduced into cultured cells by transfection, express a mixed population of RNAs, including a subset in which exon sequences internal to the inserted genomic DNA (or polyadenylation signals) are inserted into the test gene RNA. The inserted (trapped) exons can be recovered easily using PCR and further characterized. These methods will recover in principle most if not all spliced genes in a particular interval. Of importance, gene isolation is independent of the site of synthesis of the encoded gene. For complex traits for which the site of expression is unknown, this feature offers substantial benefits. Indeed it has been used successfully to isolate several mutant loci in human and mouse species, including the Huntington's disease gene and the mouse *bcg* gene (29, 30).

Mutation Detection

Each gene isolated from the nonrecombinant region is by definition a candidate for the mutant gene. Currently, the principal problem in identifying the mutations is in evaluating each of the candidate genes. In general, this entails isolation of full length cDNAs followed by a comparison of the DNA sequences between affected and unaffected individuals. Mutations can be detected using conventional DNA sequencing methods or indirect methods such as single strand conformational polymorphisms (SSCP). This method detects differences in the secondary structure of single strand DNA as a function of single base changes (31). Such differences in secondary structure are apparent after electrophoresis in acrylamide gels under nondenaturing conditions. Whereas direct DNA sequencing using the dideoxy chain terminator method is suitable for recessive mutations, which are often homozygous, SSCP offers important advantages for the identification of dominant mutations (which are heterozygous). This is because it is often difficult to distinguish a heterozygous mutation from a sequencing error. Similar difficulties in analyzing DNA sequence may also arise in compound heterozygotes.

The evaluation of each candidate gene represents a substantial investment of time and labor. It is estimated that there is one gene each 50 000 pairs in mammals (based on estimates of 100 000 genes distributed in a 3×10^9 base pair genome). Based on large-scale DNA sequencing efforts in yeast, this density of genes actually may be an underestimate, though the gene density varies in different regions of the genome (32). For example, the polycystic kidney disease gene (PKD) maps to a 500 000 base pair interval on human chromosome 4 that contains no fewer than twenty independent transcripts (Steven Reeders, personal communication). Even in the most favorable cases the search for novel genes using the technology of positional cloning may require the evaluation of upwards of five novel genes. Since this is a labor-intensive endeavor, any biologic information that might prioritize the candidate gene is of great value. Unfortunately, as indicated, for most complex traits it may be difficult to preconceive the biologic characteristics of the encoded gene. This uncertainty regarding the biologic function of the key genetic loci for common diseases makes their identification of immense clinical importance.

Resolution of Complex Traits into Single Mendelian Loci

The methodology of positional cloning allows the isolation of important genes in cases in which the gene segregates as a single locus. Operationally this means that the inheritance of a particular allele of a given gene is associated with a demonstrable and consistent phenotypic difference. For the genetic analysis of complex traits this objective represents the principal challenge, particularly in humans. It is likely that inheritance of complex traits such as obesity is both genetically heterogeneous (*i.e.,* different genes can independently contribute to an indistinguishable or similar phenotype) and polygenic (*i.e.,* many different genes act synergistically to lead to the phenotype). Although the resolution of genetically complex traits is straightforward in organisms in which animal crosses can be set up, a genetic approach to common human diseases requires the use of analytical and molecular tools that are still evolving.

GENETIC ANALYSIS IN ANIMALS

In animals, the resolution of genetically heterogeneous traits is straightforward. If test matings between similarly affected animals, mutant at a single locus, yield affected progeny, one concludes the animals carry defects in the same gene. Conversely, if such matings fail to produce mutant progeny one concludes that independent genetic loci are affected. In this way, five single loci causing obesity in mice have been localized (33). Once localized, cloning efforts can be initiated, as described, to isolate the contributing gene.

Methodology for the analysis of polygenic traits has also been recently developed. The advent of RFLPs as genetic markers has revolutionized our potential ability to dissect quantitative traits into Mendelian loci by making available dense genetic maps. The experimental strategy for mapping polygenes remains the same as initially suggested by Spickett and Thoday (34). In the 1960s, Spickett and Thoday used an intercross between two strains of *Drosophila melanogaster* that differed with regard to the number of abdominal bristles. By counting abdominal bristles among F2 flies, and looking for cosegregation of bristle number with other genetic markers, they were able to identify genetic loci that contribute to this quantitative trait. In this study, they were not able to scan the entire genome, since a sufficient number of genetic markers were not available. With the advent of microsatellites, this difficulty is no longer relevant.

To localize mammalian polygenes, crosses are established between two inbred strains that are variant for a particular trait. Genetic haplotypes at specific intervals across the genome are scored using RFLPs or SSLPs and compared with values for the quantitative trait among individual progeny of a cross. Correlations in F2 individuals between the DNA haplotype and a particular trait characteristic of one of the parental strains can be used to determine how much of the variance is contributed by a particular interval. This can then be used to localize quantitative trait loci (QTLs). The analytical tools and computer programs necessary for such calculations have been developed by Lander and Botstein (35). Several points relevant to the earlier discussion should be noted: in QTL analysis each individual is simultaneously typed for haplotype at genetic loci that span the genome as well as for the quantitative trait of interest. It is critical that the parental strains differ substantially for the trait, and that one should be able to measure the trait accurately without excessive environmental variance. The number of F2 or N2 animals necessary for this analysis bears a direct relationship to the number of QTLs that are responsible for that trait. The more contributing genes that are segregating, the lower the frequency of animals at the extremes of phenotype. In cases in which a great number of genes are segregating, a larger cross will be necessary to generate sufficiently large numbers of animals at the extremes of the distribution. However, the use of large genetic crosses may not be overwhelming. Since only the animals at the phenotypic extremes are genetically informative, haplotyping need be performed only on animals at the ends of the distribution. The number of animals that need to be scored is also a function of several other parameters that have been discussed in detail by Lander and Botstein (*i.e.,* the denser the available genetic map, the fewer F2 or N2 animals will be required) (35). Of note, such analyses do not readily distinguish between a QTL that has a large effect but that is distant from a marker locus and a QTL with a small effect but that is close to the marker locus.

The ideal situation occurs when phenotypic difference between the two parental strains is large relative to environmental (F1) variance. It is also helpful if the parental strains to be used are the result of selective breeding for the quantitative trait followed by multigenerational inbreeding to "fix" the genes responsible for the quantitative trait under study. Brief intense selection makes it likely that the "high strain" carries only high alleles and vice versa. Instances in which the inbred "high" line carried some low alleles can be discerned in retrospect, however, if there are F2 progeny whose phenotype is more extreme than either parent.

This methodology has recently been successfully applied to localize poly genes that contribute to body adiposity and diet-induced obesity

(36, 37). Efforts to isolate the contributing genes will require the development of congenic mouse lines in which subchromosomal regions are transferred genetically between the parental strains. The demonstration that a congenic segment reproducibly confers a phenotypic difference provides the requisite genetic information that will be necessary for the cloning of the contributing gene. The use of PCR-based genetic markers makes this task straightforward, albeit costly and time consuming. Identification of the contributing genes will be considerably more difficult in cases in which this criterion is not satisfied.

GENETIC ANALYSIS IN HUMANS

The analysis of complex traits in humans is confounded by the obvious requirement that all matings be analyzed retrospectively. Thus, separation of heterogeneous traits into their individual genetic components requires extensive genotyping and sophisticated analytical methods. Three such methods are available: segregation analysis, affected pedigree marker analysis, and association studies. A brief description of these methods is shown in Figure 2 and a more detailed discussion follows below.

One approach in human genetics, segregation analysis, depends on the collection and characterization of multiplex pedigrees with multiple affected individuals (38, 39). The genetic data derived from these studies is analogous to, albeit more complicated than, those derived from genetic crosses. The resulting genetic information is analyzed to localize and map the causal gene. Evidence for linkage is presented as a log-of-the-odds (LOD) score, which is a statistical determination of the likelihood that a given data set is best explained by genetic linkage. Formally, the LOD score is the log of the odds in favor of linkage divided by the log of the odds against linkage (40). This approach is often referred to as parametric. Since each family by itself is often insufficient for analysis owing to the small family size, multiple independent kindreds must be collected. Cumbersome analytical problems arise if different families are affected as a consequence of different genetic lesions (41). In addition, analysis of such pedigrees requires that one have an indication as to the mode of inheritance and penetrance of the contributing gene. For these reasons, standard pedigree analysis has not proved to be of great value for the localization of the genes for common diseases. However, this method has proved useful for the analysis of

Association Study

- association between a particular RFLP/microsatellite variant and a disease in the general population

Affected Pedigree Member Analysis

- higher than expected frequency of allele sharing at a particular locus in affected relative pairs

Pedigree Analysis

- coinheritance of particular RFLP/microsatellite variants with a disease in multiplex families

Figure 2. Analytical methods in human genetics. Three basic methods are available for studies of the inheritance of complex traits in human: pedigree analysis, affected relative pair analysis, and association studies.

syndromic obesity. Thus, both the single gene Prader-Willi locus as well as the genes for the heterogeneous Bardet-Biedl syndrome have been localized (42, 43). For reasons that will be addressed, analysis of large pedigrees may also prove necessary for the ultimate isolation of the genes that contribute to obesity in the general population.

An alternative to pedigree analysis, affected pedigree member analysis, has reemerged as a powerful method for the localization of genes contributing to complex traits (44). The power of this nonparametric method has been amplified by the recent availability of dense microsatellite maps of humans. In affected pedigree member analysis, linkage is inferred if one finds excessive allele sharing at a particular locus in a large cohort of affected relative pairs. For a given polymorphic marker, on average, two affected siblings would have a 25% chance of sharing no alleles, a 50% chance of sharing one allele and a 25% chance of sharing two alleles (Fig. 3). If DNA from each of many pairs of siblings is systematically analyzed, one can calculate, for a particular locus (or subchromosomal interval), the average number of alleles shared per sib pair. The expected result, assuming no linkage, is an average num-

Affected Sib-Pair Analysis

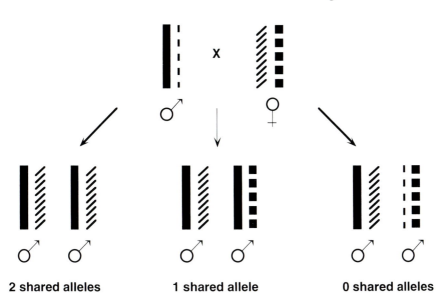

2 shared alleles   **1 shared allele**   **0 shared alleles**

Figure 3.   Allele sharing in a single sib pair. Pairs of siblings will, on average, carry both of the same parental chromosomes (on alleles) 25% of the time, share one chromosome 50% of the time, and share zero chromosomes 25% of the time. Coinheritance of chromosomes can be scored by using informative microsatellites. The systematic analysis of many such afflicted sib pairs can be used to demonstrate linkage (see Fig. 4). If the parental genotypes are available, IBD methods are used; if not, the less powerful IBS can be applied.

ber of shared alleles of one. Deviation of the average number of shared alleles to a value higher than one suggests that the locus is linked to a contributing gene. A hypothetical example of this method is shown in Figure 4. The method is best used in cases in which the genotype of the parents is known. These data ensure that the parents were heterozygous for the marker analyzed, a requirement for a meaningful result. When parental genotypes are known the analysis is known as identity by descent (IBD) (45). An alternative method known as identify by state analysis (IBS) has also been developed in which linkage can be detected without access to the parental genotype (46). This approach incorporates data estimating the heterozygosity of a particular locus in the population but is not as robust as IBD analysis.

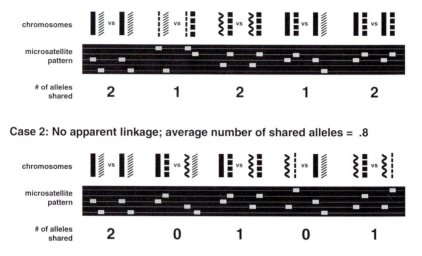

Figure 4. Hypothetical data sets from affected sib pairs. Large numbers of sibling pairs are collected in which both siblings are affected by the same disorder. The number of shared alleles for a given polymorphic locus is ascertained for each sib pair, and the average number of shared alleles per sib pair is calculated for each locus. Statistically significant deviations of the number of shared alleles above one (the average number of shared alleles expected by chance) indicates linkage.

The suitability of this approach for the analysis of complex traits rests in its ability to detect linkage independent of the mode of inheritance, or penetrance of the trait under study. Since only affected individuals are scored, reduced penetrance does not pose a problem. In addition, even a heterogeneous disorder might be effectively analyzed, since, with enough sib pairs, statistical deviations can be detected even if only a subset of the sib pairs are affected by a particular locus. Similarly, polygenic traits are detectable provided the locus contributes significantly to the variance in the measured parameters.

Mathematical modeling of the method has indicated that the likelihood of detecting linkage is a function of a parameter λ_R, the affected relative risk ratio (47, 48). This parameter is the ratio between the risk to an individual if a family member is already affected versus the risk to a general member of the population; thus $\lambda_R = Kr/K$. For example,

λs for Type I diabetes (the affected sibling relative risk ratio) is calculated as the risk of developing Type I diabetes if one has a sibling with a diagnosis of Type I diabetes (Ks) divided by the risk in the general population (K). It has been suggested that the higher the value of λ, the fewer the likely number of causal genes. This can be explained as follows: if many different genes contribute to the phenotype, the likelihood that all the relevant genes will be transmitted from parent to children in a given family is low and approaches the likelihood seen in the general population. In such cases, the gene frequency of the relevant loci would have to be quite high. Conversely, if λ is high one concludes that the number of contributing genes is low. The number of sib pairs required to detect linkage has been estimated both as a function of λ and the density of markers used for genotyping. It has been estimated that even with a relatively low affected risk ratio of 2, analysis of approximately 200 affected sib pairs would still offer a good chance of success provided that enough genetic markers were used (49). Systematic genotyping of this number of individuals with markers across the genome is possible with the application of robotic preparation of PCR reactions and automated genotyping using automated DNA sequencers. The use of this method for the analysis of obesity will require that accurate diagnosis of the phenotype (with sensible cutoffs) be made before the affected sib pairs are included in the analyses.

Although affected pedigree member analysis is suitable for detecting linkage, in its current form it is not capable of providing sufficient genetic resolution for the cloning of the causal gene. Since 25% of affected sibs will share two alleles by chance, the determination of map position based on recombination events in a given family are highly likely to give erroneous information regarding the position of the causal gene. Thus other methods, such as pedigree analysis or the use of linkage disequilibrium mapping, will have to be used in order to narrow the search for disease genes. Nevertheless, the affected pedigree member analysis method is an important first step for localizing genes to subchromosomal regions, and will have an important impact on the genetic analysis of obesity.

The last method of analysis, association study, is the simplest analytical method and depends on a demonstration that affected individuals in a population carry a particular allele with a significantly higher frequency than do unaffected members. For example, the recent demonstration that Alzheimer's patients have an increased gene frequency of the apoE4 allele of the apolipoprotein E gene suggests that apoE4 contributes to the development of Alzheimer's disease (50).

In a fully outbred population, the demonstration of a genetic association generally requires the use of candidate genes. However, in special populations, association studies may prove to be useful, particularly in cases in which long segments of linkage disequilibrium are retained in association with the causal gene. Although segments in linkage disequilibrium with single gene loci have been characterized a number of times, it is yet unclear whether or when such segments will be identifiable for common genetic diseases (51). The likelihood that one can detect linkage using this approach is highest in cases in which there has been relatively recent admixture between two different populations (52, 53). The genotypic analysis of affected members of an admixed population may reveal consistent association between a particular set of alleles (presumably from one of the founder populations) and affected status. Moreover, the boundaries of the segments may serve as guides to the subchromosomal region and ultimately lead to the cloning of the causal gene. However, this analytical method is still evolving. Thus, the precise positioning of non-Mendelian loci in humans remains a substantial problem. This challenge will have to be overcome if one hopes to isolate the contributory genes directly from humans.

In summary, the future holds the promise that many of the genes responsible for the inheritance of complex traits will be identified. The technologies with which one can identify mutant genes is available. At present, this approach requires that the genes that contribute to complex traits be resolved into Mendelian loci. This requirement is more easily satisfied for animal models of human disease. The challenge for the direct analysis of human disease rests in the continued development of the analytical tools for the genetic and physical mapping of a large number of contributing genes.

ACKNOWLEDGMENTS

I would like to thank Susan Korres for her expert assistance in preparing this manuscript. This work was supported by a grant from the National Institutes of Health (#DK41096).

REFERENCES

1. Morgan TH. Sex-limited inheritance in *Drosophila*. *Science*. 1910; 32:1.
2. Sturtevant AH. *J Exp Zool*. 1913;14:43–59.
3. Botstein D, White RL, Skolnick M, Davis RW. Construction of a genetic linkage map in man using restriction fragment length polymorphisms. *Am J Hum Genet*. 1980;32:314–331.
4. Weber JL, May PE. Abundant class of human DNA polymorphisms which can be typed using the polymerase chain reaction. *Am J Hum Genet*. 1989;44:388–396.
5. Dietrich W, Katz H, Lincoln SE, *et al*. A genetic map of the mouse suitable for typing intraspecific crosses. *Genetics*. 1992;131:423–447.
6. Olson M, Hood L, Cantor C, Botstein D. A common language for physical mapping of the human genome. *Science*. 1989;245:1434–1435.
7. Gyapay G, Morissette J, Vignal A, *et al*. The 1993–94 Genethon human genetic linkage map. *Nature Genet*. 1994;7:246.
8. Dietrick WF, *et al*. A genetic map of the mouse with 4006 simple sequence length polymorphisms. *Nature Genet*. 1994;7:220.
9. Friedman JM, Liebel RL, Bahary N. Molecular mapping of obesity genes. *Mammalian Genome*. 1991;1:130–144.
10. Abbs S, Roberts RG, Mathew CG, Bentley Dr, Bobrow M. Accurate assessment of intragenic recombination frequency within the Duchenne muscular dystrophy gene. *Genomics*. 1990;7:602–606.
11. Drumm ML, Smith CL, Dean M, Cole JL, Iannuzzi MC, Collins FS. Physical mapping of the cystic fibrosis region by pulsed-field gel electrophoresis. *Genomics*. 1988;2:346–354.
12. Reeders ST, Keith T, Green D, *et al*. Regional localization of the autosomal dominant polycystic kidney disease locus. *Genomics*. 1988;3:150–155.
13. Burke DT, Carle GF, Olson MV. Cloning of large segments of exogenous DNA into yeast by means of artificial chromosome vectors. *Science*. 1987;236:806–812.
14. Larin Z, Monaco AP, Lehrach H. Yeast artificial chromosome libraries containing large inserts from mouse and human DNA. *Proc Natl Acad Sci USA*. 1991;88:4123–4127.
15. Murray AW, Schultes NP, Szostak JW. Chromosome length controls mitotic chromosome segregation in yeast. *Cell*. 1986;45:529–536.

16. Green ED, Olson MV. Systematic screening of yeast artificial-chromosome libraries by use of the polymerase chain reaction. *Proc Natl Acad Sci USA.* 1990;87:1213–1217.

17. Stumberg N, Ruether J, de Riel K. Generation of a 50 000-member human DNA library with an average DNA insert size of 75–100 kbp in a bacteriophage P1 cloning vector. *New Biol.* 1990;2:151–162.

18. Shizuya H. Cloning and stable maintenance of 300-kilobase-pair fragments of human DNA in *Escherichia coli* using an F-factor-based vector. *Proc Natl Acad Sci USA.* 1992;89:8794–8797.

19. Leonardo ED, Sedivy JM. A new vector for cloning large eukaryotic DNA segments in *Escherichia coli. Biotechnology.* 1990;8:841–844.

20. Chumakov I, Rigault P, Guillou S, *et al.* Continuum of overlapping clones spanning the entire human chromosome 21q. *Nature.* 1992; 359:380–387.

21. Vollrath D, Foote S, Hilton A, *et al.* The human Y chromosome: a 43-interval map based on naturally occurring deletions. *Science.* 1992;258:5079.

22. Bellanne-Chantelot C, Lacroix B, Ougen P, *et al.* Mapping the whole human genome by fingerprinting yeast artificial chromosomes. *Cell.* 1992;70:1059–1068.

23. Uberbacher EC, Mural RJ. Locating protein-coding regions in human DNA sequences by a multiple sensor-neural network approach. *Proc Natl Acad Sci USA.* 1991;88:11261–11265.

24. Venter CJ, ed. *Automated DNA Sequencing and Analysis.* New York: Academic Press; 1993.

25. Parimoo S, Patanjali SR, Shukla H, Chaplin DD, Weissman SM. Efficient PCR approach for the selection of cDNAs encoded in large chromosomal DNA fragments. *Proc Natl Acad Sci USA.* 1991;88: 9623–9627.

26. Morgan JG, *et al.* The selective isolation of novel cDNAs encoded by the regions surrounding the human interleukin 4 and 5 genes. *Nucleic Acids Res.* 1992;20:5173–5179.

27. Buckler AJ, *et al.* Exon amplification: a strategy to isolate mammalian genes based on RNA splicing. *Proc Natl Acad Sci USA.* 1991; 88:4005–4009.

28. Krizman DB, Berget SM. 3'-Terminal exon trapping: identification of genes from vertebrate DNA. *Focus.* 1993;4:106–108.

29. Huntington's Disease Collaborative Research Group. A novel gene containing a trinucleotide repeat that is expanded and unstable on Huntington's Disease chromosome. *Cell.* 1993;72:971–983.

30. Vidal SM, Malo D, Vogan K, Skmene E, Gros P. Natural resistance to infection with intraecellular parasites: isolation of a candidate for Bcg. *Cell.* 1993;73:469–485.

31. Grompe M. The rapid detection of unknown mutations in nucleic acids. *Nature Genet.* 1993;5:111–117.

32. Oliver SG, *et al.* The complete DNA sequence of yeast chromosome 111. *Nature.* 1992;357(6373):38–46.

33. Friedman JM, Liebel RL. Tackling a weighty problem. *Cell.* 1992; 217–220.

34. Thoday JM. Location of polygenes. *Nature.* 1961;191:368–370.

35. Lander ES, Botstein D. Mapping Mendelian factors underlying quantitative traits using RFLP linkage maps. *Genetics.* 1989;121: 185–199.

36. Warden CH, Fisler JS, Pace MJ, Svenson KL, Lusis AJ. Coincidence of genetic loci for plasma cholesterol levels and obesity in a multifactorial mouse model. *J Clin Invest.* 1993;92:773–779.

37. West D, York B, Goudey-Lefevre J, Truett GE. Genetics and physiology of dietary obesity in the mouse. In: Bray G, Ryan D, eds. *Molecular and Genetic Aspects of Obesity.* Pennington Center Nutrition Series, 5. Baton Rouge, LA: Louisiana State University Press; 1995;5:100–119.

38. Haldane JE, Smith CAB. A new estimate of the linkage between the genes for colour-blindness and hemophilia in man. *Ann Eugen.* 1947;14:10–31.

39. Smith CAB. The detection of linkage in human genetics. *Am J Hum Genet.* 1953;7:277–318.

40. Morton NE. The detection and estimation of linkage between the genes for elliptocytosis and the Rh blood type. *Am J Hum Genet.* 1956;8:80–96.

41. Lander ES, Botstein D. Strategies for studying heterogeneous traits in humans by using a linkage map of restriction fragment length polymorphisms. *Proc Nat Acad Sci USA.* 1986;83:7353–7357.

42. Nicholls RD, Knoll JH, Butler MG, Karam S, Lalande M. Genetic imprinting suggested by maternal heterodisomy in non-deletion Prader-Willi syndrome. *Nature.* 1989;342:281–285.

43. Leppert M, *et al.* Bardet-Biedl syndrome is linked to DNA markers on chromosome 11q and is genetically heterogeneous. *Nature Genet.* 1994;7:108.

44. Penrose LS. The detection of autosomal linkage in data which consist of pairs of brothers and sisters of unspecified parentage. *Ann Eugen.* 1935;6:133–138.

45. Risch N. Assessing the role of HLA-linked and unlinked determinants of disease. *Am J Hum Genet.* 1987;40:1–14.

46. Bishop DT, Williamson JA. The power of identity-by-state methods for linkage analysis. *Am J Hum Genet.* 1990;46:254–265.

47. Risch N. Linkage strategies for genetically complex traits, I: multilocus models. *Am J Hum Genet.* 1990;46:222–228.

48. Risch N. Linkage strategies for genetically complex traits, II: the power of affected relative pairs. *Am J Hum Genet.* 1990;46:229–241.

49. Risch N. Linkage strategies for genetically complex traits, III: the effect of marker polymorphism on analysis for affected relative pairs. *Am J Hum Genet.* 1990;46:242–253.

50. Corder EH, Saunders AM, Strittmatter WJ, *et al.* Gene dose of apolipoprotein E type 4 allele and the risk of Alzheimer's disease in late onset families. *Science.* 1993;261:921–923.

51. Lehesjoki AE, *et al.* Localization of the EPM1 gene for progressive myoclonus epilepsy on chromosome 21: linkage disequilibrium allows high resolution mapping. *Hum Mol Genet.* 1993;2:1229–1234.

52. Reed TE. Caucasian genes in American negroes. *Science.* 1969;165:762–768.

53. Dean M, Stephens C, Winkler C, *et al.* Polymorphic admixture typing in human ethnic populations. *Am J Hum Genet.* 1994;55:788–808.

JANIS S. FISLER and CRAIG H. WARDEN

Detection of Genetic Loci for Obesity and Associated Phenotypes in Multifactorial Mouse Models

ABSTRACT

Rodent models provide a wide variety of resources to rapidly identify genes promoting multifactorial obesity. Those resources include many inbred strains with differing phenotypes, a highly developed genetic map, and the availability of recombinant inbred and congenic strains. These resources can be used with quantitative trait locus mapping, which is a general technique for mapping Mendelian factors underlying quantitative traits. Quantitative trait locus mapping involves the following steps: (1) two different inbred strains are crossed to produce F2 or backcross progeny; (2) all of the progeny are individually genotyped for markers that span the genome; (3) phenotypes are measured in each of the progeny; and (4) statistical associations of markers and phenotypes are performed.

We have used the multifactorial BSB mouse model to identify genetic loci for obesity and blood lipids using quantitative trait locus mapping. BSB mice, the backcross progeny of a cross between *Mus spretus* and C57BL/6J mice, range from <1% to >60% body fat. Distal chromosome 7 and proximal chromosome 6 both contain quantitative trait loci for measures of obesity that are coincident with those for plasma total cholesterol. The recessive mutants tubby (chromosome 7) and obese (chromosome 6) are located within these regions, implying that variants in these genes could be involved in polygenic obesity and, thus, could be involved in human obesity.

Mouse Models of Polygenic Obesity

Although it has been difficult to identify directly the genes underlying obesity in humans, animal models clearly have important advantages

87

for both genetic and biochemical studies. The mouse is the model of choice for genetic studies, primarily because hundreds of inbred strains exist, but also because of the availability of other powerful genetic tools. These tools include a genetic map that currently includes over 4000 mapped loci (GBase, 1994, the Jackson Laboratory), making it second only to the human map in completeness. Moreover, the homologies between mouse and human chromosomes have been well defined (1). It is frequently possible to identify the chromosomal location of a gene in humans by mapping it in mice, often with more precision than is provided by human mapping studies. Control is another major advantage of animal studies—control of heterogeneity, breeding, physiological, and biochemical studies, and control of germ line transmission in transgenics and targeted mutations for hypothesis testing. These advantages make it possible to pursue approaches to identify directly genes underlying polygenic obesity in animal models.

A number of rodent models of spontaneous obesity caused by autosomal dominant or recessive inheritance of single genes, such as *ob/ob*, *db/db*, and the yellow obese mouse, have been described (2–4). Studies of polygenic obesity in rodents are fewer (2–4) and the underlying genes not nearly so well defined. The New Zealand obese (NZO) mouse and the Japanese KK mouse are inbred strains that spontaneously develop obesity. Spontaneous obesity is also observed in hybrid models such as the Wellesley mouse (C3H × I F1 hybrid) and the BSB mouse (*Mus spretus* × C57BL/6J backcross).

The NZO mouse, selectively bred for obesity (5), can become massively obese, with weight in adult males ranging from 45 g to 89 g (up to 75% body fat). The fat is primarily stored in the abdomen (6). New Zealand obese mice are hyperinsulinemic but, depending on the age and sex, are not severely hyperglycemic. The NZO mouse is also sensitive to a high-fat diet, which converts the obesity in the NZO mouse from a primarily hypertrophic obesity to a hypertrophic-hyperplastic obesity (7). The Japanese KK mouse was also bred for large body size (8). The obesity in this strain is moderate and tends to diminish in older mice. During the period of weight gain, Japanese KK mice are hyperphagic and develop hyperinsulinemia and a moderately impaired glucose tolerance, which can be prevented by dietary restriction. Dietary fat readily induces obesity in the Japanese KK mouse (9). For a more detailed review of the metabolic characteristics of the Japanese KK mouse and the NZO mouse see Bray and York (3).

The Wellesley mouse is the F1 hybrid resulting from a cross between strains C_3H and I (10). It develops moderate spontaneous obesity with a maximum weight of about 50 g after 3 to 4 months of age. The mice are hyperinsulinemic and moderately hyperglycemic. These abnormalities are intensified by a diet containing 11% fat by weight and can be prevented by diet restriction (11). We have identified a new hybrid mouse model of polygenic obesity involving progeny of a cross between *Mus spretus* and C57BL/6J (*M. musculus*) (12). A particular advantage of the *M. musculus* $\times$ *M. spretus* cross is that these mice are widely diverged (at least three million years), making the identification of DNA polymorphisms between strains relatively straightforward. Although these mice are interfertile, the F1 males are sterile. Therefore, genetic analysis requires that F1 females be backcrossed to either parent, and it is in the progeny of the F1 females backcrossed to the C57BL/6J males that we have found the variation in obesity. We have observed that young C57BL/6J mice and F1 hybrids (*M. spretus* $\times$ C57BL/6J) have about 13% body fat, whereas young *M. spretus* are very lean. Obesity is first observed in the backcross mice, in which body fat varies from less than 1% to greater than 60% of wet carcass weight.

Although the precise mode of inheritance is not understood in any of these models, the obesity is generally thought to be polygenic (5, 13). The obesity and diabetes in the Japanese KK mouse may result from a dominant gene with incomplete penetrance and a modifier gene (14). Since obesity is first observed in the backcross mice, the simplest genetic model for BSB mice is that obesity results from the interactions of two or more genes. One locus must be homozygous for C57BL/6J alleles (BB), and another locus must be heterozygous (SB), since this is the only combination that is unique to backcross mice. Thus, obesity in the BSB mouse may be an example of a heterozygous epistasis interaction between two or more genes. This is a mechanism that might be of considerable importance in outbred populations such as humans, in whom both heterozygosity and homozygosity are common.

Approaches to Genetic Analysis of Complex Traits

The two basic approaches to identifying the underlying genes of complex diseases such as obesity can be called *phenotype down* and *genotype up* (Fig. 1). In the phenotype down approach the products of the genes underlying disease are directly isolated and protein sequences, anti-

APPROACHES TO GENETIC ANALYSIS OF POLYGENIC OBESITY

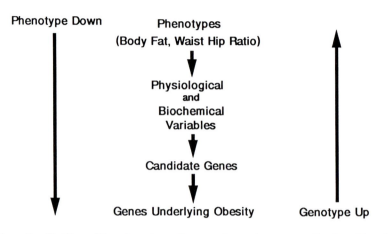

Figure 1. Outline of the phenotype down and genotype up methods to identify the genes underlying inherited metabolic diseases.

Adapted, with permission, from Figure 1 in Warden CH, Fisler JS. Identification of genes underlying polygenic obesity in animal models. In: Bouchard C, ed. *The Genetics of Obesity.* Boca Raton, FL: CRC Press, Inc.; 1994:183. Copyright CRC Press, Boca Raton, Florida.

bodies, or functions of those products are then used to isolate the underlying genes. Success with this approach usually requires that the results of the genetic variation are numerous, that tissues or cells expressing the altered gene product are accessible, and that some clues about the type of the variation can be deduced (15). Although numerous phenotypic and biochemical differences have been identified between lean and obese animals and humans, none of these differences has been conclusively shown to cause any form of obesity (16–19). The candidate gene approach is a phenotype down technique in which a candidate protein is identified and its gene is tested for genetic association with obesity phenotypes. For example, the biochemical approach has identified serum insulin and adipose tissue lipoprotein lipase (LPL) activity as candidates to cause obesity. These candidate genes have then been tested for linkage or association with obesity in humans, but to date there is no consensus on the role of either LPL or insulin in obesity. Even though the "biochemical" and "candidate gene" approaches have proved relatively useful in studies of the genetic control of cholesterol metabolism (20–22), they have not been as useful in the study of obesity. A problem with these approaches is that they require more understanding of the underlying molecular mechanisms than is currently available for obesity.

The genotype up approach is the second major approach to identify genes underlying obesity (Fig. 1). In this method one identifies genetic polymorphisms that segregate (correlate or associate) with obesity. A strength of the reverse genetics approach is that it is not dependent upon an understanding of the disease. Given the current difficulty in locating consensus candidate genes, the genotype up approach is very likely to be important in pinpointing the genes underlying obesity.

Quantitative Trait Locus Mapping

This review concentrates on quantitative trait locus (QTL) mapping, a genotype up method for the identification of loci underlying obesity and its risk factors by surveying the entire genome of experimental animal models (23, 24). The QTL method is a technique for mapping Mendelian factors underlying quantitative traits, in virtually any animal model, using genetic linkage maps (25, 26). This method requires no knowledge of, or assumptions concerning, the biological nature of the characteristics or defects being tracked. Although complete surveys of the genome for loci underlying quantitative traits is not a new concept, the method has only recently become feasible, owing to the development of both numerous highly polymorphic genetic markers that span the genome and mathematical methods for data analysis. This technique has been applied to the mapping of Mendelian factors that underlie continuous variables in tomatoes (27), and more recently the technique has been used to identify genes for obesity in the mouse (24) and hypertension in the rat (26, 28). The quantitative trait locus method can identify chromosomal regions regulating a trait in any animal model system for which two key resources are available—inbred strains and a complete linkage map of the genome (25, 26).

The methods to identify quantitative trait loci can be divided into four steps, which are illustrated for a hypothetical example in Figure 2. First, two different inbred strains are crossed to produce F2 or backcross progeny; second, all of the progeny are individually genotyped for markers that are spread throughout the genome; third, phenotypes are assayed for all of the progeny; and finally, statistical associations of markers and phenotypes are performed to identify loci underlying the

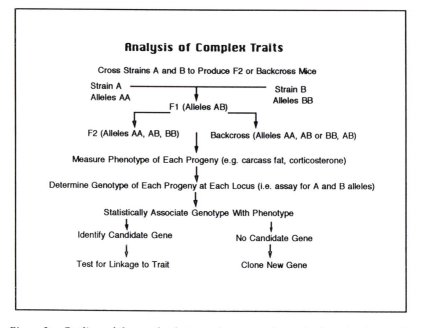

Figure 2. Outline of the methods to analyze complex traits in animal models. Strain A with genotype *AA* is crossed to strain B, with genotype *BB* to produce F1 animals with genotype *AB*. F1 animals are crossed with each other to produce F2 animals, with genotypes *AA*, *AB* or *BB*, or with one of the parental strains to produce backcross with genotypes of *AA*, *AB* or *BB*, *AB* depending on the parental strains used for the backcross. Phenotypes, genotypes, and QTLs are assayed as described in the text.

Adapted, with permission, from Figure 2 in Warden CH, Fisler JS. Identification of genes underlying polygenic obesity in animal models. In: Bouchard C, ed. *The Genetics of Obesity.* Boca Raton, FL: CRC Press, Inc.; 1994:185. Copyright CRC Press, Boca Raton, Florida.

traits. For quantitative traits these associations can reveal quantitative trait loci (QTLs), and for yes/no traits the associations can be revealed by a chi square analysis.

There are three major considerations in setting up crosses. First, the parental strains used should be inbred. The genes passed on by any one animal of an inbred strain will be identical to those of any other animal of that strain; thus animals from an inbred strain provide an invariant gene pool that can be used for all subsequent phenotyping and genotyping experiments. Second, identification of polymorphisms is simplified by the use of strains that are evolutionarily divergent.

However, many of the markers presently available, such as microsatellites or simple sequence repeats, are highly polymorphic among closely related strains of *Mus domesticus* (29). Third, identification of individual QTLs with relatively large phenotypic effects may be difficult when the means of the parental strains differ by less than two standard deviations for the trait under consideration. On the other hand, different strains may have coincidentally similar phenotypes while exhibiting substantial genetic differences. In crosses involving such parental strains, the phenotypes of the progeny are expected to span a much wider range of values than the parents. One such instance of this phenomenon is the obesity in BSB mice.

Phenotyping will depend on the trait of interest. The most specific measure available should be used. For example, percent of carcass weight as fat is a better measure of obesity than body weight or body mass index. Particular care should be taken to minimize the error of the assay, since nongenetic variation will reduce the power of the method. Quantitative trait locus mapping can be applied to any continuously variable trait. Many of the correlates and risk factors of obesity can be considered as quantitative diseases, since many of its associated markers, such as carcass lipid, waist-hip ratio, basal metabolic rate, and blood triglycerides, insulin, and glucose, are quantitative.

Genotyping means to identify which of the two parental strains has contributed alleles to a specific locus in each F2 or backcross animal (Fig. 2). The two most common methods for genotyping are polymerase chain reaction (PCR) assay of simple sequence repeats (SSRs), and restriction fragment length polymorphisms (RFLPs) of cDNA or genomic clones. The most common SSR consists of a variable number of (CA)n repeats, is present at approximately 100 000 copies per genome and is so polymorphic that any two inbred mouse strains will, on average, be polymorphic at 50% of existing SSR loci (26, 30). Genotyping with SSR primers is faster and cheaper than RFLPs, in part because reactions can be performed in 96-well PCR plates, and in part because more than 3000 mouse SSR primer pairs are available at low cost from Research Genetics (Birmingham, AL). Genotyping by RFLPs requires that one acquire and prepare cDNA or genomic clones, prepare Southern blots, and probe the blots. Genotyping by RFLPs remains useful when one needs to test a specific candidate gene for linkage to a trait.

A linear regression of phenotype on genotype, such as an analysis of variance, is the classical method for identifying if the difference between the phenotype means at the different genotypes is significantly different from zero at loci that might underlie complex traits. Finding a significant phenotypic difference between animals with different genotypes suggests that the locus, or one to which it is tightly linked, controls a measurably detectable difference in the phenotype. This approach is limited both by the number and spacing of the individual loci genotyped, since linear regression can be used only to detect linkage to each genotyped locus. The major difficulty is that one cannot distinguish a small, close QTL from a large, distant one. This technique has been improved by implementing several modifications (25).

The ability to analyze phenotype and genotype information for QTLs in model systems is combined together in the Mapmaker (31) and Mapmaker/QTL programs (25). Quantitative trait locus analysis requires the construction of genetic linkage maps of ordered markers that can be constructed from primary data using the Mapmaker program (31). This program is interactive and relatively easy to use and the linkage maps constructed can be used directly by the Mapmaker/QTL program. Mapmaker/QTL uses genetic linkage maps along with quantitative phenotype data to locate QTLs by an efficient interval mapping method that calculates log-of-the-odds (LOD) scores for each quantitative trait at 1 cm to 2 cm intervals between each marker (26). Log-of-the-odds scores provide a measure of the significance of linkage of trait and genotype. A LOD score of 3.0 or greater is considered a statistically significant evidence of linkage.

The BSB Model of Obesity

A new model of polygenic obesity has arisen by crossing two interfertile species of mice (M. spretus × C57BL/6J). Chow-fed backcross progeny (BSB mice) range from very lean to massively obese (up to 95 g body weight in older mice). Obesity in this model is associated with hyperinsulinemia, insulin resistance, and hypertriglyceridemia as is commonly seen in obese humans (12). Using quantitative trait locus mapping with RFLP and microsatellite maps, two genetic loci that are coincident for plasma cholesterol and obesity were identified (Fig. 3) (24). Statistical analysis revealed that distal mouse chromosome 7 exhibits significant linkage both to plasma total cholesterol (LOD score 5.8) and to carcass lipid (LOD score 3.8) (24). This locus accounts for 17% of the variance in plasma cholesterol in males and 5% in females.

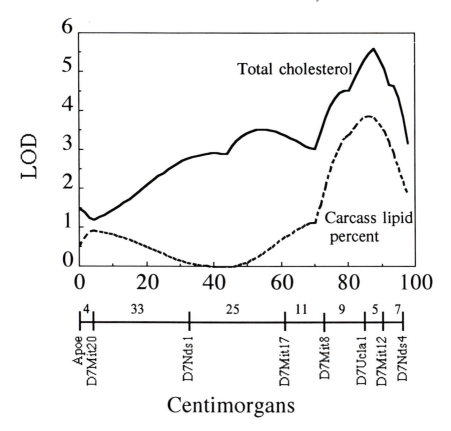

Figure 3. Log-of-the-odds (LOD) likelihood plot for plasma cholesterol levels and carcass lipid percent, adjusted for a linear effect of age, on chromosome 7. *D7Mit20, D7Nds1, D7Mit17, D7Mit12, D7Nds4,* and *D7Mit8* are simple sequence length variants (30). The *y* axis shows the LOD score calculated by the Mapmaker/QTL program at 2-centimorgan intervals. The *x* axis shows the genetic distances of markers in centimorgans. All eight loci are linked to each other with log likelihood scores of at least 5. The orders of these markers is supported by odds ratios of at least 100:1. The position of *D7Ucla1* is supported by an odds ratio > 1000:1.

Reproduced from *Journal of Clinical Investigation,* 1993, 92:776, by copyright permission of the American Society for Clinical Investigation.

The same locus explains 8% of the variance in carcass lipid. Located approximately 10 centimorgans proximal to this locus on chromosome 7 is the recessive mutation *tubby* that results in obesity in mice. A locus identified on chromosome 6 (Table 1) also shows significant linkage to

Table 1. Comparison of Subcutaneous Fat Pad and Plasma Total Cholesterol on Chromosome 6 at *D6Mit1* in *BSB* Mice

| | Statistics by Genotype | | |
	BB	*SB*	*ANOVA*
Femoral Fat (g)	0.29 ± 0.09	0.75 ± 0.10	p<0.0009
	N = 52	N = 38	
Plasma Cholesterol (mg/dl)	63 ± 1.7	74 ± 1.8	p<0.0001
	N = 115	N = 103	

Data are age adjusted means ± SE.

plasma total cholesterol (LOD score 5.6), accounting for 8% of the variance in total cholesterol, and to a subcutaneous fat pad (LOD score 2.8), accounting for 16% of the variance in the femoral fat pad, but shows no linkage to carcass lipid (24). The chromosome 6 locus is approximately 4 centimorgans from the *obese* gene. It is, therefore, possible that variations of the *tubby* and *obese* mutations are involved in these traits in BSB mice. If so, it would imply that variants in these genes could be involved in multigenic obesity and, thus, could be involved in human obesity.

Homology to Humans

Although no animal model is perfect, there is a growing number of animal models in which mutations of the same genes in animals and humans lead to homologous diseases. Ancestral mammalian chromosomes have been shuffled during evolution in identifiable segments. Thus, the same genes are in the same order in mouse and human chromosomal segments. The average length of conserved chromosomal segments between mice and humans has been calculated as 10 to 20 centimorgans (32). The basic approach to using QTLs identified in mice for human studies is to identify a human locus that is homologous to the mouse QTL and then to test for associations of the trait with the locus in humans. A locus on mouse chromosome 9 was identified in *NOD* mice as containing a gene for susceptibility to diabetes (33). The homologous human chromosome, 11q, was then tested for linkage to diabetes in diabetic pedigrees; in this case, however, no linkage was found.

Animal models are likely to be important in endeavors to understand the genetics of obesity. At present, the mapping of loci contributing to complex traits in animal models appears to be the most powerful general method for identifying new genetic factors contributing
to obesity and its associated diseases. The approach is clearly feasible
and in fact has already been applied to several diseases related to obesity in animal models.

ACKNOWLEDGMENTS

This paper was supported in part by National Institutes of Health grant
DK45066.

REFERENCES

1. O'Brien SJ, Womack JE, Lyons LA, Moore KJ, Jenkins NA, Copeland
   NG. Anchored reference loci for comparative genome mapping in
   mammals. *Nature Genet.* 1993;3:103–112.
2. Bray G, York DA. Genetically transmitted obesity in rodents. *Physiol
   Rev.* 1971;51:598–646.
3. Bray GA, York DA. Hypothalamic and genetic obesity in experimental animals: an autocrine and endocrine hypothesis. *Physiol Rev.*
   1979;59:719–808.
4. Festing MFW. The inheritance of obesity in animal models of obesity. In: Festing MFW, ed. *Animal Models of Obesity.* New York: Oxford University Press; 1979:15–37.
5. Bielschowsky M, Bielschowsky F. A new strain of mice with hereditary obesity. *Proc Otago Med School.* 1953;31:29–31.
6. Crofford OB, Davis CK. Growth characteristics, glucose tolerance
   and insulin sensitivity of New Zealand Obese mice. *Metabolism.*
   1965;14:271–280.
7. Herrberg L, Doeppen W, Major E, Gries FA. Dietary induced hypertrophic-hyperplastic obesity in mice. *J Lipid Res.* 1974;6:580–585.
8. Nakamura MA. A diabetic strain of the mouse. *Proc Jpn Acad.* 1962;
   38:348–352.
9. Taketomi S, Tsuda M, Matsuo J, Iwatska H, Suzuoki Z. Alterations
   of hepatic enzyme activities in KK and yellow KK mice with various diabetic states. *Horm Metab Res.* 1973;5:333–339.
10. Jones EE. Spontaneous hyperplasia of the pancreatic islets associ-

ated with glucosuria in hybrid mice. In: Brolin SE, Hellman B, Knutson H, eds. *The Structure and Metabolism of the Pancreatic Islets.* Oxford, Eng: Pergamon Press; 1964:189–191.

11. Gleason RE, Lauris V, Soeldner JS. Studies on experimental diabetes in the Wellesley hybrid mouse. *Diabetologia.* 1967;3:175–178.

12. Fisler JS, Warden CH, Pace MJ, Lusis AJ. BSB: a new mouse model of multigenic obesity. *Obesity Res.* 1993;1:271–280.

13. Nakamura M, Yamada K. A further study of the diabetic (KK) strain of the mouse: F1 and F2 offspring of the cross between KK and C57BL/6J mice. *Proc Jpn Acad.* 1963;39:489–493.

14. Butler L, Gerritsen G. A comparison of the modes of inheritance of diabetes in the Chinese hamster and the KK mouse. *Diabetologia.* 1970;6:163–167.

15. Goldstein JL, Brown MS. Familial hypercholesterolemia. In: Stanbury JB, Wyngaarden JB, Fredrickson DS, Goldstein JL, Brown MS, eds. *The Metabolic Basis of Inherited Disease.* New York: McGraw-Hill; 1983:672–712.

16. Bouchard C, Després J-P, Tremblay A. Genetics of obesity and human energy metabolism. *Proc Nutr Soc.* 1991;50:139–147.

17. Bouchard C. Heredity and the path to overweight and obesity. *Med Sci Sports Exerc.* 1991;23:285–291.

18. Bouchard C. Genetic factors in obesity. *Med Clin North Am.* 1989; 73:67–81.

19. Bray GA. Weight homeostasis. *Annu Rev Med.* 1991;42:205–216.

20. Breslow JL. Lipoprotein transport gene abnormalities underlying coronary heart disease susceptibility. *Annu Rev Med.* 1991;42:357–371.

21. Lusis AJ. Genetic factors affecting blood lipoproteins: the candidate gene approach. *J Lipid Res.* 1988;29:397–429.

22. Breslow JL. The genetic basis of lipoprotein disorders: introduction and overview. *J Intern Med.* 1992;231:627–631.

23. Lusis AJ, Castellani LW, Fisler J. Fitting pieces from studies of animal models into the puzzle of atherosclerosis. *Curr Opin Lipidol.* 1992;3:143–150.

24. Warden CH, Fisler JS, Pace MJ, Svenson KL, Lusis AJ. Coincidence of genetic loci for plasma cholesterol levels and obesity in a multifactorial mouse model. *J Clin Invest.* 1993;92:773–779.

25. Lander ES, Botstein D. Mapping Mendelian factors underlying

quantitative traits using RFLP linkage maps. *Genetics.* 1989;121: 185–199.

26. Jacob HJ, Lindpaintner K, Lincoln SE, *et al.* Genetic mapping of a gene causing hypertension in the stroke-prone spontaneously hypertensive rat. *Cell.* 1991;67:213–224.

27. Paterson AH, Lander ES, Hewitt JD, Peterson S, Lincoln SE, Tanksley SD. Resolution of quantitative traits into Mendelian factors by using a complete linkage map of restriction fragment length polymorphisms. *Nature.* 1988;335:721–726.

28. Hilbert P, Lindpaintner K, Beckmann JS, *et al.* Chromosomal mapping of two genetic loci associated with blood-pressure regulation in hereditary hypertensive rats. *Nature.* 1991;353:521–529.

29. Montagutelli X, Serikawa T, Guénet J-L. PCR-analyzed microsatellites: data concerning laboratory and wild-derived mouse inbred strains. *Mammalian Genome.* 1991;1:255–259.

30. Dietrich W, Katz H, Lincoln SE. A genetic map of the mouse suitable for typing intraspecific crosses. *Genetics.* 1992;131:423–447.

31. Lander ES, Green P, Abrahamson J, *et al.* Mapmaker: an interactive computer package for constructing primary genetic linkage maps of experimental and natural populations. *Genomics.* 1987;1:174–181.

32. Nadeau JH, Taylor BA. Lengths of chromosomal segments conserved since divergence of man and mouse. *Proc Natl Acad Sci USA.* 1984;81:814–818.

33. Hyer RN, Julier C, Buckley JD, *et al.* High-resolution linkage mapping for susceptibility genes in human polygenic disease: insulin-dependent diabetes mellitus and chromosome 11q. *Am J Hum Genet.* 1991;48:243–257.

DAVID B. WEST, BARBARA YORK,
JO GOUDEY-LEFEVRE, and GARY E. TRUETT

Genetics and Physiology of
Dietary Obesity in the Mouse

ABSTRACT

AKR/J and SWR/J inbred mice differ markedly in their sensitivity
to dietary obesity. Male AKR/J mice increase adiposity approximately threefold, whereas SWR/J remain relatively lean when fed
a high-fat diet for twelve weeks. At 5 weeks of age these mouse
strains have comparable body fat percentages when fed a low-fat
diet, yet they differ in a number of metabolic markers. AKR/J mice
are less physically active, have a higher rate of excretion of norepinephrine in the urine, have increased sensitivity to insulin-
stimulated glucose disposal and decreased maximally stimulated
epinephrine lipolysis in isolated adipocytes. These metabolic
markers may represent underlying physiological differences under genetic control, which partially explain the differential sensitivity to dietary obesity in these two strains. A quantitative analysis of the segregation of body adiposity in F2 and F1 $\times$ SWR/J
progeny suggests that this phenotype is under the control of a
minimum of three to four genes and that there is partial dominance of the AKR/J genotype. Molecular mapping in F2 and F1
$\times$ SWR/J populations using the quantitative trait loci mapping
approach and random simple sequence length polymorphisms has
identified several quantitative trait loci with significant likelihood
of of-the-odds scores that are linked to dietary obesity. These loci
are located on chromosomes 4, 9, and 15, and several candidate
genes are co-localized at these loci.

Interaction of Genes and Environment to Produce Obesity

Clearly, genes make a significant contribution to the risk for the development of human obesity. This evidence comes from twin studies (1),

100

as well as from an evaluation of the segregation of the trait in populations (2) and mathematical modeling of the phenotype distributions (3). The data are convincing and argue that inherited genes play an important role in human obesity development, though the magnitude of the genetic effect is debated.

Furthermore, it is generally accepted that a number of environmental factors also conspire to promote obesity in human populations. Recently, the role of dietary fat in promoting obesity has been emphasized (4). However, the data most supportive of a role for high levels of dietary fat in the development of human obesity are cross-cultural studies that are interesting but difficult to interpret (5).

In animals it is very clear that genes can play an important role in the expression of obesity. Numerous single gene models of rodent obesity exist (6), and these generally result in a profound obesity that is not modulated by diet. There also exist a number of polygenic models of rodent obesity, which reportedly do show modulation of expression by dietary effects (7). In animal studies, the data are very convincing that the level of dietary fat can have a very powerful effect on body fat content. Numerous studies have shown a significant increase in body fat content in mice (8, 9), rats (10), and dogs (11) with long-term exposure to diets containing high-fat content. It is not clear if hyperphagia is a necessary component of this dietary obesity; however, it is frequently observed with high-fat diets (12).

If obesity is the result of genetic factors predisposing for the disease and environmental factors that allow the expression of the obesity phenotype, then any analysis of the genetics of both human and animal obesity must allow for the importance of environment and should attempt to control for these environmental factors. Although attempts are under way to identify the genes responsible for human obesity, approaches such as linkage analysis and population comparisons may be difficult to apply successfully in human studies. It is likely that in human populations there are multiple genes controlling the phenotype. This genetic heterogeneity may make it difficult to identify these genes in diverse populations. Furthermore, environmental factors will certainly increase the variance in the phenotype, further complicating the genetics of human obesity.

An alternative to directly characterizing the genetics of human obesity is to develop animal models with similar phenotypes and to use these models to identify and characterize the specific genes contributing to variation. This approach may lead to specific candidate genes and/or metabolic pathways whose role in the genetics of human obesity can then be tested directly. In this report, we describe the physiological and genetic characterization of a mouse model of differential sensitivity to dietary obesity.

Development of a Mouse Model to Evaluate Genetic Factors Contributing to Dietary Obesity

Because of the well-defined genetic map in the mouse (13) and the availability of many inbred strains with differing phenotypes, it is clear that the mouse is one of the animal models of choice for mapping studies of the genes underlying complex phenotypes such as body fat content. Although a number of single gene models of obesity exist in the mouse (6), these gene defects result in massive obesity with no clear modulation of the gene effects by diet. Because of the lack of an existing mouse model that clearly shows an interaction between genetic background and diet to produce obesity, we evaluated a number of different inbred mouse strains in order to identify those sensitive or resistant to dietary obesity (8). Male mice from nine mouse strains were fed either a chow diet (Purina Rodent Chow #5001; 11.6% of calories from fat) or a diet moderately high in dietary fat (Condensed Milk Diet; 32.6% of calories from fat) for seven weeks, beginning at 5 weeks of age. The mouse strains showed a range of responses to the high-fat diet (Fig. 1). Some mouse strains, such as the AKR/J strain, significantly increased carcass fat content when fed the high-fat diet, whereas other strains, such as the SWR/J, showed no increase in carcass fat content with seven weeks of access to the high-fat diet. The AKR/J and SWR/J mouse strains were selected as the most responsive and least responsive to dietary obesity respectively, and the experiment was repeated in these two strains with twelve weeks of access to the high-fat diet, beginning at 5 weeks of age. Figure 2 shows the response of a larger number of male mice from these two strains to twelve weeks access to either a chow diet or the condensed milk, moderately high-fat diet (14). Although the AKR/J strain was fatter than the SWR/J strain at 17 weeks of age independent of diet, it was also clear that the AKR/J strain was more responsive to dietary obesity than the SWR/J strain. This strain difference was not unique to the condensed milk–based diet. When the body fat response of these two strains to a variety of defined diets

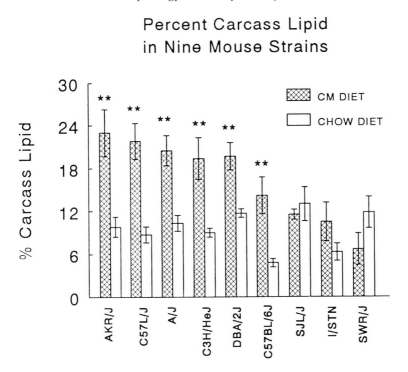

Figure 1. Percentage of carcass composed of lipid in mice from nine inbred strains fed either high-fat condensed milk (CM) diet or the low-fat Purina Rodent Chow #5001 diet. Mice (n = 5 per strain and diet group) were fed the diets beginning at five weeks of age for a total of seven weeks. Data are presented as mean values, with error bars representing standard error.
**P < .01, significant CM diet versus chow diet difference within a strain (ANOVA and Tukey's protected *t*-test).
From reference 8, with permission of the American Physiological Society.

varying in fat, carbohydrate, and protein was tested, the AKR/J strain was more responsive to the level of dietary fat in the diet and had significantly more body fat than the SWR/J strain in all dietary conditions (data not shown).

In order to study the genetic basis of a phenotype, that phenotype must be measurable with relative ease and accuracy, since genetic studies can require large numbers of animals. Although total carcass lipid content by chemical extraction was one possible phenotype to evaluate in this mouse model, it was undesirable for several reasons. First, the

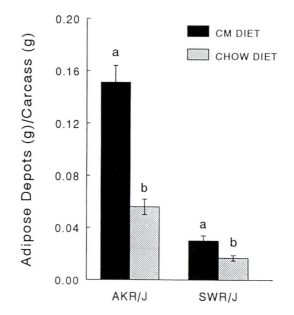

Figure 2. Adiposity index (weight of seven dissected adipose depots divided by the eviscerated carcass weight) of AKR/J and SWR/J mice (n = 15 for each strain) fed either the high-fat condensed milk diet or the low-fat chow diet for twelve weeks beginning at five weeks of age. Data are presented as means and standard errors. Within each strain, a significant difference between diet conditions is indicated by a different letter notation above the error bars.
From reference 14, with permission of the American Physiological Society.

chemical extraction procedure is tedious and time consuming. Second, the chemical extraction includes lipids stored in membranes and adipose tissue in joints and other areas that are not readily accessible energy stores. Finally, a chemical extraction of total body lipids gives no information regarding the regional distribution of body fat. Therefore, we decided to use an index of body fat derived by dividing the summed weight of seven adipose tissue depots (left and right inguinal subcutaneous, left and right epididymal, left and right retroperitoneal, and the mesenteric depot) by the eviscerated carcass weight (not including the dissected depots). This adiposity index is highly linearly correlated with total body lipid content in AKR/J and SWR/J mice fed defined diets containing a range of fat content (Fig. 3), and it can be used to accurately estimate total body fat content. In addition, the individual depot weights can be used as phenotypes to evaluate the genetic control of regional adipose tissue mass.

Metabolic Differences Between AKR/J and SWR/J Inbred Mice

The identification of two inbred mouse strains that markedly differ in their sensitivity to dietary obesity, as well as the development of a reliable and accurately measured phenotype, was the first step in the development of a useful model to study differential sensitivity to die-

Correlation: Carcass Lipid and Adiposity Index

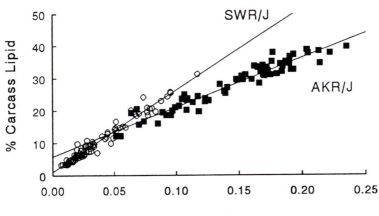

Figure 3. Correlation of carcass lipid content to adiposity index. Carcass lipid content and the adiposity index were examined in a study of the effect of diets varying in macronutrient content in AKR/J and SWR/J mice. Following twelve weeks of access to the diets, beginning at five weeks of age, the mice were euthanatized and dissected. The adiposity index was calculated as the weight of seven dissected adipose depots (left and right inguinal subcutaneous, left and right epididymal, left and right retroperitoneal, and mesenteric) divided by the eviscerated carcass weight (carcass weight did not include dissected depots). Carcass lipid content was highly correlated with the adiposity index in both AKR/J and SWR/J mice, although the regression lines for each strain were different. The $r > 0.97$ in both mouse strains.

tary obesity in the mouse. However, it was also important to determine if there were metabolic differences between these strains that might explain their different sensitivity to dietary obesity. The identification of specific metabolic differences would provide information about likely candidate genes to evaluate in future genetic studies.

We have evaluated a number of metabolic and behavioral measures in the AKR/J and SWR/J mouse strains and have identified a number of differences, which are listed in Table 1.

The greater excretion of norepinephrine in the urine of AKR/J mice over a four-hour period following intraperitoneal glucose injection, as well as a greater spontaneous twenty-four-hour urinary norepinephrine excretion in AKR/J mice (15), is similar to the findings in outbred rats that are sensitive or resistant to dietary obesity. Levin *et al.* have previously shown that some Sprague-Dawley rats become obese on a high-fat diet while others remain lean (16). They have observed that those rats that are sensitive to dietary obesity secrete more norepinephrine into the blood following the physiological stress of intravenous glucose injection and also excrete more norepinephrine in their urine over a twenty-four-hour period (17). This finding in rats, and now similar findings in mice, is paradoxical, since it would seem to reflect a greater sympathetic nervous system activity in the rats or mice that are more sensitive to dietary obesity. However, it might be explained by a greater end-organ resistance to norepinephrine in the diet-sensitive strain, resulting in greater turnover of this catecholamine and a greater release of the neurotransmitter during stress.

If this hypothesis is correct, then diet-sensitive animals should have a shifted dose response to catecholamines in a number of systems. We

Table 1.   Metabolic Differences Between AKR/J and SWR/J Mice

Metabolic Feature	Strain Difference
24-hour urinary norepinephrine excretion	AKR/J >> SWR/J
4-hour urinary norepinephrine following intraperitoneal glucose	AKR/J > SWR/J
Sensitivity of isolated adipocytes to epinephrine-stimulated lipolysis	AKR/J < SWR/J
Physical activity	AKR/J < SWR/J
Sensitivity of isolated adipocytes to insulin-stimulated glucose uptake	AKR/J > SWR/J

have evaluated this in AKR/J and SWR/J mice and found that the dose response of isolated epididymal depot adipocytes to epinephrine-stimulated lipolysis is shifted in AKR/J mice. AKR/J mice are resistant to epinephrine-stimulated lipolysis compared with the SWR/J mice. This suggests that altered basal and stimulated sympathetic control of adipocyte function may be involved in the differential sensitivity to dietary obesity in these two mouse strains.

The lower physical activity, measured by an activity monitor, in the AKR/J mice compared with the SWR/J mice is also consistent with the AKR/J mice being more sensitive to dietary obesity.

Of particular interest is the difference in adipocyte insulin sensitivity in these two strains (14). Epididymal adipocytes isolated from the two strains show markedly different sensitivity to insulin; and with short-term access to a high-fat diet this strain difference was amplified (Fig. 4). Compared with the SWR/J mice, adipocytes from the AKR/J were significantly more sensitive to insulin-stimulated glucose uptake. The greater uptake of glucose by AKR/J adipocytes would provide more precursors for lipogenesis compared with SWR/J glucose uptake and utilization. This is certainly consistent with a mechanism that would tend to preferentially shunt calories to lipid storage in AKR/J mice to a greater extent than in SWR/J mice.

Most of these studies were performed when the mice were approximately five to six weeks of age when there was only a slight difference in body fat content. Figure 5 shows the adiposity index of AKR/J and SWR/J mice between the ages of 5 and 10 weeks of age when they were maintained on a low-fat diet and clearly shows that the difference in total body fat content is minimal at the age of 5 weeks between these two strains. In addition, for the adipocyte metabolic studies, the epididymal adipocytes were of identical size in the two strains when the animals were young and were fed the low-fat diet. Therefore, in these studies, observed metabolic differences were not attributable to differences in body fat composition or adipocyte size.

These metabolic differences suggest that genes involved in the pathways modulating the response of adipocytes to insulin and catecholamines are likely candidates involved in the differential response to dietary fat by these two mouse strains. If genes involved in these metabolic pathways map to areas of the mouse genome that are linked to sensitivity to dietary obesity, then these genes should be given a high priority for further evaluation.

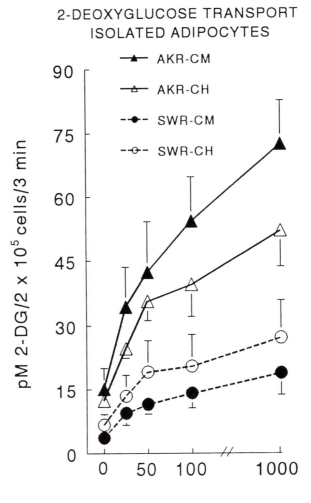

2-DEOXYGLUCOSE TRANSPORT
ISOLATED ADIPOCYTES

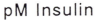

pM Insulin

Figure 4. Response of isolated epididymal adipocytes to insulin. Transport of 2-deoxy-[³H]glucose into isolated adipocytes at different levels of insulin. Adipocytes were obtained from AKR/J and SWR/J mice fed either the high-fat condensed milk (CM) for one week or maintained on chow (CH) diet. For the chow-fed AKR/J and SWR/J groups there was no significant difference in epididymal adipocyte size. In the CM-fed AKR/J and SWR/J groups, the AKR/J had significantly larger epididymal adipocytes. Data are presented as mean and standard errors. There was a significant main effect of strain with the AKR/J strain significantly more sensitive to insulin stimulated glucose uptake.

From reference 14, reproduced with permission of the American Physiological Society.

Adiposity of AKR/J & SWR/J Mice
Chow Diet

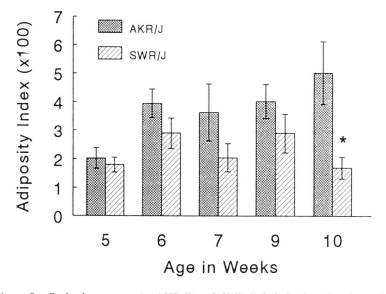

Figure 5. Body fat content in AKR/J and SWR/J fed the low-fat chow diet during the postweaning period. AKR/J and SWR/J mice were weaned at approximately four weeks of age and fed the chow diet ad libitum. The mice were sacrificed at five, six, seven, nine, and ten weeks of age and the adipose depots dissected in order to calculate the adiposity index (n = 5–8 for each diet group). There was no significant difference between the strains in adiposity until ten weeks of age ($P < .05$, *t*-test).

Segregation of Dietary Obesity in AKJR/J × SWR/J MICE

In order to determine if the AKR/J × SWR/J model of differential sensitivity to dietary obesity would be useful for molecular mapping studies, it was important to determine if the trait segregated in intercrosses between the two parental strains. First generation (F1) progeny were generated from an intercross between AKR/J and SWR/J parental animals and these F1 animals were then intercrossed to produce the F2 generation or backcrossed upon either the AKR/J or SWR/J parental strains. Male mice were weaned at approximately 3 to 4 weeks of age and fed the high-fat condensed milk diet beginning at 5 weeks of age for a twelve-week period. The animals were then sacrificed, and the adiposity index phenotype was measured at approximately 17 weeks of age.

Figure 6 shows the frequency distribution of the adiposity index in parental (AKR/J and SWR/J), F1 (AKR/J × SWR/J), F1 × SWR/J, F1 × AKR/J, and F2 (F1 × F1) animals (18). The adiposity index was clearly separated in the two parental strains with no overlap of the populations. The adiposity index of the F1 population lay between the parental phenotypes, whereas the F2 population ranged in adiposity from the leanest of the SWR/J to the fattest of the AKR/J. However, the majority of the F1 × AKR/J mice had an adiposity phenotype within the range of the parental AKR/J mice; approximately two-thirds of the F1 × SWR/J mice also had a phenotype within the range of the AKR/J parental strain. The adiposity index was clearly segregating in the F2 and the F1 × SWR/J populations. However, the observation that the majority of animals in the F1 × AKR/J group were within the phenotype range of the AKR/J parental strain suggested that the AKR/J genotype has some dominance.

These data were further analyzed using the equations of Wright (19) to calculate both dominance and the minimum number of effective loci controlling the adiposity index that were segregating in this cross. Dominance (d) was calculated to be 0.73, suggesting a significant amount of dominance of the AKR/J genotype. Assuming a dominant model, with equivalent effects on the phenotype of each segregating locus, a minimum of three to four loci are segregating in this cross. However, estimation of the number of loci involved in controlling a trait by this method is generally assumed to be an underestimate.

The observation that this complex phenotype was segregating in this intercross, and that there were a relatively small number of loci segregating, suggested that this model might be amenable to a molecular mapping study to localize the genes controlling the phenotype of sensitivity to dietary obesity.

Loci Linked to Dietary Obesity in the AKR/J × SWR/J Model

We used a mapping population of 931 male F2 progeny of an intercross between AKR/J and SWR/J mice, as well as a population of 375 F1 × SWR/J male mice. All of the mice were weaned at approximately 4 weeks of age and placed on the condensed milk high-fat diet for a

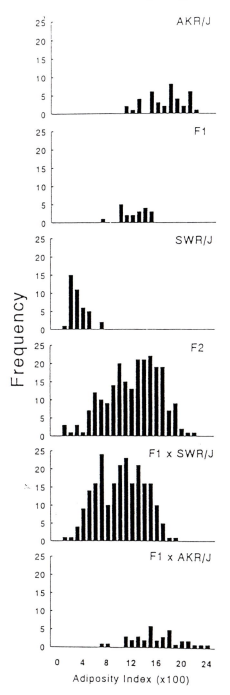

Figure 6. Segregation of the trait in F2 and backcross populations. Frequency distribution of the adiposity index measured after twelve weeks of access to the high-fat condensed milk diet beginning at five weeks of age. The adiposity index was measured as described in the text. Data are presented for AKR/J (n = 39), F1 (n = 20), SWR/J (n = 40), F2 (n = 230), F1 × SWR/J (n = 225), and F1 × AKR/J (n = 236) mice. The plotted range for this index is from .01 to .24.

From reference 18, with permission of the International Mammalian Genome Society and Springer-Verlag.

twelve-week period beginning at 5 to 6 weeks of age. The mice were then sacrificed, the adipose depots were dissected, and the adiposity index was calculated.

Mice from the 10% tails of the adiposity index phenotype distribution were genotyped at simple sequence length polymorphisms (SSLPs) using amplification by Taq polymerase. We used SSLPs that had previously been developed and mapped in the mouse (20) and are commercially available (Research Genetics, Huntsville, AL).

The statistical approach taken was the mapping of quantitative trait loci (QTL) described by Lander and Botstein (21, 22), and the program Mapmaker/QTL (23) was used to analyze the data. This approach uses a multipoint interval mapping approach to establish if there is linkage between a set of markers and a specific quantitative trait. The log of the odds (LOD) score gives the probability across a linkage group that a locus is linked to the specific quantitative trait. Generally, a LOD score of greater than 3.0 is accepted as significant evidence of linkage with this approach. Genotyping only the 10% tails of the phenotype distribution, but using the entire phenotype distribution, in the statistical treatment significantly increases the statistical power and reduces the number of animals that must be genotyped (24).

We have identified quantitative trait loci (QTLs) linked to dietary obesity (*i.e.*, the adiposity index) in the AKR/J × SWR/J model on chromosomes 4, 9, and 15 using the F2 mapping population (18, 25). These loci have been assigned the names *Do1* (chromosome 4), *Do2* (chromosome 9), and *Do3* (chromosome 15), respectively, for dietary obese 1, 2, and 3. Figure 7 gives the LOD probability plot for the chromosome 4 locus, Figure 8 gives the LOD probability plot for the chromosome 9 locus, and Figure 9 gives the plot for the chromosome 15 locus.

The peak LOD scores for the chromosomes 4, 9, and 15 loci were 4.5, 4.85, and 3.93, respectively. Data for each of these loci fit a model with additive genetics. However, the allele from the SWR/J strain at the chromosome 9 locus actually is associated with *increased* adiposity, whereas it is the alleles from the AKR/J strain at the chromosome 4 and 15 loci that are associated with greater adiposity. Since the SWR/J strain is the lean strain, it is paradoxical that its allele at the *Do2* locus should be associated with greater body fat. However, this may be explained by unmasking of the phenotype effects of the *Do2* SWR/J allele by other AKR/J loci in the F2 population, which are yet to be identified.

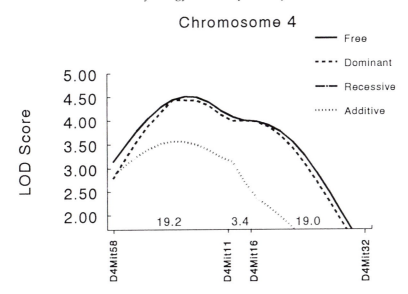

Figure 7.   Quantitative trait locus on chromosome 4. Log of the odds ratio on chromosome 4 for total body adiposity in F2 progeny of an intercross between AKR/J and SWR/J mice using unconstrained (free), AKR/J dominant, AKR/J recessive, and additive genetic models. Since the LOD score for the AKR/J recessive model does not exceed 1.5 in this interval, the AKR/J recessive model does not appear on the figure due to the restricted range of the Y-axis in this plot. The SSLPs used for the linkage analysis are indicated on the abscissa, and the map distance separating these markers is indicated in centimorgans (cM). The LOD scores were calculated at 2 cM intervals between markers. This QTL on chromosome 4, which is linked to sensitivity to dietary obesity, has been named dietary obese 1 (*Do1*).

From reference 18, with permission of the International Mammalian Genome Society and Springer-Verlag.

The locus on chromosome 15 that we found in the F2 mapping population has been confirmed in the F1 × SWR/J mapping population at the same location (data not shown). However, for the chromosome 9 locus, the F1 × SWR/J mapping population gave no evidence of the presence of a QTL at this location. This may be explained by the fact that some AKR/J alleles at presently unknown locations are necessary for the unmasking of the SWR/J allele effect at the *Do2* locus. Since three-fourths of the alleles segregating in the F1 × SWR/J population are SWR/J alleles, the appropriate combination of genes may not occur at a high enough frequency for the unmasking effect to be observed in

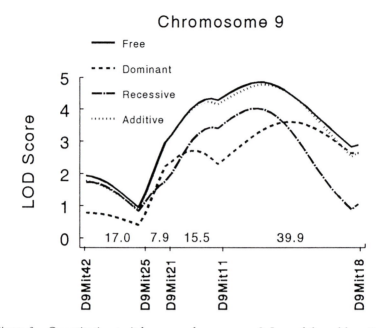

Figure 8. Quantitative trait locus on chromosome 9. Log of the odds ratio on chromosome 9 for total body adiposity in F2 progeny of an intercross between SWR/J and AKR/J mice. This QTL on chromosome 9 has been named dietary obese 2 (*Do2*). Notations as in Figure 7.

this backcross. We have not yet evaluated the F1 × SWR/J population for linkage at the *Do1* locus.

It is possible to estimate the percent of the variation in the adiposity index that is controlled by a specific QTL using the program Mapmaker/QTL. For the loci that we have described, the percent of the variation controlled ranges from approximately 4% to approximately 8% of the total variance. However, since only the tails of the phenotype distribution were genotyped, it is unlikely that all possible combinations of genotypes at these three loci (and presumably other loci not yet identified) were represented. Therefore, the estimation of the control of these loci over the phenotype may not be accurate. The identification of all of the loci having significant effects on the trait and the control of their effects in the statistical model will give a better estimate of the magnitude of their individual effects on the phenotype.

Chromosome 15

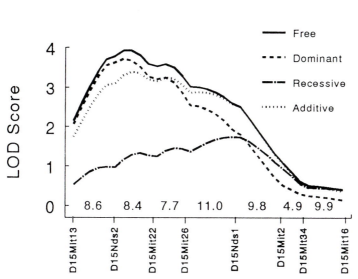

Figure 9.   Quantitative trait locus on chromosome 15. Log of the odds ratio on chromosome 15 for total body adiposity in F2 progeny of an intercross between SWR/J and AKR/J mice. This QTL on chromosome 15 has been named dietary obese 3 (*Do3*). Notations as in Figure 7.

A number of candidate genes have been mapped to the QTLs linked to dietary obesity that we have identified. On chromosome 4, at the *Do1* locus, the *GLUT1* glucose transporter has been mapped (26). This glucose transporter is constitutively expressed in adipose tissue and skeletal muscle, and mutations in this gene could certainly affect a number of phenotypes, including energy metabolism and lipid storage. On chromosome 9, at the *Do2* locus, the alpha inhibitory subunit of G protein (*Gnai-2*) has been mapped (27). This alpha inhibitory subunit is expressed in adipocytes and is important for mediating the effects of alpha-2 adrenergic stimulation (28). We have previously shown that the AKR/J epididymal adipocytes are less sensitive to epinephrine-stimulated lipolysis than adipocytes from the SWR/J mouse. This difference could certainly be mediated by altered G protein function. Finally, on chromosome 15, at the *Do3* locus, the growth hormone receptor has been previously mapped (29). Since the growth hormone receptor is expressed in adipocytes and growth hormone has an antilipogenic effect on adipocytes (30), this is a likely candidate gene. The role of these candidate genes in the control of the dietary obesity phenotype in this model are presently being evaluated.

Conclusions

The AKR/J × SWR/J model of differential sensitivity to dietary obesity may be a useful model for elaborating both the genetic and metabolic basis for dietary obesity. The difference in response of the two strains to a diet high in fat calories is robust, with the AKR/J strain clearly more responsive than the SWR/J strain. The segregation of the trait in the F2 generation and in the backcross animals, and the relatively low number of loci that are segregating, suggest that this model will be amenable to molecular mapping of the loci controlling the trait. This has been confirmed by the identification of three loci linked to dietary obesity in the F2 and F1 × SWR/J mapping populations. A significant fraction of the genome has not been scanned for linkage in this model, and it is likely that several more loci will be localized. The identification of genes previously mapped to the areas of the mouse genome that are linked to dietary obesity in this model, and that plausibly could be involved in the phenotype, provides a significant advantage over simply testing potential candidates without any evidence of linkage.

A number of metabolic differences exist between these two strains that may be causally related to the different diet sensitivity. The identification and further characterization of these metabolic differences may provide additional plausible candidate genes that may regulate this phenotype, or may target a specific candidate gene already mapped to a linked locus. For example, the resistance to epinephrine-stimulated lipolysis in the AKR/J epididymal adipocytes supports a role for the involvement of the alpha inhibitory subunit of G protein, which coincidentally was previously mapped to the *Do2* locus on chromosome 9.

Of course, the ultimate goal of this project is to identify and characterize the genes controlling the phenotype of sensitivity to dietary obesity in this mouse model. A variety of approaches must be taken in order to achieve this goal, including the evaluation of candidate gene physiology, expression, and structure based upon mapping data and physiological differences between the strains. Additionally, the evaluation of the effect of individual loci introgressed into the different background strains will provide crucial information regarding the magnitude of control of a specific locus over the phenotype. Finally, a positional cloning approach may be necessary if a locus has a large enough effect and if the evaluation of potential candidate genes in the region does not identify the gene or genes controlling the trait. It is an open question as to whether genes involved in the regulation of a complex phenotype in an animal model such as the mouse will also be functioning in human disease.

ACKNOWLEDGMENTS

This paper was supported in part by a Faculty Scholar in Nutrition Award from the Pew National Nutrition Program to David B. West and by NIH grant #DK45895. We acknowledge the excellent technical assistance of Stephanie Hancock and Jody Waguespack and statistical consulting by Dr. Pat Wozniak.

REFERENCES

1. Stunkard AJ, Foch TT, Hrubec H. A twin study of human obesity. *JAMA.* 1986;256:51–54.
2. Moll PP, Burns TL, Laver RM. The genetic and environmental sources of body mass index variability: the Muscatine ponderosity family study. *Am J Hum Genet.* 1991;49:1243–1255.
3. Price RA, Ness R, Laskarzewski P. Common major gene inheritance of extreme overweight. *Hum Biol.* 1990;62:747–765.
4. Tucker LA, Kano MJ. Dietary fat and body fat: a multivariate study of 205 adult females. *Am J Clin Nutr.* 1992;56:616–622.
5. Curb JD, Marcus EB. Body fat and obesity in Japanese Americans. *Am J Clin Nutr.* 1991;53:1552S–1555S.
6. Bray GA, York DA. Genetically transmitted obesity in rodents. *Physiol Rev.* 1971;51:598–646.
7. Festing MFW. The inheritance of obesity in animal models of obesity. In: Festing MFW, ed. *Animal Models of Obesity.* New York: Oxford University Press; 1979:15–38.
8. West DB, Boozer CN, Moody DL, Atkinson RL. Dietary obesity in nine inbred mouse strains. *Am J Physiol.* 1992;262:R1025–R1031.

9. Salmon DMW, Flatt JP. Effect of dietary fat content on the incidence of obesity among ad libitum fed mice. *Int J Obes.* 1985;9:443–449.

10. Schemmel R, Mickelsen O, Gill JL. Dietary obesity in rats: body weight and body fat accretion in seven strains of rats. *J Nutr.* 1970; 100:1041–1048.

11. Rocchini AP, Moorehead C, Wentz E, Deremer S. Obesity-induced hypertension in the dog. *Hypertension.* 1987;9(suppl 3):64–68.

12. Sclafani A. Dietary-induced overeating. *Ann NY Acad Sci.* 1989;575: 281–289.

13. Copeland NG, Jenkins NA, Gilbert DJ, *et al.* A genetic linkage map of the mouse: current applications and future prospects. *Science.* 1992;262:57–66.

14. Eberhart GP, West DB, Boozer CN, Atkinson RL. Insulin sensitivity of adipocytes from inbred mouse strains resistant or sensitive to diet induced obesity. *Am J Physiol.* 1994;266:R1423–R1428.

15. West DB, Moody DL, Boozer CN, Atkinson RL, Levin BE. Differential catecholamine response to intraperitoneal glucose injection in inbred mice susceptible or resistant to dietary obesity. *Int J Obesity.* 1991;15(suppl 3):16.

16. Levin BE, Sullivan AC. Glucose-induced norepinephrine levels and obesity resistance. *Am J Physiol.* 1987;253:R475–R481.

17. Levin BE. Sympathetic activity, age, sucrose preference and diet-induced obesity. *Obesity Res.* 1993;1:281–287.

18. West DB, Waguespack J, York B, Goudey-Lefevre J, Price RA. Genetics of dietary obesity in AKR/J × SWR/J mice: segregation of the trait and identification of a linked locus on chromosome 4. *Mammalian Genome.* 1994;5:546–552.

19. Wright S. *Evolution and the Genetics of Populations.* Vol. 1, *Genetic and Biometric Foundations.* Chicago: University of Chicago Press; 1968.

20. Dietrich W, Katz H, Lincoln SE, *et al.* A genetic map of the mouse suitable for typing intraspecific crosses. *Genetics.* 1992;131:423–447.

21. Lander ES, Botstein D. Mapping complex genetic traits in humans: new methods using a complete RFLP linkage map. *Cold Spring Harb Symp Quant Biol.* 1986;51:49–62.

22. Lander ES, Botstein D. Strategies for studying heterogeneous genetic traits in humans by using a linkage map of restriction fragment length polymorphism. *Proc Natl Acad Sci USA.* 1986;83:7353–7357.

23. Lander ES, Green P, Abrahamson J, *et al.* Mapmaker: an interactive

computer package for constructing primary genetic linkage maps of experimental and natural populations. *Genomics*. 1987;1:174–181.

24. Lander ES, Botstein D. Mapping Mendelian factors underlying quantitative traits using RFLP linkage maps. *Genetics*. 1989;121: 185–199.

25. West DB, Goudey-Lefevre J, York B, Truett GE. Dietary obesity linked to genetic loci on chromosomes 9 and 15 in a polygenic mouse model. *J Clin Invest*. 1994;94:1410–1416.

26. Bahary, N, Leibel RL, Joseph L, Friedman JM. Molecular mapping of the mouse *db* mutation. *Proc Natl Acad Sci USA*. 1990;87:8642–8646.

27. Blatt CP, Eversole-Cire VH, Cohn S, *et al*. Chromosomal localization of genes encoding guanine nucleotide-binding protein subunits in mouse and human. *Proc Natl Acad Sci USA*. 1988;85:7642–7646.

28. Begin-Heick N. Alpha-subunits of Gs and Gi in adipocyte plasma membranes of genetically diabetic (*db/db*) mice. *Am J Physiol*. 1992; 263:C121–129.

29. Eicher EM, Lee BK. Growth hormone receptor (Ghr) and hemoglobin alpha-chain pseudogene 3(Hba-ps3) map proximal to the myelocytomatosis oncogene (Myc) on mouse chromosome 15. *Mammalian Genome*. 1991;1:57–58.

30. Ng FM, Adamafio NA, Graystone JE. Effects of exogenous growth hormone on lipid metabolism in the isolated epididymal fat pad of growth hormone-deficient little mouse. *J Mol Endocrinol*. 1990;4: 43–49.

M. L. KLEBIG, J. E. WILKINSON, and R. P. WOYCHIK

Molecular Analysis of the Mouse Agouti Gene and the Role of Dominant Agouti-Locus Mutations in Obesity and Insulin Resistance

ABSTRACT

The lethal yellow ($A^y/-$) and viable yellow ($A^{vy}/-$) mouse agouti mutants have a predominantly yellow pelage and display a complex syndrome that includes obesity, hyperinsulinemia, and insulin resistance, hallmark features of some forms of type II diabetes in humans. A new dominant agouti allele, A^{iapy}, has recently been identified; like the A^{vy} allele, it is homozygous viable and confers obesity and yellow fur in heterozygotes. The agouti gene was cloned and characterized at the molecular level. The gene is expressed in the skin during hair growth and is predicted to encode a 131 amino acid protein that is likely to be a secreted factor. In both $A^y/-$ and $A^{iapy}/-$ mice, the obesity and other dominant pleiotropic effects are associated with an ectopic expression of agouti in many tissues in which the gene product is normally not produced. In A^y, a 170-kilobase deletion has occurred that causes an upstream promoter to drive the ectopic expression of the wild-type agouti coding exons. In A^{iapy}, the coding region of the gene is expressed from a cryptic promoter within the long terminal repeat of an intracisternal A-particle, which has integrated within the region just upstream of the first agouti coding exon. Transgenic mice ubiquitously expressing the cloned agouti gene under the influence of the beta-actin and phosphoglycerate kinase promoters display obesity, hyperinsulinemia, and yellow coat color. This

The submitted manuscript has been authored by a contractor of the United States government under Contract DE-AC05-84OR21400. Accordingly, the U.S. government retains a nonexclusive, royalty-free license to publish or reproduce the published form of this contribution, or allow others to do so, for U.S. government purposes.

120

demonstrates unequivocally that ectopic expression of agouti is responsible for the obese yellow syndrome.

The agouti (a) gene in mouse chromosome 2 normally functions in the production of the wild-type agouti coat color of mice. Several agouti-locus mutations, most notably lethal yellow (A^y) and viable yellow (A^{vy}), cause a number of dominant pleiotropic effects that include not only an abnormal yellow pelage, but also obesity, insulin resistance, and increased susceptibility to neoplasia (reviewed in 1–5). Because of this "obese yellow" syndrome, dominant agouti mutants have been used as experimental models in obesity and diabetes research (reviewed in 2–6). In addition to this syndrome in heterozygotes, embryos homozygous for A^y die prior to implantation in the uterus, whereas A^{vy}/A^{vy} mice are perfectly viable and display the pleiotropic disease phenotype (1). Based on our molecular analysis of the A^y allele (see below), the embryonic lethality is most likely unrelated to the agouti gene, but instead may be caused by the inactivation of another gene that is closely linked to agouti as a result of a 170-kilobase (kb) deletion.

The agouti protein normally signals hair-bulb melanocytes to switch from the production of eumelanin (black pigment) granules to phaeo-melanin (yellow pigment) granules (1). In contrast to most of the other coat color genes that have been identified, agouti exerts its effect on the melanocyte in a non–cell-autonomous manner. Skin transplantation experiments by Silvers and Russell (reviewed in 1) revealed that the agouti protein is a paracrine factor that functions from within the follicular environment, not from within the melanocyte.

Dominant Agouti Mutations (A^y and A^{vy}) and the Yellow Obese Syndrome

The many different phenotypic traits of the complex yellow obese syndrome have been defined chiefly from analyses of mice carrying the dominant agouti alleles A^y and A^{vy}. Next to yellow fur, obesity is the most obvious disorder of $A^y/-$ and $A^{vy}/-$ mice. Although these mice are hyperphagic, their obesity develops primarily as a result of their ability to more efficiently utilize their food for lipogenesis and other anabolic processes than normal mice (7, 8). Eventually, they develop body fat contents of 31% to 50% of total weight in females and 17% to

36% in males, compared with 6% to 28% in normal female and male littermates (9–13). The increase in adipose tissue is due primarily to hypertrophy rather than hyperplasia of adipocytes (14). The $A^y/-$ and $A^{vy}/-$ mice reach their peak weights between 8 and 17 months of age and may lose their excess weight in old age (15, 16).

In addition to the marked elevation in fat content, yellow mice exhibit milder increases in linear (skeletal) growth (11, 17, 18), muscle mass (18), and fat-free dry weight (12, 19). This anabolic effect occurs even in the absence of the anabolic action of endogenous testosterone in castrated males (19). In light of this effect and the more efficient weight gain of these mice, Wolff and colleagues (4) proposed that an unknown alteration of their metabolic dynamics has biased their metabolism toward anabolic reactions. These additional growth effects induced by the A^y and A^{vy} mutations have not been reported in any other rodent genetic or induced obesity disorder (20). In fact, the opposite effect on skeletal growth occurs in the *ob/ob* mouse (21).

Numerous physiological features of the obese yellow mice are consistent with a primary metabolic abnormality. These mice have a juvenile rate of lipogenesis about twice the normal rate; the juvenile rate does not decrease to the lower adult rate upon maturation, resulting in a lipogenic rate that is six times that in normal adults (10, 13). The elevated lipogenic rates can be overcome, and these mice lose weight in response to treatment with certain antiobesity compounds such as β agonists and some appetite suppressants (6, 22–24). The adipose tissue of A^{vy}/a mice has depressed basal lipolytic rates; A^{vy}/a adipocytes appear to have a defect in the signal transduction pathway for lipolysis at the level of the production or maintenance of intracellular cyclic AMP (cAMP) levels (reviewed in 6). The degree of obesity can be increased by feeding the mice high-fat diets (8, 9, 25), which likely exacerbates their abnormal lipid metabolism. Food restriction can eventually eliminate their excess body weight, but muscle mass appears to be lost preferentially to fat (18). Obese yellow mice have elevated blood lipids and ketones; fasting decreases blood ketones in obese yellow mice but increases them in normal mice (25, 26). In addition, $A^y/-$ mice, particularly females, have greater rates of cholesterogenesis in liver than controls (10), and females exhibit hypercholesterolemia (25). Adipose tissue transplantations between obese yellow A^y/a mice and normal *a/a* (C57BL/6J) littermate controls have shown that the transplanted adipocytes increase or decrease in size depending on the genotype of the host, not the genotype of the transplanted adipocyte (27). This finding suggests that the metabolic environment of A^y/a mice, not an intrinsic defect in adipocytes, may be responsible for their obesity (27).

In addition to their obesity, yellow obese $A^y/-$ and $A^{vy}/-$ mice exhibit insulin resistance of hepatic and peripheral tissues that is likely caused by post-insulin-receptor defects (28–30), pancreatic islet hypertrophy and hyperplasia (31–33), elevated plasma insulin and amylin (islet amyloid polypeptide) levels (26, 28–30, 34, 35, 36), and impaired glucose tolerance (8, 28–30). Moderate nonfasted hyperglycemia, particularly in males, has been observed in some but not all studies (25, 26, 28, 30, 33, 35). The development of overt hyperglycemia in these dominant agouti mutants appears to be dependent upon the development of both insulin resistance and beta-cell defects and on strain background, gender, and diet (6).

It is not yet known if obesity in these mice is primary or secondary to their insulin resistance. The development of increased hepatic lipogenic enzyme activity in A^{vy}/a mice correlated with the development of hyperinsulinemia (reviewed in 6). Between 5 and 6 weeks of age the plasma insulin levels of male A^{vy}/A mice rose to twice the normal level, but their weights were only slightly greater than normal (28). The development of hyperinsulinemia and obesity in A^{vy}/A females closely paralleled each other in this study (28). In another study, A^{vy}/A females developed insulin levels twice that of normal by 4 weeks of age, but they did not become significantly heavier than controls until 8 to 10 weeks of age (35). In addition, it appears that the hyperplasia of the pancreatic islets precedes changes in insulin and glucagon levels in the pancreas as well as the increase in body weight (6). These data argue that the primary defect in A^{vy}/A mice first leads to pancreatic abnormalities, then hyperinsulinemia, and, finally, obesity. Consistent with this, elevated insulin is known to stimulate lipogenesis, decrease lipolysis, and lead to obesity and insulin resistance (reviewed in 37, 38). When the obesity of A^{vy}/a mice peaked at 6 months of age, the insulin levels in males and females were 25 and 140 times greater than normal, respectively, in one study (26). These and other data indicate that adult female $A^{vy}/-$ mice are more hyperinsulinemic and have more severe islet hyperplasia and hypertrophy than males (reviewed in 6). Some compounds that improve insulin sensitivity were able to reduce plasma insulin and glucose levels of adult A^{vy}/a mice to normal without causing weight loss (26, reviewed in 6). This result suggests that the elevated insulin and insulin resistance of these mice are not required to maintain their obesity once it is established (6).

The propensity of $A^y/-$ and $A^{vy}/-$ mice to become obese and develop many of the dominant pleiotropic effects is apparently not mediated entirely by pituitary, adrenocortical, or thyroid hormones, since neither hypophysectomy (11, 30, 39), adrenalectomy (12, 36), nor genetic deficiency of growth hormone or thyrotrophin (40) is able to prevent these mice from developing some degree of obesity relative to wild-type littermate controls. However, pituitary and adrenal hormones are apparently necessary for the complete expression of the obese yellow syndrome. An intact pituitary is required to develop hyperinsulinemia in A^{vy}/A mice (30) and an increased susceptibility to hepatomas in A^y/A mice (39). Adrenalectomy decreased blood glucose levels to normal in A^{vy}/a mice (36) and is reported to prevent the development of pancreatic islet hypertrophy of $A^y/-$ mice (32). The importance of adrenal hormones in the development of the syndrome is also controversial. Plasma corticosterone levels were found to be normal or slightly less than normal in A^y/a and A^{vy}/a mice in one study (41) but elevated in A^{vy}/a mice in another study (36). In addition, adrenalectomy is reported to prevent the excessive weight gain (but not the development of larger fat pads) of A^{vy}/a mice relative to littermates in the short term (32 days) (36), but not in A^y/a mice in the long term (5–7 months) (12).

Although the reported results from parabiosis experiments with obese yellow mice have been contradictory (42, unpublished data in 32), the best controlled set of published experiments indicate that surgically uniting A^y/a and a/a littermates to each other did not make the a/a partner obese, nor did it make the A^y/a partner lean (43). In addition to confirming that circulating hormones are not directly involved in the development of obesity, these results indicate that a functional agouti protein is not shared in the circulation between the parabiotic partners. Taken together, the above observations suggest that the underlying cause of the obese yellow syndrome is an altered metabolic environment that is not mediated by hormones or other low-molecular-weight, secreted molecules that make it into general circulation.

There is indirect evidence that at least some aspects of the obese yellow phenotype may be caused by a hypothalamic defect. The hypothalamus is thought to contain a "central controller" that maintains body weight and body-fat content at a predetermined level or "set point" by modulating food intake or energy expenditure (44). The responses of obese yellow mice to different schedules of food reinforcement, fasting, and refeeding suggest that they have normal satiety mechanisms but a stronger motivation than normal to consume food (2). Also, it appears that alterations in the efficiency of food utilization, rather than in thermogenesis, are primarily involved in the changes in body weight observed in A^{vy}/a mice in response to restricted food intake (reviewed in 6). Both the excessive motivation to eat and the increased efficiency in utilizing food are consistent with a possible hypothalamic defect that results in an abnormally high set point for body weight in the yellow obese mice (2, 44, 45). Moreover, since the hypothalamus controls the hormone secretions of the pituitary and the glands under the control of the pituitary, the observations on hypophysectomized and adrenalectomized obese yellow mice suggest that hypothalamic defects in these mice could lead to their hyperinsulinemia, hyperglycemia, and increased susceptibility to tumors.

No direct evidence of anatomical or biochemical lesions of the hypothalamus has been found in obese yellow mice (2). However, Bray and colleagues (46) have found that the pituitaries of obese yellow A^{vy}/a mice have increased levels of desacetyl-melanocyte stimulating hormone (d-MSH) but lower-than-normal levels of alpha-MSH (α-MSH), which primarily stimulates eumelanin synthesis by the melanocyte. Since MSH is processed from pro-opiomelanocortin (POMC) in the hypothalamus as well as the pituitary (47), the hypothalamus may also produce elevated levels of d-MSH. Because administration of d-MSH increases food intake, body weight, and serum corticosteroid levels to a greater extent than α-MSH, it is possible that interference in the acetylation of MSH and, as a consequence, elevation of d-MSH could be involved in the hyperphagia and faster weight gain of yellow obese mice (48).

Cloning the Agouti Gene

Despite the extensive pathophysiological studies that have been conducted on $A^y/-$ and $A^{vy}/-$ mice over the past several decades, the primary molecular lesion associated with these mutations was only recently revealed as a result of the cloning of the agouti gene (49–52). In contrast to strict positional-cloning approaches that had been unsuccessful in identifying the agouti gene (53–57), the first molecular access to the agouti locus was accomplished with the use of a radiation-induced inversion mutation of agouti (an extreme nonagouti, null allele) called Is1Gso (49). Is1Gso contains an intrachromosomal inversion between the limb deformity (*ld*) and agouti loci (Fig. 1; 49), loci that are normally separated by 22 centimorgans (cM) on mouse chromosome 2. Utilizing a DNA probe that had been generated from an insertional mutation at the *ld* locus (58), Woychik and colleagues (49) were able to clone DNA associated with the Is1Gso inversion, which resulted in a molecular "jump" 22 cM directly into the agouti locus (49, 50). They were then able to use DNA probes from the agouti locus and the inversion breakpoint to ultimately identify the agouti gene (51).

Molecular Characteristics of the Agouti Gene

Woychik and colleagues (51) initially characterized the wild-type agouti gene from *A/A* mice. In the *A* allele, the gene is about 20 kb in length and is comprised of four exons, the last three of which encode the open reading frame (Fig. 2; 51). The coding region of the agouti gene is disrupted by the Is1Gso mutation and contains an intragenic deletion in the extreme nonagouti (null) allele, a^{5MNU} (Fig. 2; 51). The agouti gene gives rise to a 0.8-kb mRNA that is normally expressed in neonatal skin in a temporal manner that is consistent with its role in the production of the normal agouti pigmentation pattern (Fig. 3; 51). Molecular analysis of cDNA clones derived from neonatal skin libraries from *A/A* mice revealed that the agouti mRNA has the potential to give rise to a 131 amino acid protein (Fig. 4; 51). The predicted agouti protein contains a consensus signal peptide and a number of noteworthy features that include a highly basic region within the middle of the protein, as well as a cysteine-rich region near the carboxy terminus (Fig. 4; 51). GenBank analysis of the agouti protein sequence failed to reveal any significant homology with other previously characterized proteins. The fact that the agouti protein contains a consensus signal peptide is consistent with a scenario, originally suggested by the results of skin transplantation experiments (1), in which the agouti protein is secreted from cells in the follicular environment of the melanocyte and functions to control hair pigmentation through some form of direct or indirect intercellular communication with the melanocyte.

More recently, molecular analysis of the nonagouti black (*a*), black-

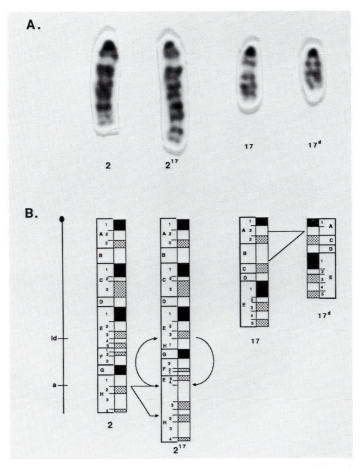

Figure 1. Structure of the rearranged chromosomes 2 and 17 in the radiation-induced mutant Is1Gso. (A) Chromosomes from Giemsa-banded mitotic metaphase karyotypes. From left to right, normal chromosome 2, rearranged chromosome 2 (designated 2^{17}), normal chromosome 17, and deleted chromosome 17 (designated 17^d). (B) G-banding diagrams illustrating the proposed structure for the radiation-induced chromosomal rearrangement involving chromosomes 2 and 17 (49). Broken, curved arrows show the position of the inverted 2E4-2H2 section of chromosome 2. Solid linear arrows between chromosomes 2 and 2^{17} show the position of the interstitial segment of chromosome 17 that has integrated into the distal portion of chromosome 2, immediately adjacent and distal to the 2E4-2H2 inversion. The probable positions of the *a* and *ld* loci relative to the banded map are shown to the left of the diagram for the normal chromosome 2.

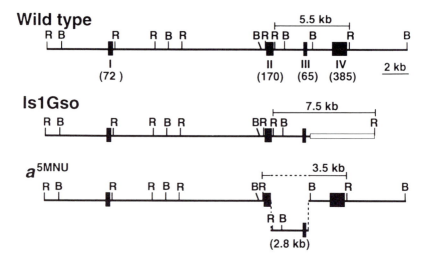

Figure 2.   Intron/exon structure of the wild-type locus and two extreme non-agouti mutations. Schematic representation of the genomic structure of the agouti gene in DNA from wild-type, Is1Gso, and a^{5MNU} mice. The four exons are depicted as solid boxes, and the introns and flanking sequences are shown as a solid line. The first exon, which is 72 bp long in the cDNA clone, is 8–10 bp longer at its 5′ end based on RNase protection experiments (data not shown). The 3′ junction of the last exon corresponds to the 3′ end of the cDNA clone, immediately upstream from the poly(A) tract. The precise location of each intron/exon junction was ascertained by identifying where genomic DNA sequences diverged from the cDNA sequence. At each splice junction, the genomic DNA sequence matched the canonical sequence for 5′ splice donor and 3′ splice acceptor sites. The open box in the Is1Gso schematic represents genomic DNA from the *ld* gene in the opposite transcriptional orientation relative to agouti. The 2.8 kb intragenic deletion in the a^{5MNU} mutation is depicted by a horizontal dashed line above the mutant locus, with the deleted region shown below the mutant locus.

and-tan (*a^t*), and white-bellied agouti (*A^w*) alleles (refer to references 1 and 5 for a description of these alleles) revealed that the agouti gene can give rise to at least two different classes of mRNA, referred to as form I and form II transcripts (Fig. 5; 59). Form I transcripts are those that arise from the *A* allele and correspond to the 0.8-kb agouti mRNA described above. Form II transcripts are also 0.8 kb in length, but they contain an alternative upstream untranslated region (59) that is encoded by exons that map over 100 kb upstream of the rest of the gene

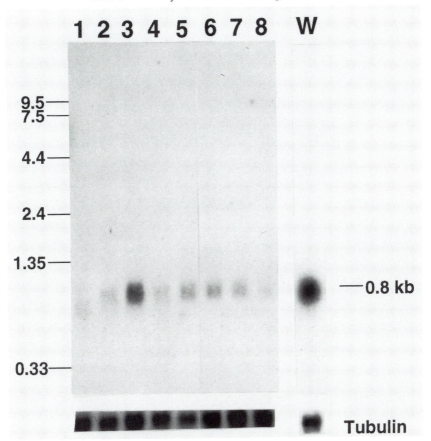

Figure 3. Northern blot analysis of wild-type (*A/A*) neonatal skin. The full-length cDNA clone (Fig. 4) was ^{32}P-labeled and hybridized to poly(A)$^+$ RNA (2.5 µg per lane) from skin of day 1 through day 8 wild-type neonates (1–8). The cDNA was also hybridized to RNA from skin of day 6 *W/W^v* neonates (W), which are devoid of hair-bulb melanocytes, to indicate that the agouti gene is expressed in cells other than melanocytes. RNA molecular weight standards are shown on the left in kb. The filter was subsequently hybridized with a tubulin probe as a control to analyze the quantity and quality of the RNA in each lane.

Reproduced with permission from reference 51.

(Fig. 5; 59, 60). Both form I and form II agouti transcripts have the same protein coding potential (59). The form II transcripts were not identified initially (51) because they are not expressed from the *A* allele. In fact, Bultman *et al.* (59) have proposed that *A* is actually not the wild-type

TTCAAGGACAGGAAAGACATTCTGGCCTGGCTTCCCTTAGGGGAGCTGATGCGGAATAGAGTC   63

ACTTGTGCTGCTTCTCAGG ATG GAT GTC ACC CGC CTA CTC CTG GCC ACC CTA   115
                    Met Asp Val Thr Arg Leu Leu Leu Ala Thr Leu   11

GTG AGC TTC CTG TGC TTC TTC ACC GTC CAC AGC CAC CTG GCA CTC GAG   163
Val Ser Phe Leu Cys Phe Phe Thr Val His Ser His Leu Ala Leu Glu   27

    PO₄   PO₄   *
GAG ACG CTT GGA GAT GAC AGG AGT CTG CGG AGT AAC TCC TCC ATG AAC   211
Glu Thr Leu Gly Asp Asp Arg Ser Leu Arg Ser Asn Ser Ser Met Asn   43

                                           PO₄
TCG CTG GAT TTC TCC TCT GTT TCT ATC GTG GCA CTG AAC AAG AAA TCC   259
Ser Leu Asp Phe Ser Ser Val Ser Ile Val Ala Leu Asn Lys Lys Ser   59

       PO₄   PO₄ PO₄
AAG AAG ATC AGC AGA AAA GAA GCC CAG AAG CGG AAG AGG TCT TCC AAG   307
Lys Lys Ile Ser Arg Lys Glu Ala Gln Lys Arg Lys Arg Ser Ser Lys   75

       PO₄
AAA AAG GCT TCG ATG AAG AAG GTG GCA AGG CCC CCG CCA CCT TCG CCC   355
Lys Lys Ala Ser Met Lys Lys Val Ala Arg Pro Pro Pro Pro Ser Pro   91

                     PO₄
TGC GTG GCC ACC CGC GAC AGC TGC AAG CCA CCC GCA CCC GCC TGC TGC   403
Cys Val Ala Thr Arg Asp Ser Cys Lys Pro Pro Ala Pro Ala Cys Cys   107

                                             PO₄
GAC CCG TGC GCC TCC TGC CAG TGC CGT TTC TTC GGC AGC GCC TGC ACC   451
Asp Pro Cys Ala Ser Cys Gln Cys Arg Phe Phe Gly Ser Ala Cys Thr   123

TGT CGA GTA CTC AAC CCC AAC TGC TGA CGCAGCTTCTTCGCTGCGCGCGCAGCT   505
Cys Arg Val Leu Asn Pro Asn Cys End   131

TCGGGAACGGGTGATTGGGCGGGGCTTCAGGGTCCCGCGCTTCTAGGCTGAGGGGCGGGTCTC   568

TGTGGGTGGGGCTTGTGGGTGGGCGTGGTCAGTGGTTGTGACTTGTGGGCGCTTTCAAAAAAC   631

CGGTTTTCTAGGAAACCTAGTGGAAGCTAAAATCAGAATACAATAATATTTTTAGGCTGCC(A)   692

Figure 4. Nucleotide and predicted amino acid sequence of agouti cDNA. The putative signal peptide sequence is underscored with a double line and the polyadenylation signal with a single line. The boxed region represents a highly basic domain that has the potential to be phosphorylated at a number of sites designated by PO₄. An asterisk denotes a potential N-linked glycosylation site, and cysteine residues are highlighted by solid circles. Arrowheads delimit the boundaries of the four individual exons.

Reproduced with permission from reference 51.

agouti allele and that it contains a mutation that blocks the expression of form II transcripts. Instead, these investigators (59) favor the possibility, proposed previously (1), that A^w, which produces both form I and form II transcripts, is actually the wild-type allele at agouti.

Molecular Analysis of the Lethal Yellow (A^y) Mutation

Northern blot analysis revealed that the wild-type agouti gene is expressed in the skin during hair growth and is not expressed in a variety of adult tissues (Fig. 6; 51). In striking contrast to wild-type, analysis of agouti expression in $A^y/-$ mice revealed that agouti mRNA is expressed in a number of adult tissues as well as neonatal skin (Fig. 6; 51). Moreover, the size of the mRNA produced from the A^y allele is about 1.1 kb, which is significantly larger than that observed for the wild-type sized 0.8-kb mRNA (51).

The nature of the A^y mutation was initially explored by isolating and characterizing cDNA clones of the size-altered A^y-specific 1.1-kb agouti transcript (51, 61). This analysis revealed that the entire coding portion of the agouti gene (exons 2–4) is intact in A^y, whereas the untranslated first exon is missing and replaced by novel sequence (Fig. 7; 51, 61). Additional experiments ultimately revealed that this novel sequence at the upstream end of the A^y-specific agouti mRNA actually corresponds to the upstream untranslated region of a gene called *Raly* (Fig. 7; 61), which normally maps 280-kb proximal to agouti on mouse chromosome 2 (Fig. 8; 60). *Raly* is expressed in a ubiquitous manner and has the potential to encode a novel member of the heterogeneous ribonuclear-protein gene family (61). Further analysis revealed that the A^y allele contains a 170-kb deletion that removes all but the first noncoding exon of *Raly* (Fig. 8; 60). Consistent with the data, Michaud and colleagues (60) proposed that the ubiquitous A^y-specific 1.1-kb mRNA's arise by a mechanism that involves transcription from the *Raly* promoter and splicing of the *Raly* upstream noncoding region to the agouti coding exons (Fig. 9).

Based on their analysis of the structure of the A^y allele, Michaud *et al.* (60) proposed that the deletion of *Raly* is responsible for the recessive embryonic lethality of the A^y mutation and that the ectopic and ubiquitous expression of the agouti gene, directed by the *Raly* promoter, is the basis for the dominant obese yellow syndrome exhibited by $A^y/-$ mice.

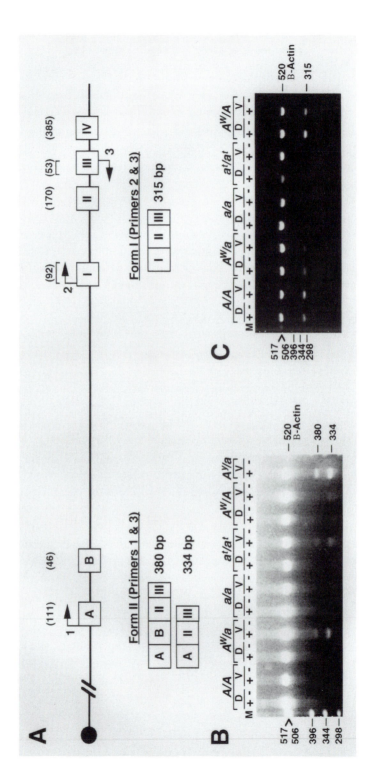

Molecular Analysis of A^{iapy}, a New Dominant Agouti Allele Similar to the Viable Yellow Allele

Animals carrying the A^{vy} allele display the same dominant syndrome as $A^y/-$ mice, but as the name implies, homozygotes are viable. Initial molecular analysis of A^{iapy}, a new dominant agouti allele that confers a phenotype almost identical to A^{vy}, revealed that, like in $A^y/-$ mice, the agouti mRNA is ectopically overexpressed in what appears to be a ubiquitous manner in $A^{iapy}/-$ mice (Fig. 10; 62). Further analysis revealed that, in the case of A^{iapy}, an intracisternal A-particle (IAP) integrated just upstream of the first agouti coding exon (Fig. 11A; 62). A cryptic promoter within the long terminal repeat (LTR) of the IAP appears to be responsible for the ectopic expression of the agouti tran-

---

Figure 5. Identification of two forms of agouti transcripts by RT-PCR. (A) A schematic map of the agouti gene showing the approximate locations of exons (boxes labeled A, B, I, II, III, and IV) and oligonucleotide primers (arrows labeled 1, 2, and 3) used in the PCR analysis. The map is shown 5' to 3' (left to right), and the position of the chromosome 2 centromere is indicated to the left. The size of each exon or portion of exon amplified with the indicated primers is given in bp enclosed in parentheses above. Each of the boxes labeled A and B may consist of one or more exons. The RT-PCR products detected are depicted schematically below the map. Primers 1 and 3 amplify 380-bp and 334-bp portions of form II transcripts that consist of the exons indicated, whereas primers 2 and 3 amplify a 315-bp segment of the form I transcript comprised of the indicated exons. (B and C) RT-PCR products amplified with primers 1 and 3 (B) or primers 2 and 3 (C) from total RNA treated with ($+$) or without ($-$) reverse transcriptase. All of the RNA samples were derived from the dorsal (D) or ventral (V) skin of 4- to 5-day-old neonatal mice of the following genotypes and strains: A/A (C3H$_f$/R1), A^w/a (A^{W-42J} stock), a/a (C57BL), a^t/a^t (original), A^w/A (C3H × 101), and A^y/a. Shown are photographs of RT-PCR products size-fractionated in agarose gels and stained with ethidium bromide. Numbers to the left of each panel indicate the sizes in bp of the 1 kb ladder molecular weight marker (lane M); numbers to the right of the panels indicate the sizes of the RT-PCR products. The 520-bp fragment was amplified using oligonucleotide primers specific for the β-actin mRNA and serves as a positive control. Although the 380-bp fragment of the form II transcript is not readily visible in the ventral skin of A^w/A (panel B), it and the other agouti-specific fragments hybridized to an agouti cDNA probe after the gel was Southern blotted to a nylon membrane (data not shown).

Reproduced with permission from reference 59.

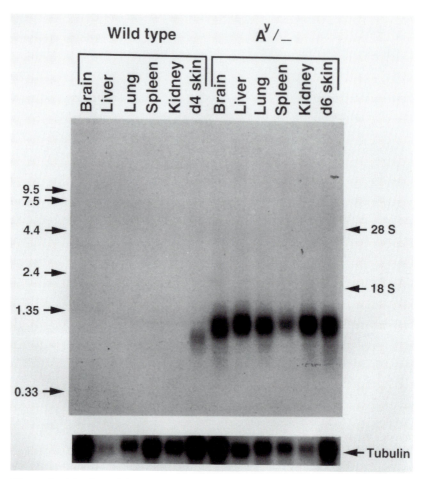

Figure 6. Northern blot analysis of adult tissues from wild-type and lethal-yellow heterozygotes. The full-length cDNA clone (Fig. 4) was ^{32}P-labeled and hybridized to poly(A)+ RNA (2.5 µg per lane) from adult tissues or neonatal skin of wild-type or $A^y/-$ mutant animals. RNA molecular weight standards are shown on the left in kb, and the positions of the 28S and 18S rRNA subunits are indicated on the right. The filter was subsequently hybridized with a tubulin probe as a control to analyze the quantity and quality of the RNA in each lane. $A^y/-$, lethal yellow heterozygotes with genotypes of A^y/a and A^y/a^e, were used in this analysis; d4 skin-day 4 postnatal skin; d6 skin-day 6 postnatal skin.

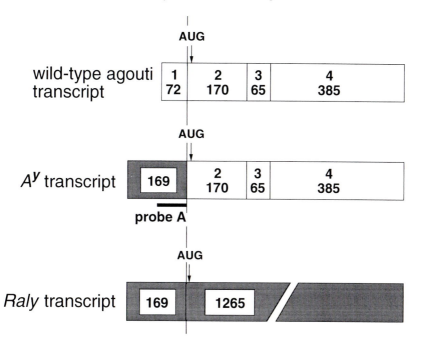

Figure 7. The A^y allele encodes a *Raly*/agouti fusion transcript. The wild-type agouti transcript is composed of a sequence derived from four exons (numbered 1–4, with their respective sizes indicated below). The A^y transcript is identical to the wild-type agouti transcript for the sequence derived from the second, third, and fourth exons (coding region), but the noncoding first exon of agouti has been removed and replaced by the noncoding first exon of *Raly* (represented by the shaded region, 169 bases in length). Probe A corresponds to a sequence that was initially identified as being unique to the 5′ end of the A^y transcript and subsequently used to isolate wild-type *Raly* cDNA and genomic clones. The vertical line indicates that the replacement of the first agouti exon with the first *Raly* exon in the A^y transcript occurs precisely at an exon-intron splice junction in both wild-type genes. The proposed sites for translation initiation in all three transcripts are indicated by AUGs.

Reproduced with permission from reference 61.

script (Fig. 11; 62). Therefore, although the transcript from the A^{iapy} allele is of normal size (0.8 kb), it actually contains a unique 5′ end upstream from the first agouti coding exon. Even with the structural changes, the A^{iapy} mRNA has the potential to encode a wild-type agouti protein (62).

Like A^{vy}, the A^{iapy} allele exhibits a variability in the pigmentation of the fur that ranges from a totally yellow pelage to various degrees of

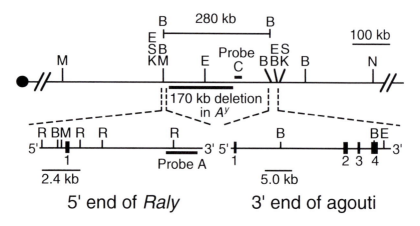

Figure 8.　Long-range restriction map of the mouse chromosome 2 region containing the *Raly* and agouti loci in the *A* and *A^y* alleles. Shown below the restriction map are expanded views of the 5′ end of the *Raly* gene (the solid box denotes the noncoding first exon) and the 3′ end of the agouti gene (numbered solid boxes indicate exons). Separate scale bars are shown for the long-range restriction map and for each of the expanded regions. The expanded agouti region is shown to scale, except for the four exons, which are enlarged for clarity. The 2.4-kb *Eco*RI (R) fragment shown at the 5′ end of *Raly* contains a CpG island with one or more of each of the following restriction enzyme recognition sites: *Eag*I (E), *Sma*I (S), *Ksp*I (K), *Bss*HII (B), and *Mlu*I (M). All of these enzyme sites are indicated on the long-range map, but only the *Bss*HII and *Mlu*I sites are shown in the expanded region because of space considerations. The probes used to detect the *A^y* deletion breakpoints (Probes A and C) are also shown. The 111-bp probe C is shown larger than scale. Only restriction enzyme sites that are cut in genomic DNA are included on the map. N-*Not*I.

mottling (yellow fur mixed with agouti-like hair) to a coat referred to as "pseudoagouti" that closely resembles wild-type agouti (1, 4, 62, 63). Interestingly, Michaud and coworkers (62) found that the level of ectopic agouti expression is closely correlated with the amount of yellow pigmentation in the coats of $A^{iapy}/-$ mice. Solid yellow mice exhibit the highest levels, pseudoagouti mice have very low levels, and mottled-yellows display intermediate levels of expression (Fig. 12). Pseudoagouti $A^{vy}/-$ mice do not become fat and insulin resistant (16, 34, 63), whereas $A^{vy}/-$ mice with only slightly increased amounts of yellow pigmentation do develop the disorder (63). Pseudoagouti $A^{iapy}/-$ mice also have normal body weights; their ability to maintain glu-

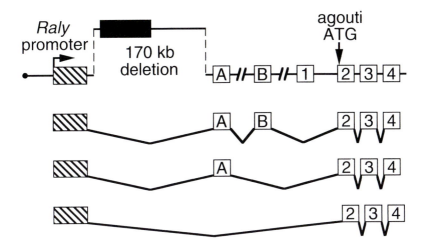

Figure 9. A model for the production of chimeric *Raly*/agouti transcripts from the A^y allele. Because of the 170-kb deletion in the A^y allele, transcriptional initiation at the *Raly* promoter is proposed to result in the transcription of the noncoding first exon of *Raly* (cross-hatched box), the intergenic sequence, and the downstream agouti gene. The processing of this novel primary transcript could result in the joining of the splice donor of the first *Raly* exon to the downstream acceptor sites of agouti. The result would be A^y transcripts consisting of the noncoding first exon of *Raly* and the three coding exons of the agouti gene (exons 2–4), with alternative splicing of agouti exons A and B, as previously described (61).

Reproduced with permission from reference 60.

cose homeostasis and their susceptibility to tumors remain to be thoroughly investigated. The level of ectopic agouti expression in $A^{iapy}/-$ mice was also found to be inversely correlated with the methylation status of the IAP 5′ LTR (62).

Ectopic Expression of Agouti Causes Obesity

The molecular analysis of the A^y and A^{iapy} alleles strongly implicated the ectopic expression of the normal agouti gene as being responsible for the obesity and other dominant pleiotropic effects exhibited by mice carrying these alleles. However, the nature of the structural changes discovered in the mRNA and genomic sequences in each of these mutations made it impossible to unequivocally determine that the ectopic expression of agouti is solely responsible for the pleiotropic effects.

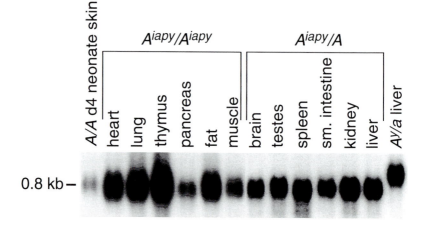

Figure 10. Ectopic overexpression of the agouti mRNA in a variety of adult tissues of mice carrying a new dominant agouti allele, A^{iapy}. A wild-type agouti cDNA clone was ^{32}P-labeled and hybridized to Northern blots containing poly(A)+ RNA ($\approx$2.5 µg per lane, except for pancreas and muscle which are underloaded) from a variety of adult A^{iapy}/A^{iapy} and A^{iapy}/A tissues, and from wild-type agouti (*A/A* day 4 neonate skin) and lethal yellow (A^y/a adult liver) controls. The size of the wild-type transcript is shown on the left in kilobases.
Reproduced with permission from references 61 and 62.

Therefore, as a direct test of the role of ectopic expression of agouti in obesity, we generated transgenic mice (64) in which a wild-type agouti cDNA was expressed under the influence of two different gene promoters that normally function in a ubiquitous manner, human beta-actin (BA) (65, 66) and mouse phosphoglycerate kinase (PGK) (67–69) (Fig. 13).

With each construct (BAPa and PGKPa), several transgenic lines were prepared, and the expression of the agouti transgene in adult mice from several of these lines was investigated by Northern-blot analysis (Fig. 14; 64). This analysis identified BAPa and PGKPa lines (*e.g.*, B20 and P8 in Fig. 14) in which the agouti transgene was expressed at levels comparable to the level of agouti expression in A^y/A mice in many tissues (64). In skeletal muscle, however, the BAPa lines expressed agouti at extremely high levels. In one BAPa line (B52 in Fig. 14), no expression was detectable in liver and very low levels of expression were found in some of the other tissues analyzed (*e.g.*, small intestine, kidneys, salivary gland), while levels of mRNA comparable to those in

A^y/A mice were detected in the remaining tissues. Moreover, after preparing F1 hybrids of the transgenics with C57BL/6J (the transgenics were prepared in the albino FVB/N inbred line), we determined that ectopic expression of the agouti transgene caused the same yellow pigmentation patterns observed in animals carrying the A^y, A^{vy}, and A^{iapy} alleles (64). The presence of the yellow pigmentation clearly indicated that the agouti transcripts derived from the transgenes in these animals were capable of giving rise to a functional agouti protein.

Sequential analysis of the weights of BAPa20 transgenic animals revealed that they become markedly obese as compared to their nontransgenic littermates (Fig. 15; 64). This is particularly true for transgenic females, which are about 1.5 times heavier than their nontransgenic controls by 4 to 5 months of age (Fig. 15). Additionally, analysis of plasma insulin and glucose values from several animals in the BAPa20 transgenic line revealed that the average insulin/glucose ratio obtained for the transgenic mice was about twice that of the nontransgenic controls (Fig. 16; 64). These results indicate that the agouti transgenics must produce higher levels of insulin to remain normoglycemic (64).

The results from the transgenic experiments have allowed us to unequivocally establish that ectopic expression of the agouti gene is responsible not only for the yellow fur, but also for the obesity and insulin resistance. Experiments are currently under way to determine whether the transgenics, like the $A^y/-$ and $A^{vy}/-$ mutants, also have an increased susceptibility to the development of spontaneous and induced tumors (4).

Models for Agouti Function in Pigmentation and Obesity

Agouti and the POMC-derived peptide α-MSH have opposing effects on pigmentation. Injection of α-MSH into A/a, $A^y/-$, and $A^{vy}/-$ mice, after hair-plucking or treating skin explants from $A^y/-$ mice with α-MSH in vitro, causes melanocytes that are producing phaeomelanin to switch to eumelanin production (70–73). Alpha-MSH exerts this effect by binding to the melanocyte stimulating hormone receptor (MSH-R) on the surface of the melanocyte (74). The MSH-R is encoded by the extension (e) locus (75) and is a member of a melanocortin subfamily of the seven-transmembrane-domain G-protein-linked receptor family (74). Alpha-MSH binding stimulates adenylate cyclase activity, thereby

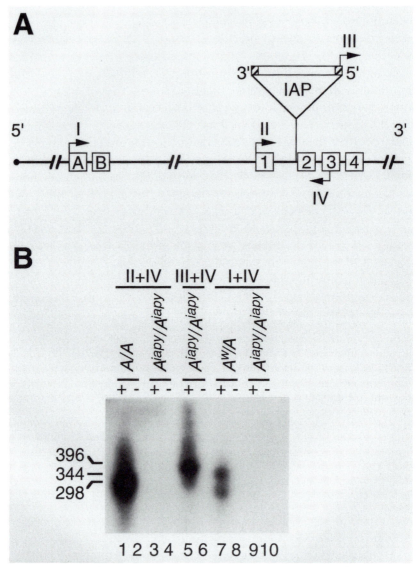

Figure 11. RT-PCR analysis reveals that transcription of agouti from the A^{iapy} allele initiates from the inserted IAP genome. (A) RT-PCR strategy used to determine the location of initiation of agouti transcription from the A^{iapy} allele. Shown is the structure of the wild-type agouti gene as it was originally described (exons 1–4; 51) and the recently identified (59, 61) additional 5′ noncoding exons A and B (the single box A actually represents two agouti exons;

(*continued*)

elevating intracellular cAMP and activating a signal transduction pathway that shifts pigment production from phaeomelanin to eumelanin (73–76).

A model for agouti protein function has been proposed in which it interferes with the binding of α-MSH to its receptor, thereby preventing the elevation of intracellular cAMP and eumelanin production (51, 73, 76–78). This model is based on the coat color phenotypes of mice that carry loss- or gain-of-function mutations of the MSH-R gene along with various agouti-locus alleles (51, 75–78). In addition, it accounts for the effects of in vivo treatment with α-MSH and dibutyryl cAMP on the coat colors of mice of different agouti-locus genotypes, as well as the effects of in vitro treatment with these agents on melanogenesis in skin explants derived from these mice (51, 75–78). In this proposed

---

60). Also shown is the IAP, its location of insertion into the agouti gene, and the 5' to 3' transcriptional orientation of agouti and the IAP. Primers I or II were each used in conjunction with primer IV to detect the normal form II or form I agouti transcripts, respectively (see Fig. 5). Primer III was used in conjunction with primer IV to detect any transcripts initiating from the IAP 5' LTR. (B) RT-PCR assay for determining the location of initiation of agouti transcription from the A^{iapy} allele. Total RNA (10 μg) from adult A^{iapy}/A^{iapy} thymus, 4-day-old A/A dorsal neonate skin (control for form I transcript), and 5-day-old A^w/A ventral neonate skin (control for form II transcripts), were reverse transcribed and subjected to PCR with different combinations of primers as indicated. The PCR products were electrophoresed through a 3% agarose gel, blotted, and hybridized with a ^{32}P-labeled agouti cDNA probe that consists primarily of the three coding exons (2–4). Each lane is numbered below, and above is shown whether reverse transcriptase was (+) or was not (−) included in the RT reaction (control for contaminating genomic DNA), the genotype of the RNA sample, and the primers used in the PCR reaction. Oligonucleotide primers from the mouse β-actin gene were used as an internal control for each PCR reaction. A β-actin fragment of the expected size was observed in all five RT+ reactions (lanes 1, 3, 5, 7, and 9) by ethidium bromide staining of the DNA in the agarose gel prior to transfer (data not shown). Primer combinations II and IV (lane 1), and I and IV (lane 7) amplified the expected sized fragments from form I and form II agouti transcripts, respectively. Two fragments are expected in lane 7 because exon B is alternately processed in ventral-specific transcripts of A^w mice (Fig. 5; 59). Only primers III and IV amplified the expected sized fragment from the A^{iapy} RT template (lane 5). DNA molecular size standards are shown at left in bp.

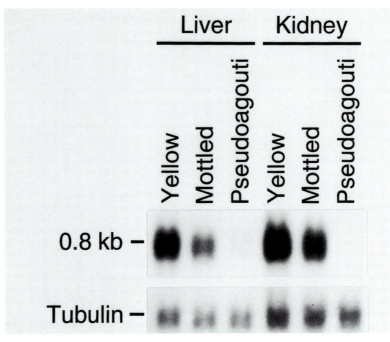

Figure 12. Northern blot analysis of agouti locus expression in adult liver and kidney from A^{iapy}/a mice with either a solid yellow, moderately mottled (yellow plus pseudoagouti mix), or completely pseudoagouti coat color. The wild-type agouti cDNA clone was ^{32}P-labeled and hybridized to poly(A)+ RNA ($\approx$2.5 µg per lane) from the kidney and liver of A^{iapy} mice exhibiting the two extremes (yellow and pseudoagouti) and an intermediate (mottled) in the spectrum of coat color phenotypes. The filter was also hybridized with a chicken tubulin probe to control for the quantity and quality of RNA in each lane. On a longer exposure of the filter to X-ray film, a signal was visible in the pseudoagouti liver lane (62).

Reproduced with permission from reference 62.

mechanism, the agouti protein antagonizes the binding of α-MSH to its receptor by either competing for the hormone-binding site of the receptor or by binding to α-MSH directly (51, 78).

An alternative model has also been proposed in which the agouti protein is a ligand for its own receptor in the melanocyte and activates a pathway that opposes the effects of α-MSH binding downstream of the MSH-R (79). However, this model does not appear to adequately explain the observed effects of α-MSH treatment and dominant MSH-

R mutations on pigment production in the presence of excess agouti protein (see discussion in 75, 78).

Our demonstration that ectopic expression of agouti is responsible for the dominant obese yellow syndrome suggests that the agouti protein may function as an activator or repressor ligand on cells other than melanocytes. In keeping with the two proposed mechanisms for agouti function in hair-bulb melanocytes, the agouti protein would exert its effect on other cells by antagonizing a ligand-receptor interaction(s) according to the first model, or by binding to its own receptor in the second model. If the first model proves to be the case, a receptor other than the MSH-R must be involved in non-melanocyte cells because the syndrome is not observed in *e/e* mice (80), which lack a functional MSH-R (75). Perhaps other melanocortin receptors are targets for antagonism by the agouti protein. These include the adrenocorticotrophic hormone (ACTH) receptor (74), as well as the recently identified melanocortin-3 (MC3) and melanocortin-4 (MC4) receptors that are expressed predominantly in the brain and placenta (81, 82). The ACTH, MC3, and MC4 receptors all elicit increased intracellular cAMP levels upon stimulation by certain POMC-derived peptides.

With the exception of low levels of expression of the MC3 receptor in the pancreas, none of the other melanocortin receptors discovered so far is reported to be expressed in those tissues in which metabolic dysfunctions are directly involved in developing obesity, insulin resistance, and hyperinsulinemia (*e.g.,* adipose tissue, skeletal muscle, liver, or pancreas; 74, 81, 82). Therefore, if no other melanocortin receptors are found in these tissues and if the agouti protein actually functions by specifically antagonizing melanocortin receptor-ligand interactions, then the defects in lipid metabolism and maintenance of glucose homeostasis observed in obese yellow mice would have to be secondary responses of agouti action. Under this scenario, the MC3 and MC4 receptors, which are expressed in the hypothalamus and other areas of the brain, would be likely candidates for ligand-receptor antagonism by agouti in these mice. It is possible, for example, that these receptors may have important roles in the hypothalamic control of weight and body fat.

Alternatively, if the hypothesis that the agouti protein has its own receptor in melanocytes proves to be true, then the dominant obese yellow syndrome would likely be mediated by the binding of the agouti protein to its own receptor in other cell types. For example, the inter-

A (BAPa)

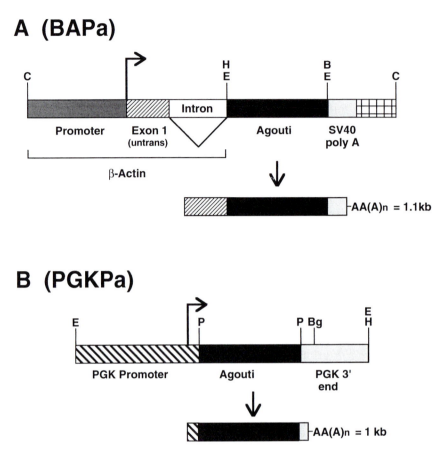

Figure 13. Transgene constructs containing the agouti cDNA under the transcriptional control of the promoters of the ubiquitously expressed genes β-actin and phosphoglycerate kinase 1 (PGK). (A) The 5.3 kb BAPa construct consists of a 700 bp *HindIII-BamHI* fragment that contains the agouti cDNA (black box labeled Agouti), under the control of the human β-actin promoter and enhancer contained within the 4.2 kb *ClaI-HindIII* fragment at the 5' end of the construct (bracketed and labeled β-actin). Restriction enzyme sites are abbreviated as follows: C = *ClaI*; H = *HindIII*; E = *EcoRI*; B = *BamHI*. The cDNA fragment is a 667 bp portion of the agouti cDNA shown in Figure 4 that contains the entire coding region but not the endogenous polyadenylation signal. The *HindIII-BamHI* agouti cDNA fragment was cloned into a modified form of the pHβ APr.2 expression vector (64, 65) to generate the BAPa construct. The dark gray box represents the 3.3 kb fragment containing the promoter and transcriptional control elements from the 5' flanking region of the β-actin gene

(*continued*)

action of ectopic agouti protein with its own receptor in the hypothalamus and/or other areas of the brain may somehow elevate the set point for body weight or fat content. Perhaps an activated agouti receptor in the brain initiates a signal that inhibits the acetylation of d-MSH to α-MSH and, thereby, results in the observed elevation of d-MSH in A^{vy}/a mice (46). The increased food intake and body weight gain that has been associated with elevated d-MSH levels (48) may then lead to some of the disorders in these mice.

The isolation of the agouti protein will be instrumental in distinguishing between the two hypotheses for agouti protein action. Once the agouti protein is available, an obvious approach is to directly test, in competitive-binding experiments, whether it binds directly to α-MSH, its receptor, or other members of the melanocortin receptor family. With the use of antibodies to purified agouti protein, it should also be possible to identify cells that produce a receptor that may interact with the agouti protein, and then isolate the receptor from these cells.

(Promoter). The other boxes represent the following: diagonally striped box, first untranslated exon of the β-actin gene (Exon 1); white box, first intron of the β-actin gene, which contains the β-actin enhancer and endogenous splice acceptor and donor sites (Intron); light gray box, the SV40 late region fragment containing a polyadenylation signal and addition site (SV40 poly A); and cross-hatched box, a small portion of the pBR322 vector. The ≈1.1 kb transcript expected to be expressed from this construct is indicated below the construct. Transcription will initiate at the position indicated by the bent arrow and terminate at the poly-A addition site, the intron will be spliced out of the primary transcript, and a poly-A tail (≈150 bp) added. (B) The 1.7 kb PGKPa construct consists of a 700 bp PstI fragment containing the same portion of agouti cDNA as in (A) (black box, labeled Agouti), under the transcriptional control of the −437 to +65 bp (numbered according to the consensus transcription initiation site located 86 bp upstream of the Pgk-1 initiation codon) Pgk-1 gene promoter/enhancer region contained within the 525 bp EcoRI-PstI fragment (diagonally striped box, labeled PGK Promoter) (66, 68). Restriction enzyme sites are abbreviated as in (A) and as follows: P = PstI; Bg = BglII. The polyadenylation signal and poly-A addition site is provided by the endogenous Pgk-1 3' flanking region (gray box labeled PGK 3' end) contained within the 470 bp PstI-HindIII fragment (67). The ≈1 kb transcript expected to be expressed from this construct is indicated below the construct. Transcription will initiate at the position indicated by the bent arrow ≈75 bp upstream of the 5' PstI site, proceed through the agouti cDNA, and terminate at the poly-A addition site 51 bp downstream of the 3' PstI site. The restriction fragments and DNA segments are not drawn to scale in either panel.

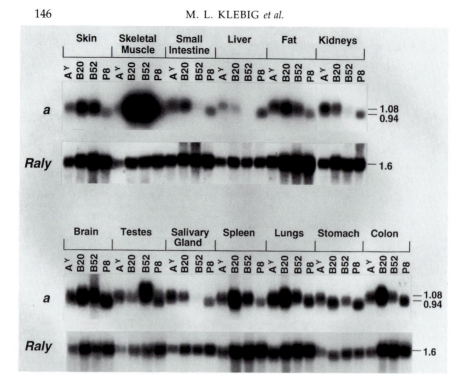

Figure 14.   Ubiquitous agouti gene expression in several tissues of adult trans-genic mice. Northern-blots containing poly(A)$^+$ RNA ($\approx$2.5 µg per lane) from tissues of adult mice hemizygous for agouti transgenes (B20, B52, and P8) and of A^y/A mice (A^y) were hybridized with a radiolabeled agouti (*a*) cDNA probe. The transgenic mice are designated as B20 (line BAPa20), B52 (BAPa52), and P8 (PGKPa8). The blots were subsequently stripped and rehybridized with a cDNA probe for the constitutively expressed *Raly* (61) gene to control for the amount of RNA in each lane. The sizes (in kb) of the transcripts detected are indicated to the right. The average transcript size of the $A^y/-$ and BAPa samples is 1.08 kb, and that of the PGKPa samples is 0.94 kb. Since *Raly* is not expressed from the A^y allele, the signal intensity from hybridization with *Raly* in $A^y/-$ samples is only half that in the transgenic samples. All of the signals in the lanes represent transgene expression, since agouti is not expressed in any of these tissues in wild-type mice (Fig. 6; 51).

In an attempt to identify the particular tissue(s) in which expression of the agouti gene causes or contributes to the syndrome, we are cur-rently investigating the effects of tissue-specific expression of agouti in transgenic mice. For example, if agouti has a primary effect in tissues directly involved in lipogenesis, lipolysis, the production of insulin and

Weight Gain-Line TgBAPa20

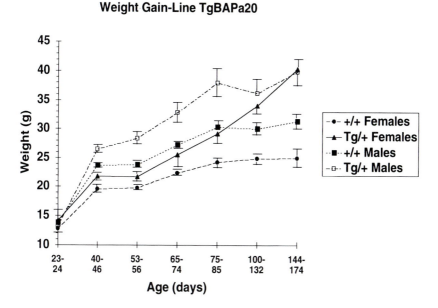

Figure 15. Weight gain of transgenic and nontransgenic mice from line BAPa20. Separate curves are shown for each sex for both transgenic (Tg/ +) and nontransgenic (+ / +) littermates according to the indicated legend. Average weights in grams of mice are plotted with respect to their ages in days. Standard error (SE) bars (indicating one SE) are shown above and below each data point. Each age point on the horizontal axis represents an age range in days, as indicated. The difference between the age points varies and the spacing indicated on the axis does not reflect these differences.

blood glucose, and glucose uptake (*i.e.,* pancreas, liver, muscle, and fat), then expression of the agouti gene specifically in one or more of these tissues should lead to some or all of the disorders of the obese yellow mouse. If, on the other hand, the agouti protein affects these processes indirectly, then expression in tissues that control them (*e.g.,* different regions of the central nervous system) should lead to the disorders.

In addition to the above analyses of the mouse agouti gene and its role in the pleiotropic effects of dominant agouti mutants, the human homolog of the agouti gene has recently been cloned in our laboratory (83). It has the potential to encode a protein of 132 amino acids that is 80% identical to the predicted mouse protein and also contains a consensus signal peptide (Fig. 17; 83). This human agouti gene maps to

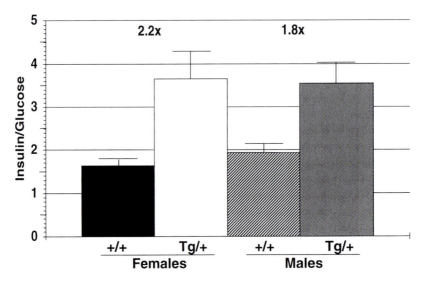

Figure 16. Plasma insulin to glucose ratios of transgenic and nontransgenic mice from line BAPa20. A bar graph is shown to compare the average insulin/ glucose (I/G) ratios for each sex of both transgenic (Tg/ +) and nontransgenic (+ / +) littermates, as indicated below the horizontal axis. Standard error bars (indicating one SE) are shown extending above each average I/G ratio. Since blood was taken from nonfasted mice, they were compared by the ratio of their insulin to glucose values to help correct for biases in the individual values due to recent feeding. The I/G ratio for each individual sample was calculated by multiplying the insulin value (in microunits/mL) by 10 and dividing the total by the glucose value (in mg/deciliter). Since no appreciable change in the insulin/glucose ratio was apparent for each group of mice over the period from 9 to 22 weeks of age, the values obtained during this period were pooled. The average I/G ratio for Tg/ + females is 2.2 times that of + / + females, and the average I/G ratio for Tg/ + males is 1.8 times that of + / + males.

chromosome 20 near one of the loci for maturity-onset diabetes of the young (MODY) (Fig. 18; 83). Experiments are in progress to study the normal function of agouti in humans and to investigate whether or not a mutation in human agouti is responsible for *MODY* or other noninsulin-dependent diabetes conditions that are associated with obesity.

The isolation and molecular analysis of the agouti gene has, therefore, set the stage for experiments that should eventually elucidate the

```
Met Asp Val Thr Arg Leu Leu Leu Ala Thr Leu Val
 .   .   .   .   .   .   .   .   .   .   .  Leu

Ser Phe Leu Cys Phe Phe Thr Val His Ser His Leu
Val  .   .   .   .   .   .  Ala Asn  .   .   .

Ala Leu Glu Glu Thr Leu Gly Asp Asp Arg Ser Leu
Pro Pro  .   .  Lys  .  Arg  .   .   .   .   .

Arg Ser Asn Ser Ser Met Asn Ser Leu Asp Phe Ser
 .   .   .   .   .  Val  .  Leu  .   .  Val Pro

Ser Val Ser Ile Val Ala Leu Asn Lys Lys Ser Lys
 .   .   .   .   .   .   .   .   .   .   .   .

Lys Ile Ser Arg Lys Glu Ala Glu Lys Arg Lys Arg
Gln  .  Gly  .   .  Ala  .   .   .   .   .   .

Ser Ser Lys Lys Lys Ala Ser Met Lys Lys Val Ala
 .   .   .   .  Glu  .   .   .   .   .   .  Val

Arg Pro Pro Pro Pro Ser  -   -  Pro Cys Val Ala
 .   .  Arg Thr  .  Leu Ser Ala  .   .   .   .

Thr Arg Asp Ser Cys Lys Pro Pro Ala Pro Ala Cys
 .   .  Asn  .   .   .   .   .   .   .   .   .

Cys Asp Pro Cys Ala Ser Cys Gln Cys Arg Phe Phe
 .   .   .   .   .   .   .   .   .   .   .   .

Gly Ser Ala Cys Thr Cys Arg Val Leu Asn Pro Asn
Arg  .   .   .  Ser  .   .   .   .  Ser Leu  .

Cys    mouse
 .     human
```

Figure 17. Comparison of the predicted amino acid sequences of the mouse and human agouti proteins. On the top line is the mouse sequence shown in Figure 4. On the bottom line is the human sequence as predicted from the open-reading frame that was deduced from homologous regions of a human genomic clone. In the human sequence, amino acids that are identical to those of the mouse sequence are represented by dots, and amino acid differences are indicated. The dashes indicate gaps introduced in the mouse sequence to maintain sequence homology with human.

Reproduced with permission from reference 83.

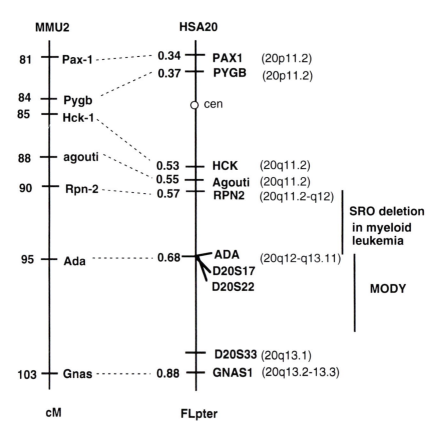

Figure 18. Assignment of the agouti gene locus to human chromosome 20q11.2 and localization of the gene on the physical map of chromosome 20 (HSA 20). The human agouti gene was assigned to band 20q11.2 by fluorescence in situ hybridization (FISH) using a lambda clone containing the coding portion of the gene (83). Utilizing FISH, the gene was localized on the physical map of the chromosome, which was constructed from length measurements also determined with FISH. This human physical map demonstrates conservation of synteny within the respective segment shown of the composite linkage map of mouse chromosome 2 (MMU2). Numbers to the left of MMU2 indicate genetic distances in centimorgans (cM) of the loci from the centromere. Numbers to the left of HSA20 indicate physical map positions of the loci as measured by FISH and expressed as fractional length from the p-terminus (FLpter; 84). The cytogenetic bands in which the human loci map are indicated in parentheses to the right of the chromosome. To the far right are indicated the locations on the cytogenetic map within which the *MODY* locus may lie and the region of the chromosome commonly deleted in patients with myeloid leukemia.

Reproduced with permission from reference 83.

biochemical and physiological roles that the ectopic agouti protein plays in the development of obesity, insulin resistance, and neoplasia in the obese yellow mice and, possibly, in humans.

NOTE ADDED IN PROOF

After this manuscript was submitted for publication, the following additional information became available. Zemel and colleagues (85) recently showed that A^{vy}/a mice have elevated levels of intracellular free calcium ($[Ca^{2+}]_i$) in their soleus muscle and that recombinant agouti protein induces elevated $[Ca^{2+}]_i$ levels in skeletal muscle myocytes in vitro. In view of the fact that skeletal muscle is the primary site of glucose disposal and that elevated $[Ca^{2+}]_i$ can lead to insulin resistance and hyperinsulinemia, which in turn can lead to obesity (discussed in 85 and 64), these findings indicate that the ectopic agouti protein in skeletal muscle could directly mediate the development of insulin resistance and consequently hyperinsulinemia and obesity in obese yellow mice by this pathogenic mechanism. At the same time, Lu and coworkers (86) have shown that recombinant agouti protein antagonizes α-MSH activation of a melanocortin receptor that is expressed in brain nuclei involved in neuroendocrine and sympathetic control (82, 86). It is conceivable that this receptor antagonism could be responsible for the reduced sympathetic tone observed in obese yellow mice (6). Since decreased adrenergic tone can lead to decreased lipolysis and increased insulin production (reviewed in ref. 6), the antagonism of the brain-specific melanocortin receptor by agouti could indirectly lead or contribute to the obesity and hyperinsulinemia of these mice.

ACKNOWLEDGMENTS

We are grateful to S. J. Bultman, E. J. Michaud, M. J. van Vugt, and H. Y. Kwon for providing previously published material and thank the members of our laboratory for helpful discussions. We are also very grateful to J. Hardin, S. Goff, and P. Besmer for providing the pBAP.2 (β-actin promoter) expression vector and to C. Stewart for providing the pKJ-1 (PGK promoter) expression vector. This research was sponsored by the Office of Health and Environmental Research, Department of Energy, under Contract DE-AC05-84OR21400 with Martin Marietta Energy System, Inc., and supported in part by an Individual National Research

Service Award to M. L. Klebig, sponsored by the Public Health Service National Institutes of Health, Department of Health and Human Services, under Grant 1 F32 DK 08880-01 BIOL1.

REFERENCES

1. Silvers WK. *The Coat Colors of Mice: A Model for Mammalian Gene Action and Interaction.* New York: Springer-Verlag; 1979:6–44.
2. Bray GA, York DA. Hypothalamic and genetic obesity in experimental animals: an autonomic and endocrine hypothesis. *Physiol Rev.* 1979;59:719–809.
3. Herberg L, Coleman DL. Laboratory animals exhibiting obesity and diabetes syndromes. *Metabolism.* 1977;26:59–99.
4. Wolff GL, Roberts DW, Galbraith DB. Prenatal determination of obesity, tumor susceptibility, and coat color pattern in viable yellow (A^{vy}/a) mice. *J Hered.* 1986;77:151–158.
5. Green MC. Catalog of mutant genes and polymorphic loci. In: Lyon MF, Searle AG, eds. *Genetic Variants and Strains of the Laboratory Mouse.* 2nd ed. Oxford, England: Oxford University Press; 1989:12–403.
6. Yen TT, Gill AM, Frigeri LG, Barsh GS, Wolff GL. Obesity, diabetes, and neoplasia in yellow $A^{vy}/-$ mice: ectopic expression of the agouti gene. *FASEB J.* 1994;8:479–488.
7. Dickerson GE, Gowen JW. Hereditary obesity and efficient food utilization in mice. *Science.* 1947;105:496–498.
8. Frigeri LG, Wolff GL, Teguh C. Differential responses of yellow A^{vy}/A and agouti *A/a* (BALB/c × VY)F$_1$ hybrid mice to the same diets: glucose tolerance, weight gain, and adipocyte cellularity. *Int J Obes.* 1988;12:305–320.
9. Fenton PF, Chase HB. Effect of diet on obesity of yellow mice in inbred lines. *Proc Soc Exp Biol Med.* 1951;77:420–422.
10. Zomzely C, Mayer J. Fat metabolism in experimental obesities, IX: lipogenesis and cholesterogenesis in yellow obese mice. *Am J Physiol.* 1959;196:611–613.
11. Plocher TA, Powley TL. Effect of hypophysectomy on weight gain and body composition in the genetically obese yellow (A^y/a) mouse. *Metabolism.* 1976;25:593–602.
12. Jackson E, Stolz D, Martin R. Effect of adrenalectomy on weight

gain and body composition of yellow obese mice (A^y/a). *Horm Metab Res.* 1976;8:452–455.

13. Yen TT, Allan JA, Yu PL, Acton MA, Pearson DV. Triacylglycerol contents and in vivo lipogenesis of *ob/ob, db/db* and A^{vy}/a mice. *Biochim Biophys Acta.* 1976;441:213–220.

14. Johnson PR, Hirsch J. Cellularity of adipose depots in six strains of genetically obese mice. *J Lipid Res.* 1972;13:2–11.

15. Dickie MM, Woolley GW. The age factor in weight of yellow mice. *J Hered.* 1946;37:365–368.

16. Roberts DW, Wolff GL, Campbell WL. Differential effects of the mottled yellow and pseudoagouti phenotypes on immunocompetence in A^{vy}/a mice. *Proc Natl Acad Sci USA.* 1984;81:2152–2156.

17. Castle WE. Influence of certain color mutations on body size in mice, rats, and rabbits. *Genetics.* 1941;26:181–191.

18. Heston WE, Vlahakis G. Elimination of the effect of the A^y gene on pulmonary tumors in mice by alteration of its effect on normal growth. *J Natl Cancer Inst.* 1961;27:1189–1196.

19. Wolff GL. Genotype-dependent modification of sarcoma 37 growth in castrated mice. *Cancer Res.* 1971;31:1570–1572.

20. Friedman JM, Leibel RL. Tackling a weighty problem. *Cell.* 1992;69: 217–220.

21. Heston WE, Vlahakis G. Genetic obesity and neoplasia. *J Natl Cancer Inst.* 1962;29:197–209.

22. Shaw WN, Schmiegel KK, Yen TT, Toomey RE, Meyers DB, Mills J. LY79771: a novel compound for weight control. *Life Sci.* 1981;29: 2091–2101.

23. Yen TT, McKee MM, Bemis KG. Ephedrine reduces weight of viable yellow obese mice (A^{vy}/a). *Life Sci.* 1981;28:119–128.

24. Coleman DL. Antiobesity effects of etiocholanolones in diabetes (*db*), viable yellow (A^{vy}), and normal mice. *Endocrinology.* 1985;117: 2279–2283.

25. Carpenter KJ, Mayer J. Physiologic observations on yellow obesity in the mouse. *Am J Physiol.* 1958;193:499–504.

26. Gill AM, Yen TT. Effects of ciglitazone on endogenous plasma islet amyloid polypeptide and insulin sensitivity in obese-diabetic viable yellow mice. *Life Sci.* 1990;48:703–710.

27. Meade CJ, Ashwell M, Sowter C. Is genetically transmitted obesity due to an adipose tissue defect? *Proc R Soc Lond.* 1979;205:395–410.

28. Frigeri LG, Wolff GL, Robel G. Impairment of glucose tolerance in

yellow (A^{vy}/A) (BALB/c × VY) F-1 hybrid mice by hyperglycemic peptide(s) from human pituitary glands. *Endocrinology.* 1983;113: 2097–2105.

29. Salem MAM, Wolff GL. Potentiation of response to insulin and anti-insulin action by two human pituitary peptides in lean agouti *A/a*, obese yellow A^{vy}/A, and C57BL/6J-*ob/ob* mice. *Proc Soc Exp Biol Med.* 1989;191:113–123.

30. Salem MAM, Lewis UJ, Haro LS *et al.* Effects of hypophysectomy and the insulin-like and anti-insulin pituitary peptides on carbohydrate metabolism in yellow A^{vy}/A (BALB/c × VY)F1 hybrid mice. *Proc Soc Exp Biol Med.* 1989;191:408–419.

31. Silberberg R, Silberberg M. Lesions in "yellow" mice fed stock, high-fat, or carbohydrate diets. *Yale J Biol & Med.* 1957;29:525–539.

32. Hausberger FX, Hausberger BC. The etiologic mechanism of some forms of hormonally induced obesity. *Am J Clin Nutr.* 1960;8:671–681.

33. Hellerstrom C, Hellman B. The islets of Langerhans in yellow obese mice. *Metabolism.* 1963;12:527–536.

34. Wolff GL. Genetic modification of homeostatic regulation in the mouse. *Am Nat.* 1971;105:241–252.

35. Wolff GL, Greenman DL, Frigeri LG, Morrissey RL, Suber RL, Felton RP. Diabetogenic response to streptozotocin varies among obese yellow and among lean agouti (BALB/c × VY)F1 hybrid mice. *Proc Soc Exp Biol Med.* 1990;193:155–163.

36. Shimizu H, Shargill NS, Bray GA. Adrenalectomy and response to corticosterone and MSH in the genetically obese yellow mouse. *Am J Physiol.* 1989;256:R494–R500.

37. Rifkin H, Porte DP, eds. *Diabetes Mellitus: Theory and Practice.* New York: Elsevier; 1990.

38. Straus DS. Growth-stimulatory actions of insulin in vitro and in vivo. *Endocr Rev.* 1984;5:356–369.

39. Heston WE. Complete inhibition of occurrence of spontaneous hepatomas in highly susceptible (C3H × YBR)F1 male mice by hypophysectomy. *J Natl Cancer Inst.* 1963;31:467–474.

40. Wolff GL. Hereditary obesity and hormone deficiencies in yellow dwarf mice. *Am J Physiol.* 1965;209:632–636.

41. Wolff GL, Flack JD. Genetic regulation of plasma corticosterone concentration and its response to castration and allogeneic tumour growth in the mouse. *Nature.* 1971;232:181–182.

42. Weitze M. *Hereditary Adiposity in Mice and the Cause of this Anomaly.* Copenhagen, Denmark: University of Copenhagen; 1940. PhD thesis.

43. Wolff GL. Growth of inbred yellow (A^y/a) and non-yellow (a/a) mice in parabiosis. *Genetics.* 1963;48:1041–1058.

44. Harris RBS. Role of set-point theory in regulation of body weight. *FASEB J.* 1990;4:3310–3318.

45. Turner ML. Hereditary obesity and temperature regulation. *Am J Physiol.* 1948;152:197–204.

46. Shimizu H, Bray GA, Retzius T, York DA. Acetylation to α-MSH in pituitary may be an important factor in the development of obesity in the yellow mice. *Clin Res.* 1986;36:193A.

47. White JD, Stewart KD, Krause JE, McKely JF. Biochemistry of peptide-secreting neurons. *Physiol Rev.* 1985;65:553–606.

48. Shimizu H, Shargill NS, Bray GA, Yen TT, Gesellchen PD. Effects of MSH on food intake, body weight and coat color of the yellow obese mouse. *Life Sci.* 1989;45:543–552.

49. Woychik RP, Generoso WM, Russell LB, *et al.* Molecular and genetic characterization of a radiation-induced structural rearrangement in mouse chromosome 2 causing mutations at the limb deformity and agouti loci. *Proc Natl Acad Sci USA.* 1990;87:2588–2592.

50. Bultman SJ, Russell LB, Gutierrez-Espeleta GA, Woychik RP. Molecular characterization of a region of DNA associated with mutations at the agouti locus in the mouse. *Proc Natl Acad Sci USA.* 1991;88:8062–8066.

51. Bultman SJ, Michaud EJ, Woychik RP. Molecular characterization of the mouse agouti locus. *Cell.* 1992;71:1195–1204.

52. Miller MM, Duhl DMJ, Vrieling H, *et al.* Cloning of the mouse agouti gene predicts a secreted protein ubiquitously expressed in mice carrying the lethal yellow mutation. *Genes Dev.* 1993;7:454–467.

53. Copeland NG, Jenkins NA, Lee BK. Association of the lethal yellow A^y coat color mutation with an ecotropic murine leukemia virus genome. *Proc Natl Acad Sci USA.* 1983;80:247–249.

54. Siracusa LD, Russell LB, Jenkins NA, Copeland NG. Allelic variation within the *Emv-15* locus defines genomic sequences closely linked to the *agouti* locus on mouse chromosome 2. *Genetics.* 1987;117:85–92.

55. Siracusa LD, Buchberg AM, Copeland NG, Jenkins NA. Recombi-

nant inbred strain and interspecific backcross analysis of molecular markers flanking the murine *agouti* coat color locus. *Genetics.* 1989; 122:669–679.

56. Barsh GS, Epstein C. Physical and genetic characterization of a 75-kilobase deletion associated with a^l, a recessive lethal allele at the mouse *agouti* locus. *Genetics.* 1989;121:811–818.

57. Barsh GS, Epstein C. The long-range restriction map surrounding the mouse agouti locus reveals a disparity between physical and genetic distances. *Genomics.* 1989;5:9–18.

58. Woychik RP, Stewart TA, Davis LG, D'Eustachio P, Leder P. An inherited limb deformity created by insertional mutagenesis in a transgenic mouse. *Nature.* 1985;318:36–40.

59. Bultman SJ, Klebig ML, Michaud EJ, Sweet HO, Davisson MT, Woychik RP. Molecular analysis of reverse mutations from nonagouti (*a*) to black-and-tan (*a^t*) and white-bellied agouti (*A^w*) reveals alternative forms of agouti transcripts. *Genes Dev.* 1994;8:481–490.

60. Michaud EJ, Bultman SB, Klebig ML, *et al.* A molecular model for the genetic and phenotypic characteristics of the mouse lethal yellow (*A^y*) mutation. *Proc Natl Acad Sci USA.* 1994;91:2562–2566.

61. Michaud EJ, Bultman SJ, Stubbs LJ, Woychik RP. The embryonic lethality of homozygous lethal yellow mice (*A^y/A^y*) is associated with the disruption of a novel RNA-binding protein. *Genes Dev.* 1993;7:1203–1213.

62. Michaud EJ, Van Vugt MJ, Bultman SJ, Sweet HO, Davisson MT, Woychik RP. Differential methylation of a new dominant agouti allele (*A^{iapy}*) is correlated with variation in the level of ectopic gene expression and is influenced by parental lineage. *Genes Dev.* 1994; 8:1463–1472.

63. Wolff GL. Body composition and coat color correlation in different phenotypes of "viable yellow" mice. *Science.* 1965;147:1145–1147.

64. Klebig ML, Wilkinson E, Geisler J, Woychik RP. Ectopic expression of the agouti gene in transgenic mice causes obesity, features of the Type II diabetes, and yellow fur. *Proc Natl Acad Sci USA.* 1995;92: 4728–4732.

65. Gunning P, Leavitt J, Muscat G, Ng S-Y, Kedes LA. Human β-actin expression vector system directs high-level accumulation of antisense transcripts. *Proc Natl Acad Sci USA.* 1987;84:4831–4835.

66. Ray P, Higgins KM, Tan JC, *et al.* Ectopic expression of a c-*kit*[W42] minigene in transgenic mice: recapitulation of *W* phenotypes and

evidence for c-*kit* function in melanoblast progenitors. *Genes Dev.* 1991;5:2265–2273.

67. Adra CH, Boer PH, McBurney MW. Cloning and expression of the mouse *pgk-1* gene and the nucleotide sequence of its promoter. *Gene.* 1987;60:65–74.

68. Boer PH, Potten H, Adra CN, Jardine K, Mullhofer G, McBurney MW. Polymorphisms in the coding and noncoding regions of murine Pgk-1 alleles. *Biochem Genet.* 1990;28:299–308.

69. McBurney MW, Sutherland LC, Adra CN, Leclair B, Rudnicki MA, Jardine K. The mouse *Pgk-1* gene promoter contains an upstream activator sequence. *Nucleic Acids Res.* 1991;19:5755–5761.

70. Geschwind II. Change in hair color in mice induced by injection of α-MSH. *Endocrinology.* 1966;79:1165–1167.

71. Geschwind II, Huseby RA, Nishioka R. The effect of melanocyte-stimulating hormone on coat color in the mouse. *Recent Prog Horm Res.* 1972;28:91–130.

72. Tamate BT, Takeuchi T. Induction of the shift in melanin synthesis in lethal yellow (A^y/a) mice in vitro. *Dev Genet.* 1981;2:349–356.

73. Tamate BT, Takeuchi T. Action of the *e* locus of mice in the response of phaeomelanic hair follicles to α-melanocyte-stimulating hormone in vitro. *Science.* 1984;224:1241–1242.

74. Mountjoy KG, Robbins LS, Mortrud MT, Cone RD. The cloning of a family of genes that encode the melanocortin receptors. *Science.* 1992;257:1248–1251.

75. Robbins LS, Nadeau JH, Johnson KR, *et al.* Pigmentation phenotypes of variant extension locus alleles result from point mutations that alter MSH receptor function. *Cell.* 1993;72:827–834.

76. Takeuchi T, Kobunai T, Yamamoto H. Genetic control of signal transduction in mouse melanocytes. *J Invest Dermatol.* 1989;92:239S–242S.

77. Jackson IJ. Color-coded switches. *Nature.* 1993;362:587–588.

78. Jackson IJ. More to color than meets the eye. *Curr. Biol.* 1993;3:518–521.

79. Conklin BR, Bourne HR. Mouse coat color reconsidered. *Nature.* 1993;364:110.

80. Hauschka TS, Jacobs BB, Holdridge BA. Recessive yellow and its interaction with belted in the mouse. *J Hered.* 1968;59:339–341.

81. Gantz I, Konda Y, Tashiro T, *et al.* Molecular cloning of a novel melanocortin receptor. *J Biol Chem.* 1993;268:8246–8250.

82. Gantz I, Miwa H, Konda Y, *et al.* Molecular cloning, expression, and gene localization of a 4th melanocortin receptor. *J Biol Chem.* 1993; 268:15174–15179.
83. Kwon HJ, Bultman SJ, Loffler C, *et al.* Molecular structure and chromosomal mapping of the human homolog of the agouti gene. *Proc Natl Acad Sci USA.* 1994;91:9760–9764.
84. Lichter P, Tang CC, Call K, *et al.* High-resolution mapping of human chromosome 11 by in situ hybridization with cosmid clones. *Science.* 1990;247:64–69.
85. Zemel MB, Kim JH, Woychik RP, *et al.* Agouti regulation of intracellular calcium: role in the insulin resistance of viable yellow mice. *Proc Natl Acad Sci USA.* 1995;92:4733–4737.
86. Lu D, Willard D, Patel IR, *et al.* Agouti protein is an antagonist of the melanocyte-stimulating-hormone receptor. *Nature.* 1994;371: 799–802.

PART II

Biology of Animal Models

GERARD P. SMITH, JOHN D. DAVIS,
and DANIELLE GREENBERG

The Direct Control of Meal Size in the Zucker Rat

ABSTRACT

Increased food intake is a characteristic phenotypical expression
of genetic obesity in rodents. To investigate the causal links between genetic mutation and increased meal size, the abnormality
in the controls of meal size must be identified. On the basis of
recent experiments on the microstructural analysis of the ingestion
of carbohydrate test meals, we proposed that the size of a meal
was determined by the relative potencies and central interactions
of the positive and negative sensory feedbacks produced by ingested food on the central network for eating that controls the rate
and duration of eating. When the increased meal size of obese (fa/
fa) rats was investigated within the framework of these feedback
controls, we found two abnormalities: increased positive, orosensory feedback of corn oil in relationship to sucrose when these two
nutrients are presented simultaneously and decreased negative
feedback by cholecystokinin in male obese rats, but not in female
obese rats. The relevance of these abnormalities to increased meal
size in obese rats in other experimental conditions and whether
they represent a phenotypic expression of the genetic mutation or
are the result of the obese state are unknown.

Hyperphagia is a characteristic phenotypical expression of genetic obesity in rodents. It usually takes the form of increased meal size. To
exploit the recent progress in the genetic analysis of obese rodents, it
is necessary to identify gene products involved in any phenotypic expression of a specific mutation. Thus, for the investigation of the causal
links between genetic mutation and increased meal size, a sequential
process of investigation is required. First, we must identify how the
normal controls of meal size are distorted in a rodent with a specific

161

genetic mutation. Second, candidate gene products of the specific mutation must be tested for their ability to mediate the abnormal controls of eating that are responsible for the increased meal size in the mutant animal.

Direct and Indirect Controls of Meal Size

What are the normal controls of meal size? With the normal rat, meal size can be changed by prior experience, ecological niche, diurnal rhythm, ambient temperature, the metabolic effects of the diet, metabolic state, and the sensory characteristics of the diet. This daunting catalog of operational manipulations that change meal size apparently defies simple investigation. Fortunately all of these controls divide into a direct sensory control system that encodes, transmits, and processes the sensory stimuli provided by food during a meal, and also indirect control systems (*e.g.,* metabolism, temperature, gonadal hormones, foraging experience) that encode, transmit, and process all of the other sensory stimuli produced by all other adequate stimuli for the control of meal size. This dichotomy of control systems is not simply a renaming of short-term controls and long-term controls because those terms usually refer to the controls of meal size and meal number (short-term controls) and the controls of food intake that serve the larger, more complex physiological system of energy balance (long-term controls).

The controls discussed here have two important characteristics. First, they are only concerned with meal size. Their relevance to meal number and energy balance is an open question, in need of systematic investigation. Second, the indirect controls of meal size operate by modulating the direct controls. This indicates that these controls are functionally sequential, not parallel. This is a necessary conclusion from the fact that we can detect the influence of the indirect controls on meal size only when the direct sensory controls are stimulated by food during eating. Although this sequential, functional relationship between indirect and direct sensory controls seems self-evident, the relevant literature does not often reflect it. That the potency of indirect controls on meal size can *only* be measured by changes in the position or the slope of the function-relating rate of eating or meal size to intensity of a specific, direct sensory control mechanism is rarely emphasized, even though this is a necessary conclusion of the sequential relationship of the direct and indirect sensory controls of eating. The report from Figlewicz and his colleagues (1) that central administration of insulin, a peptide signal for indirect control by adipose tissue, increased the satiating potency of peripherally administered cholecystokinin (CCK), a peptide signal for direct control, is an instructive exception.

The Direct Sensory Control of Meal Size

The direct sensory control of meal size begins to operate on the first postnatal day (2). Initially this control responds to oral chemical and (presumably) mechanical stimuli and to mechanical stimuli in the stomach (3). By the end of the second postnatal week, ingestion of sucrose and oils becomes a linear function of concentration (4), and chemical stimuli in the small intestine are now effective (3).

By the end of the third week, at a time when weaning can be achieved with little difficulty, the direct control system appears to be complete. In contrast, it is not until now that inhibitors of glucose or fat metabolism can be shown to increase meal size (5). The ontogenetic appearance of the other indirect controls is not well known, although temperature can change intake during the preweaning period (3).

The direct sensory control system has chemical and mechanical receptors lining the gut from the tip of the tongue to the end of the small intestine. The chemical receptors are diverse and are distinguished by their adequate stimuli, which include glucose, fatty acids, amino acids, osmolality, hydrogen ion concentration, and temperature. After transduction at the receptor, the sensory information is transmitted to the brain by cranial nerves 1, 5, 7, 9, and 10 and to the spinal cord by visceral afferent fibers of cells in the dorsal root ganglia.

Because the sensory information for the direct control of meal size is the result of the food being eaten, all of the sensory information is acting in a feedback manner. The positive or negative effect of this feedback information on eating depends on its origin. The sensory feedback from an acceptable food stimulus is transmitted from the mouth to the brain over cranial nerves 1, 5, 7, 9, and 10. The orosensory feedback stimulates the central network for eating, tending to prolong eating. In this sense it has a positive feedback effect on eating. But note that positive feedback in this context denotes a *net* stimulation of the final motor mechanisms of eating; it does not produce the characteristic increasing effect of a positive feedback in control theory (6). The sensory feedback transmitted from the stomach and small intestine to the brain and spinal cord by visceral afferent fibers inhibits the central network for eating, tending to stop eating. This postingestive sensory input provides negative feedback on eating and meal size. Thus, the size of a meal is determined by the relative potencies and central interactions of the positive and negative sensory feedbacks on the central network for eating that controls the rate and duration of eating.

Results from a recent experiment demonstrate these sensory feedbacks (7). The experiment was concerned with the increase in meal size that occurs when rats sham feed without food accumulating in the gut, instead of really feeding. Two groups of rats were tested with 0.8M sucrose after four hours of food deprivation (Fig. 1). The first group (open circles connected with dashed lines) increased their intake progressively over three sequential sham feeding (SF) trials to reach an asymptote of about 40 mL in the thirty-minute test. The second group

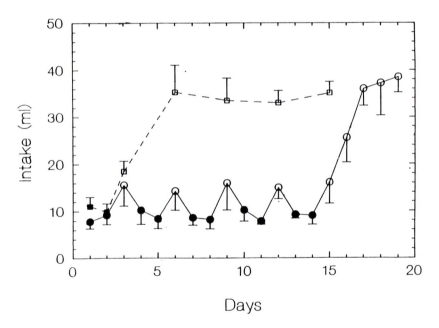

Figure 1. Mean ± SE thirty-minute intake for two groups on successive days of experiment. Closed symbols, days on which RF tests were given; open symbols, days on which SF tests were given. Circles, group 1; squares, group 2 (see text). SE bars are omitted on one side of average points to reduce clutter.

of rats (open and filled circles connected by continuous lines) were run on a different protocol. For the first fourteen tests on these rats each SF test was preceded by two real feeding (RF) tests (gastric cannula was closed). Opening the gastric cannula eliminated postingestive negative feedback information, and intake on the first SF test doubled. On subsequent SF tests interspersed between two RF tests, the same doubling of intake occurred. Because this effect did not change with repetition, we consider it to be unconditioned. Note that this doubling of intake was significantly less than the intake observed after sequential SF tests. This suggested residual negative feedback from food stimuli acting in the mouth or esophagus. This negative feedback appeared to be a conditioned process because it extinguished when sequential SF tests occurred on test days 15 through 19 (Fig. 1).

Note that intake in the fourth and fifth sequential SF tests of both groups was not significantly larger than intake in the third sequential SF test (Fig. 1). Maximal intake represents the intake when the positive feedback operates in the absence of unconditioned and conditioned negative feedback under these conditions. Although these results demonstrate the operation of positive feedback and two kinds of negative feedback, conditioned and unconditioned, meal size and intakes are only indirect measures of licking behavior in this eating situation.

To measure licking behavior directly we used a computer-assisted lickometer technique to measure every lick the rats made during these experiments. This technique not only provides a complete record of licking for analysis of rate and microstructure, but because each lick correlates with activation of the hypoglossal nuclei by the putative motor pattern generator in the caudal hindbrain (8), each lick is a measure of the final motor pathway of the central network for ingestion.

The rate and pattern of licking differed among the three test conditions in group 2 (Fig. 2). Because the initial rate of licking was not different, the difference in the rate of licking was the result of differences in the rate of decay of licking. The rate of decay of licking was most rapid during real feeding and licking essentially stopped after about sixteen minutes. This is the end of the meal. When the gastric cannula was opened the first two times, licking decayed at the same rapid rate for about the first four minutes, but then the rate was maintained above 50 licks/min until twenty minutes. This pattern of licking during SF did not change much across the five SF tests preceded by two RF tests (compare first two and last two SF tests, Fig. 2). This pat-

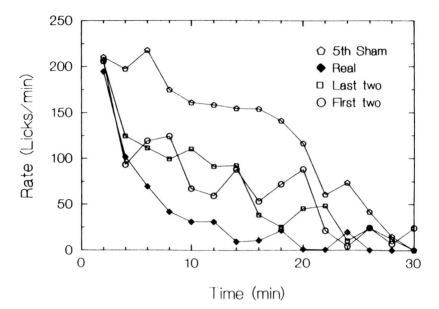

Figure 2. Rate of licking calculated at successive two-minute intervals for RF and fifth consecutive SF tests (top and bottom curves) and for average of first two and average of last two SF tests with RF tests intervening (middle two curves). Averages of first two and last two SF tests are displayed to reduce variability and are justified, because there was no significant differences between them.

tern is the result of the removal of the *unconditioned,* negative feedback effect of postingestive food stimuli.

The rapid rate of decay of licking in the first four minutes was gradually eliminated by sequential SF tests without intervening RF tests (Fig. 2). Now licking was maintained at a rapid rate for twenty minutes because the sequential SF tests extinguished the association between orosensory and postingestive stimuli that is responsible for the conditioned, rapid rate of decay of licking in the first four minutes of eating (7). The pattern of rapid, sustained licking represents the positive feedback of orosensory stimuli on licking in the absence of conditioned and unconditioned negative feedbacks.

Note that under these experimental conditions, licking stopped toward the end of the thirty-minute test when the gastric cannula was opened. The mechanism responsible for this is not accounted for by the feedback processes described above. This may represent orosensory habituation as suggested by Swithers-Mulvey and Hall (9). Whatever the mechanism, it is sensitive to deprivation because after seventeen hours of food deprivation, rats sham feed at a rapid rate for sixty minutes or longer (10).

The potency and temporal domains of the positive and negative feedbacks in these experiments are depicted schematically in Figure 3. Our working hypothesis is that the potency and the central interaction(s) of these feedbacks are operating to determine every meal in all

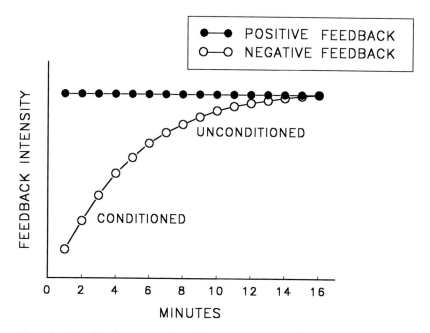

Figure 3. Idealized presentation of the positive orosensory feedback and conditioned and unconditioned negative feedbacks demonstrated during a meal of 0.8 mol sucrose. Feedback intensity refers to perceived (central) intensity of the feedback stimuli. The intensity of positive feedback is initially relatively high with this concentrated sucrose solution and is maintained constant throughout the meal in this idealized situation. The intensity of negative feedback is initially low but increases throughout the meal until it equals the positive intensity as judged by a postulated central comparator mechanism; then licking stops. The early, rapid increase in negative feedback intensity involves conditioning. The later increase in negative feedback is unconditioned. See text for relationship between this figure and figures 1 and 2.

mammals. The temporal domains of the conditioned and unconditioned negative feedbacks and the potencies of all three feedbacks are
dependent on the sensory characteristics of the food and prior experience eating it, if the indirect controls of eating are held constant. In our
view, the wide range of food intake that rats exhibit is a result of the
dynamic interactions of preabsorptive sensory feedback processes that
provide the direct control of meal size. We are aware that a major limitation of the hypothesis is that it has been generated from experiments
with sucrose and other carbohydrate solutions (7, 8, 11). Only extensive
testing can decide whether the interaction of the sensory feedback processes identified here is paradigmatic or idiosyncratic.

Direct Control of Meal Size in Zucker Rats

Obese (*fa/fa*) rats eat larger meals than lean rats under a variety of conditions, but especially on high-fat diets. This consistent phenotypical
difference should be viewed within the context of the direct control of
meal size just described. If meal size is the result of the dynamic interactions of preabsorptive sensory feedback processes, then a larger meal
size could be produced by one of three patterns of feedback interactions
(Table 1). Note that the most common interpretation of an increased
meal size as due to a decrease or absence of a postingestive, negative
feedback, satiating signal is only one of three logically equivalent possibilities. We have begun to investigate which of these possibilities is
responsible for the increased meal size in obese rats.

Postingestive Negative Feedback in Obese and Lean Rats

Small Intestine

To test the negative feedback effect of fat in the small intestine, Intralipid, a soluble mixture of long-chain fats, was infused into the duodenum through a chronically implanted catheter at a rate within the
normal range of gastric emptying of Intralipid. These duodenal infusions inhibited intake during SF with equivalent potency in obese and
lean rats (12). Because the inhibition occurred during SF, it was not
mediated indirectly through the well-known inhibition of gastric emp-

Table 1. Patterns of Changes of Sensory Feedbacks Responsible for Increased Meal Size

Feedback Potency	
Positive	Negative
Increased	No change
Increased	Decreased
No change	Decreased

tying produced by fat in the small intestine. Instead, Intralipid acts preabsorptively in the small intestine to inhibit eating (13–15). The preabsorptive signal in the rat appears to be free fatty acids rather than triglycerides (16). The signal is carried by afferent vagal fibers to the brain. The vagal afferents respond to fatty acids (17) and to CCK released from mucosal cells in the upper half of the small intestine (18). The effect of CCK is blocked by antagonists of the CCK_A receptors (18). The site of these receptors is presumably on the vagal afferent terminals (19).

Although no significant difference was detected in the inhibitory potency of intraduodenal Intralipid in these obese and lean male rats, Strohmayer and Greenberg (20) recently observed a significant difference in food intake during blockade of CCK_A receptors by devazepide. Devazepide increased meal size and meal duration significantly in lean male rats, but not in obese male rats. In fact, the meal size in lean rats after devazepide was equal to the meal size of obese rats under these conditions.

These results suggest that obese male rats have a defect in the satiating effect of CCK. The defect does not include receptor mechanisms because adult obese male rats respond to exogenous CCK in an apparently normal manner (21). This suggests that the defect involves the synthesis or release of CCK. Whatever the defect, it was only observed in males; devazepide had no effect on intake in lean and obese female rats (22). These results are the first example of a correlation between a specific satiating molecule, CCK, and the increased meal size of obese male rats. Considerably more work is required to determine the meaning of these results and whether the differential response to devazepide is seen under other experimental conditions.

Stomach

Gastric satiating mechanisms have been tested only indirectly. It is possible that gastric signals for meal termination (23) are stimulated less in obese than in lean rats. Possibly, less stimulation would occur if fat or other nutrients were emptied from the stomach more rapidly in obese rats than in lean rats. To test this possibility, the effect of intraduodenal infusion of corn oil on gastric emptying was measured. Gastric emptying was inhibited by intraduodenal corn oil at least as much in obese rats as in lean rats (24). Although this apparently eliminates less gastric stimulation as a result of faster gastric emptying as a cause of increased meal size in obese male rats, more direct tests of gastric negative feedback mechanisms are clearly warranted.

Comment

The only evidence of a decreased postingestive, negative feedback in the obese rats is the preliminary report of a loss of the satiating effect of CCK in obese male rats. We assume that this is the loss of an unconditioned negative feedback mechanism, but specific experiments to evaluate the possible role of CCK in conditioned negative feedback have not been done. It is also an open question whether this defect is a phenotypical trait of the *fa/fa* rat or whether it occurs as a result of the long experience of hyperphagia and abnormal nutrient partitioning that results in the obese state.

Orosensory Positive Feedback in Obese and Lean Rats

Single-Stimulus Sham-Feeding Tests

Obese rats ingested the same volume of sucrose or corn oil in one-bottle SF tests as lean rats (25, 26). This was true across a wide range of concentrations with two exceptions: Obese rats ingested significantly *less* (0.05 mol) sucrose and 100% corn oil than lean rats. Thus, there was no evidence in these experiments for increased positive feedback from orosensory stimulation during SF that could contribute to the increased meal size of obese rats.

PREFERENCE TESTS

Given the possible involvement of increased positive orosensory feedback for fats in the consistent reports of fat preference in obese rats, obese and lean rats were presented with specific concentrations of sucrose and corn oil simultaneously for thirty minutes of SF after they had experience with the sucrose and corn oil presented alone on alternate days. Obese male and female rats preferred corn oil to sucrose more than lean male and female rats (27, 28; Table 2).

COMMENT

The preference for corn oil over sucrose in SF tests is the only evidence of increased positive feedback in obese rats currently available that could contribute to the larger meal size and fat preference of obese rats.

Summary

When the larger meal size of obese rats was analyzed in terms of the direct control of meal size by the interaction of positive and negative feedbacks, we found two abnormalities: an increased positive, orosensory feedback of corn oil in relationship to sucrose when these two nutrients are presented simultaneously and a decreased negative feedback by CCK in male obese rats but not in female obese rats. The relevance of these abnormalities to increased meal size in other experimental conditions and whether they represent a phenotypic expression of the genetic mutation or are the result of the obese state is unknown.

The experiments we have reviewed are the only ones relevant to the investigation of the relative contribution of defects in the positive and

Table 2. Mean Sucrose Isohedonic Concentrations with 100% Corn Oil in Obese and Lean Rats

	Male	Female
Obese	30.0	17.5
Lean	20.0	2.5

The mean isohedonic concentration (%) of sucrose is the concentration that the specific groups of rats (n = 4–8) ingested a volume of which was equal to the volume of 100% corn oil ingested in a two-bowl choice test that lasted thirty minutes (27, 28).

negative feedbacks controlling meal size. It is therefore clear that much more analysis of the mechanisms of the hyperphagia of the obese rat is required in order for the relationship of this behavioral phenotype to the specific genetic mutation to be investigated effectively. Thus, one of the benefits of the recent progress of the genetic analysis of the *fa/fa* rat is that it forces more precise and detailed analyses of all of the phenotypic differences, including the behavioral, that are correlated with the genetic mutation.

ACKNOWLEDGMENTS

We thank Jane Magnetti for expert processing of this manuscript. Dr. James Gibbs made many helpful suggestions to improve it. The research was supported by National Institutes of Health grants DK41536 (JD), DK38757 (DG), MH15455, MH40010, and MH00149 (GPS) and by a grant from the International Life Sciences Institute Research Foundation to Danielle Greenberg.

REFERENCES

1. Figlewicz DP, West DB, Stern LJ, Woods SC, Porte D, Jr. Insulin alters the sensitivity of baboons to CCK-induced single meal suppression. *Am J Physiol.* 1986;250:R856–R860.
2. Hall WG. The ontogeny of feeding in rats, I: ingestive and behavioral responses to oral infusions. *J Comp Physiol Psychol.* 1979;93:977–1000.
3. Hall WG. What we know and don't know about the development of independent ingestion. *Appetite.* 1985;6:333–356.
4. Ackerman SH, Albert M, Shindledecker RD, Gayle C, Smith GP. Intake of different concentrations of sucrose and corn oil in preweanling rats. *Am J Physiol.* 1992;262:R624–R627.
5. Leshem M, Flynn FW, Epstein AN. The ontogeny of the metabolic controls of ingestion: does brain energy privation control ingestion in the rat pup? *Am J Physiol.* 1990;258:R365–R375.
6. McFarland DJ. Feedback mechanisms in animal behavior. New York: Academic Press; 1971.
7. Davis JD, Smith GP. Learning to sham feed: behavioral adjustments to loss of physiological postingestional stimuli. *Am J Physiol.* 1990;259:R1228–R1235.

8. Davis JD, Smith GP. Analysis of the microstructure of the rhythmic tongue movements of rats ingesting maltose and sucrose solutions. *Behav Neurosci.* 1992;106:217–228.

9. Swithers-Mulvey SE, Hall WG. Control of ingestion by oral habituation in rat pups. *Behav Neurosci.* 1992;106:710–717.

10. Young RC, Gibbs J, Antin J, Holt J, Smith GP. Absence of satiety during sham feeding in the rat. *J Comp Physiol Psychol.* 1974;87:795–800.

11. Davis JD, Smith GP. Analysis of lick rate measures the positive and negative feedback effects of carbohydrates on eating. *Appetite.* 1988; 11:229–238.

12. Greenberg D, Gibbs J, Smith GP. Intraduodenal infusions of fat inhibit sham feeding in Zucker rats. *Brain Res Bull.* 1986;20:779–784.

13. Greenberg D, Smith GP, Gibbs J. Intraduodenal infusions of fats elicit satiety in the sham feeding rat. *Am J Physiol.* 1990;259:R110–R118.

14. Greenberg D, Kava R, Lewis DR, Greenwood MRC. Satiation following intraduodenal Intralipid precedes appearance of [14C]-Intralipid in hepatic portal blood. *FASEB J.* 1991;5:A1451.

15. Greenberg D, Smith GP, Gibbs J. Intravenous triglycerides fail to elicit satiety in sham feeding rats. *Am J Physiol.* 1993;264:R409–R413.

16. Greenberg D, Smith GP, Gibbs J. Oleic acid inhibits sham feeding when duodenally infused while triolein does not. *Soc Neurosci Abstr.* 1988;14:1196.

17. Melone J. Vagal receptors sensitive to lipids in the small intestine of the cat. *J Auton Nerv Syst.* 1986;17:331–341.

18. Greenberg D, Torres NI, Smith GP, Gibbs J. The satiating effects of fats is attenuated by the cholecystokinin antagonist lorglumide. *Ann NY Acad Sci.* 1989;575:517–520.

19. Schwartz GJ, McHugh PR, Moran TH. Integration of vagal afferent response to gastric loads and cholecystokinin in rats. *Am J Physiol.* 1991;261:R64–R69.

20. Strohmayer AJ, Greenberg D. Devazepide alters meal patterns in lean, but not obese, male Zucker rats. In press.

21. Strohmayer AJ, Greenberg D, von Heyn R, Dornstein L, Baltman C. The integrity of cholecystokinin satiety mechanisms in genetically obese Zucker rats. *Soc Neurosci Abstr.* 1988;14:1196.

22. Strohmayer AJ, Greenberg D. CCK_A receptor antagonist devazep-

ide increased food intake in male, but not female, obese Zucker rats. *Soc Neurosci Abstr.* 1993;19:1823.

23. Deutsch JA. Food intake: gastric factors. In: Stricker EM, ed. *Handbook of Behavioral Neurobiology.* 10th ed. New York: Plenum Press; 1990:151–182.

24. Greenberg D, Gibbs J, Smith GP. Corn oil decreases gastric emptying more in obese than lean Zucker rats. *Eastern Psychol Assn Abstr.* 1987;58:48.

25. Joyner KS, Smith GP. Differential effects of four sugars on sham feeding by obese and lean Zucker rats. *Eastern Psychol Assoc Abstr.* 1986;57:65.

26. Greenberg D, Lewis DR, Philopena JM, Smith GP. Effect of dilutions of corn oil on intake and preference in lean and obese male Zucker rats. *Soc Neurosci Abstr.* 1992;18:1232.

27. Greenberg D, Weatherford SC. Obese and lean Zucker rats differ in their preferences for sham fed corn oil or sucrose. *Am J Physiol.* 1990; 259:R1093–R1095.

28. Lewis DR, Philopena JM, Greenberg D. Obese and lean male Zucker rats differ in preferences for sham fed corn oil. *Eastern Psychol Assn Abstr.* 1991;62:135.

VIOLAINE ROLLAND, ISABELLE HAINAULT,
ERIC HAJDUCH, MICHÈLE GUERRE-MILLO,
ANNIE QUIGNARD-BOULANGÉ, RAYMOND BAZIN,
ISABELLE DUGAIL, and MARCELLE LAVAU

Fatty Genotype Effect on Adipocyte Lipogenic Gene Expression: Implication of Transactivating Factors

ABSTRACT

The obesity in the Zucker rat is of autosomal and recessive inheritance and is caused by a single gene mutation (*fa* for fatty). The nature of this gene remains totally unknown. This rat develops a syndrome that shares many features with human obesity, providing a useful experimental model. An early phenotypic trait that develops in this mutant prior to hyperphagia and prior to hyperinsulinemia is an increase in fat cell size, suggesting the presence in these cells of a "metabolic pull" channeling nutrients into triglycerides. Consistently, a subset of lipid storage enzymes, lipoprotein lipase, glucose transporter GLUT4, glyceraldehyde-3-phosphate dehydrogenase, fatty acid synthase, and malic enzyme, display excessive activity. Studies of the underlying molecular mechanisms showed that the primary responsible step was an overexpression of the genes arising primarily from an increased transcriptional activity. In an attempt to clarify the mechanism by which the increased transcription of these genes is driven in obese rat adipocytes we developed a system of transiently transfected adipocytes using lipogenic gene promoters fused to gene reporters. We provide evidence that promoter activities of glyceraldehyde-3-phosphate dehydrogenase, fatty acid synthetase and glucose transporter GLUT4 were several times higher in adipocytes from obese rats than in those from lean rats, clearly indicating that the fatty mutation affected transcription factors. 5' deletion analysis of glyceraldehyde-3-phosphate dehydrogenase and GLUT4 promoters allowed us to delineate regions critical to the genotype-mediated increase in promoter activities suggesting that they

175

harbor *fa*-response element(s). The nature of the *fa*-dependent transactivating factor(s) targeting these *fa*(RE) remains to be elucidated.

Introduction

The obesity of the Zucker rat, first described by Zucker and Zucker (1) is inherited as an autosomal recessive mutation. It is caused by a single gene defect, called *fa* for fatty, that has been mapped recently to chromosome 5 (2) but remains totally obscure. These rats develop a syndrome with multiple metabolic and hormonal disorders that closely resembles human obesity. Hyperphagia, hyperinsulinemia, hypertriglyceridemia, hypertrophy and hyperplasia of fat cells, as well as insulin resistance and renal complications, are features common to both species (3). Therefore, the unraveling of the biochemical defect in fatty rats might prove to be useful to a better understanding of human obesity in cases in which genetic factors also play a major role (4–6).

Early in life, the young mutant rat pup presents few disorders. In contrast to the complex profile displayed by the adult obese rat, the only detectable phenotypic alteration in the neonate is an increase in body fat deposits (7) and fat cell size (8), which develop well in advance of the onset of hyperphagia and hyperinsulinemia. This strongly suggests that the cellular energy homeostasis is disrupted by the expression of the mutated gene occurring primarily in adipocytes.

Therefore, as an approach to the nature of the mutation, we have attempted to identify the early metabolic disorders taking place in adipocytes and to elucidate the underlying molecular events. We have provided evidence that a subset of lipid storage genes are overexpressed because of a coordinate increase in transcription rates. This coordinate overtranscription was found to be orchestrated by the presence of *fa*-dependent transacting factors, as revealed by the large increase in the capacity of obese rat adipocytes to transactivate transfected lipogenic gene promoters, indicating transfactors as a potential site of the fatty mutation.

Material and Methods

The rats used in these studies were bred in our laboratory from pairs originally provided by the Harriet G. Bird Memorial Laboratory, Stowe,

Massachusetts. Known heterozygous (*Fa/fa*) lean females and obese males (*fa/fa*) were mated. From this mating, 50% of the littermates are expected to be obese and 50% are expected to be lean and of the heterozygous (*Fa/fa*) genotype. We selected litters numbering between nine and twelve pups of both sexes.

In studies of pups younger than 16 days of age the tissues were removed by surgery under ether anesthesia in order to keep the pups alive for later genotype identification. Some litters were used for both the total lipectomy of the right inguinal fat pad and liver biopsy ($\approx$20 mg). In studies of pups 16 days old, the animals were killed and their genotype was diagnosed by plotting the fat pad weight versus body weight as previously described (9). Enzyme activity determinations, Western and Northern blot analysis, nuclear run-on transcription assays, and Southern analysis have been described previously (10).

Transfection of Isolated Rat Adipocytes

Isolated adipose cells were prepared by collagenase digestion of inguinal fat pads. Cells were washed three times and resuspended in Dulbecco's modified eagle medium (DMEM). Then 0.2 mL of cell suspension (about 4×10^5 cells) was distributed in 0.4 cm gap electroporation cuvettes (Eurogentec, Seraing, Belgium) containing plasmid DNA, and electroporation was performed at 200 V and a capacitance of 960 microforad using a gene pulser apparatus (Biorad). Cells were then transferred to 2 mL Eppendorf tubes containing 1.5 mL of DMEM supplemented with 10% fetal calf serum (Gibco), 20 mmol glucose, antibiotics (100 U/mL penicillin, 100 μg/mL streptomycin). After 24 or 40 hours at 37°C in 7.5% CO_2/92.5% humidified air atmosphere cells were then washed with phosphate buffered saline (PBS). The infranatant was removed and 100 μL of lysis buffer (0.25 mol Tris-HCl pH 8, 5 nmol dithiothreitol [DTT]) added. After sonication and centrifugation at 12 000 g for 15 minutes, a clear cell lysate was obtained and aliquots used for chloramphenicol acelyltransferase (CAT) and luciferase determinations. Gene reporter activities driven by eukaryotic promoters were normalized to the activities of cotransfected viral promoter.

Results and Discussion

An early abnormality present in adipose tissue of mutant pups is an increased activity of fatty acid synthetase (FAS), a key lipogenic enzyme that is detectable during the first days of life (7). As shown in Figure 1, this alteration precedes the onset of hyperinsulinemia. In contrast to adipose tissue the hepatic FAS overactivity develops only after weaning as a secondary manifestation of the obese state, when hyperphagia and hyperinsulinemia have been established (11).

Finding an overactivity of FAS raised the question of whether the molecular mechanism responsible for this alteration was caused by changes in structure, mass, or stability of the protein. This was an important issue, since this information had the potential to illuminate the nature of the genetic lesion. To this end we purified the enzyme from both obese and lean rat adipose tissues and raised an anti-FAS antibody. We observed that FAS electrophoretic mobility was identical in the two genotypes (migration as a single band of approximatedly 220 000 daltons molecular weight). Purified enzymes also had similar specific activities (1650 nmol of NADPH oxidized per minute per milligram protein at 35°C) and identical Km values for substrates (10); in addition, the immunoreactivity of the enzymes as assessed by immunotitration was not different. These observations suggested that FAS overactivity in adipose tissue of obese rats was mediated by an increase in enzyme mass rather than by structural changes (10). In order to further document this point we devised an absolute quantitative immunoblotting assay for FAS mass, taking advantage of the availability of highly purified FAS and monospecific antibody. Figure 2 clearly shows that there is a very close relationship between the genotype effect on FAS activity and FAS mass, with identical fold increase between the two parameters both at 16 and 30 days of age. These studies revealed that FAS, at 30 days of age, was a major protein in obese rat adipocytes amounting to 13% of total cytosolic protein, whereas it did not represent more than 2% in lean rat adipocytes. In order to clarify the mechanism involved in the overabundance of FAS protein in adipose tissue from obese as compared to lean rats, the relative rates of FAS synthesis were examined in 30-day-old rats using the pulse labeling method. We found that FAS synthesis in the mutant rat represents 17% of the synthesis of total soluble proteins, a finding in excellent agreement with the conclusion that FAS is a major cytosolic protein in adipose tissue from obese rats. The conclusion of the pretranslational level of regulation of FAS by the fatty genotype was further supported by the observation that FAS mRNA was increased four- and fourteenfold over those of lean rats at 16 and 30 days of age, respectively.

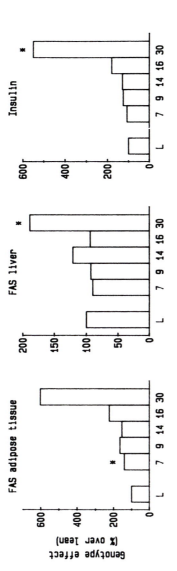

Figure 1. Fatty genotype effect on fatty acid synthetase activity in adipose tissue and liver and on insulinemia in 7- to 16-day-old suckling pups and in postweaning 30-day-old rats. Lean values are set to 100.

*Significant at the level $P = 0.05$ or less.

Computed from previously published data (11).

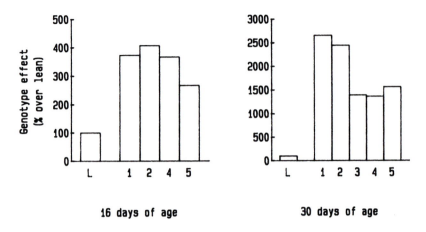

16 days of age   30 days of age

Figure 2. Fatty genotype effect on fatty acid synthetase activity (1), mass (2), synthesis rate (3), mRNA level (4), and transcription rates (5) in inguinal adipose tissue from suckling 16-day-old pups and in postweaning 30-day-old rats. Lean values are set to 100.

Computed from previously published data (10).

The question of whether transcription rate increases were the determinant of these changes in mRNA was assessed by run-on assays in isolated adipose cell nuclei. As shown in Figure 2, FAS gene transcription rates were increased in close proportion to FAS mRNA changes, providing strong evidence that the transcriptional level was the primary defective step responsible for FAS overexpression in this genetic obesity. The possibility that FAS gene overtranscription might result from large gene modifications was examined by Southern analysis of genomic DNA, which showed that after digestion with several restriction enzymes the intensities and the patterns of restriction fragments detected by using a FAS cDNA probe were strictly identical in lean and obese rats, making gene amplification or large structural alterations unlikely (10). Altogether these data suggested that FAS was a target of the mutated gene rather than the site of the mutation.

This conclusion raised the question of whether, concomitantly to FAS, other genes were overtranscribed in adipose tissue of young mutant pups. As shown in Figure 3, a number of lipid storage–related genes such as lipoprotein lipase, malic enzyme, glyceraldehyde-3-phosphate dehydrogenase (12–14), and glucose transporter GLUT4 (15) already were found to be overexpressed by 16 days of age, in close pro-

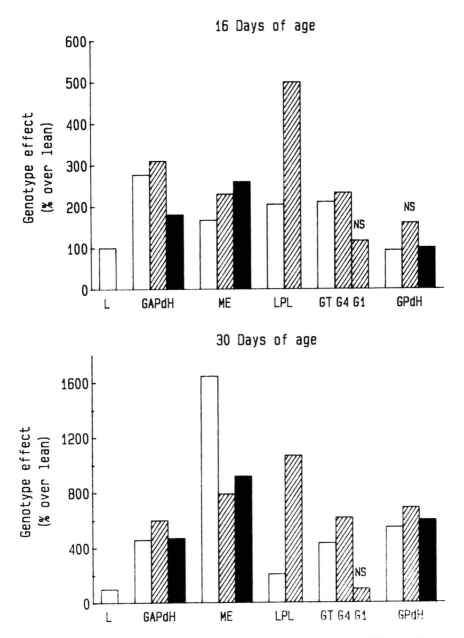

Figure 3. Fatty genotype effect on enzyme or glucose transport (GT) activities (white bars) on mRNA levels (striped bars) and transcription rates (black bars) in inguinal adipose tissue. Lean rat values are set to 100. GAPDH: glyceraldehyde-3-phosphate dehydrogenas; ME: malic enzyme; LPL: lipoprotein lipase; G4: GLUT4; G1: GLUT1; GPDH: glycerophosphate dehydrogenase; NS: not significant.

Computed from previously published data (11–15).

portion to the increase in their respective activity. In contrast there was no change in the expression of GLUT1 (15) or glycerophosphate dehydrogenase genes (13), pointing out the specificity of the genotype effect. After weaning (30 days of age), an increase in the glycerophosphate dehydrogenase (GPDH) mRNA level emerged in obese rats and genotype-mediated differences were dramatically amplified for lipoprotein lipase, malic enzyme, and GLUT4 mRNAs, suggesting an interaction between genotype and dietary carbohydrates, and/or hyperinsulinemia or other developmental factors. However, GLUT1 mRNA levels remained unchanged. Transcription rates were assessed by run-on analysis for malic enzyme, glyceraldehyde-3-phosphate dehydrogenase, and glycerophosphate dehydrogenase in lean and obese Zucker rats aged either 16 or 30 days (13). The results illustrated in Figure 3 clearly show that, at both 16 and 30 days of age, changes in transcription rates fully accounted for changes in mRNA levels. Collectively these data argued for the existence of transacting factor(s) in adipocytes of genetically obese rats that would trigger the expression of this subset of genes. In order to test this hypothesis, we transiently transfected metabolic gene promoters fused to gene reporters into primary cultured rat adipocytes (16, 17). Using pFAS-CAT, pGAPDH-CAT, or pGLUT4-luciferase plasmids electroporated into lean or obese rat adipocytes, we found that obese rat fat cells have an increased capacity to transcribe these three genes, ranging several times over that of lean rat adipocytes (Fig. 4). These data clearly establish the presence of *fa* genotype–dependent transactivating factors in adipocytes from obese rats. Deletion analysis of GAPDH and GLUT4 promoters revealed the presence of sequences critical to the genotype-mediated increases in transcription, suggesting that these regions harbored *fa*-responsive elements (16, 17). The nature of *cis* and *trans* factors involved in the fatty genotype effect is currently being approached through studies of differential polypeptide expression (18, 19) and nuclear protein-DNA interactions in adipocytes of lean and obese rats.

In conclusion, our studies with the first demonstration that *fa* gene affects adipocyte transcription factor(s) have allowed us to narrow down the primary functional effect of the *fa* mutation. Through their activation of fat storage genes these transfactors are to play a crucial pathogenic role in the disruption of the caloric homeostasis of adipocytes leading to a pull in of glucose (20). They have the potential to

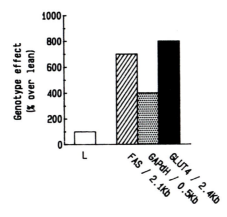

Figure 4. Fatty genotype effect on promoter activities in transiently transfected adipocytes from lean and obese rats. Lean rat values are set to 100.
Computed from previously published data (16, 17).

account for the development of obesity independently of hyperphagia, which is a salient feature of the obese Zucker rat (8, 21, 22).

ACKNOWLEDGMENTS

We are grateful to C. Guichard and X. Le Liepvre for their expert assistance. We wish to thank Drs. M. Alexander-Bridges, D. B. Jump and S. D. Clarke, and J. Pessin for their kind gifts of pGAPdH-CAT, pFAS-CAT, and pGLUT 4-luciferase plasmids, respectively.

REFERENCES

1. Zucker LM, Zucker TF. Fatty, a new mutation in the rat. *J Hered.* 1961;62:275–278.
2. Truett GE, Bahary N, Friedman JM, Leibel RL. Rat obesity gene fatty (*fa*) maps to chromosome 5: evidence for homology with the mouse gene diabetes (db). *Proc Natl Acad Sci USA.* 1991;88:7806–7809.
3. Bray GA, York DA. Hypothalamic and genetic obesity in experimental animals: an autosomic and endocrine hypothesis. *Physiol Rev.* 1979;59:719–809.
4. Stunkard AJ, Sorensen TIA, Harris G, Teasdale TN. An adoption study of human obesity. *N Engl J Med.* 1986;314:193–198.

5. Bouchard C. Genes and body fat. *Am J Hum Biol.* 1993;5:425–432.

6. Friedman JM, Leibel RL. Tackling a weighty problem. *Cell.* 1992;69:217–220.

7. Lavau M, Bazin R, Guerre-Millo M. Increased capacity for fatty acid synthesis in white and brown adipose tissues from 7-day-old obese Zucker pups. *Int J Obes.* 1985;9(suppl 1):61–66.

8. Boulangé A, Planche E, de Gasquet P. Onset of genetic obesity in the absence of hyperphagia during the first week of life in the Zucker rat *fa/fa*. *J Lipid Res.* 1979;20:857–864.

9. Lavau M, Bazin R. Inguinal fat pad weight plotted versus body weight as a method of genotype identification in 16-day-old Zucker rats. *J Lipid Res.* 1982;23:941–943.

10. Guichard C, Dugail I, Le Liepvre X, Lavau M. Genetic regulation of fatty acid synthetase expression in adipose tissue: overtranscription of the gene in genetically obese rats. *J Lipid Res.* 1992;33:679–687.

11. Bazin R, Lavau M. Development of hepatic and adipose tissue lipogenic enzymes and insulinemia during suckling and weaning on to a high-fat diet in Zucker rats. *J Lipid Res.* 1982;23:839–849.

12. Dugail I, Quignard-Boulangé A, Bazin R, Le Liepvre X, Lavau M. Adipose-tissue-specific increase in glyceraldehyde-3-phosphate dehydrogenase activity and mRNA amounts in suckling pre-obese Zucker rats. *Biochem J.* 1988;254:483–487.

13. Dugail I, Quignard-Boulangé A, Le Liepvre X, Ardouin B, Lavau M. Gene expression of lipid storage–related enzymes in adipose tissue of the genetically obese Zucker rat. *Biochem J.* 1992;281:607–611.

14. Dugail I, Quignard-Boulangé A, Brigant L, Etienne J, Noe L, Lavau M. Increased lipoprotein lipase content in the adipose tissue of suckling and weaning obese Zucker rats. *Biochem J.* 1988;249:45–49.

15. Hainault I, Guerre-Millo M, Guichard C, Lavau M. Differential regulation of adipose tissue glucose transporters in genetic obesity (fatty rat). *J Clin Invest.* 1991;87:1127–1131.

16. Hainault I, Hajduch E, Lavau M. Fatty genotype-induced increase in GLUT4 promoter activity in transfected adipocytes: delineation of two *fa*-responsive regions and glucose effect. *Biochem Biophys Res Commun.* 1995;209:1053–1061.

17. Rolland V, Dugail I, Le Liepvre X, Lavau M. Evidence of increased glyceraldehyde-3-phosphate dehydrogenase and fatty acid synthe-

tase promoter activities in transiently transfected adipocytes from genetically obese rats. *J Biol Chem.* 1995;270:1102–1106.

18. Rolland V, Le Liepvre X, Houbiguian ML, Lavau M, Dugail I. C/EBPα expression in adipose tissue of genetically obese Zucker rats. *Biochem Biophys Res Commun.* 1995;207:761–767.

19. Laurent-Winter C, Dugail I, Quignard-Boulangé A, Le Liepvre X, Lavau M. Differential polypeptide expression in adipose tissue of lean and obese Zucker rats. *Biochem J.* 1992;284:813–817.

20. Krief S, Bazin R, Dupuy F, Lavau M. Increased in vivo glucose utilization in 30-day-old obese Zucker rat: role of white adipose tissue. *Am J Physiol.* 1988;254:E342–E348.

21. Bray GA, York DA, Swerloff RS. Genetic obesity in the rat: the effect of food restriction on body composition and hypothalamic function. *Metabolism.* 1973;22:435–442.

22. Cleary MP, Vasselli JP, Greenwood MRC. Development of obesity in Zucker obese *fa/fa* rat in absence of hyperphagia. *Am J Physiol.* 1980;238:284–292.

NICOLE BÉGIN-HEICK

β-Adrenergic Receptors and G Proteins in Genetic Obesity

ABSTRACT

Lipolysis and adenylyl cyclase activation in response to β-adrenergic agents are abnormally low in white epididymal adipose tissue of the *ob/ob* mouse. The abundance of the two principal G-proteins that control the transduction of adenylyl cyclase is abnormally low in several tissues of the *ob/ob* mouse. By contrast, β-adrenergic receptor levels appear normal in adipose tissue and are elevated in liver. The relative importance of β-adrenergic receptor activity and G protein levels in the response of the *ob/ob* mouse was reassessed in view of the discovery of the β_3-adrenergic receptor and to assess the effect of hypercortiscism in the *ob/ob* mice. The results show the following: the β_3-adrenergic receptor is the major beta adrenergic receptor (βAR) isoform in mouse adipose tissue; the levels of these receptors are severely decreased in the obese mouse; adrenalectomy of the *ob/ob* mouse does not restore normal beta response in adipose tissue, though it does so in the liver; β_3-receptor function in adipose tissue is extremely sensitive to the ambient concentrations of guanosine triphosphate (GTP).

Among the many models of genetic obesity in rodents, the most extensively studied has probably been the *ob/ob* mouse. The obese-hyperglycemic syndrome in mice is associated with hyperinsulinemia, hyperglycemia, and extreme resistance of tissues to insulin. In addition, adrenal hyperplasia and hypercortiscism are present and are believed to contribute to the development of obesity (1–3). Although the principal visible outcome of the syndrome is fat accretion, especially in adipose tissues and liver, most body systems seem to be affected by the syndrome (*cf.* 4).

186

The finding of a defect in catecholamine-stimulated lipolysis and the central importance of the adipocyte in maintaining energy balance led to the study of the adenylyl cyclase system. Early studies showed that adenylyl cyclase and the downstream lipolytic machinery behaved normally in adipose tissue of the *ob/ob* mouse (*cf.* 5). By contrast, β-adrenergic stimulation elicits much lower levels of cAMP in obese-mouse adipocyte membranes than in lean-mouse adipocyte membranes. It therefore seemed appropriate to center the search for the cause of the anomaly on the signaling system responsible for the modulation of cAMP production. Guanosine triphosphate (GTP) has long been known to have a bimodal effect on adenylyl cyclase activity stimulated by β-adrenergic ligands in white adipocyte membranes of rats (*cf.* 6). This bimodal effect of GTP is also present in white adipocyte membranes of the normal lean mouse, but it is absent in the *ob/ob* mouse and only partially evident in the heterozygote (+ /*ob*) (7). Taken together, these results pointed to a role for G proteins in the lipolytic defect of the *ob/ob* mouse.

G protein Levels in Tissues of Lean and Obese Mice

Two classes of heterotrimeric (αβγ) G proteins, G_s and G_i, have been implicated in the modulation of adenylyl cyclase activity in tissues. Although initially the modulatory activity was believed to be vested in the alpha subunits, it is now clear that the beta and γ subunits, each of which exists in several isoforms, confer specificity, diversity, and versatility to the alpha subunits (8–10). There are several isoforms of the catalytic subunit of adenylyl cyclase in tissues, some of which differ in their mode of regulation by G-proteins. Types 4, 5, and 6 appear to be the most ubiquitously distributed, but the form(s) present in adipose tissues has not yet been determined (*cf.* 11).

Experiments aimed at defining the types and amounts of G proteins in several tissues of the *ob/ob* mouse revealed that in epididymal adipocytes and liver membranes, both $G_s\alpha$ and $G_i\alpha$ were present in abnormally low amounts, whereas in testis, only $G_s\alpha$ was affected (Fig. 1). Mainly the long (45 kilodaltons [kd]) form of $G_s\alpha$ and the form of $G_i\alpha$ (40 kd) corresponding to $G_i\alpha2$ were affected in adipocytes and liver (12, 13), whereas in testis, only the short form of $G_s\alpha$ was decreased (14). With the antibodies available, no difference was noted in the abundance of beta subunits either at the mRNA or at the protein level in

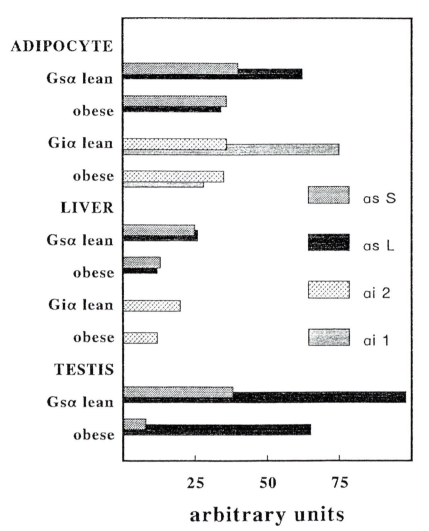

Figure 1.   Immunodetection of G$_s$ and G$_i$ alpha subunits in tissues of lean and obese mice. Immunodetection was carried out with specific antibodies as described in detail previously (13). αs S and αs L refer to the short (42 kd) and long (45 kd) forms of G$_s$; αi 2 and αi 1 refer to the two forms of G$_i$ most abundant in these tissues.

any of these tissues. A comparative study with the *db/db* mouse, another model of genetic obesity, revealed similar alterations in G-protein levels in the adipose tissue and liver of that model, without the attendant effects on adenylyl cyclase response in either tissue (15, 16). This suggested that factors other than, or in addition to, the abundance of the alpha subunit of these G proteins were at play.

β-Adrenergic Receptor Subtypes in Mouse Adipose Tissue

The presence of an "atypical" β-adrenergic receptor specific to adipose tissues had long been suspected, based on pharmacological studies (17, 18). The cloning of the β_3-adrenergic receptor in man (19), mouse (20), and rat (21, 22) has revealed that it is expressed at high levels, if not exclusively, in adipose tissue of many species. This has also allowed the structural properties (20, 23–27) and function (28–36) of the receptor to be investigated. Species differences are evident in the ability of β_3-receptor agonist to stimulate lipolysis: rat and hamster are classed as hyperresponders, rabbit and dog as hyporesponders, and man and guinea pig are considered nonresponders on the basis of their relative lipolytic response to selective β_3-agonists versus nonselective β-agonists (37). The expression of the β_3-adrenergic receptor mRNA is depressed in white and brown adipose tissue of the *fa/fa* rat compared with lean controls (21), suggesting that β_3-receptor activity is altered in obesity, and thus suggesting a mechanism for the propensity of these tissues to accumulate lipids. Although the mouse β_3-adrenergic receptor has been cloned and characterized (20) and some of its functions studied in an adipogenic murine cell line (26), until recently, β_3-adrenergic receptor function had not been studied in the mouse, and in particular, the *ob/ob* mouse.

β-Adrenergic agonists and antagonists have low potency in activating adenylyl cyclase in lean-mouse adipocyte membranes (10 μM), compared with similar preparations from other species, such as the rat, dog, or guinea pig in which the EC_{50} for isoproterenol is ≈1 μM (30, 34, 36).* Paradoxically, in obese-mouse adipocyte membranes, the intrinsic activity of epinephrine and norepinephrine relative to isoproterenol is greater than in lean-mouse membranes, though the maximal adenylyl cyclase activity that can be elicited by any agonist in these membranes is only a fraction of that obtained in lean-mouse mem-

*The potency of an agonist for adenylyl cyclase activation in membrane preparation is usually at least ten times lower than the potency of the same agonist for lipolysis or other function assessed in whole cells.

branes (Table 1). By contrast, the specific β_3-receptor agonist, CL-316,243 (38) has the highest potency of all agonists tested in lean- and obese-mouse adipocyte membranes (EC_{50} = 1 and 2 μM, respectively against 10 μM and higher for isoproterenol).

The low potency of several β_1- and β_2-adrenergic receptor selective antagonists in adipose tissue has long been recognized and, indeed, has served as the basis for the development of the concept of the β_3-receptor (18). Mouse adipose tissue is no exception. A number of β-antagonists had similar effects when assayed against half maximally active concentrations of isoproterenol (10 μM) or CL-316,243 (1 μM), suggesting that the stimulatory effect of the "classical" β-adrenergic agonists in lean-mouse membranes is due to their interaction with the β_3-adrenergic receptors.

As shown in Table 1, under conditions in which cyclase is either maximally activated (100 nM) or maximally inhibited (100 μM) by GTP, propranolol, a β_1/β_2 antagonist, has no effect on cyclase activity elicited by either isoproterenol (ISO) or by CL-316,243 (CL) in membranes from lean mice. This shows that isoproterenol elicits adenylyl cyclase activity via a β_3, rather than a β_1/β_2 effect. By contrast, in membranes from obese mice, propranolol inhibits isoproterenol-stimulated cyclase activity at high (100 μM) but not at low (100 nM) GTP and is without effect on CL-316,243-stimulated activity at either concentration. This shows that the receptor balance has been altered in the obese mouse, such that a decrease in β_3-receptor unmasks β_1/β_2 effects. Taken together, these data show that the β-adrenergic receptor complement of lean- and

Table 1. Effect of Propranolol on β-Agonist-Stimulated Adenylyl Cyclase Activity in Adipocyte Membranes

[GTP]	+/+		ob/ob	
	100 nM	100 μM	100 nM	100 μM
Ligands	pmol/mg protein/min			
ISO (100 μM)	1090 ± 81	413 ± 60	239 ± 14	450 ± 45
ISO + Pr (1 μM)	982 ± 59	323 ± 51	265 ± 8	224 ± 27*
CL (10 μM)	1140 ± 101	314 ± 12	239 ± 10	189 ± 2
CL + Pr (1 μM)	1046 ± 97	279 ± 8	228 ± 14	176 ± 9

*Significantly different from ISO alone.

obese-mouse adipocytes is different and is likely to be responsible for the resistance to lipolysis characteristic of obese-mouse adipocytes. In guinea pig adipocyte membranes, which are devoid of β_3-adrenergic receptors, 1 μM propranolol inhibits isoproterenol-stimulated activity completely at all GTP concentrations and CL-316,243 is unable to elicit cyclase activation. Currently, the lack of specific β_3 antagonists and labeled ligands impedes the precise quantification of the β_3 receptor subtype. However, it has been reported that lean-mouse adipocytes have 20% β_1/β_2- and 80% β_3-adrenergic receptors, whereas obese-mouse adipocytes express mostly the β_2, but little if any of the β_1 and β_3 receptor (39). The extremely low level of expression of the β_3 receptor mRNA reported in that study is surprising, in view of the significant functional activity elicited by β_3-agonists in obese-mouse β_2-membranes.

The Effect of GTP on β_3-Receptor-Stimulated Adenylyl Cyclase Activity

Adipose tissue adenylyl cyclase activity is regulated by GTP in a bimodal fashion; the nucleotide stimulates at low concentrations (below 100 nM) and inhibits at higher concentrations. Paradoxically, this bimodal effect of GTP is enhanced in the presence of β-adrenergic agonists and the inhibitory phase is relieved by treatment with pertussis, but not cholera, toxin (40). This was interpreted as meaning that at high GTP concentrations the β-adrenergic receptor somehow couples via the inhibitory G protein G_i. However, since these initial observations, the adenylyl cyclase signaling system has been shown to be much more complex than had then been anticipated, with diverse arrangements of G protein subunits having the potential to modulate several classes of adenylyl cyclases.

Isoproterenol, epinephrine, norepinephrine, and other β-agonists can enhance the bimodal effect of GTP in lean-mouse membranes, and relief from inhibition can be obtained by treatment with pertussis toxin. By contrast, the bimodal effect of GTP is not revealed by these agonists in obese-mouse membranes; therefore, pertussis toxin does not significantly enhance adenylyl cyclase activity at μM GTP concentrations (Fig. 2). However, the biphasic effect of GTP is evident in membranes of both the lean and obese mouse when specific β_3-agonist such as CL-316,243 and BRL-37344 are the agonists. These data taken together with the ability of propranolol to inhibit isoproterenol-stimulated activity

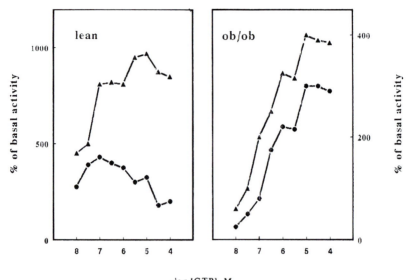

Figure 2.   The effect of pertussis toxin on agonist-stimulated activity. Adipocyte membranes pre-incubated with (triangles) or without (circles) activated
pertussis toxin were assayed for adenylyl cyclase activity using 100 μM isoproterenol and the indicated concentrations of GTP. The data are expressed as
percent stimulation over basal activity.

(an effect of its ability to antagonize β_1/β_2 receptors) at high GTP in
obese-mouse but not lean-mouse membranes (Table 1) support the
view that the bimodal effect of GTP is vested in the β_3-adrenergic receptor. The mechanism whereby this occurs is unclear. The fact that the
inhibitory phase induced by GTP in the presence of β-adrenergic activation is relieved by treatment with pertussis toxin (Fig. 2) would seem
to implicate coupling via G_i. This seems unlikely, however, in view of
the highly selective nature of the new β_3-agonists. It is more likely that
a solution to this enigma should be sought in the complex interactions
between αβγ subunits of G_s, as it couples to the β_3-adrenergic receptor
and the subsequent effect on adenylyl cyclase.

Effects of Adrenal Steroids on
β-Adrenoreceptor Function in Obesity

Corticosteroids have been demonstrated to regulate β-adrenergic receptors and thus potentially to alter cAMP production. For example,

the β$_2$-adrenergic receptor is up-regulated by dexamethasone in smooth muscle cells of the hamster (41, 42). Similarly, it has been demonstrated that exposure of the adipogenic cell, 3T3-F442A, results in up-regulation of the β$_2$- and down-regulation of the β$_3$-adrenergic receptor (26, 42, 43). It was therefore pertinent to establish whether the hypercorticism prevalent in the *ob/ob* mouse in some way alters the complement of β-adrenergic receptor present in tissues. Adenylyl cyclase activity was measured in adipose tissue and liver of the obese mouse two weeks after adrenalectomy (ADX) or sham operation (SHM) in comparison with that found in normal lean mice. Adrenalectomy did not alter the response in adipocyte membranes (Table 2). By contrast, the exaggerated β$_2$-adrenergic response of obese-mouse liver membranes is returned to normal by adrenalectomy and parallels a decrease in the number of receptor binding sites (16). This shows that correcting the hypercorticism normalizes β$_2$-adrenergic receptor activity in obese-mouse liver. The apparent lack of effect of treatment in adipose tissue from the same animals suggests that either the adipose tissue β$_2$-adrenergic receptor is not affected by adrenal steroids or that any effect is masked by the presence of other receptors. Unfortunately, specific antibodies reactive against mouse β-adrenergic receptors are not yet available to help distinguish between these possibilities. However, the finding that adrenalectomy did not improve β$_3$-adrenergic receptor function in the obese mouse supports the view that receptor regulation is not sensitive to these hormones in mature adipocytes.

Table 2. Effect of Adrenalectomy on Adenylyl Cyclase Activation in Adipocyte Membranes

	Lean	Obese SHM	Obese ADX
	Adenylyl cyclase activity pmol/mg protein/min (fold stimulation)		
Basal	52.4 ± 9.5(1)	20 ± 2.9(1)	24.5 ± 2.9(1)
GTP, 100 nM	60.9 ± 9.7(1.2)	31 ± 2.3(1.6)	31.5 ± 3.8(1.3)
GTP + ISO*	655 ± 113(13.8)	85 ± 4.6(4.5)	137 ± 8.3(5.2)
GTP + EPI	357 ± 38(7.8)	51 ± 1.1(2.8)	62 ± 8.4(2.5)
GTP + NEPI	327 ± 41(7.1)	58 ± 3.7(3.0)	76 ± 16.4(3.0)
GTP + CL	625 ± 126(12.8)	112 ± 7.7(5.9)	154 ± 20(6.3)

*All agonists used at 100 μM.

Conclusions

Although G proteins are less abundant in many tissues of obese mice compared with their lean counterparts, this phenomenon is not necessarily correlated to decreases in the transduction of hormonal signals. Indeed, in liver membranes from *ob/ob* mice, β-adrenergic stimulation of adenylyl cyclase is enhanced threefold over that obtained in lean mice, in correlation with the number of β_2-adrenergic binding sites. Adrenalectomy corrects both the exaggerated receptor number and cyclase activation, but not the abnormally low abundance of G protein. In adipocyte membranes, it appears that the abundance and type of β-adrenergic receptor are also the most important determinants. The low level of β_3-receptor responsiveness likely is the factor limiting β-adrenergic activation of adenylyl cyclase and lipolysis in the *ob/ob* mouse.

ACKNOWLEDGMENTS

Thanks are due to the Medical Research Council of Canada for grant support and to Pascale Reinhardt-Poulin for expert technical assistance.

REFERENCES

1. Saito M, Bray GA. Diurnal rhythm for corticosterone in obese (*ob/ob*), diabetes (*db/db*), and gold-thiglucose-induced obesity in mice. *Endocrinol.* 1983;113:2181–2185.
2. Bailey CJ, Day C, Bray GA, Lipson LG, Flatt PR. Role of adrenal glands in the development of abnormal glucose and insulin homeostasis in genetically obese (*ob/ob*) mice. *Horm Metab Res.* 1986; 18:357–360.
3. Shimomura Y, Bray GA, Lee M. Adrenalectomy and steroid treatment in obese (*ob/ob*) and diabetic (*db/db*) mice. *Horm Metab Res.* 1987;19:295–299.
4. Bray GA, York DA. Genetically transmitted obesity in rodents. *Physiol Rev.* 1979;51:598–646.
5. Bégin-Heick N, McFarlane-Anderson, N. G-proteins in obesity syndromes. In: Milligan G, Wakelam M, eds. *G-Proteins in Disease States.* London: Academic Press; 1992:129–156.
6. Cooper DMF, Schliegel W, Lin MC, Rodbell M. The fat cell aden-

ylate cyclase system; characterization and manipulation of its bi-modal regulation by GTP. *J Biol Chem.* 1979;256:8927–8931.

7. Bégin-Heick N. Absence of the inhibitory effect of guanine nucle-otides on adenylate cyclase activity in white adipocyte membranes of the *ob/ob* mouse. *J Biol Chem.* 1985;260:6187–6193.

8. Iñiguez-Lluhi J, Kleuss C, Gilman AG. The importance of G-protein βγ subunits. *Trends Cell Biol.* 1993;3:230–236.

9. Kleuss C, Scherübl H, Herscheler J, Schultz G, Wittig B. Different β-subunits determine G-protein interaction with transmembrane receptors. *Nature.* 1992;358:424–426.

10. Kleuss C, Scherübl H, Herscheler J, Schultz G, Wittig B. Selectivity in signal transduction determined by γ subunits of heterotrimeric G proteins. *Science.* 1993;259:832–834.

11. Iyengar R. Multiple families of Gs-regulated adenylyl cyclases. *Adv Second Messenger Phosphoprotein Res.* 1993;28:27–36.

12. McFarlane-Anderson N, Bailly J, Bégin-Heick N. Levels of G-pro-teins in liver and brain of lean and obese (*ob/ob*) mice. *Biochem. J.* 1992;282:15–23.

13. Bégin-Heick N. Quantification of the α and β subunits of the trans-ducing elements (G_s and G_i) of adenylate cyclase in adipocyte mem-branes from lean and obese (*ob/ob*) mice. *Biochem J.* 1990;268:83–89.

14. McFarlane-Anderson N, Bégin-Heick N. mRNA and protein levels of the stimulatory guanine nucleotide regulatory protein G_s are lower in the testis of the obese (*ob/ob*) mouse. *Cell Signal.* 1991;3: 233–241.

15. Bégin-Heick N. (1992) α-Subunits of G_s and G_i in adipocyte plasma membranes of genetically diabetic (*db/db*) mice. *Am J Physiol.* 1992; 263:(Cell Physiol. 32):C121–C129.

16. Bégin-Heick N. Liver β-adrenergic receptors. G-proteins and ad-enylyl cyclase activity in obesity/diabetes syndromes. *Am J Physiol.* 1994;265. In press.

17. Harms HH, Zaagsma J, Vente JD. Differentiation of beta-adreno-ceptors in rat atrium, diaphragm and adipose tissue of the rat, us-ing stereoisomers of propranolol, alprenolol, nifenalol and practo-lol. *Life Sci.* 1974;21:123–128.

18. Arch JRS, Ainsworth AT, Cawthorne MA, *et al.* Atypical beta-adrenoceptor on brown adipocytes as target for anti-obesity drugs. *Nature.* 1984;309:163–165.

19. Emorine LJ, Marullo S, Briend-Sutren M-M, *et al.* Molecular char-

acterisation of the human beta$_3$-adrenergic receptor. *Science.* 1989; 245:1118–1121.

20. Nahmias C, Blin N, Elalouf J-M, Mattei MG, Strosberg AD, Emorine LJ. Molecular characterisation of the mouse beta$_3$-adrenergic receptor: relationship with the atypical receptor of adipocytes. *EMBO J.* 1991;10:3721–3727.

21. Muzzin P, Revelli J-P, Kuhne F, *et al.* An adipose tissue specific beta-adrenergic receptor: molecular cloning and down-regulation in obesity. *J Biol Chem.* 1991;266:24053–24058.

22. Granneman JG, Lahners KN, Chaudry A. Molecular cloning and expression of the rat beta$_3$-adrenergic receptor. *Mol Pharmacol.* 1991; 40:895–899.

23. Van Spronsen A, Nahmias C, Krief S, Briend-Sutren M-M, Strosberg AD, Emorine LJ. The promoter and intron/exon structure of the human and mouse β3-adrenergic-receptor genes. *Eur J Biochem.* 1993;213:1117–1124.

24. Granneman JG, Lahners KN. Differential adrenergic regulation of β$_1$- and β$_3$-adrenoreceptor messenger ribonucleic acids in adipose tissues. *Endocrinology.* 1992;130:109–114.

25. Thomas RF, Holt BD, Schwinn DA, Liggett SB. Long term agonist exposure induces upregulation of β-adrenergic receptor expression via multiple cAMP response elements. *Proc Natl Acad Sci USA.* 1992; 89:4490–4494.

26. Fève B, Baude B, Krief S, Strosberg AD, Pairault J, Emorine LJ. Inhibition by dexamethasone of beta3-adrenergic receptor responsiveness in 3T3-F442A adipocytes: evidence for a transcriptional Mechanism. *J Biol Chem.* 1992;267:15909–15915.

27. Granneman JG, Lahners KN, Chaudhry A. Characterization of the human β$_3$-adrenergic receptor gene. *Mol Pharmacol.* 1993;44:264–270.

28. Carpéné C, Galitzki J, Collon P, Esclapez F, Dauzats M, Lafontan M. Desensitization of *beta*-1 and *beta*-2, but not *beta*-3 adrenoceptor-mediated lipolytic responses of adipocytes after long-term norepinephrine infusion. *J Pharmacol Exp Ther.* 1993;265:237–247.

29. Wheeldon NM, McDevitt DG, Lipworth BJ. Do β$_3$-adrenoceptors mediate metabolic responses to isoprenaline. *Q J Med.* 1993;86:595–600.

30. Murphy GJ, Kirkham DM, Cawthorne MA, Young P. Correlation of β$_3$-adrenoceptor-induced activation of cyclic AMP-dependent

protein kinase with activation of lipolysis in rat white adipocytes. *Biochem Pharmacol.* 1993;46:575–581.

31. Van Liefde I, Witzenburg A, Vauquelin G. Multiple *beta* adrenergic receptor subclasses mediate the *l*-isoproterenol-induced lipolytic responses in rat adipocytes. *J Pharmacol Exp Ther.* 1992;262:552–558.

32. Van Liefde I, Witzenburg A, Vauquelin G. Isoproterenol and selective agonists stimulate similar atypical β-adrenoceptors in rat adipocytes. *Biochem Pharmacol.* 1993;45:974–977.

33. Langin D, Portillo M, Saulnier-Blache J-S, Lafontan M. Coexistence of three β-adrenoceptor subtypes in white fat cells of various mammalian species. *Eur J Pharmacol.* 1991;199:291–301.

34. Langin D, Ekholm D, Ridderstrale M, Lafontan M, Belfrage P. cAMP-dependent protein kinase activation mediated by β_3-adrenergic receptors parallels lipolysis in rat adipocytes. *Biochim Biophys Acta.* 1992;1135:349–352.

35. Galitzky J, Reverte M, Carpéné C, Lafontan M, Berlan M. β3-Adrenoceptors in dog adipose tissue: studies on their involvement in the lipomobilizing effect of catecholamines. *J Pharmacol Exp Ther.* 1993;266:358–366.

36. Galitzky J, Reverte M, Portillo M, Carpéné C, Lafontan M, Berlan M. Coexistence of β_1-, β_2-, and β_3-adrenoceptors in dog fat cells and their differential activation by catecholamines. *Am J Physiol.* 1993; 264:(Endocrinol. Metab. 27):E403–E412.

37. Lafontan M, Berlan M. Fat cell adrenergic receptors and the control of white and brown fat cell function. *J Lipid Res.* 1993;34:1057–1091.

38. Bloom JD, Dutia MD, Johnson BD, *et al.* Disodium (R,R)-5-[2-[[2-(3-chlorophenyl)-2-hydroxyethyl]-amino]propyl]-1,3-benzodiozole-2,2-dicarboxylate (CL 316,243): a potent β-adrenergic agonist virtually specific for β_3 receptors; a promising antidiabetic and antiobesity agent. *J Med Chem.* 1992;35:3081–3084.

39. Collins S, Daniel KW, Rohlfs EM, Taylor IL, Gettys TW. Impaired expression and functional activity of the β_3- and β_1-adrenergic receptors in adipose tissue of congenitally obese (C57Bl/6J *ob/ob*) mice. *J Cell Biochem Suppl.* 1994;18A:177.

40. Murayama T, Ui M. Loss of the inhibitory function of the guanine nucleotide regulatory component of adenylate cyclase due to its ADP ribosylation by islet activating protein, pertussis toxin, in adipocyte membranes. *J Biol Chem.* 1983;258:3319–3326.

41. Collins S, Caron MG, Lefkowitz RJ. β_2-Adrenergic receptors in ham-

ster smooth muscle cells are transcriptionally regulated by glucocorticoids. *J Biol Chem* 1988;263:9067–9070.

42. Hadcock JR, Malbon CC. Regulation of β-adrenergic receptors by
    "permissive" hormones: glucocorticoids increase steady-state lev-
    els of receptor mRNA. *Proc Natl Acad Sci USA.* 1988;85:5021–5025.

43. Féve B, Emorine LJ, Briend-Sutren M-M, Lasnier F, Strosberg AD,
    Pairault J. Differential regulation of beta$_1$- and beta$_2$-adrenergic re-
    ceptor protein and mRNA levels by glucocorticoids during 3T3-
    F442A adipose differentiation. *J Biol Chem.* 1990;265:16343–16349.

H. DOUGLAS BRAYMER, YIBING WANG,
HUIJUN DONG, and DAVID A. YORK

Glucocorticoids in Genetic Obesity

ABSTRACT

Glucocorticoids are involved in all animal obesities. Adrenalectomy of obese (*fa/fa*) Zucker rats prevents obesity, and glucocor-
ticoid-replacement restores the obese phenotype. This dependence
on glucocorticoids is possibly due to differences in transcriptional
regulation of a group of genes involved in metabolism. We have
selected two positively regulated genes to study, malic enzyme
and tyrosine aminotransferase (TAT). We have utilized DNA from
the upstream regions of these genes to study differences in binding
of nuclear protein extracts from homozygous lean and obese animals in band-shift studies. An 882 bp upstream DNA fragment of
the malic enzyme gene and a 2950 bp upstream DNA fragment of
the TAT gene were initially utilized to find protein binding regions
from these two genes that differ between lean and obese animals.
We identified a 222 bp DNA fragment located between -491 and
-712 of the malic enzyme gene that demonstrated a difference in
the band shift pattern between the lean and obese nuclear protein
extracts. This area includes a GRE binding site and a TATA box,
but a fragment containing the GRE binding site alone did not demonstrate any differences in gel retardation with these extracts.
However, the region containing the TATA box is shifted less by
the lean than by the obese nuclear extract at the same total protein
amount, but identically if larger amounts of lean extract are added.
This suggests there is a different concentration of the retarding
protein(s) in lean and obese nuclei. In similar studies of the upstream region of the TAT gene, we have identified a 60 bp fragment containing one of the GRE elements that differs in binding
of lean and obese nuclear proteins.

Introduction

All the animal models of obesity show evidence of glucocorticoid involvement (1). The genetically obese Zucker rat is one of the most thoroughly studied of the models for which clear evidence of glucocorticoid involvement has been presented (2). If the obese Zucker rat (*fa/fa*) is adrenalectomized or type II glucocorticoid receptors are blocked, a further development of obesity is prevented (3, 4). After subsequent treatment with glucocorticoids the obesity is restored. Lean adrenalectomized rats replaced with identical steroid doses do not become obese. At this time the molecular basis for this glucocorticoid dependence of obesity is unclear.

Studies of malic enzyme and glyceraldehyde-3-phosphate dehydrogenase genes have indicated that the mRNA levels of these enzymes are elevated in the obese animals and that the levels decrease upon adrenalectomy (5). Glucocorticoid treatment resulted in an enhanced increase in the level of mRNA in rats with the obese genotype, indicating a direct or indirect role for glucocorticoids in regulating transcription in these genes. This has led to a working hypothesis that the genetic defect in the obese Zucker rat is expressed as a defective protein that is normally involved in the modulation of glucocorticoid regulation of genes. As an initial approach to investigating this hypothesis we are studying the binding of nuclear proteins to the upstream region of glucocorticoid regulated genes in lean and obese Zucker rats. Our approach has been to utilize DNA from the upstream region of the malic enzyme and the tyrosine aminotransferase (TAT) genes. We are utilizing the band shift technique to look for differences in binding of nuclear proteins from lean and obese rats to these DNA regions.

Methods

The emphasis in this paper will be on binding to the upstream region of the TAT gene. We have utilized the upstream region of DNA of TAT from a clone provided by Gunther Schutz (6). This clone contains a 2950 bp upstream DNA fragment of the TAT gene. This DNA was digested with the restriction enzymes *XbaI* and *PstI*, and the resulting 1700 bp fragment was cloned into *pUC19* and the resulting plasmid named *pTAT1.7*. The DNA was also restricted with *PstI* and *EcoRI*; the resulting 1200 bp fragment was cloned into *pUC19*. This plasmid was named *pTAT1.2*. These two plasmids have served as the source of DNA fragments for the band-shift experiments.

The binding proteins were prepared from extracts of purified nuclei of homozygous lean and obese animals. Liver tissue from 4-week-old obese (*fa/fa*) and homozygous lean (*Fa/Fa*) rats was minced and homogenized in a sucrose solution (0.32 mol) containing $MgCl_2$ (1 mmol), DTT (1 mmol), PMSF (1 mmol), Pepstatin A (1 μmol), and Leupeptin (1 μmol), and centrifuged at low speed. The pellet was resuspended in 2.4 mol sucrose containing 1 mmol PMSF and 1 mmol DTT and centrifuged at 43 000 g at 4°C. The pellet was resuspended in the same solution, and Triton X was added to a final concentration of 0.25%. This suspension was centrifuged at low speed and the pellet was used as purified nuclei. The nuclei were lysed using a 10 mmol Tris buffer (pH 8.0) containing 0.4 mol KCl, 1 mmol $MgCl_2$, 1 mmol DTT, and 1 mmol PMSF. The lysate was centrifuged at 150 000 g for one hour, and the supernatant used as nuclear extract. Protein content was assayed using the Bio-Rad dye-binding method.

Ten different restriction fragments of DNA were utilized, covering the region from −52 bp to −2562 bp of the upstream region of TAT. Two additional fragments were generated using polymerase chain reaction (PCR) technology in the region between −2562 and −2370. The DNA fragments were end-labeled using [^{32}P]-dATP and DNA polymerase I Klenow fragment, or in some instances the fragment was labeled using PCR and pairs of 20 bp primers. The PCR-generated labeled fragments were purified using polyacrylamide gel electrophoresis.

Band-shift experiments were performed by incubating protein and DNA at room temperature for 20 minutes in 20μL of 10 mmol Hepes buffer (pH7.9) containing 70 mmol KCl, 5 mmol $MgCl_2$, 0.1 mol EDTA, 0.5 mmol DTT, 15% glycerol, 0.05% NP-40, 3μg nuclear protein, and 30 000 cpm [^{32}P]-labeled DNA fragment. Binding specificity was demonstrated using competition experiments, when in addition to the experimental reaction either excess unlabeled fragment or unrelated unlabeled *Escherichia coli* DNA were added. Band-shifting was then assessed using electrophoresis through 5% polyacrylamide gel with Tris-glycine buffer (pH 8.0) containing 1 mmol EDTA.

The role of glucocorticoid receptor in the formation of the DNA-protein complex was studied using a monoclonal antibody (Affinity BioReagents Co.) against mouse glucocorticoid receptor (7) as a possible inhibitor of complex formation.

Two methods were used to purify proteins from the DNA-protein complexes that were contained in the complex. The first method was to elute the proteins from the excised gel slice using electroelution. In the second approach the proteins were purified using magnetic DNA affinity beads by the method of Gabrielsen and Huet (1993). The purified proteins in each case were analyzed by SDS-PAGE gel electrophoresis and stained using the Bio-Rad silver staining kit.

Results and Discussion

The band-shift experiments demonstrated a difference in the amount of fragment shifted between lean and obese nuclear proteins with six of the DNA fragments (Fig. 1). In every case the obese extract shifted more of the fragment. The region between -2562 and -2370 bp was selected for more thorough examination. An 83 bp and a 60 bp fragment from this region were labeled using PCR. The 83 bp fragment did not show a difference in the band-shift, whereas with the 60 bp fragment there was an increase in the amount of fragment shifted by the obese extract in comparison with the lean.

The possibility that type II glucocorticoid receptor protein was present in the 60 bp DNA-protein complex was investigated by studying the effect of a monoclonal antibody to the receptor on the gel shift. The antibody had no effect on the band-shfit pattern, suggesting that the glucocorticoid receptor protein is not necessary for formation of the complex that exhibits the band-shift difference between lean and obese nuclear proteins.

Purification of the proteins from the 60 bp DNA-protein complex by electoelution identified three bands that had molecular weights of 58, 62, and 65 kd. Since these proteins were also present when nuclear extracts were electrophoresed in the absence of DNA fragments, it was necessary to utilize a different purification method to verify that these proteins were part of the DNA-protein complex. The 60 bp DNA fragment was bound to magnetic DNA affinity beads, and these were used to purify proteins that bound to the fragment. This method of purification resulted in the isolation of the same three proteins. This indicates that these proteins are part of the complex. We are presently purifying larger quantities of these proteins in order to characterize them and identify their potential role in modulating the transcriptional responses to glucocorticoids.

TAT UPSTREAM REGION

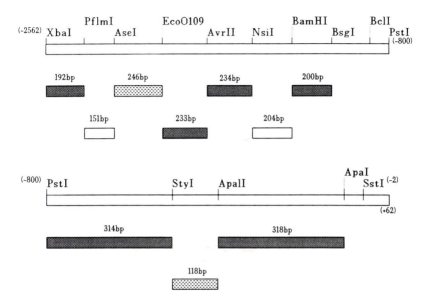

Figure 1.   Upstream DNA of the TAT gene that shows differences in band shift patterns. The shaded boxes indicate a difference in the amount of protein binding between lean and obese rats. The dotted boxes indicate a slight difference in the amount of protein binding between lean and obese rats. The white boxes show no difference in the amount of protein binding between lean and obese rats.

ACKNOWLEDGMENTS

The research for this paper was supported by the National Institute of Child Health and Human Development grant number 28997.

REFERENCES

1. Bray GA, Fisler J, York DA. Neuroendocrine control of the development of obesity: understanding gained from studies of experimental models of obesity. *Front Neuroendocrinol.* 1990;11:128–181.
2. Bray GA, York DA, Fisler J. Experimental obesity: a homeostatic fail-

ure due to defective nutrient stimulation of the sympathetic nervous system. *Vitam Horm.* 1989;45:1–125.

3. Okada A, York DA, Bray GA. Mifepristone (RU 486), a blocker of type II glucocorticoid and progestin receptors, reverses a dietary form of obesity. *Am J Physiol.* 1992;262:R1106–R1110.

4. Langley S, York D. Effects of antiglucocorticoid RU 486 on development of obesity in obese *fa/fa* Zucker rats. *Am J Physiol.* 1990;259: R539–R544.

5. Bray GA, York DA, Lavau M, Hanault I. Adrenalectomy in the Zucker fatty rat: effect on m-RNA for malic enzyme and glyceraldehyde 3-phosphate dehydrogenase. *Int J Obesity.* 1991;15:703–709.

6. Jantzen H, Strähle U, Gloss B, *et al.* Cooperativity of glucocorticoid response elements located far upstream of the tyrosine aminotransferase gene. *Cell.* 1987;49:29–38.

7. Gametchu B, Harrison R. Characterization of a monoclonal antibody to the rat liver glucocorticoid receptor. *Endocrinology.* 1984;114:274–279.

GÖKHAN S. HOTAMISLIGIL and BRUCE M. SPIEGELMAN

Mechanisms of TNF-α Mediated Insulin Resistance: Inhibition of Insulin Receptor Tyrosine Kinase

ABSTRACT

Insulin resistance is a central component of non–insulin-dependent diabetes mellitus. Obesity is associated with insulin resistance and represents a major risk for the development of non–
insulin-dependent diabetes. We have previously demonstrated
that the adipose tissue of obese-diabetic animals expresses elevated levels of tumor necrosis factor-α (TNF-α) and that neutralization of TNF-α dramatically improves the sensitivity of these animals to insulin-stimulated glucose intake. Although these results
suggest that TNF-α may be a key component linking obesity and
diabetes, it is not clear how TNF-α interferes with insulin action.
We show here that chronic exposure of adipocytes to very low
concentrations of TNF-α strongly inhibits insulin-stimulated glucose uptake. Treatment with TNF-α causes a moderate decrease
in the insulin-stimulated autophosphorylation of the insulin receptor and a dramatic decrease in the phosphorylation of IRS-1,
the major substrate of the insulin receptor in vivo. The degree of
inhibition of these tyrosine phosphorylations depends upon the
concentration of both TNF-α and insulin. The insulin receptor isolated from TNF-α–treated cells is defective in the ability to auto-
phosphorylate and phosphorylate IRS-1. These results show that
TNF-α directly interferes with the signaling of insulin through its
receptor and could play an important role in noninsulin-dependent diabetes mellitus.

Introduction

Non–insulin-dependent diabetes mellitus (NIDDM) is among the most
common metabolic diseases of the industrial world, affecting more than
twenty million in the United States alone (1). Despite its high incidence

and overwhelming health implications, the pathological basis of NIDDM remains largely elusive. It has been demonstrated that the major defects in NIDDM are at the level of insulin secretion and in the peripheral responses to insulin (1). The latter is usually referred to as insulin resistance, a less than normal biological response to a given dose of insulin. Obesity is the major predisposing factor for the development of insulin resistance and NIDDM, and again, little is understood about the mechanisms by which obesity is linked to insulin resistance and diabetes at the molecular level (1, 2).

It has been hypothesized that there may be molecules produced by adipose tissue during the course of obesity that are capable of interfering with insulin action at target tissues, such as fat, muscle, and liver (3, 4). Since adipose tissue expands greatly in obesity, it may become a major source for such molecules. In addition, obesity leads to infiltration of tissues, such as muscle tissue, by adipose cells, thereby enhancing the accessibility of these sites to secreted products of fat. Recent studies on adipocytes have provided valuable information toward identification of such fat-derived molecules.

In rodents, obesity is associated with abnormalities in circulating immune molecules (4, 5). This observation was based on studies showing that adipsin, a fat-specific serine protease, is a key enzyme in the alternative pathway of complement (5). Adipsin expression is metabolically regulated, and several different rodent models of obesity exhibit a severe adipsin deficiency in fat tissue (4). Besides adipsin, cultured adipocytes can produce many other necessary components and activate the proximal portion of the alternative pathway of complement in the absence of infection (6). However, this activation requires the presence of a cytokine (TNF-α, or IL-1). In contrast to cultured cells, the pathway runs spontaneously in fat tissue in vivo, suggesting the presence of an endogenous cytokine.

Obesity-Related Expression of TNF-α from Adipose Tissue and Its Role in Insulin Resistance

Our earlier work examining the presence of an endogenous cytokine has demonstrated that both TNF-α mRNA and protein are expressed in adipose tissue. Surprisingly, TNF-α expression in fat tissue was found to be elevated in genetic as well as transgenic models of rodent obesity (7, 8, 9). It also appeared that adipocytes are the major source of TNF-α production in adipose tissue (7). The expression was evident as early as 3 to 4 weeks of age in *fa/fa* rats and 6 to 7 weeks of age in *db/db* mice.

Analysis of several different models of rodent obesity indicated that TNF-α overexpression is a general phenomenon, and all models of severe obesity and insulin resistance examined so far seem to have elevated levels of TNF-α production from fat tissue (7–9). These include (in the order of expression levels), KKA[y], *db/db*, *ob/ob*, and *tub/tub* mice and *fa/fa* rats (Fig. 1). Mice with monosodium glutamate–induced obesity did not display this pattern of TNF-α expression at early stages of mild obesity and no insulin resistance (7). Similarly, rats treated with streptozotocin to induce type I diabetes did not have elevated levels of TNF-α expression. These observations suggested a possible correla-

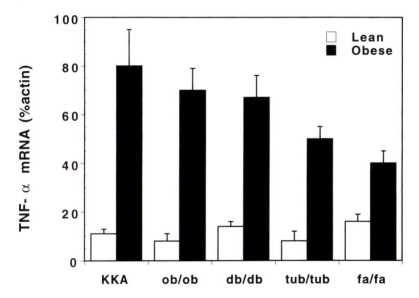

Figure 1. TNF-α mRNA expression in adipose tissue in different rodent models of obesity. Total RNA (20 μg) from epididymal fat pads of different animal models was subjected to Northern blot analysis, as described (7). All animals were males, KKA[y], *ob/ob*, *db/db*, and *tub/tub* mice and their respective controls were 12–13 weeks old, *fa/fa* rats were 7–8 weeks old. The mRNA levels are quantitated by digital densitometry and normalized to % β-actin mRNA in adipose tissue. The values represent mean ± SE from four to six independent measurements.

tion between TNF-α production and severe obesity and insulin resistance.

The biological role of TNF-α overexpression in obesity became apparent in studies in which TNF is neutralized in obese animals using a soluble TNF receptor–IgG (TNFR-IgG) fusion protein. Obese *fa/fa* rats treated with this fusion protein showed significant increases in their peripheral insulin sensitivity (7–8). The peripheral glucose utilization in response to insulin increased two- to threefold in obese animals compared with controls (Fig. 2). No significant changes were observed in the rates of hepatic glucose output. Although neutralization of TNF-α did not restore the insulin sensitivity completely, it clearly demonstrated that this molecule is a key player in linking obesity to insulin resistance.

Mechanisms of TNF-α Mediated Insulin Resistance in NIDDM

Defects in the quantity and function of the insulin-regulated glucose transporter (GLUT4) have been demonstrated in insulin resistant rodents and humans with NIDDM (10, 11). Earlier studies showing that TNF-α can specifically reduce the expression of GLUT4 mRNA in cultured adipocytes (7, 12, 13) suggested that this mechanism could be at least partly responsible for the TNF-mediated insulin resistance observed in animal models of obesity (7). However, when regulation of GLUT4 protein by TNF-α was examined in adipocytes, no direct correlation was observed between gross GLUT4 down-regulation and TNF-α-mediated inhibition of insulin-stimulated glucose transport (14). Moreover, expression of GLUT4 mRNA in fat or muscle tissues of *fa/fa* rats was not affected by neutralization of TNF-α, though this treatment significantly enhanced insulin sensitivity in these animals. These observations suggested that TNF-α must affect more proximal steps in insulin signaling.

Upon binding to its cell surface receptor, insulin starts its biological actions by activating the tyrosine kinase in the beta subunit of the insulin receptor, leading to autophosphorylation of the beta subunit on tyrosine residues (15). This in turn enables the receptor to phosphorylate its cellular substrates such as IRS-1 and 4PS (16–18). The effects of TNF-α on this part of the insulin receptor (IR) signal transduction pathway was examined by immunoprecipitation of the IR and IRS-1 from extracts of 3T3-F442A or -L1 adipocytes treated with low doses of TNF-

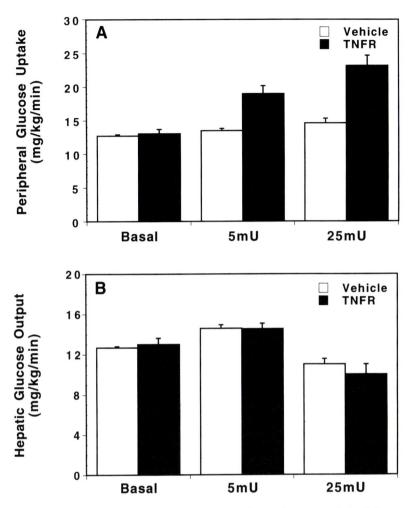

Figure 2. Effects of TNF-α neutralization on glucose homeostasis in *fa/fa* rats, as measured by hyperinsulinemic-euglycemic clamps (7). (A.) Peripheral glucose utilization. (B.) Hepatic glucose output. Peripheral glucose utilization (Rd) and hepatic glucose uptake (HGO) were measured at 2 doses of insulin and calculated, as described (7). Peripheral glucose utilization increased 45.65 and 78.26% over basal upon 5 and 25mU/kg/min insulin infusion, respectively, in TNFR-treated animals. The same doses of insulin infusions resulted in 13.84% and 31.02% increase over basal in controls. The values represent the mean ± SE of Rd and HGO of all animals in each group.

α followed by immunoblottings with antiphosphotyrosine antibodies (14). These experiments demonstrated that TNF-α treatment dramatically suppressed insulin-stimulated IR and IRS-1 phosphorylation, in a dose-dependent manner (14). Treatment of cells with 0.5–5 ng/mL of TNF-α resulted in a 15% to 50% reduction in the tyrosine phosphorylation of IR and a 20% to 85% decrease in phosphorylation of IRS-1 (Fig. 3). Chronic treatment (at least three days) was necessary to observe the effects of TNF-α on insulin-stimulated phosphorylations as well as insulin-stimulated glucose transport and adipocytes completely recovered from this insulin-resistant state, three days after the termination of TNF-α treatments (14).

The decreases in insulin-stimulated phosphorylations occurred without significant changes in the quantity of IR or IRS-1 protein at the same dose range of TNF-α (Fig. 3). However, at TNF doses higher than 5 ng/mL some reduction in the IR protein was also observed. Finally, increasing doses of insulin could improve but not completely overcome the inhibition of the insulin-stimulated phosphorylation of IR and IRS-1. The extent of tyrosine phosphorylation of IR and IRS-1 in TNF-α–treated cells was 40% and 20% of that in controls, respectively, at saturating concentrations of insulin (14). In order to further characterize the TNF-induced defect(s), we partially purified IR from TNF-α–treated adipocytes by wheat germ agglutinin (WGA) affinity chromatography and measured the kinase activity in vitro (14, 19). These experiments demonstrated a 40% to 50% overall decrease in insulin-stimulated autophosphorylation and a 20% to 50% decrease in phosphorylation of IRS-1 in material from TNF-α–treated cells compared with controls. These results indicated defective action of the IR from TNF-α–treated cells (14). The detailed analysis of the nature of the TNF-induced defect(s) in insulin signaling machinery is currently under way.

Effects of TNF-α on IR Signaling in Obesity

Defects in IR signaling, similar to those observed in cultured adipocytes following TNF-α treatment, have been demonstrated in NIDDM. Studies have shown decreased IR tyrosine kinase activity in human adipose tissue (20). Recently, reductions in insulin-stimulated tyrosine phosphorylation of IRS-1, as well as decreased IRS-1-associated PI 3-kinase activity, have been demonstrated in rodent models of obesity (21–24). To test whether TNF-α expression plays a role in this defective IR sig-

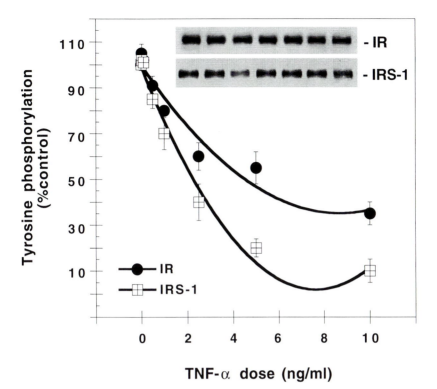

Figure 3. Effect of TNF-α on insulin-stimulated tyrosine phosphorylation of the IR and IRS-1 in murine cultured adipocytes. Murine 3T3-F442A adipocytes were cultured and differentiated in 10% FCS and 100 ng/mL insulin, and treated with 0, 0.1, 0.5, 1, 2.5, 5, and 10 ng/mL TNF-α for total of 5 days, as described (14). The extent of tyrosine phosphorylation or protein quantity was determined by immunoprecipitation of IR and IRS-1 from cellular extracts followed by immunoblotting with antiphosphotyrosine, anti-IR or anti-IRS-1 antibodies. The insert shows protein levels of IR and IRS-1, and the graph represents changes in tyrosine phosphorylation in extracts from cells treated with indicated doses of TNF-α. Quantitations were done by digital densitometry and the values (mean ± SE) represent tyrosine phosphorylation (presented as % control) corrected for protein quantity.

naling observed in the insulin resistance of obesity-diabetes syndromes, we analyzed IR tyrosine kinase activity in the Zucker (*fa/fa*) rat model of obesity after neutralizing TNF-α with a soluble TNFR-IgG fusion protein. This neutralization resulted in a significant improvement in insulin-stimulated autophosphorylation of IR, as well as phosphorylation of insulin receptor substrate 1 (IRS-1) in muscle and fat tissues of the *fa/fa* rats without affecting the protein levels for either IR or IRS-1 (24). No significant change was observed in IR signaling in liver. These results demonstrated that the mechanism by which TNF-α mediates insulin resistance in obesity is through its ability to inhibit IR tyrosine kinase in vivo, by affecting both muscle and fat tissues.

Discussion

Insulin resistance is a ubiquitous correlate of obesity and a central component of NIDDM (1). It has been demonstrated that a postreceptor abnormality develops during the course of insulin resistance, in addition to the decrease in the number of insulin receptors during the initial phases of obesity (1, 2). Several potential cellular targets, such as glucose transporter systems and IR signaling pathways have been extensively analyzed for identifying such postreceptor defects. Although quantitative and functional deficiencies in insulin regulated glucose transporters (GLUT4) have been described, the relative contribution of these defects to the overall insulin resistance of obesity has not been clear (10, 11).

On the other hand, recent studies have demonstrated that insulin signaling is defective in both human and rodent models of obesity-related insulin resistance (20–23). Studies on insulin-stimulated auto-phosphorylation of IR and phosphorylation of IRS-1 have demonstrated dramatic decreases in obesity/diabetes syndromes (20–23). Current evidence indicates that the tyrosine kinase activity of the insulin receptor is critical for insulin action, and IRS-1 is an important molecule in connecting the IR tyrosine kinase with a variety of cellular processes through its structural capability of interacting with proteins containing the SH2 domains, such as phosphatidyinositol-3-kinase (PI3K) (15–18, 25, 26). In support of this, it has been recently demonstrated that stimulation of PI3K activity by insulin is also decreased in rodent models of obesity and insulin resistance (22–23). These studies thus indicate that insulin signaling is altered at multiple steps in obesity. A challenging question, however, is the mechanism by which obesity imposes such an inhibitory effect on insulin action.

Our previous work demonstrated that TNF-α has an important role in linking insulin resistance and obesity through its obesity-related overexpression from adipose tissue (7–9). This role has been demonstrated by neutralization studies of TNF-α that resulted in significant increases in peripheral insulin sensitivity in *fa/fa* rats. In addition, TNF-α administration to normal rats was shown to induce insulin resistance (28).

Studies directed toward understanding the molecular mechanisms of action demonstrated that TNF-α–mediated insulin resistance is the result of alterations in IR signal transduction cascades both in cultured cells and whole animals (14, 24). Treatment of cultured adipocytes with TNF-α resulted in a marked decrease in the catalytic efficiency of the IR tyrosine kinase activity, as measured by insulin-stimulated autophosphorylation of the beta subunit as well as phosphorylation of IRS-1 (14). The IR isolated from TNF-α–treated adipocytes was also defective in its kinase activity. Similar inhibition of insulin signaling was also demonstrated in intact hepatoma cells, in which a dramatic decrease has been observed in IR autophosphorylation and phosphorylation of IRS-1, upon treatment with TNF-α (27).

Finally, neutralization of TNF-α in *fa/fa* rats resulted in dramatic increases in insulin-stimulated tyrosine kinase activity of the IR, in adipose tissue and skeletal muscle, indicating that insulin signaling is a direct target for TNF-α in obese animals, as it is in cultured cells (24). In addition, neutralization of TNF-α in *fa/fa* rats resulted in a better control of glucose homeostasis at the basal state compared with animals treated with vehicle alone. Another important point is the fact that the most significant improvements (close to levels observed in lean controls) were observed in muscle tissue following TNF-α neutralization (24). This observation is critical, since skeletal muscle plays the primary role in insulin-stimulated glucose uptake. It also became apparent that TNF-α can act on muscle tissue in vivo, possibly through endocrine or paracrine ways.

In contrast, TNF-α neutralization did not result in significant changes in insulin signaling in liver (24). This is similar to previous observations in which no effect of TNF-neutralization has been demonstrated on hepatic glucose output in *fa/fa* rats, despite a significant increase in insulin-stimulated glucose disposal (24). The reason(s) for this is not currently clear, but it is possible that different mechanisms are involved in hepatic insulin resistance. Alternatively, the neutralization protocol used in these studies may not be optimal. Complete inactivation of TNF-α or its receptors using genetic approaches should resolve the entire spectrum of TNF-α action in obesity.

REFERENCES

1. Moller DE. *Insulin Resistance.* John Wiley & Sons Ltd; 1993.
2. Moller DE, Flier JS. Insulin resistance: mechanisms, syndromes, and implications. *N Eng J Med.* 1992;325:938–948.
3. Faust IM, Johnson PR, Hirsch J. Surgical removal of adipose tissue alters feeding behavior in genetic and acquired obesity. *Science.* 1977;197:391–393.
4. Flier JS, Cook SK, Usher P, Spiegelman BM. Severely impaired adipsin expression in genetic and acquired obesity. *Science.* 1987;237:405–408.
5. Rosen BS, Cook KS, Yaglom J, *et al.* Adipsin and complement factor D activity: an immune-related defect in obesity. *Science.* 1989;244:1483–1487.
6. Choy LN, Rosen BS, Spiegelman BM. Adipsin and an endogenous pathway of complement from adipose cells. *J Biol Chem.* 1992;267:12736–12741.
7. Hotamisligil GS, Shargill NS, Spiegelman BM. Adipose expression of tumor necrosis factor-alpha: direct role in obesity-linked insulin resistance. *Science.* 1993;259:87–91.
8. Hotamisligil GS, Spiegelman BM. Through thick and thin: wasting, obesity, and TNF-alpha. *Cell.* 1993;73:625–627.
9. Hofmann C, Lorenz K, Braithwaite SS, *et al.* Altered gene expression for tumor necrosis factor-α and its receptors during drug and dietary modulation of insulin resistance. *Endocrinology.* 1994;134:264–270.
10. Pederson O, Kahn CR, Kahn BB. Divergent regulation of the GLUT1 and GLUT4 glucose transporters in isolated adipocytes from Zucker rats. *J Clin Invest.* 89:1964–1973.
11. Garvey WT, Maianu L, Huecksteadt TP, Birnbaum MJ, Molina JM, Ciaraldi TP. Pretranslational suppression of a glucose transporter protein causes insulin resistance in adipocytes from patients with non–insulin-dependent diabetes mellitus and obesity. *J Clin Invest.* 1991;87:1072–1081.
12. Cornelius P, Lee MD, Marlowe M, Pekala PH. Monokine regulation of glucose transporter mRNA in L6 myotubes. *Biochem Biophys Res Commun.* 1989;165:429–436.
13. Stephens JM, Pekala PH. Transcriptional repression of the GLUT4 and C/EBP genes in 3T3-L1 adipocytes by tumor necrosis factor-alpha. *J Biol Chem.* 1991;266:21839–21845.

14. Hotamisligil GS, Murray DL, Choy LN, Spiegelman BM. TNF-α inhibits signaling from insulin receptor. *Proc Natl Acad Sci USA.* 1994;91:4854–4858.

15. Kasuga M, Karlsson FA, Kahn CR. Insulin stimulates the phosphorylation of the 95 000-dalton subunit of its own receptor. *Science.* 1982;215:185–187.

16. White MF, Maron R, Kahn CR. Insulin rapidly stimulates tyrosine phosphorylation of a Mr-185 000 protein in intact cells. *Nature.* 1985;318:183–186.

17. Sun XJ, Rothenberg P, Kahn CR, *et al.* Structure of the insulin receptor substrate IRS-1 defines a unique signal transduction protein. *Nature.* 1991;352:73–77.

18. White MF, Kahn CR. The insulin signaling system. *J Biol Chem.* 1994; 269:1–4.

19. White MF. In: Siddle K, Hutton JC, eds. *Peptide Hormone Action: A Practical Approach.* Oxford, Eng; 1990:223–250.

20. Thies RS, Molina JM, Ciaraldi TP, Freidenberg GR, Olefsky JM. Insulin-receptor autophosphorylation and endogenous substrate phosphorylation in human adipocytes from control, obese, and NIDDM subjects. *Diabetes.* 1990;39:250–259.

21. Saad MJA, Araki E, Miralpeix M, Rothenberg PL, White MF, Kahn CR. Regulation of insulin receptor substrate-1 in liver and muscle of animal models of insulin resistance. *J Clin Invest.* 1992;90:1839–1849.

22. Folli F, Saad MJ, Backer JM, Kahn CR. Insulin stimulation of phosphatidylinositol-3-kinase activity and association with insulin receptor substrate 1 in liver and muscle of the intact rat. *J Biol Chem.* 1992;267:22171–22177.

23. Heydrick SJ, Jullien D, Gautier N, *et al.* Defect in skeletal muscle phosphatidylinositol-3-kinase in obese insulin-resistant mice. *J Clin Invest.* 1993;91:1358–1366.

24. Hotamisligil GS, Murray DL, Budavari A, Spiegelman BM. Reduced tyrosine kinase activity of the insulin receptor in obesity-diabetes central role of tumor necrosis factor-α. *J Clin Invest.* 1994; 94:1543–1549.

25. Myers MG Jr, Backer JM, Sun XJ, *et al.* IRS-1 activates phosphatidylinositol 3'-kinase by associating with src homology 2 domains of p85. *Proc Natl Acad Sci USA.* 1992;89:10350–10354.

26. Wilden PA, Siddle K, Haring E, Backer JM, White MF, Kahn CR.

The role of insulin receptor kinase domain autophosphorylation in receptor-mediated activities: analysis with insulin and anti-receptor antibodies. *J Biol Chem.* 1992;267:13719–13727.

27. Feinstein R, Kanety H, Papa MZ, Lunenfeld B, Karasik A. Tumor necrosis factor-α suppresses insulin-induced tyrosine phosphorylation of insulin receptor and its substrates. *J Biol Chem.* 1993;268: 26055–26058.

28. Lang CH, Dobrescu C, Bagby GJ. Tumor necrosis factor impairs insulin action on peripheral glucose disposal and hepatic glucose output. *Endocrinology.* 1992;130:43–52.

PART III

Regulation of Food Intake

SATYA P. KALRA, ABHIRAM SAHU, MICHAEL G. DUBE,
JUAN J. BONAVERA, and PUSHPA S. KALRA

Neuropeptide Y and Its Neural Connections in the Etiology of Obesity and Associated Neuroendocrine and Behavioral Disorders

ABSTRACT

Current evidence suggests that neuropeptide Y (NPY) is a physiological appetite transducer. Neuropeptide Y infusion centrally produces unsatiated appetite, sustained hyperphagia, and body weight gain, with little evidence of development of tolerance to NPY. Appetite stimulation is evoked by increased secretion and action of NPY in the paraventricular nucleus and other hypothalamic and extrahypothalamic sites. Changes in eating behavior induced by insulin and estradiol-17β are also mediated by altered NPY release from the paraventricular nucleus nerve terminals. Additional results show that hypothalamic obesity is associated with either high abundance (diabetes) or low abundance (VMH-lesioned and Zucker obese rats) of NPY in the paraventricular nucleus, the latter resulting from postsynaptic supersensitivity caused by a deficit in NPY. Morphological evidence shows the existence of an interconnected orexigenic network (NPY–Galanin–β-endorphin) in the hypothalamus, thereby raising the possibility that NPY may be an important component of the hypothalamic-orexigenic circuitry. Thus, disruption in hypothalamic NPY function at any one of these levels may underlie a variety of eating disorders and obesity.

Introduction

Obesity is a multivariate disease that can occur with or without hyperphagia. The prevailing view holds that imbalances in metabolic, sympathetic, and endocrine systems are important factors contributing

219

to obesity. Additionally, it is believed that elimination or subnormal operation of inhibitory (satiety) pathways may result in up-regulation of feeding either directly or indirectly by changing the functions of metabolic, sympathetic, and endocrine pathways. Although the cause and effect relationships among these contributing factors continue to be controversial (1–6), the converging evidence suggests that information relayed by imbalances in metabolic and endocrine signals and elimination of inhibitory pathways is processed by a network in the brain that is ultimately responsible for sustenance of energy homeostasis.

Disruption of hypothalamic function has long been suspected as an underlying cause in the etiology of hyperphagia and increase in body weight, progressively leading to obesity (1–6). Consequently, several questions arise. Is there a neurochemical basis for hypothalamic obesity? Is there a distinct network in the hypothalamus that plays a role in energy homeostasis? What are the components of the hypothalamic circuitry that stimulate food intake? Are the neurotransmitters/neuromodulators in this excitatory circuitry altered in experimental and genetic models of obesity?

The hypothalamus produces an array of neuropeptides to regulate neuroendocrine and sympathetic systems and ingestive and sexual behaviors. Some of these peptides richly innervate hypothalamic sites previously implicated in the control of feeding and sites where neural damage produces obesity (7–14). An emerging view is that there are at least three classes of peptides that stimulate feeding in a reliable fashion. These are neuropeptide Y (NPY), galanin (GAL), and the opioids, β-endorphin (β-END) and dynorphin (DYN). These peptides stimulate feeding in satiated rats after injection either into the cerebroventricular system or into various hypothalamic sites. A comparative analysis indicates that in terms of stimulating food intake, the rank order of potency is: NPY > GAL > opioids.

Our recent studies revealed intriguing connectivities among these three classes of peptidergic neurons, both in the arcuate nucleus (ARC) and in the paraventricular nucleus (PVN) of the hypothalamus (15, 16). We found that NPY nerve terminals synapse with immunopositive β-END and GAL perikarya and dendrites in the ARC and with GAL perikarya in the PVN. Additionally, GAL-immunopositive fibers were found in synaptic contact with a population of β-END neurons in the ARC. Since all three neuronal systems innervate the PVN and neighboring sites at which microinjection of peptides stimulated feeding, this morphological evidence implied that, in addition to stimulating appetite on its own, the NPY network may regulate feeding by controlling the release of GAL and β-END. Indeed, we have recently observed that NPY stimulated the release of β-END (17). This finding, together with the earlier report of Levine and Billington (18) that NPY-induced feeding can be attenuated by opiate receptor antagonists, strongly suggests that the orexigenic effects of NPY may, in part, be mediated by increased opioid release. Likewise, the synapses between GAL and β-END imply that GAL may stimulate food intake on its own and via stimulation of β-END release. Supporting this modality of GAL involvement are studies showing that the opiate receptor antagonist naloxone attenuated GAL-induced feeding (19). Collectively, it appears that an interconnected orexigenic network composed of at least these three classes of neuropeptides exists in the hypothalamus. Because NPY is the most potent orexigenic signal and NPY neurons synapse with GAL and opioid-producing neurons, we speculate that NPY may be one of the primary orexigenic signals in the hypothalamus orchestrating ingestive behavior.

Additional research emanating from our laboratory and that of others showed that NPY may also be crucially involved in regulation of neuroendocrine and behavioral functions (20, 21). These revelations raise the intriguing possibility that an imbalance in the production, release, and action of NPY may underlie eating disorders and the well-known accompanying neuroendocrine disturbances (2, 6, 20, 21). This article summarizes the orexigenic effects, site, and mode of action and factors regulating the synthesis and release of NPY when feeding is normally desired. In addition, the pattern of NPY secretion in experimental and genetic models of obesity is described. Finally, the orexigenic, neuroendocrine, and behavioral effects of NPY are integrated into a unifying hypothesis to account for the neuroendocrine disturbances accompanying hypothalamic-induced hyperphagia and obesity.

Is NPY a Physiological Appetite Transducer?

Since continuous hypothalamic NPY Y_1 receptor stimulation elicited a sustained episodic hyperphagic response and accelerated body weight gain with little evidence of tolerance to NPY (22, 23), it clearly raised the possibility that an abnormal rate of NPY secretion may produce hyperphagia and obesity. If this is the case, then one suspects that NPY receptor activation must be a physiological neural event in the daily pattern of eating behavior in the rat. Experimental evidence to date has shown that NPY secretion is up-regulated when feeding is normally desired. Our studies showed that in food-deprived rats NPY content and release were selectively elevated and following food consumption NPY secretion returned rapidly to the range seen in the satiated state (24–26). Neuropeptide Y synthesis is apparently augmented, since preproNPY mRNA levels were elevated in the ARC of these rats (27). Since depletion of the brainstem source of hypothalamic NPY did not adversely affect feeding, it is likely that a distinct ARC-PVN NPY pathway in the hypothalamus regulates eating in the rat (28). In a more physiological setting involving a scheduled feeding paradigm, our results showed that NPY release in the PVN and synthesis in the ARC increased at the onset of scheduled feeding time, and then as rats consumed food NPY release in the PVN decreased (25). Seemingly, an increase in the rate of NPY secretion in the PVN is responsible for the daily pattern of feeding, a notion further supported by immunoneutralization studies (29). Immunoneutralization of endogenously released NPY by central infusion of NPY antisera suppressed nighttime feeding by 75% and the cumulative 24-hour food intake by 60%. This substantial decrease in food intake may be interpreted to suggest that normally an increase in NPY neurotransmission in the PVN and in neighboring sites is required to elicit and maintain feeding during the nighttime (29, 30). The additional evidence that a partial suppression of NPY gene expression in the ARC that caused a decrease in NPY PVN stores resulted in a significant decrease in food intake (31) and, conversely, that there is an increase in NPY release in the PVN of experimentally induced hyperphagic, diabetic rats (32) is in accord with the notion that NPY may be a physiological appetite transducer.

Despite the demonstration of a tight relationship between NPY release in the PVN and the state of hunger and satiety, the NPY target sites in the brain remain to be identified. Microinjection of NPY in various hypothalamic sites was shown to readily elicit feeding (9, 33). Although there is also evidence for an extra-hypothalamic site of NPY action in the brainstem (34), it should be noted that transections of efferent and afferent fibers between the hypothalamus and brainstem failed to disrupt normal feeding pattern in the rat (28).

On the other hand, evaluation of c-fos protein, an early marker of neuronal gene activation, showed that receptive elements involved in the NPY-induced feeding may reside primarily in the hypothalamus (35). Intraventricular injections of NPY enhanced c-fos-like immuno-reactivity in the medial parvicellular (MP) and posterior magnocellular regions of the PVN. Interestingly, intense fos-like staining, confined to the MP region of the PVN, was seen even in the absence of food consumption. Evidently, a discrete population of neurons in the MP region of the PVN are likely NPY targets and may be involved in stimulation of feeding.

NPY and Ovarian Steroid- and d-Fenfluramine–Induced Hypophagia

Ovarian steroids modulate food intake and body weight gain during the course of reproductive cycles in rodents and other mammals. Hypoestrogenic conditions, such as those produced by ovariectomy, increase food intake and body weight gain, whereas estrogen-replacement therapy counteracts these effects of ovariectomy (36). Since NPY-producing neurons in the ARC may be the targets of estrogen (37), it is possible that the effects of ovarian steroids on food consumption may be mediated by altered NPY output in relevant hypothalamic sites. Indeed, long-term estrogen treatment of ovariectomized rats decreased NPY release selectively in the PVN, along with significant suppression of daily food intake and body weight (38). However, estrogen treatment failed to alter hypothalamic β-END in these rats. Seemingly, the anorectic effects of estrogen may involve decreased NPY release in the PVN, and conversely, estrogen deficiency may promote NPY release leading to hyperphagia and a gradual increase in the rate of body weight gain.

Serotonergic drugs, such as d-fenfluramine (FEN), inhibit feeding in both rodents and man. The anorectic effects of FEN are rapid and sustained for several hours (39). Our studies showed that FEN injection failed to acutely suppress NPY release in the PVN of food-deprived rats (40). However, NPY concentration in the PVN and ARC was significantly decreased two hours after FEN administration in conjunction with suppression of intake. We speculate that the acute anorectic effects of FEN may not be related to NPY release in the PVN, but on a long-term basis FEN is likely to decrease the availability of NPY for release and, like estrogens, suppress food consumption.

NPY, Insulin, Hyperphagia, and Obesity

Another revealing aspect of the research on hypothalamic NPY is that the NPY network may itself be the neural substrate in regulation of energy homeostasis by insulin. A large body of evidence is in line with the view that an interplay between circulating insulin and NPY secretion in the hypothalamus may be crucially involved in the etiology of hyperphagia and obesity in diabetes. Neuropeptide Y levels in various hypothalamic sites, including the PVN, were found to be elevated in diabetic rats (41). Neuropeptide Y release increased selectively in the PVN after the destruction of pancreatic β-cells with streptozotocin (10, 32), and insulin replacement restored the normal pattern of NPY release. Further, insulin per se and not blood glucose levels appeared to exert a regulatory control on PVN NPY efflux (41). Based on this and previous evidence that food-deprivation–induced suppression of insulin levels also up-regulated the ARC-PVN NPY axis (24–26), it is possible to envision a tight relationship between circulating insulin levels and NPY secretion in the hypothalamic integration of energy homeostasis.

The action of insulin in the brain in regulation of energy balance and body weight gain has been examined for many years (42, 43). Although an increase in peripheral insulin levels invariably resulted in hyperphagia and increase in body weight, central injections of insulin were shown to suppress food intake and body weight (42–45). Consequently, the source of insulin that controls centrally mediated ingestive behavior and body weight regulation has been controversial for several years (45). Since insulin levels in several hypothalamic sites, including the PVN, invariably increase along with increases in circulating insulin levels (46), the possibility that peripheral insulin may also be involved in suppressing food intake cannot be ruled out (42–45).

Since insulin deficiency up-regulates hypothalamic NPY (10, 32), it became possible to address the long-standing questions of how and where insulin acts in the hypothalamus. Woods and colleagues (45) showed that long-term central insulin infusion suppressed the fasting-induced increase in preproNPY mRNA, thereby implying that receptive elements on NPY perikarya and dendrites in the ARC may be insulin targets. An investigation of the effects of insulin on NPY release showed that even peripheral injections of extremely low doses of insulin, which failed to change blood glucose levels, decreased PVN NPY release in vivo (47). The site of insulin action appeared to be the PVN itself because insulin also suppressed the in vitro NPY release from PVN and not ARC fragments. These results demonstrated for the first time that insulin may act either directly or through interneurons to decrease NPY release from nerve terminals in the PVN and may not act in ARC and median eminence, the sites located outside the blood brain barrier. Furthermore, since insulin levels in the PVN vary in accordance with the peripheral concentrations (46), and since extremely low concentrations inhibit NPY release (47), it is likely that the site of insulin action in the control of food intake and body weight gain may reside either on PVN NPY nerve terminals or on interneurons that communicate directly with the PVN NPY nerve terminals.

The putative candidates for the intermediary role between insulin and NPY nerve terminals may be the insulin-like growth factors (IGF). We observed that IGF-2, and not IGF-1, inhibited NPY release in vitro from the PVN (47). In fact, suppression of PVN NPY release by insulin and IGF-2 was quantitatively quite similar. Since IGF-2 is anorectic (48, 49), our results suggested that the hypothalamic IGF-2 neural network may be the signaling pathway in regulation of PVN NPY release by insulin. Presumably, a deficit in insulin feedback, as seen in diabetic rats, initiates a chain of neural events that culminate in up-regulation of NPY, hyperphagia, and obesity.

NPY, Hyperphagia, and Obesity Induced by Ventromedial Hypothalamic Lesions

Destruction of a considerable amount of neural tissue in the ventromedial hypothalamus (VMH) invariably induces hyperphagia and obesity (1, 2, 4, 6). Contrary to expectations, we observed that PVN NPY levels and release and preproNPY mRNA in the ARC were decreased in the VMH-lesioned rats (50, and unpublished observations). The diminution in NPY release and synthesis occurred in conjunction with hyperphagia and increase in body weight in these rats. Consequently, both high abundance of NPY found in food-deprived and diabetic rats (10, 25, 26, 32) and low abundance of NPY as found in the VMH-lesioned rats (50) appeared associated with hyperphagia and obesity. There are several possible ways by which low abundance of NPY can result in hyperphagia and obesity. It is possible that VMH-lesions destroy the inhibitory satiety pathways to allow uninterrupted NPY efflux in the PVN, albeit at low rates because of the existing hyperinsulinemia. This unregulated NPY release may then result in an increase in food consumption. Our additional findings showing that immunoneutralization of NPY drastically suppressed food intake in VMH-lesioned rats is in accord with this possibility. Another plausible explanation currently under investigation is that because of a loss of regulatory control on other orexigenic signals (opioids and GAL), VMH-lesioned rats may show unregulated, exaggerated ingestive behavior.

NPY and Hyperphagia in Genetically Obese Zucker Rats

Another variant in the relationship between hypothalamic NPY and hyperphagia is seen in genetic models of obesity. General consensus is that NPY stores in the PVN are elevated in genetically obese, homozygous Zucker rats (*fa/fa*) (51, 52). However, these findings are not replicated in other models of genetic obesity (53). Similarly, considerable differences in preproNPY mRNA levels in ARC have been reported in various genetic models of obesity. Our studies show that as in the VMH-lesioned rats (50), in vitro NPY release from the PVN of genetically obese Zucker rats was significantly lower than that from the lean littermates (54). Although the pattern of NPY secretion in the PVN of other genetic models of obesity has not been examined, our findings in the VMH-lesioned and Zucker obese rats suggest that unregulated, albeit reduced, NPY efflux in the PVN may be responsible for the hyperphagic behavior. The identity of the cellular and subcellular neural events that result in exaggerated feeding in response to low abundance of NPY remains to be ascertained.

Neuroendocrine and Behavioral Effects of NPY

Increasing evidence shows that NPY is a pleiotropic neurotransmitter/neuromodulator messenger molecule in the hypothalamus. Besides playing a role in the hypothalamic control of ingestive behavior, NPY is reported to be involved in the hypothalamic control of anterior and posterior pituitary hormones (20, 21). In particular, NPY is an excitatory signal in the hypothalamic regulation of luteinizing hormone–releasing hormone, corticotropin-releasing hormone, oxytocin, vasopressin, and somatostatin. Also, central injections of NPY stimulated insulin release, and considerable evidence exists to show that insulin can feed back to regulate NPY secretion (45, 47, 55). Neuropeptide Y injections centrally inhibited female and male sex behavior (56). Therefore, increases in NPY neurotransmission in diabetic rats (32) are most likely responsible for suppressed sexual behavior reported in these rats (56). Abnormalities in pituitary hormone secretions, reduced sex behavior, and increased glucocorticoid secretions often accompany obesity and eating disorders in experimental and genetic models and in diabetics (1–5). Consequently, it is highly likely that altered production, release, and action of NPY in the hypothalamus may underlie the spectrum of concurrent abnormalities in ingestive and sexual behaviors and neuroendocrine deficits.

Concluding Remarks: A Hypothesis

The discovery of the potent appetite-stimulating effects of NPY and its morphological and functional relationships with other orexigenic signals has enriched our conceptual schemes about the pathology of eating disorders, obesity, and associated neuroendocrine and behavioral abnormalities. The evidence to date allows the formulation of a unifying hypothesis regarding the participation of hypothalamic NPY in the etiology of eating disorders and obesity. We hypothesize that an orexigenic network exists in the hypothalamus wherein NPY may play a primary regulatory role by stimulating food intake on its own and through opioids and GAL. The major receptive sites for these peptidergic signals probably reside in the PVN, though other hypothalamic and extra-hypothalamic sites may be involved under certain conditions. Insulin and estrogen have so far been identified as signals in the internal milieu to regulate NPY release from nerve terminals in the PVN. Apparently, both high abundance and low abundance of NPY in the PVN may underlie hyperphagia, abnormal body weight gain, and eventual development of obesity. High abundance of NPY is likely to produce sustained stimulation of postsynaptic NPY Y_1 receptors to induce hyperphagia and abnormalities in neuroendocrine control. The hypothalamic NPY network may operate in this manner in some genetic models of obesity. On the other hand, a deficit in NPY synthesis and release, possibly caused by hyperinsulinemia, as in VMH-lesioned rats and genetically obese Zucker rats, is likely to disrupt NPY neurotransmission to other orexigenic signals, GAL, and opioids. This deficit may lead to unregulated feeding, hyperphagia, and increased body weight gain. A detailed study of the interaction of NPY with other hypothalamic signals at the cellular and molecular levels should shed light on the pathophysiology of eating disorders.

ACKNOWLEDGMENTS

Thanks are due Sally McDonell for secretarial help. The research reported in this article was supported by the National Institutes of Health grant number DK-37273.

REFERENCES

1. Keesey RE, Powley TL. The regulation of body weight. *Annu Rev Psychol.* 1986;37:109–113.
2. Bray GA, Fisler J, York DA. Neuroendocrine control of the development of obesity: understanding gained from studies of experimental animals. *Front Neuroendocrinol.* 1990;11:128–181.
3. Han PW. Hypothalamic obesity in rats without hyperphagia. *Trans NY Acad Sci.* 1967;30:229–243.
4. Grossman S. Role of the hypothalamus in the regulation of food and water intake. *Psychol Rev.* 1975;82:200–224.
5. Hoebel BG. Neurotransmitters in the control of feeding and its rewards: monoamines, opiates and brain-gut peptides. In: Stunkard AJ, Stellar E, eds. *Eating and Its Disorders.* New York: Raven Press; 1984:15–38.
6. Bray GA. Genetic, hypothalamic and endocrine features of clinical and experimental obesity. *Prog Brain Res.* 1992;93:333–341.
7. Kalra SP, Kalra PS. Steroid-peptide interaction in the endocrine brain: reproduction. In: Motta M, ed. *Brain Endocrinology.* New York: Raven Press, Ltd; 1991:177–216.
8. Hökfelt T, Johansson O, Goldstein M. Chemical anatomy of the brain. *Science.* 1984;225:1326–1334.
9. Morley JE. Neuropeptide regulation of appetite and weight. *Endocr Rev.* 1987;8:256–287.
10. Sahu A, Kalra SP. Neuropeptidergic regulation of feeding behavior: neuropeptide Y. *Trends Endocrinol Metab.* 1993;4:217–224.
11. Clark JT, Kalra PS, Crowley WR, Kalra SP. Neuropeptide Y and human pancreatic polypeptide stimulate feeding behavior in rats. *Endocrinology.* 1984;115:427–429.

12. Khatchaturian H, Lewis ME, Schafer MH, Watson SJ. Anatomy of CNS opioid systems. *Trends Neurosci.* 1985;8:111–119.

13. Merchenthaler I, Lopez FJ, Negro-Vilar A. Anatomy and physiology of central galanin-containing pathways. *Prog Neurobiol.* 1993; 40:711–769.

14. Everitt BJ, Hökfelt T. The coexistence of neuropeptide Y with other peptides and amines in the central nervous system. In: Mutt V, Füxe K, Hökfelt T, Lundberg J, eds. *Neuropeptide Y.* New York: Raven Press; 1989:61–72.

15. Horvath TL, Naftolin F, Kalra SP, Leranth C. Neuropeptide Y innervation of β-endorphin-containing cells in the rat mediobasal hypothalamus: a light- and electronmicroscopic double-immunostaining analysis. *Endocrinology.* 1992;131:2461–2467.

16. Horvath TL, Kalra SP, Naftolin F, Leranth C. Evidence for a neuropeptide Y → Galanin → β-endorphin pathway in the rat hypothalamus. *Annu Meet Soc Neurosci.* 1993;19:1693.

17. Kalra PS, Kalra SP. Neuropeptide Y (NPY) stimulates hypothalamic β-endorphin (β-END) release in vivo: modulation by gonads. *Annu Meet Soc Neurosci.* 1993;19:847.

18. Levine AS, Billington CJ. Opioids, are they regulators of feeding? *Ann NY Acad Sci.* 1989;575:209–219.

19. Dube MG, Horvath TL, Leranth C, Kalra PS, Kalra SP. Naloxone suppresses the feeding evoked by intracerebroventricular galanin injection. *Physiol Behav.* 1994;56:811–813.

20. Kalra SP, Crowley, WR. Neuropeptide Y: a novel neuroendocrine peptide in the control of pituitary hormone secretion, and its relation to luteinizing hormone. *Front Neuroendocrinol.* 1992;13:1–36.

21. Kalra SP, Allen LG, Clark JT, Crowley WR, Kalra PS. Neuropeptide Y: an integrator of reproductive and appetitive function. In: Moody TW, ed. *Neural and Endocrine Peptides and Receptors.* New York: Plenum Press; 1986:353–366.

22. Kalra SP, Dube MG, Kalra PS. Continuous intraventricular infusion of neuropeptide Y evokes episodic food intake in satiated female rats: effects of adrenalectomy and cholecystokinin. *Peptides.* 1988;9: 723–728.

23. Catzeflis C, Pierroz DD, Rohner-Jeanrenaud F, Rivier JE, Sizonenko PC, Aubert ML. Neuropeptide Y administered chronically into the lateral ventricle profoundly inhibits both the gonadotropic and the

somatotrophic axis in adult female rats. *Endocrinology.* 1993;132: 224–234.

24. Sahu A, Kalra PS, Kalra SP. Food deprivation and ingestion in-duced reciprocal changes in neuropeptide Y concentrations in the paraventricular nucleus. *Peptides.* 1988;9:83–86.

25. Kalra SP, Dube MG, Sahu A, Phelps C, Kalra PS. Neuropeptide Y secretion increases in the paraventricular nucleus in association with increased appetite for food. *Proc Natl Acad Sci USA.* 1991;88: 10931–10935.

26. Dube MG, Sahu A, Kalra PS, Kalra SP. Neuropeptide Y release is elevated from the microdissected paraventricular nucleus of food-deprived rats: an in vitro study. *Endocrinology.* 1992;131:1195–1201.

27. Berelowitz M, Bruno JF, White JD. Regulation of hypothalamic neu-ropeptide expression by peripheral metabolism. *Trends Endocrinol Metab.* 1992;3:127–133.

28. Sahu A, Dube MG, Kalra SP, Kalra PS. Bilateral neural transections at the level of mesencephalon increase food intake and reduce la-tency to onset of feeding in response to neuropeptide Y. *Peptides.* 1988;9:1269–1273.

29. Dube MG, Xu B, Crowley WR, Kalra PS, Kalra SP. Evidence that neuropeptide Y is a physiological signal for normal food intake. *Brain Res.* 1994;646:341–344.

30. Kalra SP, Kalra PS. Neuropeptide Y: a novel peptidergic signal for the control of feeding behavior. In: Pfaff DW, Ganten D, eds. *Current Topics in Neuroendocrinology.* Berlin:Springer-Verlag; 1990;10:192–217.

31. Akabayashi A, Wahlestedt C, Alexander JT, Leibowitz SF. Specific inhibition of endogenous neuropeptide Y synthesis in arcuate nu-cleus by antisense oligonucleotides suppress feeding behavior and insulin secretion. *Mol Brain Res.* 1994;21:55–61.

32. Sahu A, Sninsky CA, Phelps CP, Dube MG, Kalra PS, Kalra SP. Neuropeptide Y release from the paraventricular nucleus increases in association with hyperphagia in streptozotocin-induced diabetic rats. *Endocrinology.* 1992;131:2979–2985.

33. Stanley BG, Chin AS, Leibowitz SF. Feeding and drinking elicited by central injection of neuropeptide Y: evidence for hypothalamic sites of action. *Brain Res Bull.* 1985;14:521–524.

34. Corp ES, Melville LD, Greenberg D, Gibbs J, Smith CP. Effect of

fourth ventricular neuropeptide Y and peptide YY on ingestive and other behaviors. *Am J Physiol.* 1990;159:R317–R323.

35. Li B-H, Xu B, Rowland NE, Kalra SP. c-Fos expression in the rat brain following central administration of neuropeptide Y and effects of food consumption. *Brain Res.* 1994;665:277–284.

36. Wade GN, Schneider JE. Metabolic levels and reproduction in female mammals. *Neurosci Biobehav Rev.* 1992;16:235–272.

37. Sar M, Sahu A, Crowley WR, Kalra SP. Localization of neuropeptide Y (NPY) immunoreactivity in estradiol concentrating cells in the hypothalamus. *Endocrinology.* 1990;127:2752–2756.

38. Bonavera JJ, Dube MG, Kalra PS, Kalra SP. Anorectic effects of estrogen may be mediated by decreased neuropeptide Y release in the hypothalamic paraventricular nucleus. *Endocrinology.* 1994;134: 2367–2370.

39. Rowland NE, Carlton, J. Neurobiology of an anorectic drug: fenfluramine. *Prog Neurobiol.* 2986;27:13–62.

40. Dube MG, Sahu A, Phelps CP, Kalra PS, Kalra SP. Effect of d-fenfluramine on neuropeptide Y concentration and release in the paraventricular nucleus of food-deprived rats. *Brain Res Bull.* 1992;29: 865–89.

41. Sahu A, Sninsky CA, Kalra PS, Kalra SP. Neuropeptide Y concentration in microdissected hypothalamic regions and in streptozotocin-diabetic rats with and without insulin substitution therapy. *Endocrinology.* 1990;126:192–198.

42. Nicolaidis S. Mechanisme nerveux de l'equilibre energetique. *Journ Annu Diabetol Hotel Dieu.* 1978;1:152–156.

43. Woods SC, Stein LJ, McKay LD, Porte D Jr. Chronic intracerebroventricular infusion of insulin reduces food intake and body weight of baboons. *Nature.* 1979;282:503–505.

44. Baskin DG, Wilcox BJ, Figlewicz DP, Dorsa DM. Insulin and insulin-like growth factors in the CNS. *Trends Neurosci.* 1988;11:107–111.

45. Schwartz MW, Figlewicz DP, Baskin DG, Woods SC, Porte D Jr. Insulin in the brain: a hormonal regulator of energy balance. *Endocr Rev.* 1992;13:387–414.

46. Gerozissis K, Orosco M, Rouch C, Nicolaidis S. Basal and hyperinsulinemia-induced immunoreactive hypothalamic insulin changes in lean and genetically obese Zucker rats revealed by microdialysis. *Brain Res.* 1993;611:258–263.

47. Sahu A, Dube MG, Phelps CP, Sninsky CA, Kalra PS, Kalra, PS. In

vivo and in vitro evidence that neuropeptide Y (NPY) secretion in the paraventricular nucleus (PVN) is regulated by peripheral insulin. *Annu Meet Soc Neurosci.* 1993;19(3):1821. Abstract #743.16.

48. Lauterio TJ, Marson L, Daughaday WH, Bailey CA. Evidence for the role of insulin-like growth factor II (IFG-II) in the control of food intake. *Physiol Behav.* 1987;40:755–758.

49. Lauterio TJ, Aravich PF, Rotwein P. Divergent effects of insulin or insulin-like growth factor II gene expression in the rat hypothalamus. *Endocrinology.* 1990;126:392–398.

50. Dube MG, Sahu A, Phelps CP, Kalra PS, Kalra SP. Neuropeptide Y (NPY) concentration is decreased in the paraventricular nucleus (PVN) of rats exhibiting excessive weight gain produced by ventromedial hypothalamic (VMH) lesions. *Annu Meet Soc Neurosci.* 1992;18(2):937. Abstract #396.6.

51. Sanacora G, Kershaw M, Finkelstein JA, White, JD. Increased hypothalamic content of preproNeuropeptide Y messenger ribonucleic acid in genetically obese Zucker rats and its regulation by food deprivation. *Endocrinology.* 1990;127:730–737.

52. Beck B, Burlet A, Nicolas JP, Burlet C. Hypothalamic neuropeptide Y (NPY) in obese Zucker rats: implications in feeding and sexual behaviors. *Physiol Behav.* 1990;47:449–453.

53. Wilding JPH, Gilbey SG, Bailey CJ, *et al.* Increased neuropeptide Y messenger ribonucleic acid (mRNA) and decreased neurotensin mRNA in the hypothalamus of the obese (ob/ob) mouse. *Endocrinology.* 1993;132:1939–1944.

54. Kalra SP, Dube MG, Finkelstein J, Sahu A. Neuropeptide release from the paraventricular nucleus (PVN) of genetically obese and lean Zucker rats. In: Proceedings of the 2nd independent meeting of the Society for the Study of Ingestive Behavior; August 16–20, 1994; McMaster Univ., Hamilton, Ontario, Canada. P-A18.

55. Moltz JH, McDonald JK. Neuropeptide Y: direct and indirect action on insulin secretion in the rat. *Peptides.* 1985;6:1155–1159.

56. Clark JT, Kalra PS, Crowley WR, Kalra, SP. Neuropeptide Y stimulates feeding, but inhibits sexual behavior in rats. *Endocrinology.* 1985;117:2435–2442.

57. Dudley SD, Ramirez I, Wade GN. Estrous behavior and pituitary and brain cell nuclear retention of [3H] estradiol in chronically insulin-deficient female rats. *Neuroendocrinology.* 1981;33:7–11.

SARAH FRYER LEIBOWITZ and AKIRA AKABAYASHI

Brain Peptides in Normal Biological Rhythms and Obesity

ABSTRACT

The brain peptides neuropeptide Y and galanin, which potentiate food intake, are highly specific in their physiological actions related to nutrient and energy balance. They produce very different effects on the behavioral process of eating, as well as on certain endocrine and metabolic systems, and they are differentially responsive to physiological and biochemical signals. Moreover, they can be distinguished by the temporal specificity of their actions, which can be linked to different natural periods of the daily feeding cycle and different stages of development. The neuroanatomical substrates involved in these actions of neuropeptide Y and galanin, as well as the experimental conditions under which these peptides are disturbed, can also be distinguished, supporting their involvement in different physiological processes.

The available information on the multiple and distinct actions and interactions of neuropeptide Y and galanin suggests the following working hypotheses. The behavioral and endocrine actions of neuropeptide Y are focused on processes related to carbohydrate intake and carbohydrate metabolism, when this nutrient constitutes the primary energy source for preserving or enhancing body weight. This peptide, working in conjunction with the circulating adrenal steroid corticosterone, operates through a specific hypothalamic circuit involving the arcuate nucleus where the neuropeptide Y–synthesizing cell bodies exist and the paraventricular nucleus to which these cell bodies project. This neurocircuit is most strongly activated at the start of the active feeding cycle or early in development, between the stages of weaning and puberty. In contrast to neuropeptide Y, galanin appears to act preferentially on the ingestion of fat and may enhance fat deposition through a reduction in energy expenditure. It operates through neurons in the paraventricular nucleus and medial preoptic area, which project locally as well as to the median eminence. Galanin gene expression and synthesis are strongly activated under conditions associated with increased fat intake and fat deposition; these include the mid-to-late hours of the active feeding cycle and the developmental period just after puberty when galanin-synthesizing neurons are positively activated by the gonadal steroids estrogen and progesterone. These peptide systems provide excellent models for investigating how the brain coordinates separate neurochemical systems that, in the presence of differential physiological and environmental challenges, contribute to the overall maintenance of body weight.

Neurotransmitters and neuromodulators synthesized within the brain have potent effects on nutrient intake, as well as on nutrient partitioning and energy expenditure. In addition, these actions are associated with physiological changes that, in turn, signal the brain to alter the activity of these neurochemicals. These feedback loops are critical for maintaining an avenue of communication between the brain and the body and also between the internal and external environments. Thus, the activity of these brain transmitters and their regulatory factors varies greatly under different physiological and environmental conditions, and consequently, the nature and extent of their contribution to nutrient homeostasis and body weight gain also fluctuates. A more complete understanding of this natural process and of condition-specific changes will elucidate the mechanisms underlying any disturbances in the body's energy and nutrient balance. This understanding will be greatly advanced by a more precise definition of the neuronal cell groups and brain systems involved in these phenomena.

This review will focus on two peptide systems of the hypothalamus. They are neuropeptide Y (NPY) and galanin (GAL), which exist in high concentrations within the hypothalamus, together with their receptor sites, and which have profound effects on behavioral and physiological processes essential to nutrient and energy balance (1, 2). Although similarly geared toward enhancing ingestion and body weight gain, these peptides have markedly different physiological actions and operate through different mechanisms. Moreover, they are differentially responsive to the feedback actions of various endocrine and biochemical signals and, thus, are believed to act under different physiological conditions.

Physiological Actions of the Neuropeptides

The physiological actions of NPY and GAL include effects on eating behavior, metabolism, and hormone secretion. Both peptides have a stimulatory effect on eating behavior (3–6). Moreover, they act in part through a structure of the hypothalamus, the paraventricular nucleus (PVN) (7–9), that controls both the endocrine and behavioral processes related to nutrient homeostasis (10–12). Their specificity of action is reflected in studies of nutrient intake, showing NPY to enhance preferentially the ingestion of carbohydrate-rich diets (13–17), while GAL produces greater intake of fat (18, 19). Whereas protein intake is generally unaffected or may be reduced by either peptide, these predominant effects on carbohydrate or fat intake may be altered under different conditions, for example, at higher peptide doses, with chronic peptide stimulation, or in animals with different dietary preferences.

The potency of these peptides is reflected in their effectiveness at low picogram doses, their potency in causing animals to consume in a brief period the amount they normally consume over 24 hours, and their long duration of action of up to 24 hours after a single injection (13, 14, 20). With its long duration of action, repeated administration of NPY into the hypothalamus is effective in potentiating daily food intake and even body weight gain, in part, by inhibiting satiety mechanisms preferentially for carbohydrate (13, 15, 21, 22). A structure-function analysis of the peptides' feeding stimulatory action shows the critical amino acid sequence for NPY to be the N-terminal amino acids 1 through 12 (23, 24) and the first 16 N-terminal amino acids for GAL (25). Although the specific receptor involved in GAL's action remains to be characterized, the NPY receptor is believed to be a variant of the Y_1 subtype, with an uncharacteristically high responsiveness to the NPY_{2-36} fragment (2, 13, 14, 23).

In addition to their impact on nutrient ingestion, NPY and GAL differentially modulate the metabolism of nutrients. In the PVN, NPY dose-dependently increases respiratory quotient without affecting overall energy expenditure (26), and GAL reduces energy expenditure without altering substrate utilization (27). This NPY-induced increase in respiratory quotient, reflecting a diversion of metabolism toward carbohydrate utilization to support fat synthesis, is consistent with other evidence showing NPY to promote white fat lipid storage, reduce sympathetic activation of interscapular brown adipose tissue, and decrease brown fat thermogenesis (28, 29). Through these metabolic actions, as well as the daily hyperphagia for carbohydrate and to a lesser extent fat, chronic NPY stimulation increases fat deposition and body weight gain and mimics the hormonal and metabolic changes associated with obesity (15, 21, 30, 31).

These different effects of the peptides on nutrient intake and metabolism may be related to their differential impact on the release of hormones which, themselves, influence food ingestion and energy metabolism. These hormones include corticosterone (CORT), insulin, and vasopressin (AVP), and the site of peptide action, once again, includes the PVN, which has a primary function in controlling the secretion of these hormones as well as responding to their feedback signals (12, 32, 33). Through hypothalamic injection studies, the effects of NPY on the release of CORT, insulin, and AVP are found to be stimulatory in nature (34–36), whereas GAL inhibits the secretion of each of these hormones (37–39).

These stimulatory effects of NPY on the endocrine systems support its potential role in maintaining carbohydrate balance, through processes of ingestion and metabolism. Both CORT and insulin are well known for their glucoregulatory functions, with CORT working to maintain blood glucose levels and insulin controlling cellular uptake of glucose (33, 40, 41), and the peptide AVP also has prominent effects on carbohydrate metabolism (42, 43). Thus, together with its preferential effect on the ingestion of carbohydrate, NPY may provide the necessary endocrine milieu for utilizing and/or storing the ingested carbohydrates. In support of this idea (41), the physiological state of low carbohydrate stores is associated with a rise in circulating CORT and NPY levels in the PVN (44–46) just prior to the onset of a natural carbohydrate meal (47, 48). In addition, a carbohydrate-rich meal is followed by a pronounced rise in circulating glucose and insulin (49, 50), which, together, should provide a negative feedback signal for peptide activity (33, 51, 52). Similar conditions, associated with enhanced carbohydrate ingestion as well as CORT and AVP secretion, can be mimicked pharmacologically by compounds that induce hypoglycemia or block glucose utilization (53–56).

These endocrine, metabolic, and behavioral patterns associated with NPY and carbohydrate-rich meals contrast markedly with those seen with GAL. As described above, this peptide inhibits the secretion of CORT and insulin, has little impact on carbohydrate metabolism, and preferentially enhances the ingestion of fat. A functional relation between these diverse actions of GAL is supported by additional evidence showing the behavioral actions of PVN-injected GAL to occur under conditions of very low circulating levels of CORT (57) and the levels of endogenous PVN GAL to rise when CORT levels are sharply declining and to shift inversely in relation to circulating insulin (see below). During acute episodes of high-fat meals, circulating insulin levels are generally low (49), though insulin resistance and hyperinsulinemia may develop under conditions of chronic high-fat diets (58). Similarly, low levels of CORT are sufficient to maintain processes underlying fat intake and fat deposition, whereas higher CORT levels are required for glucoregulatory functions (41, 59).

In relation to the reproductive hormones, the predominant effect of NPY and GAL on their secretion is believed to be excitatory in nature, with both enhancing circulating levels of luteinizing hormone (LH) (60, 61). However, differences between these hypothalamic peptides may be reflected in the additional inhibitory effect of NPY on LH secretion in ovariectomized animals (60), and in the inhibitory (62) versus excitatory (63) effects of NPY and GAL, respectively, on mating behavior. In understanding the relationship between the brain peptides and these reproductive hormones, it is important to consider the potent effects of the gonadal steroids themselves on carbohydrate and lipid metabolism (64), in addition to their differential activity at various stages of development and body weight gain (see below).

Signals Controlling Neuropeptide Gene Expression

Biochemical investigations of neurotransmitter activity in the brain, in relation to peptide gene expression, synthesis, release, and receptor binding, have helped to elucidate the physiological significance of these peptide actions. These studies have allowed the identification of several regulatory signals that modulate peptide activity, which is the focus of this section, and they have also provided essential information on their natural state of activity, a topic reviewed in subsequent sections. An integral part of these studies is the analysis of localized brain areas, which has given insight into the specific hypothalamic nuclei, neuronal cell groups, and neural projections involved in their actions. In the case of NPY, for example, a neurocircuit involved in modulating carbohydrate balance is believed to originate in the arcuate nucleus (ARC), which has a large population of NPY-synthesizing cells, and to terminate in the medial portion of the PVN (mPVN), which is densely innervated by NPY projections from the ARC as well as the brainstem (2, 65). In contrast, there is evidence that GAL-containing neurons involved in fat balance are concentrated in the lateral portion of the PVN (lPVN), in addition to the medial preoptic area (MPO), where interconnecting circuits and local innervation exist and contribute to the dense GAL projection to the mPVN as well as the median eminence (ME) (1).

ADRENAL STEROIDS

Distinct differences between NPY and GAL, in terms of their endocrine actions and neuroanatomical substrates, suggest further that they may be differentially responsive to the feedback actions of the steroids. This is true in the case of the adrenal steroids—in particular CORT, which interacts closely with NPY at all levels of the ARC-PVN projection system that has a dense concentration of glucocorticoid receptors (66), but interacts less clearly or minimally with the PVN GAL neurons that have few glucocorticoid receptors (67).

The feedback actions of CORT on the NPY projection system are stimulatory in nature and apparently mediated via glucocorticoid (type II) receptors. They include an effect at the level of the cell body, where NPY gene expression is enhanced by CORT and glucocorticoid stimulation, and also at the level of the terminal and receptor site, where CORT potentiates NPY transport, release, and receptor function (e.g., 41, 68–74). These steroid actions on NPY message level may involve intracellular genomic processes, mediated through a glucocorticoid responsive element upstream of the NPY gene (75), in addition to more rapid changes in cell-surface receptors that, in turn, affect the density and intracellular handling of the PVN Y_1-like receptors (68). Functional consequences of this positive feedback action may be the enhancement, in the mPVN, of the NPY-elicited carbohydrate feeding, which is dependent upon glucocorticoid receptor activation (41, 57), and of NPY-stimulated release of CORT, which may enable this steroid to rise to peak levels required under certain physiological conditions (44, 72).

In contrast to NPY, GAL in the PVN feeding circuit can function at low levels or independently of the adrenal steroid. The GAL-containing neurons of PVN exhibit little glucocorticoid-receptor immunoreactivity (67), and their expression of the GAL gene and production of the peptide is either unaffected by ADX and CORT replacement (76) or perhaps transiently enhanced by the loss of CORT (77). Moreover, the stimulatory effect of PVN GAL on fat ingestion remains intact in ADX animals and is unaffected by the administration of CORT or selective steroid agonists and antagonists (41, 57). Although CORT may influence GAL production in other neural systems of the brain that contain glucocorticoid receptors (76), there is a relative independence of GAL production and circulating CORT in this PVN system that acts to inhibit the release of CORT (39) and potentiate the ingestion of fat (18).

Gonadal Steroids

Similar to CORT, the gonadal steroids, estrogen (E_2), perhaps in combination with progesterone, and also testosterone, have excitatory effects on the hypothalamic peptides which, once again, are highly anatomically localized. Strong activational changes in NPY gene expression and peptide production are detected in the ARC, where nuclear steroid receptors and NPY immunoreactivity are colocalized; however, they are not seen in other hypothalamic areas, including the PVN, where peptide release stimulates feeding and NPY levels are either minimally affected or depressed by gonadal steroid manipulations (60, 78–81).

Although endogenous GAL is also activated by the gonadal steroids, this peptide or its gene expression, in contrast to NPY, is most responsive within the PVN and MPO, where some GAL-synthesizing neurons concentrate E_2, and also the ME, to which GAL axons project, but is unaffected in the ARC (82–88). This is seen in studies of ovariectomized animals receiving steroid replacement, as well as in immature females injected with pregnant mare serum gonadotropin to raise circulating E_2 levels. Although the mechanism of this phenomenon is unknown, it is possible that an E_2 responsive element exists in the 5' untranslated region of the GAL gene (89).

INSULIN

In contrast to the adrenal and gonadal steroids, which generally enhance NPY and GAL gene expression, circulating insulin has an inhibitory action on these hypothalamic peptides. In streptozotocin-diabetic rats, NPY immunoreactivity is enhanced in the PVN, ARC, and certain other hypothalamic nuclei, whereas NPY mRNA is increased specifically in the ARC (*e.g.*, 90–93). This enhancement in NPY activity in diabetic rats, apparently unrelated to their hyperglycemia, is reversed by chronic insulin replacement. Insulin administration also reverses the increase in NPY message and peptide levels produced by dexamethasone injections (94) or by food deprivation (95) and the changes in NPY receptor binding sites that occur in diabetic rats consequent to their increased synthesis and release of NPY (96). Although the mechanism of insulin's action remains unknown, the existence of insulin-receptor binding sites in the area of the NPY-synthesizing cell bodies of the ARC (97) suggests that it may act directly on these NPY neurons, through either genomic or nongenomic actions (33, 97). An additional possibility, discussed below, is that the critical signal for NPY gene expression, rather than insulin itself, is a deficiency in circulating insulin and a disturbance in glucose uptake (56, 98).

An inverse relationship between GAL-synthesizing neurons and circulating insulin also exists. Although originally detected in the pancreas where GAL levels are reduced under conditions of hyperinsulinemia (99), a negative feedback action of insulin on GAL immunoreactivity and GAL gene expression has been seen in the hypothalamus and anatomically localized to the PVN (100–102). Measurements of circulating insulin and hypothalamic peptide levels across the natural feeding cycle (see below) also suggest a reciprocal relationship between this metabolic hormone and GAL.

NUTRIENTS AND THEIR METABOLISM

In addition to circulating hormones, changes in nutritional state have clear impact on peptide gene expression, synthesis, and release in the brain. For example, an increase in NPY content, NPY-positive innervation, NPY release, or NPY mRNA has been described in studies of food-restricted or food-deprived animals (*e.g.*, 97, 103–109). These changes occur most consistently and dramatically in the NPY projection from the ARC to PVN, where NPY message and peptide levels rise naturally just prior to the initiation of the active feeding cycle (44, 46), and they can be reversed by a few hours of food ingestion (46, 103, 104). Although fewer studies have been conducted with GAL, the available evidence indicates that this peptide, its levels (110) or gene expression (111), may be less responsive to total food deprivation, though an increase in hypothalamic GAL message in food-deprived animals has been seen in obese Zucker rats (112). The possibility that chronic food restriction may have greater impact on this peptide, causing a decline in GAL message in the ARC (111), needs to be explored.

An important question to address at this point is whether these changes in hypothalamic peptides, associated with a reduction in food availability, reflect alterations in circulating hormones and/or possibly a direct effect of the nutrients and their metabolism on brain peptide function. The most likely answer to this question is that both factors play a role, as evidenced by in vitro experiments showing potent effects of nutrients as well as endocrine manipulations on gene expression (113). The importance of hormones in mediating the deprivation-induced rise in NPY gene expression and peptide levels is reflected in the loss of this response in ADX rats and its restoration after CORT replacement (72) and its attenuation after central or peripheral administration of insulin (95, 97, 114).

Although these effects of CORT and insulin may indicate their direct action on NPY gene expression, as suggested above, they may also reflect the well-known reciprocal actions of these hormones on glucose availability or utilization (40), which, in turn, may provide an important signal in the activation of NPY-synthesizing neurons and ultimately in the stimulation of appetite for carbohydrate. Evidence for this possibility is provided by the finding that NPY levels, specifically in the ARC, are increased by administration of 2-deoxy-D-glucose (2-DG), which blocks glucose utilization and preferentially enhances the ingestion of carbohydrate; however, NPY is unaffected by another metabolic inhibitor, mercaptoacetate, which blocks fatty acid oxidation and potentiates the consumption primarily of protein (54, 56, 115). Although these findings identify glucose rather than fatty acids as the key metabolic fuel affecting NPY production, they do not provide information as to whether the interactions between the nutrients and brain peptides are direct or whether they are indirect involving endocrine factors. Again, whereas both associations likely play a role under physiological conditions, further analyses under conditions of food deprivation, insulin-deficient diabetes, insulin-resistant obesity, and intense physical exercise, as well as after 2-DG administration, suggest that the enhancement of NPY gene expression and peptide levels is more closely associated with the state of negative carbohydrate balance, rather than to specific changes in either blood CORT or insulin levels (*e.g.*, 56, 90, 93, 104, 107–109, 111, 116–119). Thus, the possibility that the NPY gene in the ARC neurons responds directly to cellular glycopenia needs to be explored.

Hypothalamic GAL, once again, is distinguished from NPY in being unresponsive to alterations in glucose utilization after 2-DG (115). This peptide, however, is clearly responsive to another compound, mercaptoacetate, which blocks β-oxidation of fatty acids in the mitochondria. This metabolic inhibitor reduces GAL levels, specifically in the lPVN but not other hypothalamic areas, and it also suppresses the ingestion of fat (115). The relationship between these metabolic, neurochemical, and behavioral changes needs to be investigated.

INTRACELLULAR SIGNALS

The intracellular mechanisms regulating NPY and GAL gene expression are not understood. In addition to intracellular glucocorticoid receptors, there is recent evidence that second messenger signals generated by membrane-bound receptors, including nucleotides, may be involved. In vitro studies demonstrate a potentiation of NPY synthesis after administration of substances that stimulate the production of cyclic adenosine 3′,5′-monophosphate (cAMP) (120–122). In an in vivo study, central injections of dibutyryl cAMP are also found to cause an increase in NPY levels (123). This effect, once again, is detected exclusively in the ARC and mPVN, and it occurs in the absence of any alterations in circulating hormones or hypothalamic levels of GAL. These findings implicate cAMP as having regulatory functions within specific hypothalamic NPY-synthesizing neurons involved in energy homeostasis.

Natural Dietary Preferences and Endogenous Neuropeptides

The evidence described above relates NPY and GAL, in specific hypothalamic projection systems, to the behavioral process of carbohydrate or fat ingestion and to physiological or endocrine systems controlling the metabolism of these nutrients. This is reflected by the ability of hypothalamic peptide injections to alter the ingestion and metabolism of carbohydrate or fat and affect the release of specific hormones, and also by the responsiveness of peptide gene expression, synthesis or release, in specific hypothalamic neuronal systems, to changes in circulating hormone levels and glucose or fat oxidation. The primary question here is, Can endogenous NPY and GAL in the hypothalamic neurons be related to an animal's natural appetite for carbohydrate or fat?

Recent studies have demonstrated that Sprague-Dawley rats exhibit considerable individual differences in their appetite for the macronutrients carbohydrate and fat, with approximately 50% of the population showing a strong preference for carbohydrate (>45% of total diet) and an additional 35% consuming relatively large amounts of fat (>30%) and exhibiting greater fat deposition and body weight gain (47, 48). Analyses of rats exhibiting differential preference for these two nutrients suggest that NPY and GAL may, in fact, be related to these natural preferences and that these relationships may be highly site-specific (124–126). With NPY, a strong positive correlation exists between the daily intake of carbohydrate and peptide levels in specific hypothalamic nuclei (124). This relationship is anatomically localized, to the ARC and mPVN as well as the dorsomedial nucleus, and it is nutrient specific, unlike fat or protein. Together with other evidence associating NPY and circulating CORT at the beginning of the natural feeding cycle when carbohydrate is strongly preferred (44, 47), these results provide support for a role of endogenous NPY, and its projection from the ARC to the mPVN, in controlling natural appetite for carbohydrate.

In studies of GAL, a different relationship is found to exist between this peptide and the animals' natural appetite for specific nutrients. Consistent with the above evidence showing GAL to preferentially enhance fat intake and respond to changes in fatty acid oxidation, a convergence of evidence links GAL-synthesizing neurons, in specific hypothalamic nuclei, to the behavioral process of fat ingestion and, consequently, to body weight gain (126, 127; Leibowitz, Alexander, and Akabayashi, unpublished results). A strong positive correlation is detected between GAL mRNA or peptide levels and the amount of fat consumed, and this relationship is highly localized to GAL-synthesizing neurons in the lPVN, as well as in the MPO of female rats. Rather than related to circulating levels of CORT, these measurements of endogenous GAL in the PVN, in animals that consume variable amounts of daily fat, reveal an inverse relation between insulin and either PVN GAL levels or fat ingestion (126).

Biological Rhythms and Neuropeptide Action

The behavioral process of nutrient intake and levels of circulating hormones exhibit clear temporal rhythms, both across the light/dark cycle and in relation to reproductive activity. In light of recent evidence revealing distinct rhythms of the hypothalamic peptides NPY and GAL, the above information on peptide actions and the signals that modulate peptide gene expression provide some basis for formulating certain hypotheses concerning the physiological conditions under which these peptides and hormones normally act.

In relation to the light/dark cycle, a diurnal rhythm of nutrient intake exists, characterized by a strong preference for carbohydrate in the early hours of the feeding period and a rise in fat consumption three to four hours later (47, 48, 128). This is accompanied by a rhythm of circulating hormones, showing peak CORT levels prior to the onset of the natural feeding cycle that decline to basal levels over the next few hours (44, 45) and highest levels of insulin in association with the initial carbohydrate-rich meal and somewhat lower levels during subsequent meals (129). A possible relation between these behavioral and endocrine patterns and the hypothalamic peptides is suggested by the evidence that NPY levels, in the ARC and PVN, peak at the onset of the feeding cycle, subsequent to a rise in circulating CORT and NPY mRNA in the ARC (44, 46). Thus, the proposed interaction between CORT, acting via glucocorticoid receptors, and NPY neurons of the ARC-PVN projection may have special significance in determining the daily rhythm of carbohydrate ingestion, CORT release, and related physiological processes (*e.g.*, 10, 19, 44, 130, 131). This is further supported by the evidence showing a preferential effect of NPY on carbohydrate ingestion (14, 17), its greater potency at the onset of the feeding cycle (19), and its dependence on circulating CORT and the activation of glucocorticoid receptors (57, 132).

A contrasting pattern observed with GAL supports a differential role for this peptide across the natural feeding cycle. Whereas most hypothalamic areas exhibit no diurnal rhythm for endogenous GAL, levels of this peptide in the lPVN area show a single peak across the daily cycle, and the suprachiasmatic nucleus exhibits bimodal peaks at the light/dark transitions (133). This GAL peak in the lPVN, rather than occurring at the onset of feeding as detected for NPY, develops toward the middle of the nocturnal feeding cycle, between the third and sixth hours. This temporal rhythm is remarkably similar to that described for spontaneous fat intake (47, 48), suggesting that PVN GAL may contribute to this behavioral pattern. This does not preclude a possible additional role of endogenous GAL in the feeding of carbohydrate (18).

Contrary to NPY, this GAL rhythm shows no relation to circulating CORT, which peaks several hours before PVN GAL rises and has minimal effect on GAL's feeding response, its message or peptide content in the PVN (57, 133). However, an inverse relation exists between PVN GAL and insulin, both across the light/dark cycle (133) and in animals on macronutrient diets (126). This agrees with the above evidence for an inhibitory effect of GAL on insulin secretion and also for a negative feedback effect of insulin on GAL production. Thus, GAL is more active under conditions in which the levels of insulin, and perhaps its central satiety action (33), are relatively low. The smaller increase in carbohydrate intake produced by GAL injection, which is strongest at the onset of the feeding cycle, may be differentially affected by circulating CORT (18, 57).

In addition to the diurnal rhythm of nutrient intake, NPY and GAL, in conjunction with circulating steroids, may contribute differentially to developmental patterns of feeding behavior. For example, together with the hypothalamo-pituitary-adrenal axis, the hypothalamic NPY system, in the area of its cell bodies (ARC) and terminals (PVN), and the NPY receptors rise to approximately adult levels by postnatal day 16 (134-136). Moreover, females also have higher levels of hypothalamic NPY than males (137) and show greater adrenal responsiveness and increased basal CORT levels (138, 139). With this schedule of maturation and sex differences, the NPY system may be functionally active at this early stage and able to provide the necessary signals for controlling the intake of carbohydrate, which is strongly preferred (50% of total diet) relative to fat (5%-15%) in weanling animals and in females relative to males (140, 141). Although this sex difference in hypothalamic NPY may become even stronger at puberty, due to the rise in gonadal steroids (60, 137, 139), it is clearly evident before puberty, by postnatal day 28, along with the hypersecretion of CORT and higher carbohydrate intake (137, 140). This prepubertal pattern of development may be contrasted with a dramatic shift in eating patterns, peptide production, and endocrine status that occurs after puberty. Levels of GAL, in the whole hypothalamus and, in particular, the PVN, MPO, and ME, show a sharp rise shortly after puberty (142, 143). This rise is greater in female rats than in males, presumably because of the excitatory effects of E_2 (87), and the incidence of colocalization of GAL in luteinizing hormone–releasing hormone neurons is five-fold higher in females because of E_2 (1, 144). The postpubertal increase in GAL occurs around the same time as the natural burst in fat intake and body weight (140), suggesting a possible relationship between these neurochemical and behavioral phenomena. Since GAL also facilitates copulatory behavior (63) in addition to fat ingestion (18), this peptide may be involved in a broader array of postpubertal behaviors that are essential for reproduction. This is in contrast to NPY, which inhibits sexual behavior (62) and preferentially stimulates the ingestion of carbohydrate (14), which is preferred by prepubertal subjects. Although the relative activity of these two peptide systems may be developmentally determined, their functions in adult animals will be dictated by an array of internal, environmental, and genetic factors that affect each animal's endocrine and metabolic profile.

Pharmacological Studies of Neuropeptide Function in Relation to Feeding

Natural rhythms of eating behavior, circulating hormones, and hypothalamic peptides reveal a close relationship between these different physiological measures. Results obtained with various pharmacological manipulations, which modulate endogenous activity of NPY and GAL or their receptors, provide critical evidence for a causal relation between these peptides and the physiological responses. The compounds used include peptide receptor antagonists, antisera, and antisense oligonucleotides (ODNs), which reveal the importance of NPY and GAL for the expression of normal feeding patterns, hormone secretion, and metabolism.

Specifically, when administered into the ventricles or PVN, antisera to NPY reliably suppresses daily food intake (23, 145). Studies with macronutrient diets, as well as with GAL antiserum, have yet to be performed. With antagonists of NPY (146) and GAL (147), feeding is also suppressed. Specificity of action is revealed through a preferential effect of the NPY antagonist on carbohydrate ingestion and a strong reduction in fat intake with the GAL antagonist. Their specificity is further demonstrated by the effectiveness of these antagonists in blocking the action of their respective peptides (146, 147).

Of particular importance are recent studies using peptide antisense ODNs. This new technique has proved particularly useful in linking alterations in endogenous peptides, in localized brain areas, to changes in specific behavioral and endocrine processes. After administration of NPY antisense ODNs directly into the ARC, carbohydrate as well as fat ingestion is reduced, in association with a 30% decrease in NPY levels of the ARC and a decline in insulin (148). In contrast, a strong and selective reduction in fat ingestion has been observed after injection of GAL antisense ODNs directly into the PVN, accompanied by a decline of PVN GAL levels and a small increase in circulating insulin (126). In both studies, the essential nature of hypothalamic NPY and GAL, for normal patterns of feeding and insulin secretion, is supported by other evidence showing no effect of sense ODNs on either peptides, hormones, or behavior.

Hypothalamic Peptides in Relation to Obesity and Diabetes

A number of investigations implicate NPY and GAL in the development of abnormal eating patterns, obesity, and diabetes. Endogenous activity of these hypothalamic peptide systems is significantly increased in different obese and diabetic models. This is seen in genetically obese fatty (*fa/fa*) Zucker rats, which compared with their lean counterparts exhibit increased hypothalamic NPY levels, especially in the ARC and PVN (117, 149), enhanced NPY mRNA concentrations in the ARC (107), and increased GAL levels in the PVN (110) or hypothalamic GAL mRNA (112). Higher NPY levels in the ARC or NPY release in the PVN has also been detected in another spontaneously obese rat, the corpulent (*cp/cp*) JCR-LA (150), as well as in diabetic animals (33). These similar changes in obese and diabetic rats may be attributed, in part, to a decline in insulin secretion or insulin sensitivity, respectively.

Whether this increase in NPY production is, in fact, causally related to the hyperphagia and obesity of these animal models remains to be established. As described above, acute injections of NPY or GAL enhance white fat lipid storage or reduce energy expenditure, and chronic

NPY administration causes severe overeating and increased fat deposition and produces a full syndrome of diabetes, hypercholesterolemia, and hypertension associated with obesity (15, 21, 30, 31). Moreover, recent evidence indicates that the hypothalamic NPY system may be disturbed at an early age in genetically obese rats (151, 152). However, this change in NPY still may be a consequence of disturbances in adiposity and energy expenditure at birth (153, 154), and other findings in genetically obese rats reveal a decrease in NPY receptor number, an attenuated feeding response to hypothalamic NPY injections, and a decrease in NPY release (155, 156). Thus, close examination of the dynamic changes that occur very early in the development of obesity or diabetes is needed to assess whether the increase in hypothalamic NPY activity has functional significance.

Also, preliminary evidence in humans links brain peptide function to the pathophysiology of clinical eating disorders. For example, in bulimic patients, disturbances in cerebrospinal fluid (CSF) content of peptide YY (PYY), a pancreatic polypeptide closely related to NPY, have been detected (157). A dramatic increase in CSF PYY in bulimics who had abstained from bingeing has led to the proposal that these subjects, when initiating a binge, may be responding to heightened levels of PYY. This is consistent with the evidence in animals (14), showing this peptide to be even more potent than NPY in the stimulation of food consumption.

ACKNOWLEDGMENTS

Some of the research described in this review was supported by United States Public Health Service grant MH 43422 to Sarah Fryer Leibowitz and by a fellowship from the Naito Foundation to Akira Akabayashi.

REFERENCES

1. Merchenthaler I, Lopez FJ, Negro-Vilar A. Anatomy and physiology of central-galanin containing pathways. *Prog Neurobiol.* 1993;40:711–769.
2. Dumont Y, Martel J-C, Fournier A, St-Pierre S, Quirion R. Neuropeptide Y and neuropeptide Y receptor subtypes in brain and peripheral tissues. *Prog Neurobiol.* 1992;38:125–167.
3. Stanley BG, Leibowitz SF. Neuropeptide Y: stimulation of feeding

and drinking by injection into the paraventricular nucleus. *Life Sci.* 1984;35:2635–2642.

4. Clark JT, Kalra PS, Crowley WR, Kalra SP. Neuropeptide Y and human pancreatic polypeptide stimulate feeding behavior in rats. *Endocrinology.* 1984;155:427–429.

5. Levine AS, Morley JE. Neuropeptide Y: a potent inducer of consummatory behavior in rats. *Peptides.* 1984;5:1025–1029.

6. Kyrkouli SE, Stanley BG, Leibowitz SF. Galanin: stimulation of feeding induced by medial hypothalamic injection of this novel peptide. *Eur J Pharmacol.* 1986;122:159–160.

7. Corwin RL, Robinson JK, Crawley JN. Galanin antagonists block galanin-induced feeding in the hypothalamus and amygdala of the rat. *Eur J Neurosci.* 1993;5:1528–1533.

8. Kyrkouli SE, Stanley BG, Seirafi RD, Leibowitz SF. Stimulation of feeding by galanin: anatomical localization and behavioral specificity of this peptide's effects in the brain. *Peptides.* 1990;11:995–1001.

9. Stanley BG, Magdalin W, Seirafi A, Thomas WJ, Leibowitz SF. The perifornical area: the major focus of (a) patchily distributed hypothalamic neuropeptide Y-sensitive feeding system(s). *Brain Res.* 1993;604:304–317.

10. Leibowitz SF. Neurochemical-neuroendocrine systems in the brain controlling macronutrient intake and metabolism. *Trends Neurosci.* 1992;15:491–497.

11. Leibowitz SF. Hypothalamic paraventricular nucleus: interaction between α2-noradrenergic system and circulating hormones and nutrients in relation to energy balance. *Neurosci Biobehav Rev.* 1988;12:101–109.

12. Luiten PGM, Ter Horst GJ, Steffens AB. The hypothalamus, intrinsic connections and outflow pathways to the endocrine system in relation to the control of feeding and metabolism. *Prog Neurobiol.* 1987;28:1–54.

13. Leibowitz SF, Alexander JT. Analysis of neuropeptide Y-induced feeding: dissociation of Y1 and Y2 receptor effects on natural meal patterns. *Peptides.* 1991;12:1251–1260.

14. Stanley BG, Daniel DR, Chin AS, Leibowitz SF. Paraventricular nucleus injection of peptide YY and neuropeptide Y preferentially enhance carbohydrate ingestion. *Peptides.* 1985;6:1205–1211.

15. Stanley BG, Anderson KC, Grayson MH, Leibowitz SF. Repeated

hypothalamic stimulation with neuropeptide Y increases daily carbohydrate and fat intake and body weight gain in female rats. *Physiol Behav.* 1989;46:173–177.

16. Welch CC, Grace MK, Billington CJ, Levine AS. Preference and diet affect macronutrient after morphine, NPY, norepinephrine, and deprivation. *Am J Physiol.* 1994;266:R426–R433.

17. Morley JE, Levine AS, Gosnell A, Kneip J, Grace M. Effect of neuropeptide Y on ingestive behaviors in the rat. *Am J Physiol.* 1987; 252:R599–R609.

18. Tempel DL, Leibowitz KJ, Leibowitz SF. Effects of PVN galanin on macronutrient selection. *Peptides.* 1988;9:309–314.

19. Tempel DL, Leibowitz SF. Diurnal variations in the feeding responses to norepinephrine, neuropeptide Y and galanin in the PVN. *Brain Res Bull.* 1990;25:821–825.

20. Stanley BG, Chin AS, Leibowitz SF. Feeding and drinking elicited by central injection of neuropeptide Y: evidence for a hypothalamic site(s) of action. *Brain Res Bull.* 1985;14:521–524.

21. Stanley BG, Kyrkouli SE, Lampert S, Leibowitz SF. Neuropeptide Y chronically injected into the hypothalamus: a powerful inducer of hyperphagia and obesity. *Peptides.* 1986;7:1189–1192.

22. Lynch WC, Hart P, Babcock AM. Neuropeptide attenuates satiety: evidence from a detailed analysis of patterns ingestion. *Brain Res.* 1994;636:28–34.

23. Stanley BG, Magdalin W, Seirafi A, Nguyen MM, Leibowitz SF. Evidence for neuropeptide Y mediation of eating produced by food deprivation and for a variant of the Y1 receptor mediating this peptide's effect. *Peptides.* 1992;13:581–587.

24. Kalra SP, Dube MG, Fournier A, Kalra PS. Structure-function analysis of stimulation of food intake by neuropeptide Y: effects of receptor agonists. *Physiol Behav.* 1991;50:5–9.

25. Crawley JN, Austin MC, Fiske SM, *et al.* Activity of centrally administered galanin fragments on stimulation of feeding behavior and on galanin receptor binding in rat hypothalamus. *J Neurosci.* 1990;10:3695–3700.

26. Menendez JA, McGregor IS, Healey PA, Atrens DM, Leibowitz SF. Metabolic effects of neuropeptide Y injections into the paraventricular nucleus of the hypothalamus. *Brain Res.* 1990;516:8–14.

27. Menendez JA, Atrens DM, Leibowitz SF. Metabolic effects of gal-

anin injections into the paraventricular nucleus of the hypothal-amus. *Peptides.* 1992;13:323–327.

28. Billington CJ, Briggs JE, Levine AS. Effects of intracerebroventric-ular injection of neuropeptide Y on energy metabolism. *Am J Phys-iol.* 1990;260:R321–R327.

29. Egawa M, Yoshimatsu H, Bray GA. Neuropeptide Y suppresses sympathetic activity to interscapular brown adipose tissue in rats. *Am J Physiol.* 1990;260:R238–R334.

30. Zarjevski N, Cusin I, Vettor R, Rohner-Jeanrenaud F, Jeanrenaud B. Chronic intracerebroventricular neuropeptide-Y administration to normal rats mimics hormonal and metabolic changes of obesity. *Endocrinology.* 1993;133:1753–1758.

31. Zarjevski N, Cusin I, Vettor R, Rohner-Jeanrenaud F, Jeanrenaud B. Intracerebroventricular administration of neuropeptide Y to normal rats has divergent effects on glucose utilization by adipose tissue and skeletal muscle. *Diabetes.* 1994;43:764–769.

32. Swanson LW, Sawchencko PE. Hypothalamic integration: orga-nization of the paraventricular and supraoptic nuclei. *Annu Rev Neurosci.* 1983;6:275–325.

33. Schwartz MW, Figlewicz DP, Baskin DG, Woods SC, Porte D Jr. Insulin in the brain: a hormonal regulator of energy balance. *En-docr Rev.* 1992;13:387–414.

34. Leibowitz SF, Sladek C, Spencer L, Tempel D. Neuropeptide Y, epinephrine and norepinephrine in the paraventricular nucleus: stimulation of feeding and the release of corticosterone, vasopres-sin and glucose. *Brain Res Bull.* 1988;21:905–912.

35. Abe M, Saito M, Shimazu T. Neuropeptide Y and norepinephrine injected into the paraventricular nucleus of the hypothalamus ac-tivate endocrine pancreas. *Biomed Res.* 1989;10:431–436.

36. Wahlestedt C, Skagerberg G, Edman R, Heilig M, Sundler F, Hak-anson R. Neuropeptide Y (NPY) in the area of the paraventricular nucleus activates the pituitary-adrenocortical axis in the rat. *Brain Res.* 1987;417:33–38.

37. Koenig JI, Hooi SC, Maiter DM, *et al.* On the interaction of galanin within the hypothalamo-pituitary axis of the rat. In: Hokfelt T, Bartfai T, Jacobowitz D, Ottoson DT, eds. *Galanin: A New Multi-functional Peptide in the Neuroendocrine System.* New York: Mac-millan Press; 1991:331–342.

38. Kondo K, Murase T, Otake K, Ito M, Oiso Y. Centrally adminis-

tered galanin inhibits osmotically stimulated arginine vasopressin release in conscious rats. *Neurosci Lett.* 1991;128:245–248.

39. Tempel DL, Leibowitz SF. Galanin inhibits insulin and corticosterone release after injection into the PVN. *Brain Res.* 1990;536:353–357.

40. McMahon M, Gerich J, Rizza R. Effects of glucocorticoids on carbohydrate metabolism. *Diabetes Metab Rev.* 1988;4:17–30.

41. Tempel DL, Leibowitz SF. Adrenal steroid receptors: interactions with brain neuropeptide systems in relation to nutrient intake and metabolism. *J Neuroendocrinol.* 1994;6:479–501.

42. Hems DA, Whitton PD. Control of hepatic glycogenolysis. *Physiol Rev.* 1980;60:1–50.

43. Rofe AM, Williamson DH. Metabolic effects of vasopressin infusion in the starved rat: reversal of ketonanemia. *Biochem J.* 1983;212:231–239.

44. Akabayashi A, Levin N, Paez X, Alexander JT, Leibowitz SF. Hypothalamic neuropeptide Y and its gene expression: relation to light/dark cycle and circulating corticosterone. *Mol Cell Neurosci.* 1994;5:210–218.

45. Kreiger DT. Rhythms in CRF, ACTH and corticosteroids. In: Kreiger DT, ed. *Endocrine Rhythms.* New York: Raven Press; 1979:123–141.

46. Jhanwar-Uniyal M, Beck B, Burlet C, Leibowitz SF. Diurnal rhythm of neuropeptide Y–like immunoreactivity in the suprachiasmatic, arcuate and paraventricular nuclei and other hypothalamic areas. *Brain Res.* 1990;536:331–334.

47. Shor-Posner G, Ian C, Brennan G, *et al.* Self-selecting albino rats exhibit differential preferences for pure macronutrient diets: characterization of three sub-populations. *Physiol Behav.* 1991;50:1187–1195.

48. Shor-Posner G, Brennan G, Ian C, Jasaitis R, Madhu K, Leibowitz SF. Meal patterns of macronutrient intake in rats with particular dietary preferences. *Am J Physiol.* 1994;266:R1395–R1402.

49. Van Amelsvoort JMM, Van Stratum P, Kraal JH, Lussenburg RN, Houtsmuller UMT. Effects of varying carbohydrate: fat ratio in a hot lunch on postprandial variables in male volunteers. *Br J Nutr.* 1989;61:267–283.

50. Acheson KJ, Schutz Y, Bessard T, Ravussin E, Jequier E, Flatt JP.

Nutritional influences on lipogenesis and thermogenesis after a carbohydrate meal. *Am J Physiol.* 1984;246:E62–E70.

51. Strubbe JH, Steffens AB. Neural control of insulin secretion. *Horm Metab Res.* 1993;25:507–512.

52. Rowland NE. Peripheral and central satiety factors in neuropeptide Y–induced feeding in rats. *Peptides.* 1988;9:83–86.

53. Baylis PH, Robertson GL. Vasopressin response to 2-deoxy-D-glucose in the rat. *Endocrinology.* 1980;107:1970–1974.

54. Kanarek R, Marks-Kauffman R, Ruthazer R, Gualitieri L. Increased carbohydrate consumption by rats as a function of 2-deoxy-D-glucose administration. *Pharmacol Biochem Behav.* 1983;18:47–50.

55. Kanarek R, Marks-Kauffman R, Lipeles BJ. Increased carbohydrate intake as a function of insulin administration in rats. *Physiol Behav.* 1980;25:779–782.

56. Akabayashi A, Zaia CTBV, Silva I, Chae HJ, Leibowitz SF. Neuropeptide Y in the arcuate nucleus is modulated by alterations in glucose utilization. *Brain Res.* 1993;621:343–348.

57. Tempel DL, Leibowitz SF. Glucocorticoid receptors in the PVN: interactions with norepinephrine, neuropeptide Y and galanin in relation to feeding. *Am J Physiol.* 1993;265:E794–E800.

58. Pedersen O, Kahn CR, Flier JS, Kahn BB. High-fat feeding causes insulin resistance and a marked decrease in the expression of glucose transporters (GLUT4) in fat cells of rats. *Endocrinology.* 1991;129:771–777.

59. Devenport L, Knehans A, Sundstrom A, Thomas T. Corticosterone's dual metabolic actions. *Life Sci.* 1989;45:1389–1396.

60. Kalra SP, Crowley WR. Neuropeptide Y: a novel neuroendocrine peptide in the control of pituitary hormone secretion, and its relation to luteinizing hormone. *Front Neuroendocrinol.* 1992;13:1–46.

61. Lopez FJ, Meade EH Jr, Negro-Vilar A. Endogenous galanin modulates the gonadotropin and prolactin proestrus surges in the rat. *Endocrinology.* 1993;132:795–800.

62. Clark JT, Kalra PS, Kalra SP. Neuropeptide Y stimulates feeding but inhibits sexual behavior in rats. *Endocrinology.* 1985;117:2435–2442.

63. Bloch GJ, Butler PC, Kohlert JG, Bloch DA. Microinjection of galanin into the medial preoptic nucleus facilitates copulatory behavior in the male rat. *Physiol Behav.* 1993;54:615–624.

64. Wade GN, Schneider JE. Metabolic fuels and reproduction in female mammals. *Neurosci Biobehav Rev.* 1992;16:235–272.

65. Bai FL, Yamano M, Shiotani Y, *et al.* An arcuate-paraventricular and -dorsomedial hypothalamic neuropeptide Y–containing system which lacks noradrenaline in the rat. *Brain Res.* 1985;331:172–175.

66. Harfstrand A, Cintra A, Fuxe K, *et al.* Regional differences in glucocorticoid receptor immunoreactivity among neuropeptide Y immunoreactive neurons of the rat brain. *Acta Physiol Scand.* 1989;135:3–9.

67. Cintra A, Fuxe K, Solfrini V, *et al.* Central peptidergic neurons as targets for glucocorticoid action: evidence for the presence of glucocorticoid receptor immunoreactivity in various types of classes of peptidergic neurons. *J Steroid Mol Biol.* 1991;40:93–103.

68. Akabayashi A, Watanabe Y, Wahlestedt C, McEwen BS, Paez X, Leibowitz SF. Hypothalamic neuropeptide Y, its gene expression and receptor activity: relation to circulating corticosterone in adrenalectomized rats. *Brain Res.* 1994;665:201–212.

69. Corder R, Pralong F, Turnill D, Saudan P, Muller AF, Gaillard RC. Dexamethasone treatment increases neuropeptide Y levels in rat hypothalamic neurons. *Life Sci.* 1988;43:1879–1886.

70. Dean RG, White BD. Neuropeptide Y expression in rat brain: effects of adrenalectomy. *Neurosci Lett.* 1990;114:339–344.

71. White BD, Dean RG, Edwards GL, Martin RJ. Type II corticosteroid receptor stimulation increases NPY gene expression in basomedial hypothalamus of rats. *Am J Physiol.* 1994;266:R1523–R1529.

72. Ponsalle P, Srivastava L, Unt R, White JD. Glucocorticoids are required for food-deprivation induced increases in hypothalamic neuropeptide Y expression. *J Neuroendocrinol.* 1992;4:585–591.

73. Larsen PJ, Mikkelsen JD. Chronic dexamethasone administration elevates levels of preproneuropeptide Y and neuropeptide Y1-receptor mRNA levels in the hypothalamic arcuate nucleus. In: Abstracts of the Neuropeptide Y Meeting; 1993; University of Cambridge.

74. Leibowitz SF, Akabayashi A, Levin N, Roberts J, Watanabe Y, Paez X. Circulating corticosterone and hypothalamic neuropeptide Y: analysis of gene expression, peptide levels and receptor binding sites. *Soc Neurosci Abs.* 1993;19:1703.

75. Misaki N, Higuchi H, Yamagata K, Miki N. Identification of glucocorticoid responsive elements (GREs) at far upstream of rat NPY gene. *Neurochem Int.* 1992;21:185–189.

76. Akabayashi A, Watanabe Y, Gabriel SM, Chae HJ, Leibowitz SF. Hypothalamic galanin-like immunoreactivity and its gene expression in relation to circulating corticosterone. *Mol Brain Res.* 1994; 25:305–312.

77. Hedlund PB, Koenig JI, Fuxe K. Adrenalectomy alters discrete galanin mRNA levels in the hypothalamus and mesencephalon of the rat. *Neurosci Lett.* 1994;170:77–82.

78. Bonavera JJ, Dube MG, Kalra PS, Kalra SP. Anorectic effects of estrogen may be mediated by decreased neuropeptide-Y release in the hypothalamic paraventricular nucleus. *Endocrinology.* 1994; 134:2367–2370.

79. Sar M, Sahu A, Crowley WR, Kalra SP. Localization of neuropeptide-Y immunoreactivity in estradiol-concentrating cells in the hypothalamus. *Endocrinology.* 1990;127:2752–2756.

80. Urban JH, Bauer-Dantoin AC, Levine JE. Neuropeptide Y gene expression in the arcuate nucleus: sexual dimorphism and modulation by testosterone. *Endocrinology.* 1993;132:139–145.

81. Urban JH, Bauer-Dantoin AC, Levine JE. Effects of steroid replacement on neuropeptide Y (NPY) gene expression in the arcuate nucleus (ARC) of ovariectomized (OVX) rats. *Soc Neurosci Abs.* 1992;18:110.

82. Bloch GJ, Surth SM, Akesson TR, Micevych, PE. Estrogen-concentrating cells with cell groups of the medial preoptic area: sex differences and co-localization with galanin-immunoreactive cells. *Brain Res.* 1992;595:301–308.

83. Bloch GJ, Eckersell C, Mills R. Distribution of galanin-immunoreactive cells within sexually dimorphic components of the medial preoptic area of the male and female rat. *Brain Res.* 1993;620:259–268.

84. Brann DW, Chorich LP, Mahesh VB. Effect of progesterone on galanin mRNA levels in the hypothalamus and the pituitary: correlation with the gonadotropin surge. *Neuroendocrinology.* 1993;58: 531–538.

85. Levin MC, Sawchenko PE, Howe PR, Bloom SR, Polak JM. Organization of galanin-immunoreactive inputs to the paraventric-

ular nucleus with special reference to their relationship to catech-olaminergic afferents. *J Comp Neurol.* 1987;261:562–582.

86. Marks SL, Smith MS, Vrontakis M, Clifton DK, Steiner RA. Reg-ulation of galanin gene expression in gonadotropin-releasing hor-mone neurons during the estrous cycle of the rat. *Endocrinology.* 1993;132:1836–1844.

87. Gabriel SM, Koenig JI, Kaplan LM. Galanin-like immunoreactivity is influenced by estrogen in peripubertal and adult rats. *Neuroen-docrinology.* 1990;51:168–173.

88. Gabriel SM, Washton DL, Roncancio JR. Modulation of hypotha-lamic galanin gene expression by estrogen in peripubertal rats. *Peptides.* 1992;13:801–806.

89. Kaplan LM, Abrazczinkas D, Davidson M, Chin WW. Estrogen regulation of rat galanin transcription is mediated by sequences in the 5'-flanking region of the galanin gene. *Soc Neurosci Abs.* 1989;15:646.

90. White JD, Olchovsky D, Kershaw M, Berelowitz M. Increased hy-pothalamic content of preproneuropeptide Y messenger ribonu-cleic acid in streptozotocin-diabetic rats. *Endocrinology.* 1990;126:765–770.

91. Sahu A, Sninsky CA, Kalra PS, Kalra SP. Neuropeptide Y concen-trations in microdissected hypothalamic regions and in vitro re-lease from medial basal hypothalamus-preoptic area of strepto-zotocin-diabetic rats with and without insulin substitution therapy. *Endocrinology.* 1990;126:192–198.

92. Sahu A, Sninsky CA, Phelps CP, Dube MG, Kalra PS, Kalra SP. Neuropeptide Y release from the paraventricular nucleus in-creases in association with hyperphagia in streptozotocin-induced diabetic rats. *Endocrinology.* 1992;131:2979–2985.

93. Williams G, Gill JS, Lee YC, Cardoso HM, Okpere BE, Bloom SR. Increased neuropeptide Y in specific hypothalamic nuclei of the streptozotocin-diabetic rat. *Diabetes.* 1989;38:321–327.

94. Wilding JPH, Gilbey SG, Lambert PD, Ghatei MA, Bloom SR. In-creases in neuropeptide Y content and gene expression in the hy-pothalamus of rats treated with dexamethasone are prevented by insulin. *Neuroendocrinology.* 1993;57:581–587.

95. Malabu UH, McCarthy HD, McKibbin PE, Williams G. Peripheral insulin administration attenuated the increase in neuropeptide Y

concentrations in the hypothalamic arcuate nucleus of fasted rats. *Peptides.* 1992;13:1097–1102.

96. Frankish HM, McCarthy HD, Dryden S, Kilpatrick A, Williams G. Neuropeptide Y receptor numbers are reduced in the hypothalamus of streptozotocin-diabetic and food-deprived rats: further evidence of increased activity of hypothalamic NPY-containing pathways. *Peptides.* 1993;14:941–948.

97. Marks JL, Li M, Schwartz M, Porte D Jr, Baskin DG. Effect of fasting on regional levels of neuropeptide Y mRNA and insulin receptors in the rat hypothalamus: an autoradiographic study. *Mol Cell Neurosci.* 1992;3:199–205.

98. McKibbin PE, McCarthy HD, Shaw P, Williams G. Insulin deficiency is a specific stimulus to hypothalamic neuropeptide Y: a comparison of the effects of insulin replacement and food restriction in streptozotocin-diabetic rats. *Peptides.* 1992;13:721–727.

99. Timmers K, Coleman DL, Voyles NR, Powell AM, Rokaeus A, Recant L. Neuropeptide content in pancreas and pituitary of obese mutant mice: strain and sex differences. *Metabolism.* 1990;39:378–383.

100. Williams G, Steel JH, Cardoso H, *et al.* Increased hypothalamic neuropeptide Y concentrations in diabetic rat. *Diabetes.* 1988;37:763–772.

101. Tang C, Akabayashi A, Manitiu A, Leibowitz SF. Insulin modulates galanin gene expression in the hypothalamic paraventricular nucleus. *Soc Neurosci Abs.* 1994;20:99.

102. Bachus SE, Jhanwar-Uniyal M. Gene expression of neuropeptides in the paraventricular (PVN) and supraoptic (SON) hypothalamic nuclei of streptozotocin (STZ)-diabetic rat. *Soc Neurosci Abs.* 1993;19:1821.

103. Kalra SP, Dube MG, Sahu A, Phelps CP, Kalra PS. Neuropeptide Y secretion increases in the paraventricular nucleus in association with increased appetite for food. *Proc Natl Acad Sci USA.* 1991;88:10931–10935.

104. Beck B, Jhanwar-Uniyal M, Burlet A, Chapleur-Chateau M, Leibowitz SF, Burlet C. Rapid and localized alterations of neuropeptide Y in discrete hypothalamic nuclei with feeding status. *Brain Res.* 1990;528:245–249.

105. Calza L, Giardino L, Battistini N, *et al.* Increase of neuropeptide

Y-like immunoreactivity in the paraventricular nucleus of fasting rats. *Neurosci Lett.* 1989;104:99–104.

106. Chua SC, Leibel RL, Hirsch J. Food deprivation and age modulate neuropeptide gene expression in the murine hypothalamus and adrenal gland. *Mol Brain Res.* 1991;9:95–101.

107. Sanacora G, Kershaw M, Finkelstein JA, White JD. Increased hypothalamic content of preproneuropeptide Y messenger ribonucleic acid in genetically obese Zucker rats and its regulation by food deprivation. *Endocrinology.* 1990;127:730–737.

108. White JD, Kershaw M. Increased hypothalamic preproneuropeptide Y mRNA following food deprivation. *Mol Cell Neurosci.* 1990; 1:41–48.

109. Sahu A, Kalra PS, Kalra SP. Food deprivation and ingestion induce reciprocal changes in neuropeptide Y concentrations in the paraventricular nucleus. *Peptides.* 1988;9:83–86.

110. Beck B, Burlet A, Nicolas J-P, Burlet C. Galanin in the hypothalamus of fed and fasted lean and obese Zucker rats. *Brain Res.* 1993; 623:124–130.

111. Brady LS, Smith MA, Gold PW, Herkenham M. Altered expression of hypothalamic neuropeptide mRNAs in food-restricted and food-deprived rats. *Neuroendocrinology.* 1990;52:441–447.

112. Jhanwar-Uniyal M, Chua SC Jr. Critical effects of aging and nutritional state on hypothalamic neuropeptide Y and galanin gene expression in lean and genetically obese Zucker rats. *Mol Brain Res.* 1993;19:195–202.

113. Bernadier CD, Hargrove JL, eds. *Nutrition and Gene Expression.* Boca Raton, FL: CRC Press; 1993.

114. Schwartz MW, Marks J, Sipols AJ, *et al.* Central insulin administration reduces neuropeptide Y mRNA expression in the arcuate nucleus of food-deprived lean (*Fa/Fa*) but not obese (*fa/fa*) Zucker rats. *Endocrinology.* 1991;128:2645–2647.

115. Manitiu A, Nascimento J, Akabayashi A, Leibowitz SF. Inhibition of fatty acid oxidation via injection of mercaptoacetate decreases fat intake and galanin levels in the paraventricular nucleus. *Int Behav Neuroci Soc Abs.* 1994;3:67.

116. Abe M, Saito M, Ikeda H, Shimazu T. Increased neuropeptide Y content in the arcuato-paraventricular hypothalamic neuronal cells in both insulin-dependent and non-insulin-dependent diabetic rats. *Brain Res.* 1991;539:223–227.

117. McKibbin PE, Cotton SJ, McMillan S, *et al.* Altered neuropeptide Y concentrations in specific hypothalamic regions of obese (*fa/fa*) Zucker rats: possible relationship to obesity and neuroendocrine disturbances. *Diabetes.* 1991;40:1423–1429.

118. Williams G, Bloom SR. Regulatory peptides, the hypothalamus and diabetes. *Diabetic Med.* 1989;6:472–485.

119. Lewis DE, Shellard L, Koeslag DG, *et al.* Intense exercise and food restriction cause similar hypothalamic neuropeptide Y increases in rats. *Am J Physiol.* 1993;264:E279–E284.

120. Higuchi H, Yang H-YT, Sabol SL. mRNA structure, tissue distribution, and regulation by glucocorticoids, cyclic AMP, and phorbol ester. *J Biol Chem.* 1988;263:6288–6295.

121. Barnea A, Cho G, Hajibeigi A, Aguila MC, Magni P. Dexamethasone-induced accumulation of neuropeptide-Y by aggregating fetal brain cells in culture: a process dependent on the developmental age of the aggregates. *Endocrinology.* 1991;129:931–938.

122. Sabol SL, Higuchi H. Transcriptional regulation of the neuropeptide Y gene by nerve growth factor: antagonism by glucocorticoids and potentiation by adenosine 3′,5′-monophosphate and phorbol ester. *Mol Endocrinol.* 1990;4:384–392.

123. Akabayashi A, Zaia CTBV, Gabriel SM, Silva I, Cheung WK, Leibowitz SF. Intracerebroventricular injection of dibutyryl cyclic adenosine 3′,5′-monophosphate increases hypothalamic levels of neuropeptide Y. *Brain Res.* 1994;660:323–328.

124. Jhanwar-Uniyal M, Beck B, Jhanwar YS, Burlet C, Leibowitz SF. Neuropeptide Y projection from arcuate nucleus to parvocellular division of paraventricular nucleus: specific relation to the ingestion of carbohydrate. *Brain Res.* 1993;631:97–106.

125. Beck B, Stricker-Krongrad A, Burlet A, Nicolas J-P, Burlet C. Specific hypothalamic neuropeptide Y variation with diet parameters in rats with food choice. *NeuroReport.* 1992;3:571–574.

126. Akabayashi A, Koenig JI, Watanbe Y, Alexander JT, Leibowitz SF. Galanin-containing neurons in the paraventricular nucleus: a neurochemical marker for fat ingestion and body weight gain. *Proc Natl Acad Sci USA.* 1994;91:10375–10379.

127. Tucker SJ, Jhanwar-Uniyal M, Chua SC Jr, Grinker J, Leibowitz SF. Hypothalamic galanin gene expression is associated with preferential fat intake, insulin levels and body weight. *Soc Neurosci Abs.* 1992;18:1427.

128. Larue-Achagiotis C, Martin C, Verger P, Louis-Sylvestre J. Dietary self-selection vs complete diet: body weight-gain and meal pattern in rats. *Physiol Behav.* 1992;51:995–999.

129. Van Cauter E, Desir D, Decoster C, Fery F, Balasse EO. Nocturnal decrease in glucose tolerance during constant glucose infusion. *J Clin Endocrinol Metab.* 1989;69:604–611.

130. Albers HE, Ferris CF. Neuropeptide Y: role in light-dark entrainment of hamster circadian rhythms. *Neurosci Lett.* 1984;50:163–168.

131. Moore RY, Card JP. Neuropeptide Y and the circadian system. In: Mutt V, Hokfelt T, Fuxe K, Lundberg JM, eds. *Neuropeptide Y.* New York: Raven Press; 1989:293–301.

132. Stanley BG, Lanthier D, Chin AS, Leibowitz SF. Suppression of neuropeptide Y–elicited eating by adrenalectomy or hypophysectomy: reversal with corticosterone. *Brain Res.* 1989;501:32–36.

133. Akabayashi A, Zaia CTBV, Koenig JI, Gabriel SM, Silva I, Leibowitz SF. Diurnal rhythm of galanin-like immunoreactivity in the paraventricular and suprachiasmatic nuclei and other hypothalamic areas. *Peptides.* 1994;15:1437–1444.

134. Allen JM, McGregor GP, Woodhams PL, Polak JM, Bloom SR. Ontogeny of a novel peptide, neuropeptide Y (NPY) in rat brain. *Brain Res.* 1984;303:197–200.

135. Kagotani Y, Hashimoto T, Tsuruo Y, Kawano H, Daikoku S, Chihara K. Development of the neuronal system containing neuropeptide Y in the rat hypothalamus. *Int J Dev Neurosci.* 1989;7:359–374.

136. Sapolsky RM, Meaney MJ. Maturation of the adrenocortical stress response: neuroendocrine control mechanisms and the stress hyporesponsive period. *Brain Res Rev.* 1986;11:65–76.

137. Sutton SW, Mitsugi N, Plotsky PM, Sarkar DK. Neuropeptide Y (NPY): a possible role in the initiation of puberty. *Endocrinology.* 1988;123:2152–2154.

138. Kant GJ, Lenox RH, Bunnell BN, Mougey EH, Pennington LL, Meyerhoff JL. Comparison of stress response in male and female rats: pituitary cyclic AMP, and plasma prolactin, growth hormone and corticosterone. *Psychoneuroendocrinology.* 1983;8:421–428.

139. Lesniewska B, Miskowiak B, Nowak M, Malendowicz LK. Sex differences in adrenocortical structure and function, XXVII: the effect of ether stress on ACTH and corticosterone in intact, gonad-

ectomized, and testosterone- or estradiol-replaced rats. *Res Exp Med (Berl)*. 1990;190:95–103.

140. Leibowitz SF, Lucas DJ, Leibowitz KL, Jhanwar YS. Developmental patterns of macronutrient intake in female and male rats from weaning to maturity. *Physiol Behav*. 1991;50:1167–1174.

141. Drewnowski A, Kurth C, Holden-Wilste J, Saari J. Food preferences in human obesity: carbohydrates versus fats. *Appetite*. 1992; 18:207–221.

142. Gabriel SM, Kaplan LM, Martin JB, Koenig JI. Tissue-specific sex differences in galanin-like immunoreactivity and galanin mRNA during development in the rat. *Peptides*. 1989;10:369–374.

143. Alexander JT, Akabayashi A, Gabriel SM, Thomas BE, Leibowitz SF. Galanin and neuropeptide Y immunoreactivity in brain nuclei of female and male rats in relation to puberty. *Soc Neurosci Abs*. 1994;20:99.

144. Merchenthaler I, Lopez FJ, Lennard DE, Negro-Vilar A. Sexual differences in the distribution of neurons coexpressing galanin and luteinizing hormone–releasing hormone in the rat brain. *Endocrinology*. 1991;129:1977–1986.

145. Shibasaki T, Oda T, Imaki T, Ling N, Demura H. Injection of anti-neuropeptide Y τ-globulin into the hypothalamic paraventricular nucleus decreases food intake in rats. *Brain Res*. 1993;601:313–316.

146. Leibowitz SF, Xuereb M, Kim T. Blockade of natural and neuropeptide Y-induced carbohydrate feeding by a receptor antagonist, PYX-2. *NeuroReport*. 1992;3:1023–1026.

147. Leibowitz SF, Kim T. Impact of a galanin antagonist on exogenous galanin and natural patterns of fat ingestion. *Brain Res*. 1992;599: 148–152.

148. Akabayashi A, Wahlestedt C, Alexander JT, Leibowitz SF. Specific inhibition of endogenous neuropeptide Y synthesis in arcuate nucleus by antisense oligonucleotides suppresses feeding behavior and insulin secretion. *Mol Brain Res*. 1994;21:55–61.

149. Beck B, Burlet A, Nicolas JP, Burlet C. Hypothalamic neuropeptide Y (NPY) in obese Zucker rats: implications in feeding and sexual behaviors. *Physiol Behav*. 1990;47:449–453.

150. Williams G, Shellard L, Lewis DE, *et al*. Hypothalamic neuropeptide Y disturbances in the obese (*cp/cp*) JCR:LA corpulent rat. *Peptides*. 1992;13:537–540.

151. Chua S, LaChaussee JL. Molecular pathogenesis of obesity in the fatty rat. *Appetite.* 1993;21:303.
152. Sanacora G, Finkelstein JA, White JD. Developmental aspect of differences in hypothalamic preproneuropeptide Y messenger ribonucleic acid content in lean and genetically obese Zucker rats. *J Neuroendocrinol.* 1992;4:353–357.
153. Boulange A, Planche E, deGasquet P. Onset of genetic obesity in the absence of hyperphagia during the first week of life in the Zucker rat (*fa/fa*). *J Lipid Res.* 1979;20:857–864.
154. Moore BJ, Armbruster SJ, Horwitz BA, Stern JS. Energy expenditure is reduced in preobese 2-day Zucker *fa/fa* rats. *Am J Physiol.* 1985;249:R262–R265.
155. McCarthy HD, McKibbin PE, Holloway B, Mayers R, Williams G. Hypothalamic neuropeptide Y receptor characteristics and NPY-induced feeding responses in lean and obese Zucker rats. *Life Sci.* 1991;49:1491–1497.
156. Kalra SP, Duke MG, Finkelstein J, Sahu A. Neuropeptide Y (NPY) release from the paraventricular nucleus of genetically obese and lean Zucker rats. *Soc Study Ingestive Behav Abs.* 1994;A18.
157. Kaye WH, Berrettini W, Gwirtsman H, George DT. Altered cerebrospinal fluid neuropeptide Y and peptide YY immunoreactivity in anorexia and bulimia nervosa. *Arch Gen Psychiatry.* 1990;47:548–556.

BARTLEY G. HOEBEL, PEDRO RADA, GREGORY P. MARK,
MARCO PARADA, MARINA PUIG DE PARADA,
EMMANUEL POTHOS, and LUIS HERNANDEZ

Hypothalamic Control of Accumbens Dopamine: A System for Feeding Reinforcement

ABSTRACT

Results from this laboratory are reviewed that suggest identified neurotransmitter systems in the hypothalamus can reinforce feeding behavior in part by controlling dopamine release in the nucleus accumbens. Six findings are presented: 1) When mildly food-deprived rats performed an instrumental response for food pellets, dopamine was released in the accumbens and prefrontal cortex; 2) Conditioned taste stimuli excited or inhibited dopamine release in the accumbens depending on the meaning for the animal; 3) Basal extracellular dopamine in the accumbens was low in underweight rats; 4) Galanin in the hypothalamus that stimulated feeding activated a system for dopamine release in the accumbens; 5) Hypothalamic dopamine inhibited accumbens dopamine, as judged from the actions of local sulpiride, which blocked hypothalamic dopamine receptors and activated a circuit that released dopamine in the accumbens; and 6) Rats self-injected hypothalamic sulpiride. The results imply that when galanin or sulpiride causes an animal to eat, it also causes dopamine release in an accumbens system that reinforces ongoing operant behavior; thus it reinforces eating. If the food provides nutrition, as opposed to illness, then the flavor becomes a conditioned stimulus that can release dopamine in the accumbens and theoretically reinforce ingestion of that flavor in the future. It is speculated that animals will work to raise extracellular dopamine in the accumbens by ingesting appropriate flavors and eating, especially if they are underweight when their nucleus accumbens dopamine is low.

1. Eating Can Release Dopamine in the NAc and Dopamine Can Reinforce Instrumental Behavior

A stimulus is a positive reinforcer if its presentation increases the frequency or force of associated behavior (1). Positive reinforcers such as food, water, most drugs of abuse, and lateral hypothalamic stimulation can all increase extracellular dopamine in the nucleus accumbens (NAc) under certain conditions (2, 3). This is illustrated by Figure 1, which shows dopamine in the nucleus accumbens (NAc) during lever pressing for food pellets. The stimuli and behaviors engaged by the meal also released dopamine in the NAc and prefrontal cortex (4). As a control for anatomical selectivity dopamine did not change detectably in the region of the dorsal striatum that was sampled (3). Thus in vivo microdialysis suggests that the mesolimbic dopamine projections are involved in self-administration of natural rewards, drug rewards, and electrical rewards. This has been corroborated with dopamine antagonists administered systemically, or directly into the NAc, to block locomotion, behavior output, instrumental behavior, and sucrose sweetness (5–7). Neural recordings from dopamine cells in the ventral tegmental area of awake monkeys confirm that some of the neurons that project in part to the NAc increased their firing rate during eating (8). As the monkeys gained practice at the feeding task, neural activity in the ventral tegmental area occurred in advance of food presentation and coincided instead with discriminative stimuli that signaled the forthcoming food. Although dopamine release in the NAc is clearly involved in learning instrumental behavior, it is not always necessary for feeding as illustrated in dopamine-depleted or decerebrated rats (9). In summary the evidence from microdialysis, psychopharmacology, and electrophysiology strongly suggests that dopamine release in parts of the NAc is involved in various aspects of eating in vertebrates with intact brains.

One of the effects of dopamine in the NAc is positive reinforcement. Dopamine injected directly into the NAc is a positive reinforcer by operational definition, as shown by the fact that rats repeated operant responses, such as lever presses, that triggered self-injection of dopamine in the NAc (10). They also eat food that can release dopamine in the NAc (Fig. 1), self-inject amphetamine that releases dopamine in the NAc (11), and self-stimulate their lateral hypothalamus, which releases dopamine in the NAc (3). This suggests that the positive reinforcement

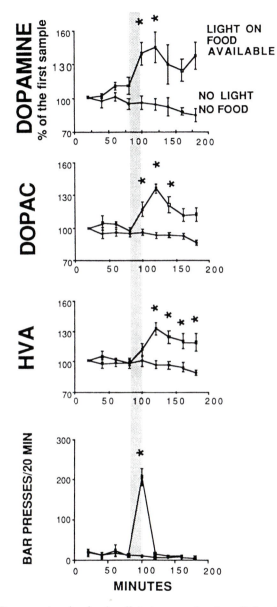

Figure 1. Bar pressing for food pellets increased extracellular dopamine and its metabolites (*P < 0.05) in the NAc (3).

effects generated in the NAc may form the basis of augmented food intake during bulimia, psychostimulant abuse, and unabated self-stimulation (12).

Microdialysis shows that stress and negative reinforcers such as foot shock or associated warning signals can also release dopamine in the NAc; thus dopamine's role is not limited to positive reinforcement but extends to aspects of negative reinforcement as well (13, 14). Normal behavior patterns that involve the release of dopamine in the NAc include approach behaviors, such as feeding, drinking, and mating, and escape behaviors elicited by stress or pain. Apparently dopaminergic modulation of the NAc is related in part to the reinforcement of instrumental behavior, its antecedents and perhaps its aftermath (2, 15–19).

The rest of this chapter is built on the premise that when extracellular dopamine increases in the NAc, this event can reinforce ongoing instrumental behavior. There may be exceptions to this principle when dopamine is counteracted by other processes, such as high levels of acetylcholine in the NAc (20), but normally an acute rise in extracellular NAc dopamine is a proven reinforcer that can contribute to the increased frequency or force of instrumental behavior for food.

2. Dopamine Release in the NAc Can Be Increased or Decreased by Classically Conditioning with Food Flavors as the Conditioned Stimuli

Rats will press a lever to self-inject food in the stomach and can control their calorie intake in a manner that maintains a stable body weight; thus postingestional effects of food can be a positive reinforcer and can be metered in the absence of taste (21). A flavor associated with intragastric feeding can become a preferred flavor (22). It is clear that neural mechanisms for classical conditioning associate the food flavor with the postingestional effects of the food.

In rats with both an oral catheter for infusing flavors and a gastric catheter for infusing food, a taste associated with intragastric carbohydrate infusion released dopamine in the NAc (23). Thus dopamine release can be classically conditioned (Fig. 2). Conversely, a flavor paired with nausea is later avoided, and it can cause extracellular dopamine to decrease instead of increase (24).

Scott and Mark (25) showed that the nucleus tractus solitarius (NTS)

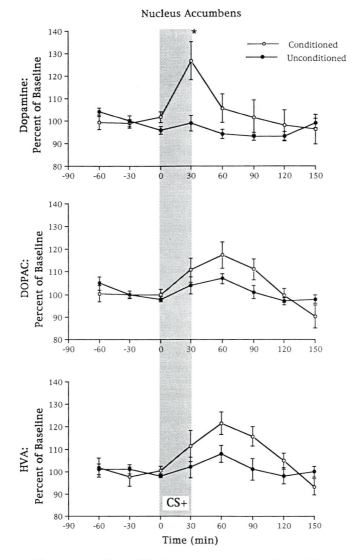

Figure 2.   The taste of a flavor (CS +) associated on prior days with intragastric infusion of nutritious polycose increased extracellular dopamine (*$P < 0.01$) in the NAc (23). This is an example of conditioned neurotransmitter release.

codes taste not just for its physical-chemical effects on the tongue, but also for its quality as a flavor on a dimension of nutrition versus poison. Apparently this learned dimension is reflected in learned release of dopamine in the NAc. The effect of the meal is the unconditioned stimulus, and the food flavor becomes a conditioned stimulus that influences dopamine release (23, 24). We hypothesize that increased dopamine is part of the flavor preference and decreased dopamine is part of the flavor aversion.

3. Basal Dopamine in the NAc Is Low in Underweight Animals

A serendipitous observation by microdialysis revealed that basal extracellular dopamine is 50% to 75% of normal in underweight rats. This was replicated using male rats that were food restricted until they reached 80% of their starting weight (Fig. 3). When the underweight animals were allowed to eat a meal of standardized size (7.5 gs), eating released dopamine, but the increase was not as big a percentage as seen in the control animals even though the baseline was lower (26).

Amphetamine (1.5 mg/kg) also increased extracellular dopamine, but in the underweight animals dopamine just reached normal levels, not the high levels seen in the control group. Morphine (20 mg/kg i.p) also increased NAc dopamine (27), but when given to underweight rats it had a relatively small effect (26). To achieve high levels of dopamine, underweight rats would need to augment their intake of food or drug. It is well known that this is precisely what they do (28). Meal taking, drug abuse, and lateral hypothalamic self-stimulation are all augmented in underweight rats (28, 29). We now theorize that this is due in part to the fact that their NAc dopamine is low and that they work to raise extracellular dopamine until some other factor provides negative feedback that stops the process. In the case of feeding, negative feedback might come from a factor associated with increasing body weight.

Figure 3.   Food restriction that caused body weight loss to 80% of start weight (top graph) was associated with a decrease of basal extracellular dopamine in the NAc (middle graph; *$P < 0.01$). Serotonin at the same site was not depressed. Dopamine was not restored by weight gain back to the starting weight, but in the meantime the control group had grown much heavier; so perhaps more time was needed for the experimental group to regain weight and basal dopamine (26).

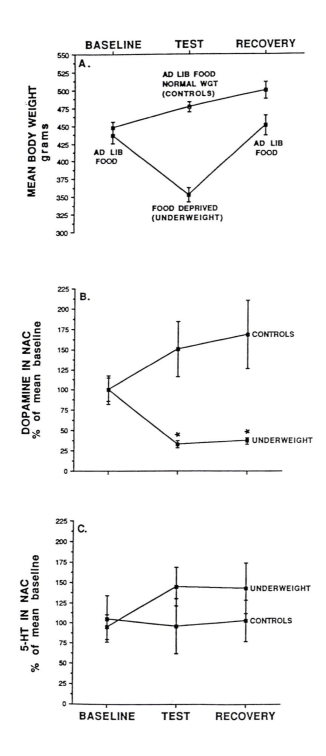

To begin testing this idea, rats were given ventromedial hypothalamic lesions that would reset body weight to a higher level (30). Microdialysis revealed elevated dopamine in the NAc during the dynamic phase of hypothalamic hyperphagia (31). On the basis of these experiments we suggest there is an interaction between some aspect of dopaminergic function and body weight. Animals that are below their preferred weight plateau tend to eat more and to raise their extracellular dopamine. Perhaps body weight plays a role in controlling mesolimbic dopamine, or mesolimbic dopamine plays a role in controlling body weight.

4. When Galanin in the Hypothalamus Stimulates Feeding, It Also Activates a System That Releases Dopamine in the NAc

The power of peptides to release mesolimbic dopamine is discussed elsewhere (32). Galanin is particularly interesting in the present context because it is involved in the regulation of fat intake and thereby plays a major role in the control of body weight (33). Galanin injections into the hypothalamic paraventricular nucleus (PVN) induce feeding, and if the animals have a choice of macronutrients, they tend to choose fat (33). The PVN galanin injections activate a natural hypothalamic mechanism as shown by radioimmunoassay for galanin, in situ hybridization for the galanin message, and local injections of galanin receptor antagonists or antisense oligonucleotides (34).

When galanin (300 picomoles) was injected in the PVN of rats equipped with a microdialysis probe in the NAc, there was a significant increase in dopamine in six of nine animals, even in the absence of food. Subsequent behavioral tests uncovered that these were the only six animals that ate food pellets in response to identical galanin injections (Fig. 4). We conclude on the basis of these results that when galanin is injected in the right place to induce eating, the peptide activates a neural circuit that release dopamine in the NAc.

The implications of this are interesting. Galanin may induce feeding behavior partly by activating the mesolimbic dopamine system and in part by its effects on the taste system, leading the animal to choose food with fat in it, and the surge in dopamine may reinforce ongoing behavior. Given that galanin induces feeding, it is feeding behavior that is likely to be reinforced. Galanin specifically induces a preference for

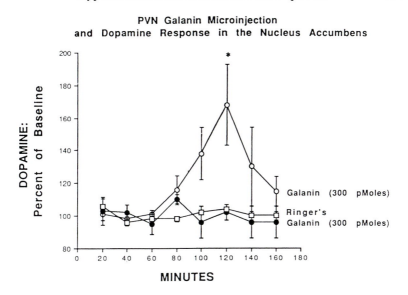

Figure 4. Local injection of galanin into the PVN increased extracellular dopamine in the NAc, but only in rats that later ate in response to identical galanin
injections (*P < 0.01). This demonstrates control of accumbens dopamine by a
hypothalamic peptide.

fat late in the daily feeding cycle; therefore, it is fat intake at times such
as these that will be reinforced by galanin-induced dopamine release.

A synthesis of result number two above (conditioned dopamine release with flavors) and result number four (galanin-induced release of
dopamine) leads to the suggestion that when an animal eats a fatty
food under the influence of PVN galanin, the flavor of that food will
become a conditioned stimulus for dopamine release. Given that dopamine can be a reinforcer (10), the conditioned stimulus flavor may
become a secondary reinforcer in this way.

If we extend this line of reasoning to humans, the new calorie-free
fat-tasting foods will be consumed as secondary reinforcers because of
conditioned dopamine release. Knowing that mesolimbic dopamine release is part of the addiction process, it is easy to speculate that galanin
in the PVN could foster an addiction to fatty food if the process were
not curbed. The next section presents new evidence of a neural mechanism that normally stops eating from releasing dopamine in the NAc
so that the individual usually does not succumb to galanin-induced
"dopamine addiction" and become overweight or bulimic.

5. Evidence That Hypothalamic Dopamine Exerts Chronic Inhibition of NAc Dopamine Release

What stops the dopamine reinforcement process? In the case of amphetamine and cocaine that act directly in the dopamine terminal regions there is little or nothing to prevent the person from boosting extracellular dopamine to the point of self-induced psychosis. However, in normal feeding behavior, the digestion of food provides negative feedback that stops eating and defines a meal by ending it. One of the many hypothalamic neurochemicals that cause satiety is dopamine. Amphetamine's ability to release dopamine partially explains why animals are willing to self-inject it into the NAc (11, 35) and manifest anorexia when it is put in their lateral hypothalamus (36, 37). The effect of lateral hypothalamic amphetamine on extracellular levels of three monoamines is shown in Figure 5 (38). All three monoamines suppress feeding when injected in the lateral hypothalamus. Excess norepinephrine released from the ventral noradrenergic bundle (39) by amphetamine in the lateral hypothalamus can act at β-adrenergic receptors (36, 40) to suppress food intake. Excess serotonin is most effective in the PVN (41), but it is also released in the lateral hypothalamus by the anorectic drug d-fenfluramine, by conditioned taste aversion, and before and during a meal (42–44); therefore, serotonin, possibly in combination with postingestional satiety peptides, may contribute to anorexia in the lateral hypothalamus as well as the PVN (2). Excess dopamine in the lateral hypothalamus is known to cause anorexia (45), even though other effects can be seen with the amounts that are iontophoresed in electrophysiological studies (46).

The overall satiety effect of dopamine in the lateral hypothalamus has been substantiated by dopamine receptor antagonists. Sulpiride was originally tested because it caused overeating and weight gain during chronic treatment in schizophrenic patients. When injected in rats, this relatively specific D_2 receptor antagonist caused hyperphagia and obesity (47, 48). The effect was localized in the medial and lateral hypothalamus where sulpiride injection could disinhibit locomotion and feeding (2, 48). This suggested that D_2 receptors in the lateral hypothalamus exert tonic inhibition of exploration and eating and contribute to the control of body weight. Since lateral hypothalamus stimulation also causes locomotion and eating and can lead to obesity (19, 49), the next question was whether or not dopamine receptor block in the lat-

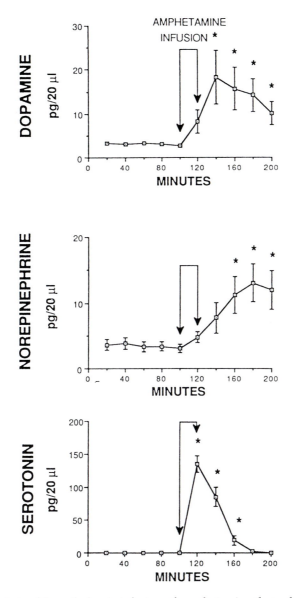

Figure 5. Lateral hypothalamic infusion of amphetamine through a microdialysis probe increased extracellular levels of the three monoamines simultaneously measured, dopamine, norepinephrine, and serotonin (20 μL of 10 μg/μL amphetamine in Ringer's solution = 200 μg amphetamine in the probe = approximately 20 μg diffusing out to the neural tissue; *$P < 0.01$). All three can suppress feeding by an action in the lateral hypothalamus.

274   BARTLEY G. HOEBEL *et al.*

eral hypothalamus would release dopamine in the NAc in a manner analogous to lateral hypothalamus stimulation.

Animals were prepared with guide shafts in the lateral hypothalamus for sulpiride injection and also in the NAc for microdialysis. The result of local lateral hypothalamus sulpiride (4, 8, or 16 μg/0.3 μl) was an increase in extracellular dopamine in the NAc. As a control, injections between the lateral hypothalamus and ventral tegmental area were not as effective as injections directly into the lateral hypothalamus. Therefore, it was concluded that one of dopamine's normal actions in the lateral hypothalamus is to inhibit dopamine release in the NAc (50).

6. Rats Self-Inject Hypothalamic Sulpiride

It followed logically that any behavior that diminished the inhibitory effect of dopamine in the lateral hypothalamus would release dopamine in the NAc and thereby be reinforced. In a preliminary experiment, this was tested by giving rats access to a lever that turned on a pump to deliver sulpiride into the lateral hypothalamus (10 ng/nL; 21 nL/2 sec/self-injection) (Fig. 6). The result was reinforcement of lever pressing as defined by self-injection (50). One can speculate that rats self-inject sulpiride in the lateral hypothalamus to disinhibit some of the same cell types that they excite by lateral hypothalamus self-stimulation; both sulpiride and electrical stimulation release dopamine in the NAc, and both are reinforcers.

In summary, there is a similarity between lateral hypothalamus injections of galanin, sulpiride, and stimulation. When any of the three are capable of inducing eating, they are apparently capable of releasing dopamine in the NAc. When any of the three release dopamine in the NAc, they are reinforcers; the animal's behavior is strengthened. The most likely anatomical route for this effect is from the lateral hypothalamus, directly or indirectly, to the ventral tegmental area and from there via the mesolimbic projection to the NAc (19). The relevant source

---

Figure 6. The dopamine receptor antagonist sulpiride (8 μg/0.3 μL) injected unilaterally in the perifornical lateral hypothalamus (pf-LH) caused an increase in extracellular dopamine far away in the NAc (symbols = $P < 0.05$). The text suggests that dopamine in the lateral hypothalamus exerts tonic inhibition on the release of dopamine in the NAc.

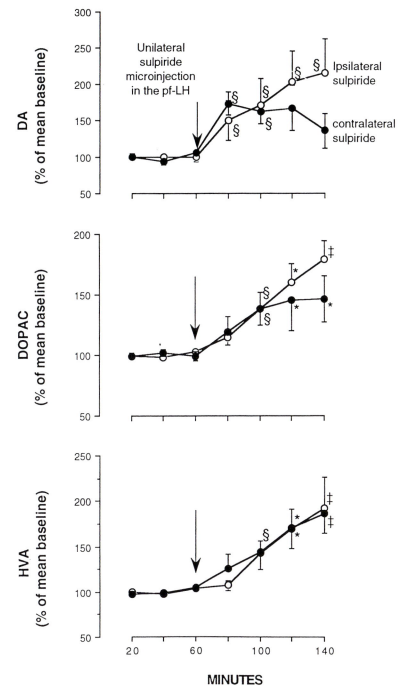

NUCLEUS ACCUMBENS

of dopamine in the hypothalamus is not known; it may come from the mesolimbic system or intrinsic hypothalamic dopamine sources. Given result number three above, that mesolimbic dopamine is low in underweight rats, we propose that this creates a potential for eating extra meals that are reinforced with dopamine in the NAc. This would continue until factors such as dopamine in the lateral hypothalamus are elevated to the point of inhibiting the mesolimbic system. Judging by the effect of ventromedial hypothalamic lesions, this region normally inhibits feeding reward and helps contribute to the control of mesolimbic dopamine. In the PVN and related hypothalamic nuclei, galanin is a natural source of stimulation leading to dopamine release in the NAc; lateral hypothalamic dopamine may counteract this effect. The balance of such factors is central to the control of foraging, eating, and satiety through the reinforcement, positive and negative, of feeding-related behaviors, including reactions to conditioned stimuli for dopamine release.

REFERENCES

1. Skinner BG. *Science and Human Behavior.* New York: The MacMillan Company; 1953.
2. Hoebel BG, Rada P, Mark G, Parada M, Puig de Parada M. Control of the mesolimbic reward system: PVN galanin and LH dopamine. In: Proceedings of the 7th International Congress of Obesity. *J Obesity.* In press.
3. Hernandez L, Hoebel BG. Feeding and hypothalamic stimulation increase dopamine turnover in the accumbens. *Physiol Behav.* 1988; 44:599–606.
4. Hernandez L, Hoebel BG. Feeding can enhance dopamine turnover in the prefrontal cortex. *Brain Res Bull.* 1990;25:975–979.
5. Smith GP. Dopamine and food reward. In: Morrison A, Fluharty S, eds. *Progress in Psychobiology and Physiological Psychology.* New York: Academic Press. In press.
6. Koob GF, Goeders NE. Neuroanatomical substrates of drug self-administration. In: Liebman JM, Cooper SJ, eds. *The Neuropharmacological Basis of Reward.* Oxford, Eng.: Oxford University Press; 1989:214–263.
7. Wise RA, Spindler J, DeWit H, Gerber GJ. Neuroleptic-induced "an-

hedonia" in rats: pimozide blocks the reward quality of food. *Science.* 1978;201:262–264.

8. Schultz W, Apicella P, Ljungberg T. Responses of monkey dopamine neurons to reward and conditioned stimuli during successive steps of learning a delayed response task. *J Neurosci.* 1993;13:900–913.

9. Grill HJ, Kaplan JM. Caudal brainstem participates in the distributed neural control of feeding. In: Stricker EM, ed. *Handbook of Behavioral Neurobiology.* New York: Plenum Press; 1990;10:125–149.

10. Dworkin SI, Goeders NE, Smith JM. The reinforcing and rate effects of intracranial dopamine administration. *Natl Inst Drug Abuse Res Monogr Ser.* 1985;67:242–248.

11. Hoebel BG, Monaco AP, Hernandez L, Aulisi EF, Stanley BG, Lenard L. Self-injection of amphetamine directly into the brain. *Psychopharmacology (Berl).* 1983;81:158–163.

12. Hoebel BG, Leibowitz SF, Hernandez L. Neurochemistry of anorexia and bulimia. In: Anderson H, ed. *The Biology of Feast and Famine: Relevance to Eating Disorders.* London: Oxford University Press; 1992:21–45.

13. Abercrombie ED, Keefe KA, DiFrischa DS, Zigmond MJ. Differential effect of stress on in vivo dopamine release in striatum, nucleus accumbens and medial frontal cortex. *J Neurochem.* 1989;52:1655–1658.

14. Young AMJ, Joseph MH, Gray JA. Latent inhibition of conditioned dopamine release in rat nucleus accumbens. *Neuroscience.* 1993;54:5–9.

15. Salamone JD. Behavioral pharmacology of dopamine systems: a new synthesis. In: Willner P, Scheel-Kruger J, eds. *The Mesolimbic Dopamine System: From Motivation to Action.* New York: John Wiley & Sons Ltd; 1991:599–613.

16. Berridge KC, Valenstein ES. What psychological process mediates feeding evoked by electrical stimulation of the lateral hypothalamus? *Behav Neurosci.* 1991;105:3–14.

17. Wise RA. The brain and reward. In: Liebman JM, Cooper SJ, eds. *The Neuropharmacological Basis of Reward.* New York: Oxford University Press; 1989:377–424.

18. Hoebel BG, Hernandez L, Mark GP, *et al.* Brain microdialysis as a molecular approach to obesity: serotonin, dopamine, cyclic-AMP.

In: Bray G, Ricquier D, Spiegleman B, eds. *Obesity: Towards a Molecular Approach.* New York: Alan R. Liss; 1990:45–61.

19. Hoebel BG. Neuroscience and motivation: pathways and peptides that define motivation. In: Atkinson RC, Herrnstein RJ, Lindzey G, Luce RD, eds. *Stevens' Handbook of Experimental Psychology.* New York: John Wiley & Sons; 1988:547–625.

20. Mark GP, Rada P, Pothos E, Hoebel BG. Effects of feeding and drinking on acetylcholine release in the nucleus accumbens, striatum and hippocampus of freely behaving rats. *J Neurochem.* 1992; 58:2269–2274.

21. Epstein AN, Teitelbaum P. Regulation of food intake in the absence of taste, smell, and other oropharyngeal sensations. *J Comp Physiol Psychol.* 1962;55:753–759.

22. Sclafani A. Nutritionally based learned flavor preferences in rats. In: Capaldi E, Powley TL, eds. *Taste, Experience and Feeding.* Washington, DC: American Psychological Association; 1990:139–56.

23. Smith SE, Mark GP, Rada PV, Hoebel BG. An appetitively conditioned taste elicits a preferential increase in mesolimbic dopamine release. *Pharmacol Biochem Behav.* In press.

24. Mark GP, Blander DS, Hoebel BG. A conditioned stimulus decreases extracellular dopamine in the nucleus accumbens after development of a learned taste aversion. *Brain Res.* 1991;551:308–310.

25. Scott TR, Mark GP. The taste system encodes stimulus toxicity. *Brain Res.* 1987;414:197–203.

26. Pothos E, Hernandez L, Auerbach SB, Creese I, Hoebel BG. Changes in body weight can alter the mesolimbic dopamine system and its response to food and drugs. *Neuropsychopharmacology.* 1993; 9:30–31S.

27. Rada P, Mark GP, Pothos E, Hoebel BG. Systemic morphine simultaneously decreases extracellular acetylcholine and increases dopamine in the nucleus accumbens of freely moving rats. *Neuropharmacology.* 1991;30:1133–1136.

28. Carroll ME, France CP, Meisch RA. Food deprivation increases oral and intravenous drug intake in rats. *Science.* 1979;205:319–321.

29. McClelland RC, Hoebel BG. d-Fenfluramine and self-stimulation: loss of inhibitory effect in underweight rats. *Brain Res Bull.* 1991;27: 341–345.

30. Hoebel BG, Teitelbaum P. Weight regulation in normal and hypothalamic hyperphagic rats. *J Comp Physiol Psychol.* 1966;61:189–193.

31. Hernandez L, Parada MA, Puig de Parada MP. Ventromedial hypothalamic lesions enhance dopamine turnover in the nucleus accumbens: an in vivo brain microdialysis study. *Int J Obes.* 1990; 14:54.

32. Hoebel BG, Rada P, Mark GP, Hernandez L. The power of integrative peptides to reinforce behavior by releasing dopamine. In Strand FL, Beckwith BE, Chronwall B, Sendman CA, eds. *Models of Neuropeptide Action.* New York: The New York Academy of Sciences; 1995:36–41.

33. Leibowitz SF. Hypothalamic galanin in relation to feeding behavior and endocrine systems. In: Hokfelt T, Bartfai T, eds. *Galanin: A New Multifunctional Peptide in the Neuro-Endocrine System.* New York: Macmillan Press; 1990.

34. Akabayashi A, Koenig JI, Watanabe Y, Alexander JT, Leibowitz SF. Galanin-containing neurons in the paraventricular nucleus: a neurochemical marker for fat ingestion and body weight gain. *Proc Natl Acad Sci USA.* 1994;91:10375–10379.

35. Hoebel BG, Hernandez L, Mark GP, Pothos E. Microdialysis in the study of psychostimulants and the neural substrate for reinforcement: focus on dopamine and serotonin. In: Frascelli J, Brown RM, eds. *Neurobiological Approaches to Brain-Behavior Interaction.* Rockville, MD: National Institute on Drug Abuse; 1992:1–34.

36. Leibowitz SF. Neurochemical systems of the hypothalamus in control of feeding and drinking behavior and water-electrolyte excretion. In: Morgane PJ, Panksepp J, eds. *Handbook of the Hypothalamus.* New York: Marcel Dekker; 1980;3a:299–437.

37. Hoebel BG, Leibowitz SF. Brain monoamines in the modulation of self-stimulation, feeding, and body weight. In: Weiner H, Hofer MA, Stunkard AJ, eds. *Brain, Behavior, and Bodily Disease.* New York: Raven Press; 1981:103–142.

38. Parada MA, Hernandez L, Schwartz D, Hoebel BG. Hypothalamic infusion of amphetamine increases extracellular serotonin, dopamine and norepinephrine. *Physiol Behav.* 1988;44:607–610.

39. Ahlskog JE, Randal PK, Henandez L, Hoebel BG. Diminished amphetamine anorexia and enhanced fenfluramine anorexia after midbrain 6-hydroxydopamine. *Psychopharmacol.* 1984;82:118–121.

40. Margules DL. Beta-adrenergic receptors in hypothalamus for learned and unlearned taste aversions. *J Comp Physiol Psychol.* 1970; 73:13–21.

41. Leibowitz SF, Weiss GF, Shor-Posner G. Hypothalamic serotonin: pharmacological, biochemical, and behavioral analyses of its feeding-suppressive action. *Clin Neuropharmacol.* 1988;11:S51–S71.

42. Schwartz D, Hernandez L, Hoebel BG. Fenfluramine administered systemically or locally increases extracellular serotonin in the lateral hypothalamus as measured by microdialysis. *Brain Res.* 1989; 482:261–270.

43. Schwartz DH, Hernandez L, Hoebel BG. Serotonin release in lateral and medial hypothalamus during feeding and its anticipation. *Brain Res Bull.* 1990;25:797–802.

44. West HL, Mark GP, Hoebel BG. Effects of conditioned taste aversion on extracellular serotonin in the lateral hypothalamus and hippocampus of freely moving rats. *Brain Res.* 1991;556:95–100.

45. Leibowitz SF, Rossakis C. Pharmacological characterization of perifornical hypothalamic dopamine receptors mediating feeding inhibition in the rat. *Brain Res.* 1979;172:115–130.

46. Fukuda M, Ono T, Nakamura K, Tamura R. Dopamine and ACh involvement in plastic learning by hypothalamic neurons in rats. *Brain Res Bull.* 1990;25:109–114.

47. Parada MA, Hernandez L. Sulpiride obesity is mediated by the ventro-medial but not by the lateral hypothalamus. *Int J Obes.* 1990; 14:53.

48. Parada MA, Hernandez L, Parada MP, Paez X, Hoebel BG. Dopamine in the lateral hypothalamus may be involved in the inhibition of locomotion related to food and water seeking. *Brain Res Bull.* 1990;25:961–968.

49. Hoebel BG. Brain-stimulation reward and aversion in relation to behavior. In: Wauquier A, Rolls ET, eds. *Brain-Stimulation Reward.* Amsterdam: Elsevier Science Publishing; 1976:335–372.

50. Parada MA, Puig de Parada M, Hoebel BG. Rats self-inject a dopamine antagonist in the lateral hypothalamus where it acts to increase extracellular dopamine in the nucleus accumbens. *Pharmacol Biochem Behav.* 1995;51. In press.

DAVID A. YORK and LING LIN

Enterostatin: A Peptide Regulator of Fat Ingestion

ABSTRACT

Enterostatin is the activation pentapeptide of procolipase, a 101
amino acid peptide that is synthesized in the exocrine pancreas
and stomach of rats. Differences in endogenous secretion may determine the variable selection of dietary fat within and between
different rat strains. After either peripheral or central intracerebroventricular administration, enterostatin selectively inhibits the
intake of dietary fat in a number of experimental feeding paradigms and during the normal daily feeding cycle. The peripheral
effects appear to be dependent upon the hepatic vagal afferents
through which signals activate specific brain nuclei, including the
paraventricular and supraoptic nucleus and the nucleus tractus
solitarius. Ingestion of dietary fat increases the production and
secretion of pancreatic colipase. Studies with a range of analogues
suggest that all the biological activity and selectivity toward dietary fat may be contained in the cyclodiketopiperazine ring structure of cyclo-aspartyl-proline (cycloDP). The dose-response curves
to enterostatin and cycloDP are U-shaped, suggesting the presence
of two receptor subtypes. Maximum inhibition of food intake occurs between 0.1 and 1.0 nanomoles intracerebro-ventricular administration, whereas at doses above 10 nanomoles food intake is
increased. The low affinity stimulating site is also activated by β-
casomorphin$_{1-7}$. Enterostatin does not bind to either galanin or
neuropeptide Y–Y$_1$ receptors. However, studies with kappa-
opioid agonist and antagonist suggest that enterostatin inhibits a
kappa-opioid feeding system that is selective for dietary fat. Enterostatin may also have independent effects on insulin and corticosterone secretion. It is hypothesized that enterostatin, or its
biologically active product, may act as a signal to regulate fat appetite and be an important determinant of the susceptibility to
develop obesity on high-fat diets.

281

Feeding and drinking have been the most intensively studied behaviors with respect to obesity because they are relatively easy to measure, quantify, and analyze. Studies of the systems that regulate feeding behavior have identified a complex of central and peripheral pathways that respond to a variety of metabolic, neural, and endocrine signals to alter food intake and feeding-associated behaviors. There have been numerous excellent reviews of this field (1–3).

Although initial studies concentrated upon dissecting the systems that control hunger and satiety, it is now recognized that the intake of specific micro- and macronutrients may be individually controlled. Numerous examples of this are listed in Table 1. To date, the best characterized of these effects are those of angiotensin and neuropeptide Y (NPY). Salt-depleted rats will preferentially select salty solutions to drink to replace their salt deficit. Angiotensin mediates this salt appetite (4). Neuropeptide Y, the most potent neuropeptide stimulator of feeding, will preferentially stimulate carbohydrate feeding when rats are allowed to choose from individual macronutrients (5). The insulin suppression of feeding and carbohydrate intake may be affected through NPY's inhibitory effects on transcription of the prepro-NPY gene (6, 7). Dietary protein intake may be increased by growth hormone–releasing hormone and suppressed by glucagon (8, 9). The systems that might regulate fat intake are of particular interest, since excessive intake of dietary fat favors the development of obesity, which increases morbidity from diabetes, hypertension, cardiovascular disease, and certain cancers (10, 11).

Table 1. Peptide Effects on Specific Nutrients

Nutrient	Increase	Decrease
Fat	Galanin Opioids (kappa)	Enterostatin Vasopressin CRH CCK
Carbohydrate	NPY Insulin	CCK
Protein	GRF	Glucagon CRH
Sodium	Angiotensin	—

See text for references.

Enterostatin is the amino-terminal pentapeptide released from pancreatic procolipase by tryptic hydrolysis after pancreatic secretions have been stimulated by the presence of fat in the proximal duodenum (Fig. 1) (12). Colipase serves as an essential cofactor to enable pancreatic lipase to digest dietary triacylglycerols in the presence of bile salts. The structure of the activation peptide enterostatin is well conserved across a range of animal species, particularly with regard to its bridged proline sequence (13–17) (Table 2). Our extensive studies over the last four years suggest that enterostatin has a selective effect to inhibit the intake of fat and may act as a feedback regulator or endogenous signal to determine fat intake and selection. Some of these studies are reviewed below.

Enterostatin and Intake of Dietary Fat

We have investigated the effects of enterostatin in rats maintained on three different feeding paradigms: no-choice high-fat or low-fat diets, two-choice selection between high-fat and low-fat diets, or three-choice

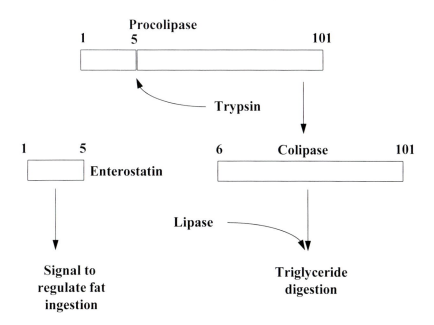

Figure 1.   Schematic representation of the formation of enterostatin.

Table 2. Amino Acid Sequences of Enterostatin and B-Casomorphins from a Range of Animal Species

Species	Sequence	Source
Rat	Val-Pro-Asp-Pro-Arg	AA
Rat	Val-Pro-Gly-Pro-Arg	cDNA
Human	Asp-Pro-Gly-Pro-Arg	cDNA/AA
Dog	Val-Pro-Asp-Pro-Arg	cDNA
Pig	Val-Pro-Asp-Pro-Arg	cDNA/AA
Horse	Val-Pro-Asp-Pro-Arg	AA
Chicken	Asp-Pro-Gly-Pro-Arg	AA
Hagfish	Asp-Pro-Gly -Arg	AA
β-casomorphin$_{1-7}$	Tyr-Pro-Phe-Pro-Gly-Pro-Ile	
β-casomorphin$_{1-5}$	Tyr-Pro-Phe-Pro-Gly	
β-casomorphin$_{1-4}$	Tyr-Pro-Phe-Pro	

Enterostatin sequences from rat (13, 15), dog (14), human (16), pig, horse (17), chicken, hagfish (13). Source refers to sequence obtained by either cDNA or amino acid analysis. All β-casomorphin sequences are bovine.

selection between individual carbohydrate, protein, and fat macronutrients. In each paradigm the effects of enterostatin are selective toward fat. It inhibits food intake in rats maintained on high-fat but not low-fat diets (18), it reduces the intake of high-fat but not low-fat diets in the two-choice selection protocol (19, 20), and it inhibits fat but not carbohydrate or protein intake in the three-choice experimental paradigm (21). In the choice paradigms there is no compensatory increase in intake of the alternative foods. The enterostatin response is evident both after overnight starvation and during the normal daily ad libitum feeding cycles (18).

Two sets of evidence suggest that the endogenous secretion of enterostatin may regulate fat appetite. First, the response to enterostatin is dependent upon the rat strain (21). Osborne-Mendel (OM) rats respond to enterostatin as do Sprague-Dawley and obese Zucker rats, whereas neither S5B/Pl nor lean Zucker rats do. Osborne-Mendel and S5B/Pl rats differ in their selection of macronutrients, OM preferring fat and S5B/Pl rats preferring carbohydrate (21). Pancreatic colipase activity and mRNA levels are lower in OM than in S5B/Pl rats. Further, the intake of dietary fat by individual rats of OM and S5B/Pl strains was negatively correlated to the endogenous level of pancreatic colipase, a marker of enterostatin secretion. In a second study on obese Zucker *fa/fa* rats, the increase in procolipase mRNA levels that followed adrenalectomy was associated with a reduction in food intake and the loss of the response to exogenous enterostatin (22). Thus, in two situations, response to exogenous peptide and high-fat selection or high levels of high-fat diet intake have been evident only when colipase levels (and presumably enterostatin secretion) have been low. A definitive demonstration that enterostatin acts as a feedback regulator of fat intake awaits the development of a specific assay for the circulating peptide. However, pancreatic colipase activity and mRNA levels are increased when rats are fed a high-fat diet, changes which should reflect an increase in enterostatin release (21–23). Further evidence that enterostatin may act as a signal to regulate food intake and/or body weight was provided by a preliminary experimental study of the response of rats to the chronic intracerebroventricular (icv) infusion of enterostatin. Rats receiving enterostatin had attenuated weight gains and a small reduction in food intake (24).

Is Enterostatin the Biologically Active Peptide?

Enterostatin has the amino acid sequence of valine-proline-aspartic acid-proline-arginine (VPDPR) in rats (13). The sequence obtained from cDNA analysis suggests that the central aspartic acid may be replaced by glycine (15). Studies with a series of peptide analogues of enterostatin have suggested that full biological activity is retained by both the shorter tripeptide proline-aspartic acid-proline (PDP) and the cyclodiketopiperazine form cyclo-aspartyl-proline (cycloDP) (25). In contrast the linear dipeptide aspartyl-proline was ineffective. Both PDP and cycloDP retained the selective effects of enterostatin toward both high-fat diets and fat macronutrients, and both were effective after central and peripheral administration, as is enterostatin. Further, both enterostatin and cycloDP have characteristic U-shaped dose-response curves (25). Two possible interpretations of this data are either that cycloDP and PDP have the appropriate three-dimensional structures to interact with an enterostatin receptor or that enterostatin is hydrolysed and cyclized to cycloDP in situ to express its biological effect. The presence of two prolines in enterostatin and cyclization of aspartyl-proline both provide rigid structures (Fig. 2).

Cyclo-Aspartyl-Proline

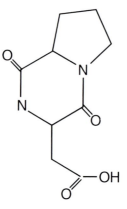

Figure 2.   Cyclo-aspartyl-proline.

SITE OF ACTION

The inhibitory effect of enterostatin has been demonstrated after various routes of administration: intraperitoneal, intracerebroventricular,
and intravenous (18, 49, 37, 38, 40). Enterostatin is produced in the
pancreas as the activation peptide of procolipase (12). We have also
identified procolipase mRNA in the pyloric region of the stomach and
the duodenum (23), but we could not identify any procolipase mRNA
signals in a range of other tissues, including brain. The response to
peripheral enterostatin was abolished by transection of the hepatic
branch of the vagus nerve, suggesting that signals generated in response to enterostatin from either the liver, stomach, or proximal duod-
erum pass to the central nervous system (CNS) via afferent vagal nerves
(25). In this case, enterostatin would be similar to a number of other
peripheral feeding signals, for example, cholecystokinin, glucagon, pyruvate, that are mediated via the afferent vagus (27, 28).

The recognition that chronic stimulation of nerve cells leads to the
activation of immediate early genes and the expression of their proteins, for example, fos (29), has provided a method to identify which
central neurons are activated by peripheral administration of enterostatin (26). Using immunohistochemical analysis of fos we identified
several hypothalamic and brain stem sites that were activated in response to peripherally administered enterostatin. Particularly strong

signals were evident in the nucleus tractus solitarius (NTS), paraventricular nucleus (PVN), supraoptic nucleus (SON), suprachiasmatic (SCN) and pontine nuclei, and the dorso-motor nucleus of the vagus (DMN). This pattern of response was quite different from that induced by the lipoprivic feeding stimulus of β-mercaptoacetate (26). More recently Qian and York (unpublished observations) have studied the fos response to icv administration of enterostatin using both immunohistochemistry and in situ hybridization of c-fos mRNA. Once again high levels of staining for fos-like immunoreactivity were observed in the PVN, SON, and NTS in enterostatin-treated rats but not in the saline controls. In situ hybridization of the c-fos mRNA confirmed this distribution. The combined data are consistent with the suggestion that the PVN and SON are important sites in modulating the effects of enterostatin and that the NTS and DMN are components of the afferent and efferent signaling pathways, respectively.

The above data do not provide definitive evidence that any of these brain regions is the site at which enterostatin regulates fat intake. Although the metabolic effects of enterostatin have not been intensively studied, evidence suggests that it may also inhibit insulin secretion (24, 30), elevate corticosterone levels, possibly through a central stimulation of corticotropin-releasing hormone (CRH) release (24), and stimulate the sympathetic drive to brown adipose tissue (Nagase, York, and Bray, unpublished results). Although CRH has anorectic properties and shows some selectivity toward fat and protein, it is not a component of the enterostatin response, since the CRH antagonist γ-helical CRH$_{9-41}$ does not block the enterostatin inhibition of food intake (24). Corticotropin-releasing hormone is distributed widely within the CNS, including the PVN, from which site pituitary corticotropin (ACTH) secretion is controlled (32). The PVN is also the site at which galanin is reported to selectively stimulate fat feeding in the studies of Liebowitz and colleagues (33), though we have been unable to demonstrate such a strong selective enhancement of fat intake by galanin (34). Our recent observation that the 5HT:5HIAA ratio was decreased in a number of brain regions including the PVN thirty minutes after injection of peripheral enterostatin (35) strongly suggests that enterostatin may influence a serotoninergic system within the PVN. Although this may explain the activation of the hypothalamic-pituitary-adrenal axis, its possible influence on feeding behavior is unclear. Serotoninergic systems have previously been linked to carbohydrate rather than fat feeding (36).

RECEPTOR SYSTEMS FOR ENTEROSTATIN

Enterostatin has been shown to have a U-shaped dose-response effect on food intake in rats and baboons (25, 37, 38). In rats, maximal inhibition is achieved after icv administration of 0.1 to 1.0 nanomoles. In contrast, high doses (10 nmols) increase intake of high-fat diets. A similar U-shaped response curve is also evident for the enterostatin analogue, cycloDP. The U-shaped dose-response curve to enterostatin is most easily explained by the hypothesis that there are two receptor subtypes with which enterostatin interacts, a high affinity receptor that modulates the inhibitory response and a lower affinity receptor through which enterostatin may enhance fat feeding at high concentrations. At this time evidence to support this hypothesis is limited. β-Casomorphin$_{1-7}$ has a similar bridged proline structure to enterostatin (Table 2). After icv administration it stimulates intake of dietary fat, as do high doses (> 10 nmols) of enterostatin (25, 39). Low doses of β-casomorphin$_{1-7}$ do not have enterostatin-like inhibitory effects on fat intake. Preliminary Scatchard binding studies with [^{3}H]-enterostatin indicate the presence of two binding sites on crude preparations of brain membranes (40). Our own studies indicate that β-casomorphin$_{1-7}$ will displace [^{3}H]-enterostatin from low affinity binding sites (Fig. 3) on brain membranes. However, neither the low nor high affinity binding sites have been characterized or isolated. Enterostatin does not displace either galanin from its specific binding sites or NPY from Y_1 binding sites (41), ruling out the possibility of direct interaction with either the galanin or NPY feeding receptor systems.

Opioidergic systems have long been recognized to be important in feeding behavior, but their precise role has been difficult to define (42, 43). Opioids increase food intake in the short term. Several reports have implicated opioidergic systems, particularly the kappa opioids, as stimulators of fat ingestion (44, 45). Over the last several months we have accumulated evidence that enterostatin may act as a kappa-opioid antagonist to affect fat indigestion. Among this evidence we have shown that:

1. The enterostatin inhibition of high-fat diet selection is blocked by a kappa-opioid agonist U-50488. More recently we have extended

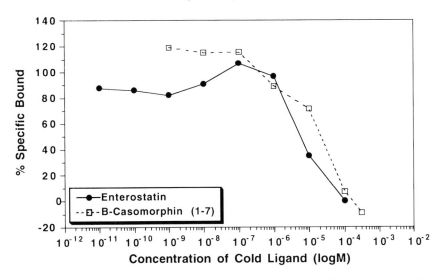

Figure 3. Displacement of [³H]-pro-enterostatin from binding sites on brain membranes by enterostatin and β-casomorphin₁₋₇. Brain membranes were incubated with 30 nmol [³H]-enterostatin and the displacement doses of enterostatin and β-casmorphin₁₋₇ shown.

this observation to show that U-50488 will block the enterostatin effect at low doses, which by themselves do not affect feeding behavior (Barton and York, unpublished observations).

2. Kappa-opioid antagonists, such as nor-binaltorphimine (norBNI), mimic the effects of enterostatin in selectively inhibiting the intake of high-fat diets in experimental paradigms in which rats may choose between high-fat and low-fat diets (Barton and York, unpublished observations).

3. Kappa-opioid agonists have opposing effects to enterostatin and will selectively increase intake of high-fat diets in rats that are satiated (Barton and York, unpublished observations).

4. Naloxone, the general opioid antagonist, inhibits the galanin feeding response. A similar finding has been reported recently by Kalra and colleagues (46).

From these and other experimental data we have suggested that a kappa-opioidergic pathway modulates the ingestion of dietary fat and that this system is activated by galanin but inhibited by enterostatin, which may act as a kappa-opioid antagonist. The relationship of this system to the lower affinity site for enterostatin and β-casomorphins is unclear at this time. Opioidergic systems also appear to be a component of the NPY feeding system (47), but the receptor subtype has not been clarified. A further question, the answer to which is unknown at this time, is how the rat recognizes fat in the diet. The enterostatin inhibition of fat intake has a rapid response time, within fifteen minutes of icv injection and the presentation of food. It is unlikely that there are major metabolic changes associated with the digestion, absorption, and metabolism of dietary fat within this time frame. It is quite possible that fat is recognized by its texture and/or palatability as a learned behavior. This suggestion is supported by recent experiments (Lin and York, unpublished observations) in which rats maintained on low-fat diets were tested with enterostatin on their first exposure to high-fat diets. In this situation, enterostatin was ineffective, indicating that prior exposure to dietary fat was necessary.

The Physiological Role of Enterostatin

Many questions remain to be answered before a clear picture of the physiological role of enterostatin in the regulation of fat intake and fat appetite can be obtained. Both peripheral and central sites of action have been identified (Fig. 4). The peripheral response appears to require afferent vagal activity, which probably originates in the liver or stomach. The afferent vagal information activates a number of central sites known to be involved in feeding regulatory behavior. It is not yet clear if the central sites are activated in response to circulating enterostatin (or its active analogue) released from central sites. Efferent pathways affect fat intake, the hypothalamic-pituitary-adrenal axis, and sympathetic activity to brown adipose tissue, and there is also a direct inhibitory effect on insulin secretion.

Levine and Billington have previously reviewed the criteria necessary for establishing a physiological role of a peptide in ingestive behavior (48). At this time few of these criteria have been answered for enterostatin. Enterostatin will decrease fat intake in the normal home environment during the normal feeding cycle without producing any obvious alternative behavioral responses (49). The peptide is not aversive (50). Indeed the behavioral sequence resembles the normal satiety sequence (49). The site of action of enterostatin appears to be at both the central and the gastrointestinal-hepatic level, this latter effect being

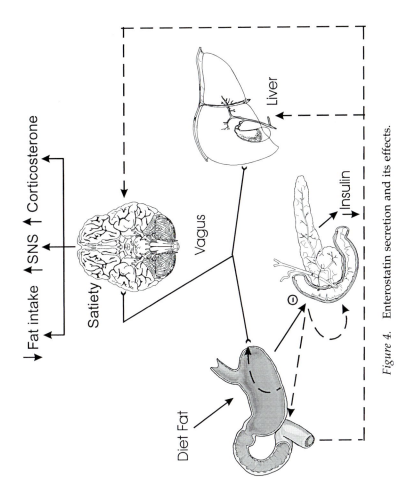

↓ Fat intake ↑ SNS ↑ Corticosterone

Satiety

Vagus

Liver

↓ Insulin

Diet Fat

Figure 4. Enterostatin secretion and its effects.

blocked by transection of the hepatic vagus. Although it is clear that enterostatin is secreted into the duodenal lumen (51), definitive evidence for its presence in the circulation awaits the development of a specific, sensitive assay. We shall need to show that enterostatin is effective on feeding behavior and that it is so within the physiological peptide concentration. Currently available assays detect enterostatin-like immunoreactivity in serum at concentrations that appear to be unrealistic for a circulating peptide. The enterostatin-like immunoreactivity is also highly labile, a fact that is difficult to relate to the biological response to exogenous enterostatin, which may be prolonged for several hours. Nevertheless, Bowyer *et al.* have suggested that enterostatin-like immunoreactivity is increased after a meal containing fat, but that this response may be absent in morbidly obese subjects (50).

If enterostatin is present in the circulation, it could arise as a peptide absorbed across the intestine, as a peptide secreted directly from the exocrine pancreas, or as a peptide derived from some other unknown source. In vitro studies suggest that enterostatin may be transported across rabbit ileum (52). We could obtain no evidence for synthesis of procolipase in the brain, though the high sensitivity of the central response and the presence of specific binding sites on brain membranes (4) suggest that enterostatin or a related peptide is effective at that level. In this case, the question to be addressed is whether the central system responds to a circulating signal or whether there is a biological form of enterostatin secreted in the brain. Thus, we have yet to show that the locus of action of the peptide is at a site where the peptide is known to be released endogenously. The half-life of enterostatin or of enterostatin's effect is, however, quite long. In studies in which we investigated the effects of delaying the presentation of food after enterostatin injection (Fig. 5) we were able to show that the inhibitory response was still evident if food availability to rats starved overnight was delayed for up to two hours after enterostatin injection.

Changes in dietary fat intake have been related to increased synthesis of the parent procolipase mRNA (23) and protein (21), partially satisfying the requirement to show that changes in the intake of the dietary component affect the synthesis and secretion of the peptide. Further studies are needed to identify the specific receptors for enterostatin and to investigate receptor regulation in response to changes in dietary fat intake. Thus, though the studies to date support the possibility that enterostatin, or a similar peptide, may regulate the intake of fat and

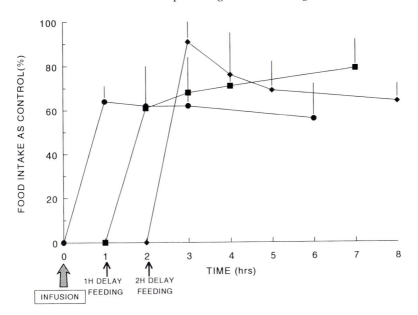

Figure 5. The effect of delayed food presentation on the feeding response to enterostatin. Enterostatin was injected intracerebroventricularly into overnight-starved rats at Time 0. Food was presented either immediately, after one hour, or after two hours as shown. Data are expressed as percentage of control rats that received saline injections.

alter fat appetite, more detailed investigations are needed to confirm that it is a physiological mediator of these behaviors.

ACKNOWLEDGMENTS

Research for this paper was supported by National Institutes of Health National Institute of Diabetes and Digestive and Kidney Diseases grant number 45278.

REFERENCES

1. Blundell J. Pharmacological approaches to appetite suppression. *TIPS.* 1991;12:147–157.
2. Stricker E, Verbalis JY. Control of appetite and satiety: insites from biologic and behavioral studies. *Nutr Rev.* 1990;48:18–25.

3. Bray GA, York DA, Fisler JS. Experimental obesity: a homeostatic failure due to defective nutrient stimulation of the sympathetic nervous system. *Vitam Horm.* 1990;45:1–125.

4. Fluharty SJ, Epstein AN. Sodium appetite elicited by intracerebroventricular infusion of angiotensin II in the rat: synergistic interaction with systemic mineralocorticoids. *Behav Neurosci.* 1983;97: 746–758.

5. Stanley BG, Daniel DR, Chin AS, Leibowitz SF. Paraventricular nucleus injections of peptide YY and neuropeptide Y preferentially enhance carbohydrate ingestion. *Peptides.* 1985;6:1205–1211.

6. Mitsushi A, Masayuki S, Hitoshi I, Takashi S. Increased neuropeptide Y content in the arcuato-paraventricular hypothalamic neuronal system in both insulin-dependent and non-insulin–dependent diabetic rats. *Brain Res.* 1991;539:223–227.

7. Schwartz MW, Sipols AJ, Marks JL, *et al.* Inhibition of hypothalamic neuropeptide Y gene expression by insulin. *Endocrinology.* 1992;130: 3608–3616.

8. Vaccarino FJ, Hayward M. Microinjections of growth hormone–releasing factor into the medial preoptic area/suprachiasmatic nucleus region of the hypothalamus stimulate food intake in rats. *Regul Pept.* 1988;21:21–28.

9. Nagai K, Thibault L, Nishikawa K, Hashida A, Ootani K, Nakagawa H. Effect of glucagon in macronutrient self-selection: glucagon-enhanced protein intake. *Brain Res Bull.* 1991;27:409–415.

10. Schutz Y, Flatt JP, Jequier E. Failure of dietary fat to provide fat oxidation: a factor favoring the development of obesity. *Am J Clin Nutr.* 1992;55:5085–5155.

11. Sjostrom L. Morbidity of reversing obese subjects. *Am J Clin Nutr.* 1992;55:5085–5155.

12. Erlanson-Albertson C. Pancreatic colipase. *Biochimica Biophysica Acta.* 1992;1125:1–7.

13. Larsson A. Pancreatic procolipase. *Secretion and Effect of Trypsin Activation.* Sweden: University of Lund; 1987. Thesis.

14. Fukuoka S, Taniguchi Y, Kitagawa Y, Scheele G. Full length cDNA sequence encoding canine pancreatic colipase. *Nucleic Acids Res.* 1990;18:5549.

15. Wicker C, Puigserver A. Rat pancreatic colipase mRNA: nucleotide sequence of a cDNA clone and nutritional regulation by a lipidic diet. *Biochem Biophys Res Commun.* 1990;167:130–136.

16. Lowe ME, Rosenblum JL, McEwen P, Strauss AW. Cloning and characterization of the human colipase cDNA. *Biochem J.* 1990;29: 823–828.

17. Chapus C, Rovery M, Sarda L, Verger R. Minireview on pancreatic lipase and colipase. *Biochimie.* 1988;70:1223–1234.

18. Okada S, York DA, Bray GA, Erlanson-Albertsson C. Enterostatin, (VAL-PRO-ASP-PRO-ARG), the activation peptide of procolipase selectively reduces fat intake. *Physiol Behav.* 1991;49:1185–1189.

19. Erlanson-Albertsson C, Jie M, Okada S, York DA, Bray GA. Pancreatic procolipase propeptide-enterostatin specifically inhibits fat intake. *Physiol Behav.* 1991;49:1191–1194.

20. Barton C, York DA, Bray GA. Opioid involvement in enterostatin induced satiety. *Obesity Res.* 1993;1(suppl 2):100s.

21. Okada S, York DA, Bray GA, Erlanson-Albertsson C. Differential inhibition of fat intake in two strains of rat by the peptide enterostatin. *Am J Physiol.* 1992;262:R1111–R1116.

22. Okada S, Onai T, Kilroy G, York DA, Bray GA. Adrenalectomy of the obese Zucker rat: effects on the feeding response to enterostatin and specific mRNA levels. *Am J Physiol.* 1993;265:R21–R27.

23. Okada S, York DA, Bray GA. Procolipase mRNA: tissue localization and effects of diet and adrenalectomy. *Biochem J.* 1993;292:787–789.

24. Okada S, Lin L, York DA, Bray GA. Chronic effects of intracerebral ventricular enterostatin in Osborne-Mendel rats fed a high fat diet. *Physiol Behav.* 1993;45:325–329.

25. Lin L, Okada S, York DA, Bray GA. Structural requirements for the biological activity of enterostatin[1]. *Peptides.* 1994;15:849–854.

26. Tian Q, Nagase M, York DA, Bray GA. Vagal-central nervous system interactions modulate the feeding response to peripheral enterostatin. *Obesity Res.* 1994;2:527–534.

27. York DA. Metabolic regulation of food intake. *Nutr Rev.* 1990;48 (Marabou Symp suppl):64–70.

28. Langhans W, Egli Y, Scharrer E. Selective hepatic vagotomy eliminates the hypophagie effect of different metabolites. *J Auton Nerv Syst.* 1985;9:207–220.

29. Morgan JI, Curran T. Stimulus-transcription coupling in neurons: role of cellular immediate early genes. *TINS.* 1989;12:459–462.

30. Mei J, Cheng Y, Erlanson-Albertsson C. Enterostatin: its ability to inhibit insulin secretion and to decrease high-fat food intake. *Int J Obes.* 1993;17:701–704.

31. Lin L, York DA, Bray GA. Acute effects of intracerebroventricular corticotropin releasing hormone (CRH) on macronutrient selection. *Int J Obes.* 1992;16(suppl 1):52.

32. Petrusz P, Merchenthaler I, Maderdrut JL, Heitz PU. Central and peripheral distribution of corticotropin-releasing factor. *Fed Proc.* 1985;44:229–235.

33. Tempel DL, Leibowitz KJ, Leibowitz SF. Effects of PVN galanin on macronutrient selection. *Peptides.* 1988;9:309–314.

34. Smith B, York DA, Bray GA. Galanin stimulates fat intake in both the paraventricular nucleus and the amygdala. *Clin Res.* 1993;41(4):757A.

35. York DA, Waggoner J, Bray GA. Brain amine responses to peripheral enterostatin. *Int. J. Obesity.* 1994;18(suppl. 2):102.

36. Leibowitz SF, Weiss GF, Shor-Posner G. Hypothalamic serotonin: pharmacological, biochemical, and behavioral analyses of its feeding-suppressive action. *Clin Neuropharmacol.* 1988;11:S51–S71.

37. Weatherford SC, Lattemann DF, Sipols AJ, *et al.* Intraventricular administration of enterostatin decreases food intake in baboons. *Appetite.* 1992;19:225.

38. Shargill NS, Tsujii S, Bray GA, Erlanson-Albertsson C. Enterostatin suppresses food intake following injection into the third ventricle of rats. *Brain Res.* 1991;544:137–140.

39. Lin L, York DA, Bray GA. The effect of enterostatin in β-casomorphin induced feeding responses in three strains of rat. *FASEB J.* 1993;7:A89.

40. Sohede M, Mei J, Erlanson-Albertsson C. Enterostatin: a gut-brain peptide regulating fat intake in rat. *J Physiol (Lond).* 1993;87:273–275.

41. Lin L, Gehlert DR, York DA, Bray GA. Effect of enterostatin on the feeding responses to galanin and NPY. *Obesity Res.* 1993;1:186–192.

42. Morley JE. Neuropeptide regulation of appetite and weight. *Endocr Rev.* 1987;8:256–390.

43. Cooper SJ, Jackson A, Kirkham TC. Endorphins and food intake: kappa opioid receptor agonists and hyperphagia. *Pharmacol Biochem Behav.* 1985;23:889–901.

44. Romsos DR, Gosnell BA, Morley JE, Levine AS. Effects of kappa opiate agonists, cholecystokinin and bombesin on intake of diets varying in carbohydrate-to-fat ratio in rats. *J Nutr.* 1986;117:976–985.

45. Shor-Posner G, Azar AP, Filart R, Tempel D, Leibowitz SF. Morphine-stimulated feeding: analysis of macronutrient selection and paraventricular nucleus lesions. *Pharmacol Biochem Behav.* 1986;24: 931–939.

46. Kalra PS, Kalra SP. Neuropeptide Y stimulates hypothalamic β-endorphin release in vitro: modulation by opioids. In: Abstracts of the 23rd annual meeting of the Society of Neurological Sciences. November, 1993; Washington, DC.

47. Schick RR, Schusdziarra V, Nussbaumer C, Classen M. *Brain Res.* 1991;552:232–239.

48. Levine AS, Billington CJ. Selected criteria for peptides as regulators of feeding: an overview. In: Bray GA, Ryan DH, eds. *The Science of Food Regulation: Food Intake, Taste, Nutrient Partitioning, and Energy Expenditure.* Pennington Center Nutrition Series, 2. Baton Rouge, La: Louisiana State University Press; 1992:210–223.

49. Lin L, McClanahan S, York DA, Bray GA. The peptide enterostatin may produce early satiety. *Physiol Behav.* 1993;53:789–794.

50. Mei J, Erlanson-Albertsson C. Effect of enterostatin given intravenously and intracerebroventricularly on high-fat feeding in rats. *Regul Pept.* 1992;41:209–218.

51. Bowyer RC, Rowston WM, Jehanli AMT, Lacey JH, Hermon-Taylor J. Effect of a satiating meal on the concentrations of procolipase propeptide in the serum and urine of normal and morbidly obese subjects. *Gut.* 1993;34:1520–1525.

52. Huneau JF, Erlanson-Albertsson C, Tomé D. Absorption of enterostatin across the rabbit ileum in vitro. *FASEB J.* 1993;7:A89.

HANS-RUDOLF BERTHOUD

The Vagus and Enteric Nervous System

ABSTRACT

The abdominal vagus nerve is the major neural link between the brain and the metabolic effector organs such as the gastrointestinal tract, pancreas, and liver. Emerging evidence suggests that the function of the vagus nerve is not just to produce a generalized parasympathetic activation, but rather to selectively stimulate specific visceral functions through its efferent fibers and to detect specific chemical and mechanical signals generated by these organs through its sensory fibers. Therefore, the task will be to establish a functional neuroanatomy of the vagal system, including its inputs and outputs at both the peripheral interface with the enteric nervous system and the central interface with the brain.

Recent methodological advances make it possible to collect the morphological as well as functional data that are necessary for the construction of structure/function relationships. We have concentrated on characterizing the distribution and structure of vagal afferent and efferent fibers and terminals in the various relevant abdominal organs by using the lipophilic, fluorescent carbocyanine dyes DiI and DiA as anterograde tracers and the optical sectioning strategy offered through laser scanning confocal microscopy. Combining this tracing with immunocytochemical detection of transmitters and peptides in neurons of the enteric nervous system allows us to associate specific functional roles to morphologically identified vagal endings. On the sensory side, we have thus far identified the gastric tension receptor, potential nutrient receptors in the duodenal mucosa, and metabolic sensors in the portal hepatic space, and on the motor side, the vagal inhibitory nitrergic innervation to the circular smooth muscle of gastric fundus and pylorus.

A sufficient and balanced supply of nutrients, vitamins, and minerals is one of the fundamental requirements of an organism. Severe reduction, imbalance, or increase of this supply not only creates specifically nutrition-related disease states like obesity, but can also contribute to a variety of other diseases and conditions. Through evolution, organisms have developed elaborate mechanisms to control or regulate this supply function. Because this balanced supply was already a fundamental requirement of phylogenetically ancient organisms, some of the control mechanisms are likely to be very old. However, the transition from cold to warm bloodedness, and the evolution of the central nervous system, which put even more emphasis on energy supply, must have added important new layers to the control system (1). This fact may be one of the reasons that intense research over more than fifty years has not resulted in a comprehensive understanding but has merely increased the list of possible contributing mechanisms. Over the years, attention has shifted from a focus on the hypothalamus to other areas of the nervous system, such as the brain stem and the autonomic nervous system. The autonomic nervous system monitors most of the crucial bodily functions and links the brain with the enteric nervous system (Fig. 1). The enteric nervous system has all the components to regulate the motility, secretory, and absorptive functions of the gut. Why then does it need connections to the brain? The main evolutionary pressures to develop the autonomic nervous system may have been to facilitate the coordination of visceral events with behaviors such as feeding. We think that a thorough understanding of these perhaps more basic and/ or phylogenetically older mechanisms will greatly facilitate an understanding of the overall regulation of feeding.

Both the vagus nerve (through its largely anabolic responses) and the sympathetic nerves (through their predominantly catabolic effects) operate to control the partitioning of energy stores in the body. As a consequence, the two divisions of the autonomic nervous system exert considerable control over the balance of energy stores. The power of the dual autonomic drive can be seen in the ventromedial hypothalamus (VMH) obesity syndrome. A large body of literature supports the interpretation that VMH-lesioned rats exhibit a decreased sympathetic and perhaps an increased parasympathetic tone. In contrast to vagotomized rats, these animals show the same feeding pattern during the day (inactive phase) as during the night, namely, frequent large meals. The diurnal elimination of lipolysis and fat oxidation, replaced by fat

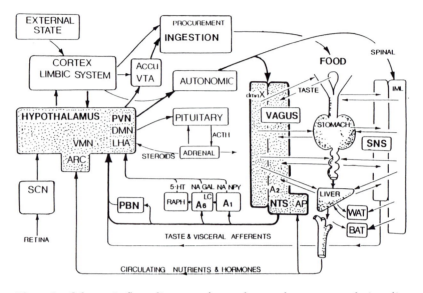

Figure 1. Schematic flow-diagram of neural control system regulating digestion, nutrient metabolism, food intake, and body weight, with special emphasis
on the autonomic nervous system. For simplicity, olfactory input and endocrine
systems such as the pancreas and thyroid have been omitted. Note the prominent reciprocal connections between the dorsal vagal complex in the brainstem
with visceral areas in the hypothalamus and other forebrain sites. Abbrevia-
tions: nucleus accumbens (ACB), area postrema (AP), arcuate nucleus (ARC),
association cortex (ASSN CTX), midbrain central gray (CG), dorsal motor nucleus of vagus (dmnX), dorsomedial nucleus hypothalamus (DMN), globus
pallidus (GP), intermediolateral column (IML), locus coeruleus (LC), nucleus
of solitary tract (NTS), parabrachial nucleus (PBN), reticular formation (RF),
substantia nigra (SN), sympathetic nervous system (SNS), striatum (STR), suprachiasmatic nucleus (SCN), ventral tegmental area (VTA), ventromedial nucleus hypothalamus (VMN), lateral hypothalamic area (LHA), raphé nucleus
(Raph), white adipose tissue (WAT), brown adipose tissue (BAT), A1, A2, A6
noradrenergic cell groups of brainstem and midbrain.

synthesis, creates this 24-hour overeating and obesity. Both the sympathetic and/or parasympathetic innervation of the pancreas, liver, adrenal gland, and gastrointestinal tract play a major role in the execution
of the metabolic shift.

The sensations of emptiness and fullness of the stomach have been
suspected for a long time to have a direct effect on the hunger and
satiety system (2). In humans, these sensations are reduced following

truncal vagotomy (3). The sensations from an empty stomach may stem from tension receptors reacting to the phasic contractions. In food-deprived rats, gastric vagal afferent tension receptors are not quiescent, but spontaneously discharge (4). Another possibility is that the sensation stems from mucosal receptors, triggered by gastric folds rubbing against each other in the absence of food.

In undeprived, free-feeding rats, it has been observed that a small transient decline of blood glucose levels precedes each meal (5), and some believe that this is the necessary signal for meal initiation (6). It is thought that the transient decline is the result of a temporary imbalance between small intestinal/hepatic glucose production and tissue glucose uptake, and that it could be detected by vagal afferents either in the liver or duodenum or, alternatively, directly by the brain (6). Vagal hepatic afferents that increase their firing rate with decreasing glucose concentration in the portal-hepatic circulation had been reported earlier (7).

More important, rats increase their food intake in response to anti-metabolites that block hepatic fuel oxidation in the liver (8–10). Although one laboratory reported this effect to depend on the integrity of the hepatic branch of the vagus nerve (9), both gastric vagal branches had to be transected to abolish the intake stimulatory effect of mercaptoacetate in another study (11, 12). These latter authors concluded that the vagal receptors for lipoprivic feeding are either diffusely distributed in the abdominal viscera or are located in the proximal duodenum, which is innervated by all divisions of the abdominal vagus, as shown by us earlier (13). Furthermore, considerable evidence shows that, once feeding has started, cephalic phase reflexes originating mainly from gustatory afferents and involving vagal efferents to the stomach and pancreas play an important role in sustaining ingestion (14–16).

Possibly the quantitatively major role of the abdominal vagus nerve is in local and vago-vagal reflexes that are primarily of a "housekeeping" nature, and may only secondarily influence feeding and body weight. The most prominent vago-vagal reflexes are receptive relaxation of the stomach, distension-induced gastric acid secretion, slowing of gastric emptying by duodenal distension, and the entero-pancreatic reflexes (Fig. 2).

Little is yet understood about the functional role of local vagal reflexes involving different axon collaterals of vagal afferent fibers. In analogy to the spinal cord dorsal root afferents, it is suspected that they

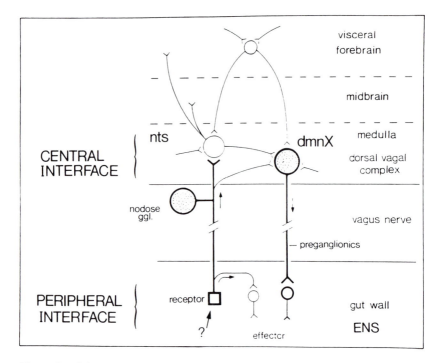

Figure 2. Schematic representation of efferent and afferent vagal system including its peripheral interface with the enteric nervous system (ENS) and its central interface (for specific central connections, see Fig. 1).

mainly serve protective functions. For example, it has been shown that destruction of vagal afferents with capsaicin facilitates ethanol-induced damage to the gastric mucosa (17). Furthermore, the close anatomical relationship between enteric neural elements and immunocytes such as mast cells and lymphocytes, the release of histamine and other messengers from mast cells, and the demonstration of functional receptors for substance P on mast cells suggest an involvement of visceral efferents in immune functions (18–20). Such neural-immune interactions are likely to play a role in inflammatory bowel disease, irritable bowel syndrome, food allergies, and parasitic infections (21, 22). More detailed information on the morphological and histochemical interrelationship between terminals of the autonomic nervous system, the enteric nervous system, and such immunocytes is crucial for a better understanding of their functional interactions.

Evidence also suggests a role of vagal afferents in nausea and vomiting. Vomiting induced by irradiation and systemic or food-related toxins can be reduced or abolished by subdiaphragmatic vagotomy (23) and electrical stimulation of the central end of the abdominal vagus induces emesis in the ferret (24). The effectiveness of 5-HT-3 receptor antagonists as anti-emetic drugs suggests an action of 5-HT on vagal afferents.

This brief review has shown that visceral afferents and efferents in general, and vagal afferents in particular, play crucial roles in 1) the control of feeding behavior and the regulation of body weight, 2) in the daily "housekeeper-functions" of the gastrointestinal tract, and 3) in the body's defense against inflammation and toxic substances. Structural research on visceral afferents, particularly vagal afferents, is lagging behind functional and behavioral analyses because of the lack of an identifying histochemical marker. In lieu of such a marker, we have used the carbocyanine dyes DiI and DiA to anterogradely label vagal afferents and efferents, respectively, and in a few cases we have combined this tracing with histochemical or immunocytochemical methods in order to identify the neurochemical makeup and functional role of the enteric targets of vagal terminals.

Materials and Methods

Carbocyanine dyes are highly lipophilic fluorescent probes that have a high affinity for the lipid bilayer of neuronal membranes. They have been extensively used in fixed tissue, where they very slowly spread over the entire neuronal membrane by passive diffusion. We have used these probes in vivo. Once inserted into the membrane, the dyes are internalized by endocytosis and more rapidly transported by fast axonal transport mechanisms.

The most critical step in evaluating their usefulness as vagal markers was to selectively label afferents or efferents (Fig. 2). When DiI is injected into the nodose ganglia in order to label vagal afferents, the dye will also come in contact with vagal efferent fibers of passage, and if it is internalized it could be transported to their terminals in the gut. We have, therefore, injected DiI into the nodose ganglia of rats that had undergone a supranodose vagotomy twelve days earlier. In these animals, the severed axonal processes of vagal efferents should die and degenerate, whereas the vagal afferents remain attached to their cell bodies and thus should survive. We have verified the successful elimination of efferents by using the retrograde tracer Fluorogold injected intraperitoneally. Comparing the distribution and structure of labeled vagal terminals between sham-vagotomized and supranodose-vagotomized rats revealed no qualitative difference, suggesting that DiI is not internalized and/or transported by efferent fibers of passage (25, 26).

In the other case, when DiA is injected into the dorsal motor nucleus, it is unavoidable to also impregnate the overlying solitary nucleus. If the central processes of vagal afferents would take the dye up and transport it transganglionically (*i.e.,* through the nodose ganglion), unwanted co-labeling of afferents would occur. We made at least three observations that rule out such nonspecific labeling. First, we did not observe labeled fibers and terminals in the gut that looked like the ones labeled with DiI injected into the nodose ganglia. Second, when DiA and DiI were injected into the dorsal motor nucleus and nodose ganglia, respectively, of the same animal, no double-labeled fibers and terminals were found throughout the gut. Third, DiA injections into the nodose ganglia did not label any vagal fibers. Therefore, we were able to selectively label vagal efferents with DiA injected into the dorsal motor nucleus and vagal afferents with DiI injected into the nodose ganglia.

Another important tool in our approach was the use of Fluorogold to stain the enteric nervous system in toto. This compound is typically used as a retrograde tracer, but we have discovered that when injected into the peritoneum, it is selectively taken up by neurons of the enteric and autonomic ganglia and by supporting cells forming the perineural sheath of autonomic nerves throughout the organism (27). Enteric neurons accumulate the fluorescent tracer in the cytoplasm and the nucleolus, but the nucleus remains unstained. This is, therefore, a convenient method to produce a fluorescent counterstain of the enteric nervous system. Additionally, the tracer is taken up by the terminals of both vagal efferent preganglionics and vagal afferents and transported to their cell bodies in the dorsal motor nucleus and the nodose ganglia. Since this retrograde transport takes place only in neurons with intact axons, it also allows us to estimate the number of fibers damaged by the injection procedures and to verify different types of selective branch vagotomies.

Another key methodological breakthrough was to combine visualization of the carbocyanine dyes with immunocytochemical and histochemical detection of neuropeptides and transmitters. The problem is that any use of alcohol or strong detergents such as Triton X-100 will completely abolish DiI and DiA label. In most immunocytochemistry protocols, Triton X-100 is essential to guarantee antibody penetration. If anything, the problem is aggravated in the case of whole mounts and relatively thick sections we are using most often. In our hands, there seems not to be one single solution for all tissues and antibodies. For each situation, a specific protocol has to be developed. For example, on thick sections (60 μm) of the pyloric sphincter we were able to simultaneously visualize DiI and calcitonin gene–related peptide (CGRP)-positive nerve fibers using a low concentration of the mild detergent Tween 20 and FITC conjugated second antibody (28). However, even with this mild detergent, the more delicately DiI-labeled elements seemed to be compromised, so that we left out detergents completely and increased incubation time in the primary antiserum. When investigating nitric oxide synthesizing enteric neurons, we were faced with the fact that the NADPH diaphorase histochemical reaction, even in the absence of Triton X-100, completely abolished DiA and DiI label. This forced us to search for an alternative approach, which we call the two-step procedure. Rather than compromise the quality of either dye visualization or histochemical staining by combining them, we photographically document the DiA- and/or DiI-labeled vagal fibers in relation to the Fluorogold-labeled elements of the enteric nervous system in the absence of any detergents or other chemicals in a first step. The cover slip is then removed, the tissue sample processed for NADPH diaphorase under optimal conditions, and the area is rephotographed in a second step. The most important part of this two-step procedure is the ability to find the same area in a given tissue sample. After using this indirect double-labeling method successfully for NADPH diaphorase staining, we extended it to immunocytochemical detection of various peptides such as galanin, enkephalin, VIP, and GRP. Although there is no penetration problem for the NADPH diaphorase histochemical reaction in whole-mounted muscularis externa peels from the stomach wall, the two smooth muscle layers represent a formidable barrier for peptide antisera even in the presence of Triton X-100 and with long incubation times. This problem was overcome by stripping the relatively thick circular muscle layer from the preparation, resulting in an open-faced myenteric plexus attached only to the longitudinal muscle layer. This stripping of the circular muscle layer for samples from the antral wall is difficult because of the presence of an additional oblique muscle layer and tougher connective tissue bonds. In this case, we obtained frozen sections tangentially at a very shallow angle to the plane of the myenteric plexus and carried out the two-step documentation.

A final important element in our method is the morphological analysis by means of laser scanning confocal microscopy. The major advantages over conventional epifluorescence microscopy are the rejection of out of focus light (pinhole), the high sensitivity (photomultiplier tube), and the capability of three-dimensional rendering of multiple optical sections. These advantages allow analysis of whole mounts and thick sections, and result in a more comprehensive visualization of nerve fibers and the anatomical relationship with their targets in the enteric nervous system. Typically, several optical sections are scanned at Z-axis intervals of 0.5–5 µm to encompass an area of interest that can extend through up to 200 µm of tissue. This "stack" of individual images can be stored and used to create stereoimages and/or to perform volume rendering. Most often, however, the individual images are superimposed on an imaginary horizontal plane, resulting in a so-called extended focus composite image. In order to simultaneously capture the Fluorogold, FITC, and DiI or DiA signal, separate stacks of optical sections were collected through the two channels, using a short (488 nm) and a longer (568 nm) wavelength excitation laser line and appropriate detection filters. Additional image processing was performed by subtracting the images collected through the two channels from each other, and using pseudo-Nomarski filter functions for edge enhancement.

Results and Discussion

VAGAL EFFERENT INNERVATION OF THE STOMACH

We had originally observed that in the myenteric plexus of the rat stomach, nearly every ganglion receives some degree of vagal preganglionic input (13). Since it is not unambiguous to define the borders of myenteric ganglia, and since the size of these ganglia varies tremendously, the percentage of contacted enteric neurons rather than ganglia is a better estimate of the density of innervation. In a group of three animals with the most successful DiA labeling of vagal efferents, we have counted the total number of enteric neurons and the number of such neurons contacted by varicose vagal fibers in representative portions of the gastric fundus. For that half of the fundic wall closer to the greater curvature, we found that roughly 50% of the neurons received vagal efferent contacts (Fig. 3A,B). For the other half of the fundic wall closer to the cardia, the number was even higher, but we were unable to do a quantitative analysis because the large number of labeled axons merely passing by the ganglia obscured the "real" contacts.

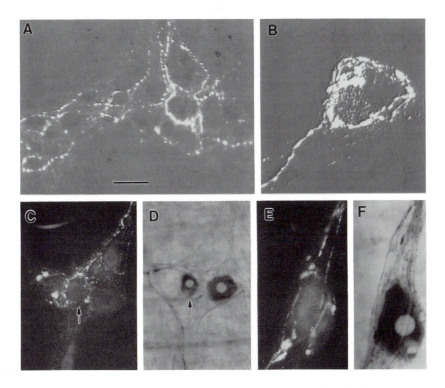

Figure 3. Vagal efferent innervation of myenteric plexus of rat fundic stomach. *A, B:* Confocal microscope images of DiA-labeled varicose vagal efferent fibers (bright white) forming ringlike terminals around myenteric neurons. *C–F:* Two examples demonstrating vagal efferent contacts with nitrergic (NADPH diaphorase–positive) neurons. In *C*, four of the six Fluorogold-labeled neurons (grayish) are contacted to some degree by DiA-labeled varicose endings (bright white). One of the contacted neurons (arrow) is NADPH diaphorase–positive as shown in *D*. In *E* and *F*, one single NADPH diaphorase–positive neuron (*F*, black) is contacted by varicose vagal efferents (*E*, bright white). Scale bar: 30 μm for *A*, *C*, and *D*; 15 μm for *B*, *E*, and *F*.

One of the functions of vagal efferent input to the fundic stomach is receptive relaxation to accommodate ingested food. Recent pharmacological evidence suggests the involvement of nitric oxide synthesizing enteric neurons (29) in this relaxation of smooth muscle. We have, therefore, analyzed the vagally contacted enteric neurons as to their content of NADPH diaphorase, which is one of the nitric oxide synthases (30). One-third of all vagally contacted neurons were NADPH diaphorase positive (Fig. 3C–F). Of the approximately 30% of all myenteric neurons that were nitrergic, about half received direct vagal efferent contacts and the other half did not. It is therefore likely that this vagal preganglionic-nitrergic postganglionic pathway represents the nonadrenergic, noncholinergic, vagal inhibitory input to the fundic stomach.

We have also started to analyze the anatomical relationship between vagal preganglionic terminals and nitrergic neurons in the pyloric sphincter, another gut area that has noncholinergic nonadrenergic inhibitory vagal input. We have reported earlier the location of vagal efferent terminals in subserosal, myenteric, intramuscular, and submucosal ganglia of the gastroduodenal junction (28). At each of these locations, there are some NADPH diaphorase–positive neurons, and we have seen DiA-labeled vagal efferent contacts with such nitrergic neurons in myenteric and intramuscular ganglia. Additionally, we have also found vagal contacts with galanin- and enkephalin-positive neurons in myenteric ganglia of the pyloric sphincter region. Systematic and quantitative analyses of the chemical phenotypes of vagal postganglionic neurons in other components of the gastrointestinal tract and the pancreas are under way.

Vagal Afferent Innervation of the Stomach

The most prominent terminal structures formed by DiI-labeled vagal afferents are the intraganglionic laminar endings (IGLEs) in the myenteric plexus (Fig. 4A, B). These endings have a more complex architecture than their efferent counterparts and typically cover in a domelike fashion parts of, or entire, ganglia (Fig. 4B). These IGLEs are not limited to the stomach, but are also found in the esophagus (31) and the small and large bowel (25). We estimate that in a rat stomach there may be as many as 2000 IGLEs. The function of these intriguing structures is not known, but several hypotheses have been formulated. It has been

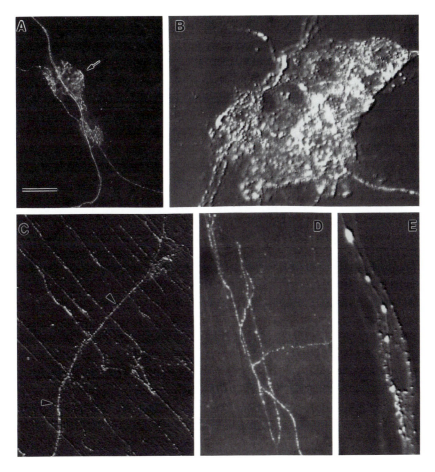

Figure 4. Vagal afferent innervation of myenteric plexus and external smooth muscle layer of rat fundic stomach. *A:* Conventional micrograph illustrating DiI-labeled vagal afferent fibers forming intraganglionic laminar ending (IGLE, arrow) in myenteric plexus. *B:* Higher magnification, extended focus confocal image of IGLE covering entire ganglion. *C:* Extended focus image of external muscle layer showing one DiI-labeled fiber running in myenteric plexus from upper right to lower left (arrowheads), and many labeled fibers running in right angle from upper left to lower right, within the longitudinal muscle layer. *D:* Individual vagal afferent fiber climbing from myenteric plexus to longitudinal muscle layer and forming intramuscular ending (tension receptor). *E:* High magnification detail of DiI-labeled varicose vagal afferent fiber clinging to interstitial cells that are part of the connective tissue matrix surrounding the muscle bundles. Scale bar: 100 μm for *A* and *C;* 30 μm for *B* and *D;* 10 μm for *E.*

suggested that these terminals are at the same time sensory and efferent, possibly transducing local tension or chemical signals into a local
effector function (31). Since we have observed earlier that single vagal
axons can possess at the same time collaterals in the external smooth
muscle layers and in the myenteric plexus (IGLEs), we have speculated
that the IGLE collaterals are closing local axon reflexes originating from
intramuscular in-series tension receptors (25). Experiments on in vitro
preparations using electrophysiological and pharmacological methods
will be necessary to test these hypotheses.

As mentioned above, in the circular and more so the longitudinal
smooth muscle layer, there were many DiI-labeled vagal afferent fibers
running parallel to the muscle bundles for long distances (25 and Fig.
4C, D). The fact that these putative in-series tension receptors are running parallel to the muscle bundles is not a contradiction. The fibers
run within the connective tissue matrix surrounding the muscle bundles (Fig. 4E), and this matrix serves as the analogue of the tendon in
skeletal muscle. As the muscle bundles are passively stretched by distension or actively contract, the connective tissue matrix containing the
sensory fibers is distorted (32).

Since the earliest experimental analysis of food intake, it has been
recognized that distension of the stomach by food or even nonnutritive
bulk acts through vagal afferents to inhibit ingestion (2). Moran and
McHugh (33) found that subthreshold doses of cholecystokinin (CCK)
and isotonic saline loads, that by themselves did not suppress food
intake, apparently potentiate each other's action to suppress intake in
monkeys. Converging electrophysiological evidence supported the
presence of CCK-sensitive gastric vagal mechanoreceptors (34–36).

Vagal Afferent Innervation of Duodenal Mucosa

Intestinal mucosa is too thick to be whole mounted, and we made thick
(50–90 μm) cryostat sections in a plane perpendicular to the serosal
surface. In the proximal duodenum, there were a considerable number
of DiI-labeled vagal afferent fibers that formed arborizations around
the crypts of Lieberkühn and within the lamina propria of the villi (Fig.
5A–C). These fibers were often found to be in intimate anatomical contact with fibrocytelike or interstitial cells (Fig. 5D). Cell bodies of interstitial cells were typically occupying the spaces between the crypts and
throughout the lamina propria. The highly varicose character of the

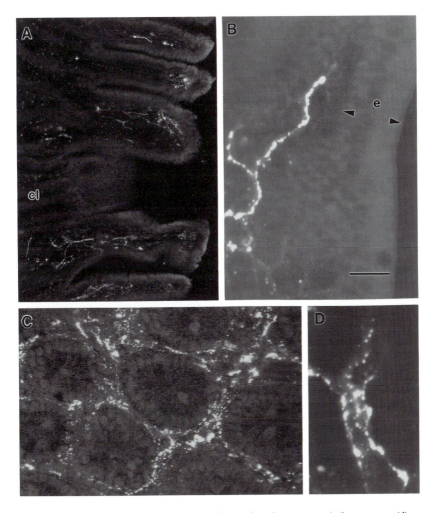

Figure 5. Vagal afferent innervation of duodenal mucosa. *A:* Low magnification conventional photomicrograph showing terminal network of DiI-labeled vagal afferents (bright white) in lamina propria of duodenal villi (cl = crypts of Lieberkühn). *B:* Higher magnification of varicose vagal afferent terminal (bright white) reaching close to the epithelial cell layer (e). *C:* Confocal image of cross section through crypts of Lieberkühn, showing dense network of DiI-labeled varicose vagal afferents (bright white) surrounding crypts. *D:* Higher magnification detail of varicose vagal afferent fiber associated with interstitial cell in lamina propria. Scale bar: 200 μm for *A;* 25 μm for *B;* 50 μm for *C;* 15 μm for *D.*

labeled vagal fibers suggested the presence of synaptic contacts with interstitial cells. Terminal vagal branches also came into close contact with epithelial cells (Fig. 5B) but were not seen to penetrate between epithelial cells toward the lumen. Because the submucosa and external muscle layers were cross sectioned, continuity of labeled fibers beyond the mucosa could rarely be established. However, from submucosa and muscularis externa peels of the same area, it appeared that vagal afferents destined to the mucosa first run in the myenteric plexus from the mesenteric pole toward the antimesenteric pole. At various distances between these two poles, the fibers penetrate the circular muscle layer, then run in the plane of the submucosal plexus where they produce several primary branches. Each of the branches then further penetrates into the lamina propria of the villi. It is also likely that the same parent fibers produce collaterals (IGLEs) in the myenteric plexus. This will, however, be difficult to prove because it is unlikely to capture the entire terminal tree in one section.

Visualization of vagal afferent fibers in the mucosa is only the first step in identifying the anatomical substrate of sensory signal transduction. A widely held view is the presence of free nerve endings that are stimulated by mechanical distortion, which is the result of either smooth muscular contraction, luminal distension, or osmotic forces (37). It has also been shown that vagal afferent fibers possess receptors for certain peptides, such as CCK (38). Such peptides would be released from epithelial endocrine cells in a nutrient specific fashion and would excite vagal endings by local paracrine action (39). A breakthrough in the demonstration of intestinal satiety came with the gastric fistula, sham-feeding rat preparation (40). In the absence of gastric food accumulation and passage to the duodenum, rats will sham feed for hours. As soon as glucose is directly infused into the duodenum, animals will stop eating. Subsequently, this preparation has been used by several investigators to assess the vagal contribution to intestinal satiety. It was shown that representatives of all the macronutrients, such as glucose, maltose, fatty acids, triglycerides and amino acids, suppress sham feeding if infused introduodenally as isotonic solutions (41–45, 39). Certain metabolizable substances, however, suppress sham-feeding very little, suggesting the existence of nutrient specific receptor mechanisms (39). Both subdiaphragmatic vagotomy and previous treatment with capsaicin, which apparently selectively destroys visceral afferents but leaves efferents intact (12), abolished intestinal maltose and oleic

acid–induced suppression of sham feeding, but only partially eliminated L-phenylalanine–induced suppression (39). In a series of earlier
studies, it was demonstrated that systemic administration of exogenous
CCK suppresses food intake (46) and that the effect depended on the
integrity of the subdiaphragmatic vagus, particularly the gastric
branches (47). More to the point, using either a surgical approach to
selectively eliminate vagal afferents or efferents (48), or capsaicin (10),
only deafferentation abolished the satiating effect of CCK. It was therefore possible that intestinal nutrients terminate a meal and suppress
food intake through the mediation of CCK. Indeed, administration of
CCK-A receptor antagonists abolished maltose and oleic acid–induced
suppression of sham feeding, but not that induced by L-phenylalanine
(49). All these observations suggest that certain metabolizable nutrients
are detected by intestinal vagal afferents through the mediation of endogenous CCK. However, since there is virtually no correlation between the capacity of a particular metabolite to suppress sham feeding
and to release CCK into the circulation, the source of CCK might not
be the mucosal endocrine cells but rather some CCK–producing enteric
neurons. Alternatively, it is possible that not all epithelial hormone–
producing cells act in a purely endocrine, but rather paracrine, fashion.
Therefore, at present, we do not know the nature and site of signal
transduction from specific nutrients to vagal afferent fibers, nor do we
know the source of peptide participation in the sensory process. The
possibility to make vagal sensory endings visible will help in elucidating the various steps in signal transduction.

ACKNOWLEDGMENTS

The skillful technical assistance of Qinwu Lin and the secretarial assistance of Marilyn LaSalle is much appreciated. This work was supported
by National Institutes of Health grant DK 47348.

REFERENCES

1. Young JZ. Influence of the mouth on the evolution of the brain. In:
   Biology of the Mouth. American Assoc. for the Advancement of Science, 1968:21–35.
2. Cannon WB, Washburn AL. An explanation of hunger. *Am J Physiol.*
   1912;29:441–454.

3. Kral JG. Behavioral effects of vagotomy in humans. In: Kral JG, Powley TL, Brooks CM, eds. *Vagal Nerve Functions: Behavioral and Methodological Considerations.* Amsterdam: Elsevier; 1983:273–281.

4. Andrews PLR, Grundy D, Scratcherd T. Vagal afferent discharge from mechanoreceptors in different regions of the ferret stomach. *J Physiol (Lond).* 1980;298:513–524.

5. Campfield LA, Smith FJ. Functional coupling between transient declines in blood glucose and feeding behavior; temporal relationships. *Brain Res Bull.* 1986;17:427–433.

6. LeMagnen J. *Neurobiology of Feeding and Nutrition.* San Diego: Academic Press; 1992.

7. Niijima A. Afferent discharges in chemoreceptors in the liver of the guinea-pig. *Science.* 1969;104:151.

8. Friedman MI, Tordoff MG, Ramirez I. Integrated metabolic control of food intake. *Brain Res Bull.* 1986;17:855–859.

9. Langhans W, Scharrer E. Evidence for a vagally mediated satiety signal derived from hepatic fatty acid oxidation. *J Auton Nerv Syst.* 1987;18:13–18.

10. Ritter S, Calingasan NY, Hutton B, Dinh TT. Cooperation of vagal and central neural systems in monitoring metabolic events controlling feeding behavior. In: Ritter S, Ritter RC, Barnes CD, eds. *Neuroanatomy and Physiology of Vagal Abdominal Afferents.* Boca Raton: CRC Press; 1992:249–277.

11. Ritter S, Hutton BW, Dinh TT. Neurons required for lipoprivic feeding are not limited to a single vagal branch. *Neurosci Abstr.* 1990; 16:295.

12. Ritter S, Dinh TT. Capsaicin-induced neuronal degeneration: silver impregnation of cell bodies, axons and terminals in the central nervous system of the adult rat. *J Comp Neurol.* 1988;271:79–90.

13. Berthoud H-R, Carlson NR, Powley TL. Topography of efferent vagal innervation of the rat gastrointestinal tract. *Am J Physiol.* 1991; 260 (Regulatory Integrative Comp. Physiol. 29):R200–R207.

14. Louis-Sylvestre J, LeMagnen J. Palatability and preabsorptive insulin release. *Neurosci Biobehav Rev.* 1980;4(suppl 1):43–46.

15. Louis-Sylvestre J, Giachetti J, LeMagnen J. Vagotomy abolishes the differential palatability of food. *Appetite.* 1983;4:295–299.

16. Berthoud H-R. Cephalic phase insulin response as a predictor of body weight gain and obesity induced by a palatable cafeteria diet. *J Obesity Weight Reg.* 1985;4:120–128.

17. Holzer P, Sometz W. Gastric and mucosal protection against ulcer-ogenic factors in the rat mediated by capsaicin sensitive afferent neurons. *Gastroenterology.* 1986;91:975–981.

18. Collins SM. Neural-immune interactions: pathophysiological and clinical implications. *Dig Dis Sci.* 1992;37:966.

19. Wallace JL, McKnight GW, Befus AD. Capsaicin-induced hypere-mia in the stomach: possible contribution of mast cells. *Am J Physiol.* 1992;263:G209–G214.

20. Befus D. Regulation of gastrointestinal mast cells. *Dig Dis Sci.* 1992; 37:967.

21. Mayer EA, Raybould HE. Role of visceral afferents in functional bowel disorders. *Gastroenterology.* 1990;99:1688–1704.

22. Andrews PLR. Modulation of visceral afferent activity as a thera-peutic possibility for gastrointestinal disorders. In: Read NW, ed. *Irritable Bowel Syndrome.* London: Blackwell Scientific; 1991:91–121.

23. Andrews PLR, Lawes INC. A protective role for vagal afferents: an hypothesis. In: Ritter S, Ritter RC, Barnes CD, eds. *Neuroanatomy and Physiology of Abdominal Vagal Afferents.* Boca Raton, FL: CRC Press; 1992:280–302.

24. Andrews PLR, Bingham S, Davis CJ. Retching evoked by stimula-tion of abdominal vagal afferents in anesthetized ferrets. *J Physiol (Lond).* 1985;358:103P.

25. Berthoud H-R, Powley TL. Vagal afferent innervation of the rat fundic stomach: morphological characterization of the gastric ten-sion receptor. *J Comp Neurol.* 1992;319:261–276.

26. Berthoud H-R, Kressel M, Neuhuber W. An anterograde tracing study of the vagal innervation of rat liver, portal vein and biliary system. *Anat Embryol (Berl).* 1992;186:431–442.

27. Powley TL, Berthoud H-R. A fluorescent tracer strategy for staining the enteric nervous system. *J Neurosci Methods.* 1991;36:9–15.

28. Kressel M, Berthoud H-R, Neuhuber WL. Vagal innervation of the rat pylorus: an anterograde tracing study using carbocyanine dyes and laser scanning confocal microscopy. *Cell Tissue Res.* 1994;275: 109–123.

29. Desai KM, Zembowicz A, Sessa WC, Vane JR. Nitroxergic nerves mediate vagally induced relaxation in the isolated stomach of the guinea pig. *Proc Natl Acad Sci USA.* 1991;88:11490–11491.

30. Hope BT, Michael GJ, Knigge KM, Vincent SR. Neuronal NADPH

diaphorase is a nitric oxide synthase. *Proc Natl Acad Sci USA.* 1991; 88:2811–2814.

31. Neuhuber WL, Clerc N. Afferent innervation of the esophagus in cat and rat. In: Zenker W, Neuhuber WL, eds. *The Primary Afferent Neuron: A Survey of Recent Morpho-Functional Aspects.* New York: Plenum Press; 1990:93–107.

32. Grundy D. Speculations on the structure/function relationship for vagal and splanchnic afferent endings supplying the gastrointestinal tract. *J Auton Nerv Syst.* 1988;22:175–180.

33. Moran TH, McHugh PR. Cholecystokinin suppresses food intake by inhibiting gastric emptying. *Am J Physiol.* 1982;242:R491–R497.

34. Davison JS, Clarke GD. Mechanical properties and sensitivity to CCK of vagal gastric slowly adapting mechanoreceptors. *Am J Physiol.* 1988;255:G55–G61.

35. Raybould HE, Davison JS. Perivagal application of capsaicin abolishes the response of vagal gastric mechanoreceptors to CCK. *Neurosci Abstr.* 1989;15:973.

36. Schwartz GJ, McHugh PR, Moran TH. Integration of vagal afferent responses to gastric loads and cholecystokinin in the rat. *Am J Physiol.* 1992;261:R64–R69.

37. Mei N. Intestinal chemosensitivity. *Physiol Rev.* 1985;65:221.

38. Moran TH, Smith GP, Hostetler AM, McHugh PR. Transport of cholecystokinin (CCK) binding sites in subdiaphragmatic vagal branches. *Brain Res.* 1987;415:149–152.

39. Ritter RC, Brenner L, Yox DP. Participation of vagal sensory neurons in putative satiety signals from upper gastrointestinal tract. In: Ritter S, Ritter RC, Barnes CD, eds. *Neuroanatomy and Physiology of Abdominal Vagal Afferents.* Boca Raton, FL: CRC Press; 1992:221–248.

40. Smith GP, Gibbs J. Cholecystokinin: a putative satiety signal. *Pharmacol Biochem Behav.* 1975;3:135–138.

41. Novin D, Sanderson J, Gonzalez M. Feeding after nutrient infusion: effects of hypothalamic lesions and vagotomy. *Physiol Behav.* 1979; 22:107–113.

42. Gibbs J, Smith GP. The neuroendocrinology of postprandial satiety. In: Martini L, Ganong WF, eds. *Frontiers in Neuroendocrinology.* New York: Raven Press; 1984;8:245.

43. Greenberg D, Gibbs J, Smith GP. Introduodenal infusions of fat inhibit sham feeding in Zucker rats. *Brain Res Bull.* 1986;17:599–604.

44. Welch IM, Sepple CP, Read NW. Comparisons of the effects on satiety and eating behavior of infusion of lipid into the different regions of the small intestine. *Gut.* 1988;29:306–311.

45. Yox DP, Ritter RC. Capsaicin attenuates suppression of sham feeding induced by intestinal nutrients. *Am J Physiol.* 1988;255:R569–R574.

46. Gibbs J, Young RC, Smith GP. Cholecystokinin decreases food intake in rats. *J Comp Physiol Psychol.* 1973;84:488–495.

47. Smith GP, Jerome C, Cushin BJ, Eterno R, Simansky KJ. Abdominal vagotomy blocks the satiety effect of cholecystokinin in the rat. *Science.* 1981;213:1036–1037.

48. Smith GP, Jerome C, Norgren R. Afferent axons in abdominal vagus mediate satiety effect of cholecystokinin in rats. *Am J Physiol.* 1985;249:R638–R641.

49. Yox DP, Brenner L, Ritter RC. CCK receptor antagonists attenuate suppression of sham feeding by intestinal nutrients. *Am J Physiol.* 1992;262:R554–R561.

MARK I. FRIEDMAN, NANCY E. RAWSON, and
MICHAEL G. TORDOFF

Hepatic Signals for Control of Food Intake

ABSTRACT

Substantial evidence indicates that the liver conveys metabolic information to the brain to control food intake. Hepatic metabolic signals from the liver can restrain and initiate feeding behavior. Studies using physiological infusions of glucose into the hepatic portal vein suggest that hepatic satiety signals operate under normal eating conditions. Experiments using the fructose analogue, 2,5-anhydro-D-mannitol, indicate that a decrease in liver adenosine triphosphate may generate a hunger signal. Metabolic signals from the liver that control food intake appear to be carried at least in part by vagal afferent fibers. The occurrence of obesity is associated with a shift in the partitioning of metabolic fuels toward storage that is independent of changes in food intake. Because the liver plays a central role in the processing of metabolic fuels, overeating in obesity may result in part from a perturbation in liver metabolism that affects the generation of hepatic signals that control food intake.

Different types of sensory information control various aspects of feeding behavior (1). Olfaction and taste are used to recognize and select food, and gastrointestinal stimuli modulate the size of a meal. Signals associated with the metabolism of nutrients are involved in initiating and terminating eating, and determining energy consumption over longer intervals. This metabolic control of food intake is of relevance to the problems of overeating and obesity because it can provide a link between energy balance and feeding behavior.

Progress in unraveling mechanisms for the metabolic control of food intake depends on the solution to four related questions: 1) Where does the metabolic stimulus originate? 2) What is the biochemical nature of the stimulus? 3) How is the stimulus transduced into a signal that is monitored by the nervous system? and 4) How is this signal transmitted to or within the nervous system to control the behavior?

Solutions to the last three questions depend in large measure on the answer to the first. Because different tissues have different metabolic and biochemical characteristics, one needs to know where to look in order to identify and characterize the metabolic stimulus. In order to identify the mode and pathway of transmission of the metabolic signal in and to the nervous system, the receptor site must be located.

This paper deals with the crucial question of the anatomical origin of the metabolic signals that control food intake. In particular, it focuses on the liver as a source for these signals and in doing so also addresses the biochemical nature of the stimulus and the route of signal transmission to the brain. The liver is uniquely suited to monitor changes in energy metabolism, given its central position in the processing of metabolic fuels during both feeding and fasting (2). Russek first proposed such a role for the liver in the control of food intake more than thirty years ago (3). Since then, considerable evidence has accumulated to suggest that changes in liver metabolism generate signals that modulate feeding behavior. In this paper we review our laboratory's contribution to this body of evidence (for other reviews and perspectives, see 4–6).

Satiety

Changes in hepatic metabolism influence both the initiation and termination of feeding behavior. Much of the early work in this area dealt with the liver's role in satiety, most likely because the organ is obviously in a good position to assess the consequences of ingestion and provide a negative feedback signal. The most straightforward test of hepatic involvement in food intake, therefore, is to compare the satiating effect of hepatic portal and systemic nutrient infusions. Although early studies of this sort produced equivocal results (7), more recent experiments have shown clearly that, with appropriate experimental designs and procedures, infusion of physiological amounts of glucose into the hepatic portal vein reduces food intake of freely feeding rats more effectively than do infusions into the jugular vein.

PHYSIOLOGICAL SATIETY AND LEARNED FLAVOR PREFERENCES

Our first experiment examined the effects of hepatic portal vein infusion of glucose on both food intake and learned food preference. We were prompted to assess the possibility that conditioning effects influenced the feeding response to portal glucose infusion based on anecdotal observations in the literature and in our laboratory, suggesting that the suppression of food intake during portal glucose infusion carried over to control conditions associated with testing (7). The results (Fig. 1) showed that infusion of glucose into the hepatic portal vein suppressed food intake and also created a preference for the food flavor

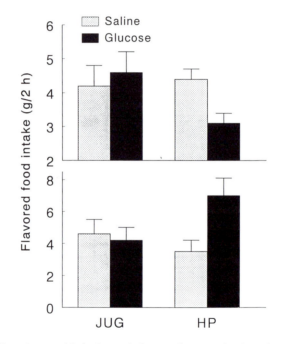

Figure 1. Hepatic portal infusions of glucose decrease food intake and increase food flavor preference. Top graph shows food intake of rats infused via the jugular (JUG) or hepatic portal (HP) vein with isotonic glucose or saline. In this intake test, rats consumed a diet to which flavors were added such that infusion of glucose or saline was paired with one of the two flavors. Bottom graph shows the intake of the flavored diet paired with saline infusion versus the flavored diet paired with glucose infusion in a later choice test when no infusions were given. Jugular vein infusion of glucose had no effect on food intake or preferences (7). Values shown are means ± SEM.

paired with glucose infusion. Jugular infusions of the same amount of glucose had no effect on either food intake or food flavor preference.

Because suppression of food intake during portal vein glucose infusion was observed using a concentration and rate of delivery of glucose well within the range seen after a meal, the results indicated that hepatic portal vein glucose may provide a physiological signal for satiety. The tests were conducted during the normal nighttime feeding period under otherwise typical feeding conditions. This suggests that the hepatic satiety signal may operate normally to control food intake.

The observation that portal vein glucose infusion produced a learned flavor preference is important for two reasons: First, it shows that suppression of food intake was not due to illness because if it were the rats would have avoided the flavor paired with glucose. Second, it indicates that delivery of glucose into the hepatic portal vein provides an unconditioned stimulus for learned flavor preference. This suggests that a hepatic mechanism may be involved in the ability to learn about the caloric consequences of food and may help to shape food selection patterns.

METABOLIC BASIS FOR THE SATIATING EFFECT OF HEPATIC PORTAL GLUCOSE

In subsequent experiments we examined the relationship between the metabolic effects of hepatic portal glucose infusions and the suppression of food intake (8). In these studies rats were infused with different concentrations of glucose into either the hepatic portal or jugular vein under otherwise normal feeding conditions. Infusion of glucose into the liver suppressed food intake, whereas infusion into the jugular vein was without effect. These differential effects of hepatic portal and jugular infusion on food intake were mirrored in the metabolic response to glucose infusions (Fig. 2). Jugular infusions raised peripheral glucose levels much more than did hepatic portal vein infusions, whereas liver glycogen increased only in rats given glucose via the portal vein.

How does an increase in portal vein glucose produce satiety? The suppression of eating behavior does not appear to be caused by the concentration of glucose in the portal blood or liver. First, infusion of different concentrations of glucose produced an equivalent 30% decrease in food intake. Second, in these studies, hepatic portal glucose infusion suppressed food intake whether infusions were given while

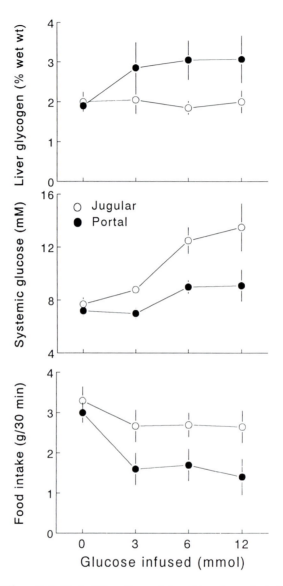

Figure 2.   Differential effect of hepatic portal and jugular vein infusion of different concentrations of glucose on food intake, plasma glucose, and liver glycogen in rats (8). Values shown are means ± SEM.

the rats were eating normally during the first hours of the night or just prior to this feeding period. This latter observation indicates that some metabolic consequence of glucose infusion may underlie the decrease in intake.

The difference in peripheral glucose concentrations between rats given hepatic portal and jugular vein infusions appeared to be attributable at least in part to a greater uptake of glucose into the liver, as evidenced by the increase in liver glycogen shown only by rats infused via the portal vein. Also, as with the suppression of food intake, hepatic portal glucose infusion had the same effect on liver glycogen regardless of the amount infused. Although a causal relationship between liver glycogen level and food intake seems unlikely to us (9), it is possible that the increase in glycogen may reflect a switch in hepatic metabolism from glucose output to glucose uptake and that some aspect of this reversal in liver metabolism provides the signal for satiety.

HEPATIC FUELS AND SATIETY

Another approach to investigate the role of the liver in satiety takes advantage of the capability of different tissues to utilize different metabolic fuels. If changes in hepatic metabolism control eating behavior, it should be possible to alter food intake by providing metabolic substrates that are preferentially utilized in the liver.

This strategy was used originally to examine the role of the liver versus the brain in the eating response to injection of insulin (10). Insulin-induced eating was prevented by infusion of fructose, which is utilized readily and primarily by the liver but, because it does not cross the blood brain barrier, is not utilized by the brain. Subsequent experiments showed that intravenous infusion of fructose also suppresses food intake under ad libitum feeding conditions (11). In some experiments, infusion of isotonic fructose more effectively decreased eating behavior when given via the hepatic portal than via the jugular route, whereas in others fructose was equally effective by either route (Fig. 3). In contrast, infusion of isotonic glucose was only effective by the hepatic portal route regardless of the testing protocol. One might expect to see no difference between hepatic portal and jugular routes of infusion of fructose under some conditions if the liver is the main site of fructose utilization. The effect of fructose infusion on liver glycogen

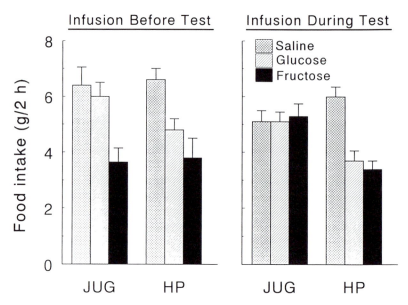

Figure 3.   Effects of intravenous glucose and fructose infusion on food intake in rats. In two separate experiments, glucose or fructose was infused into the jugular or hepatic portal vein either two hours before or for the first two hours during the normal nighttime feeding period. Glucose suppressed food intake only when infused via the portal vein regardless of the timing of infusion. Hepatic portal infusion of fructose suppressed food intake regardless of the timing of infusion; however, jugular infusions were also effective if given prior to the feeding period (11). Values shown are means ± SEM.

was consistent with this scenario in that fructose raised liver glycogen levels when given either via the hepatic portal or jugular vein.

Both glucose and fructose infusion redirects hepatic metabolism away from glucose output to uptake. It is possible therefore that infusion of either glucose or fructose shifts hepatic metabolism from a catabolic to an anabolic state. Under normal conditions this shift occurs as a result of food ingestion. The substrate infusions accelerate this metabolic process and, as a result, the behavioral process of satiety as well.

Hunger

Relative to the work on hepatic satiety, fewer studies have investigated the role of the liver in initiating eating behavior. The possibility that hepatic signals trigger hunger was first examined using 2-deoxy-D-glucose (2DG), a glucose analogue that stimulates food intake; however, experiments to localize the behavioral effect of 2DG to the liver produced equivocal results (12, 13). One likely reason for the discrepancies is that the action of 2DG is not confined to the liver. Even when 2DG is infused into the hepatic portal vein significant amounts enter the brain, where it can stimulate feeding (14).

A PROBE TO STUDY HEPATIC HUNGER SIGNALS

We have recently used a fructose analogue, 2,5-anhydro-D-mannitol (2,5-AM), to study the hepatic mechanism for initiation of feeding. The analogue 2,5-AM is structurally identical to the furanose form of fructose except for the lack of the C-2 hydroxyl group. We examined this fructose analogue for its effect on food intake because it had been shown to have marked effects on liver metabolism and, as fructose does not cross the blood brain barrier, was not expected to affect cerebral metabolism as glucose analogues do. The 2,5-AM is metabolized like fructose to the mono- and then bisphosphate forms, but is not further metabolized through glycolysis (15, 16).

The analogue 2,5-AM stimulates feeding in rats without producing overt nonspecific behavioral effects or unusual changes in circulating metabolic fuels of the sort seen when rats are given glucose analogues (17). The absence of behavioral and metabolic signs of a cerebral energetic emergency suggests that, like fructose, 2,5-AM is not taken up into the brain and instead has a peripheral site of action. Direct evidence that 2,5-AM acts in the liver to elicit eating behavior stems from the finding that infusion of 2,5-AM into the hepatic portal vein elicits eating at lower doses and more rapidly than does jugular vein infusion of the analogue (18; Fig. 4). A hepatic site of action is further supported by the observation that, at a dose that elicits feeding, the analogue is taken up mainly in the liver but is undetectable in the brain (18). Additional evidence that 2,5-AM acts in the liver to produce the feeding response comes from results of vagotomy experiments in which hepatic branch vagotomy abolished the eating response to a low dose of 2,5-AM (18; see below).

These results provide convincing evidence that 2,5-AM acts in the liver to trigger eating. Identification of the liver as the site of action for the effect of 2,5-AM on eating makes this analogue an extremely useful

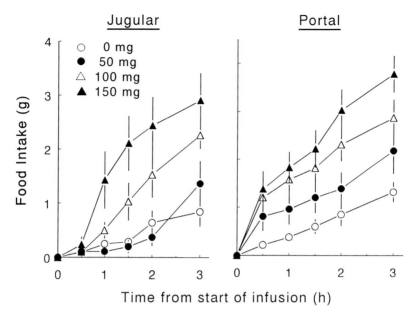

Figure 4. Hepatic portal vein infusion of 2,5-AM elicits feeding behavior more effectively than does jugular vein infusion (18). Values shown are means ± SEM.

probe for studying the control of feeding behavior. Recently, we have taken advantage of this tool to investigate several aspects of the hepatic mechanism for control of feeding, including the biochemical nature of the hepatic metabolic stimulus for feeding and the neural basis of the hepatic mechanism for feeding.

BIOCHEMICAL BASIS OF A HEPATIC SIGNAL FOR HUNGER

For many years, food intake was thought to be controlled in a coordinated fashion by signals generated by the metabolism of fat and glucose (19). Direct evidence for a mechanism that integrates information from fat and glucose metabolism in the control of feeding came from studies showing that combined blockade of fatty acid and glucose utilization with metabolic inhibitors results in a greater eating response than would be expected from separate inhibition of the metabolism of each fuel (20, 21). Such a synergistic increase in food intake would not be observed if signals from glucose and fat metabolism controlled feeding independently. This indicates that different aspects of metabolism influence feeding via a common biochemical and/or neural mechanism.

Because adenosine triphosphate (ATP) production is a final common pathway for the metabolism of both glucose and fatty acids, changes in ATP could serve at a biochemical level as an integrated signal in the metabolic control of feeding (22–24). In vitro studies with hepatocytes have shown that 2,5-AM is phosphorylated in the C1 and then C6 positions and that it decreases ATP (15, 16, 25). To determine whether 2,5-AM is phosphorylated and decreases ATP in vivo under conditions in which it elicits feeding behavior, we conducted a series of experiments (26) that examined hepatic phosphate metabolism in 2,5-AM–treated rats using in vivo ^{31}P nuclear magnetic resonance (NMR) spectroscopy. The results showed that administration of 2,5-AM decreases inorganic phosphate (Pi) and ATP during a period when the eating response would normally occur (Fig. 5). The decline in Pi and, subsequently ATP,

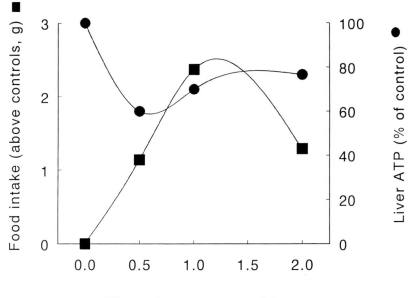

Figure 5.   The analogue 2,5-AM increases food intake and decreases liver ATP with a similar time course. Food intake shown as change from baseline is non-cumulative; ATP measured in vivo with NMR spectroscopy is shown as change from pre-injection baseline (26).

appeared to be due to trapping of phosphate in the phosphorylated forms of 2,5-AM.

These results, showing that doses of 2,5-AM that elicit eating also produce changes in high-energy, phosphate-carrying compounds in the liver, provide the first evidence that changes at this level of energy metabolism in the liver provide a stimulus for the control of feeding behavior. To determine whether low Pi levels after 2,5-AM treatment cause the reduction in hepatic ATP and are a factor in the eating response, we examined the effects of exogenous phosphate on liver ATP and feeding behavior after injection of the analogue (27).

As summarized in Figure 6, phosphate administration prevented both the increase in feeding and decrease in hepatic ATP produced by 2,5-AM injection. Sodium chloride had no effect on either the eating response or hepatic ATP. This suggests that the effect was not due to the osmotic load and was specific to the phosphate anion. Phosphate injection did not affect the eating response to acute insulin treatment or 2DG, nor did it alter water intake during the period it prevented the eating response to 2,5-AM. These results indicate that the effect of phosphate injection is behaviorally specific; that is, the effect on the eating response to 2,5-AM is not due to malaise or elicitation of competing behaviors.

These findings indicate that trapping and depletion of Pi is a critical intracellular factor in the mechanism by which 2,5-AM triggers feeding behavior. It seems unlikely that decreased Pi is the signal to eat because Pi in the liver increases during fasting (28, 29) when the need to eat is high. Rather, it appears that a decrease in hepatic Pi due to phosphorylation of 2,5-AM suppresses ATP production, which then may generate a signal for hunger. Accordingly, changes in phosphate would not be expected to play a part in the initiation of feeding under all circumstances (*e.g.*, insulin-induced eating), even though theoretically a decrease in ATP may stimulate eating. Thus, phosphate administration should be effective only when the ATP depletion is caused by a lack of Pi, and in this way can be used to counteract the mechanism of action of 2,5-AM.

FURTHER EVIDENCE THAT DECREASED ATP STIMULATES EATING

L-ethionine (Eth), an analogue of the amino acid methionine, also decreases ATP levels in liver (28, 29). However, unlike 2,5-AM, which

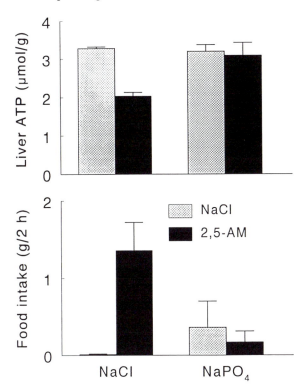

Figure 6. Pretreatment with exogenous phosphate prevents the decrease in liver ATP and the increase in food intake produced by 2,5-AM. Rats were injected with either sodium phosphate (NaPO$_4$) or isosmotic sodium chloride prior to injection with either saline (NaCl) or 2,5-AM. Liver ATP measures (from extracts of freeze-clamped livers) were made 30 minutes after 2,5-AM injection in a separate experiment following the food intake test (see 27). Values shown are means ± SEM.

reduces ATP by trapping phosphate, Eth reduces ATP by trapping the adenine moiety of ATP when it reacts with ATP to form S-adenosyl-ethionine, which is not further metabolized. As an independent means of testing the hypothesis that decreases in hepatic ATP generate a signal to eat, we examined the effect of Eth on food intake in rats. As shown in Figure 7, cumulative food intakes were markedly greater three to eight hours after rats were given ethionine compared with those given saline. Intakes decreased subsequently, such that twenty-four-hour intakes were unchanged. Under these conditions, Eth reduced hepatic

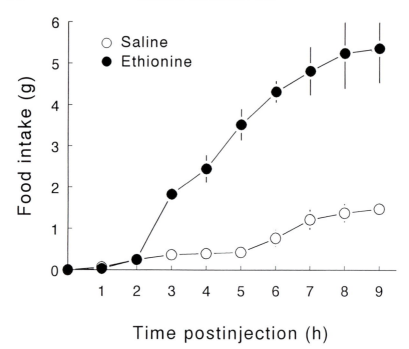

Figure 7. L-ethionine (1 gm/kg, p.o.) increases food intake in rats. Values shown are means ± SEM.

ATP content by about 30% but had no effect on plasma fuel levels. Comparison of the effect of Eth on food intake with that on hepatic ATP measured by in vivo ^{31}P NMR in anesthetized rats given the same dose (29) suggests that the change in behavior follows a time course similar to that in hepatic ATP.

Because ethionine depletes ATP in a different way than does 2,5-AM, these results provide independent evidence that decreased ATP triggers feeding, and they also lend considerable support to the hypothesis that changes in ATP provide a signal controlling feeding behavior. Additional studies are needed to determine whether the effects of Eth on food intake, like those of 2,5-AM, are due to a hepatic action of the amino acid analogue. Nevertheless, from a theoretical point of view, the effect of Eth on feeding behavior is notable. No other current theory on the control of food intake predicts it would stimulate feeding.

Transduction of Hepatic Signals for Eating Behavior

Little can be said about how metabolic events in the liver are trans-duced into signals that the nervous system uses to control eating be-havior. In general, there are several possibilities, including the presence of hepatic afferent nerves with special sensitivities to a certain meta-bolic parameter or special connections to the neural circuitry that con-trols food intake. Alternatively, hepatocytes may serve as secondary receptor cells similar to those used in other sensory systems, such as taste. The function of such hepatocytes would need to be specialized in some manner, for example, in respect to their spatial relationship to the nervous system or ability to secrete a neuroactive substance. We are intrigued by the possibility that perturbations in intracellular ATP might alter the ionic environment of the hepatocyte (30). This could operate through changes in the sodium-potassium pump (31) or, as has been demonstrated in other tissues, through alterations in mitochon-drial or cell membrane potassium channels (32, 33). A clearer knowl-edge of the hepatic stimulus for feeding and transmission of these sig-nals to the brain will surely advance our understanding of this crucial step in the hepatic mechanism that controls food intake.

Vagal Transmission of Hepatic Signals

How hepatic metabolic signals are transmitted to the nervous system to control feeding behavior is an important and unsolved question. Most attention has been focused on the role of vagal afferent nerves because of studies showing that interruption of the hepatic branch of the vagus alters ad libitum feeding behavior (34) and eliminates the effects of treatments that modify food intake (11, 31, 35, 36). Recent studies, which have shed new light on the organization of the abdom-inal vagal branches (37–39), force a reinterpretation of these findings. It is now clear that the hepatic branch of the vagus innervates other tissue besides the liver (37, 40) and that the vagal afferents from the liver travel in both the hepatic and celiac branches of the vagus (38). Thus, cutting the hepatic branch of the vagus nerve produces neither a specific denervation nor complete deafferentation of the liver. Also, because the hepatic branch contains both afferent and efferent fibers (41), behavioral effects of hepatic branch vagotomy could be due to interruption of a sensory signal from the liver or to interruption of an efferent control of hepatic metabolism (42). In short, hepatic vagotomy by itself does little to identify the liver as the site of action of experimental treatments or as a source of afferent signals for control of feeding behavior.

When combined with other treatments that affect feeding by their action in the liver, hepatic branch vagotomy can be used to provide strong confirmatory support for involvement of a hepatic mechanism in the control of eating behavior. This approach has been taken in the analysis of the suppression of feeding. For instance, the inhibitory effect of fructose infusion on insulin-induced eating is blocked by hepatic branch vagotomy (11). Similarly, the suppression of food intake in response to hepatic portal infusion of glucagon, which is more effective than systemic infusion, is prevented by hepatic vagotomy (43). Because 2,5-AM acts in the liver to elicit feeding behavior, we have begun to use the fructose analogue to pinpoint the origin of the hepatic afferent signal(s) for feeding and to examine the neural substrate of a hepatic mechanism for feeding.

Our earlier studies (18) showed that hepatic branch vagotomy blocks the feeding response to relatively low doses of 2,5-AM, but had no effect when rats were given a higher dose of the analogue. Recently, in collaboration with Dr. Sue Ritter, we have examined induction of fos-like immunoreactivity (fos-LI) in the brain after injection of 2,5-AM in rats with and without vagotomy (44). The nuclear protein fos increases in response to afferent neural input and thus can be used as an indicator of a neural activation.

Intravenous injection of 2,5-AM induced fos-LI in the area postrema (AP) and in the nucleus of the solitary tract (NTS) (Fig. 8, top), which are known to receive visceral sensory input, and in the lateral parabrachial nucleus (PBN) (Fig. 8, bottom), which receives input from the visceroceptive areas of the NTS. The effects of vagotomy on the induction of fos-LI after 2,5-AM paralleled the effects on feeding behavior. Hepatic branch vagotomy, which prevented the eating response to a relatively low dose of 2,5-AM (300 mg/kg), largely eliminated induction of fos-LI after administration of the low dose. Hepatic branch vagotomy, which did not prevent the feeding response to a higher dose of 2,5-AM (500 mg/kg), reduced but did not eliminate induction of fos-LI. In contrast, total subdiaphragmatic vagotomy virtually eliminated both induction of fos-LI and the feeding response to the high dose.

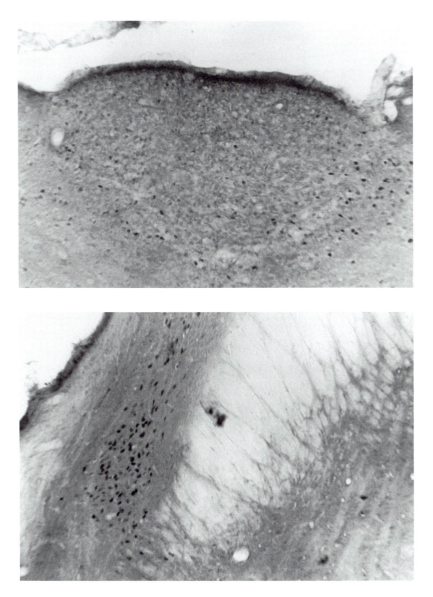

Figure 8. The analogue 2,5-AM induces fos-LI in the NST and AP (top) and in the LPN (bottom). Fos-like immunoreactivity appears as block precipitate within nuclear areas. A NiSO₄ DAB chromogen was used. Taken with a 16X objective (44).

These results indicate that 2,5-AM activates vagal afferent nerves and that this activation is associated with the eating response to the analogue. The finding that hepatic vagotomy prevents feeding and induction of fos-LI only at a relatively low dose whereas total vagotomy prevents both responses at a high dose is intriguing because it provides clues to the functional organization of the vagal branches with respect to their role in feeding behavior. Apparently, either the hepatic signal is transmitted over different vagal branches or high doses of 2,5-AM have other peripheral sites of action besides the liver.

Analysis of fos-LI in the brain after administration of 2,5-AM suggested that the behavioral response is mediated by afferent vagal input that involves both the AP/NTS region and the PBN, which receives input from the NTS. To further determine whether the PBN is involved in the eating response to 2,5-AM, we examined the effects of ibotenic acid lesions of the PBN in collaboration with Drs. Harvey Grill, Ralph Norgren, and Randy Seeley (45). Lesioned and control rats were tested for their eating responses to 2,5-AM and 2DG. Both groups of rats increased food intake in a dose-related manner after injection of 2DG, but only control animals increased feeding in response to 2,5-AM (Fig. 9). The results are consistent with the hypothesis that a vagal afferent signal reaching the level of the PBN triggers the eating response to 2,5-AM, whereas the response to 2DG is mediated by a different neural mechanism (46). Taken together with the results of vagotomy and immunohistochemistry experiments, the results begin to suggest the route by which hepatic hunger signals travel to the brain to elicit eating behavior.

Conclusions

Controlling food intake is both a problem and a solution in obesity. Although obesity can occur without hyperphagia, increased food intake is an important contributing factor in the progression of weight gain. Exerting control over food intake is the most common therapy for obesity. Elucidation of the physiological mechanisms for control of food intake, therefore, is crucial to our understanding of the etiology of obesity and to the development of strategies to treat it.

In most animal models of obesity, there is a shift in fuel partitioning toward storage of fat that is independent of any increase in food intake. At an organismic level, the hyperphagia that is seen during the devel-

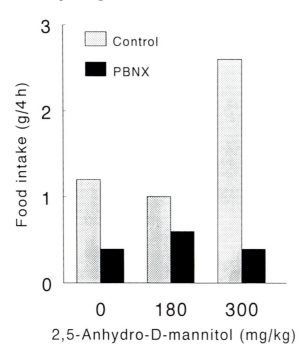

Figure 9. Rats with lesions of the parabrachial nucleus (PBNX) do not eat in response to injection of 2,5-AM. Lesions were made with ibotenic acid (45).

opment of obesity can be viewed in terms of a "loss" of oxidizable fuels into fat stores (47). Overeating compensates for this loss much as the increase in food intake in the cold compensates for the loss of energy in heat production. At a biochemical level, changes in fuel flux between oxidation and storage have been shown to affect food intake. For example, inhibition of carnitine palmitoyltransferase I, which is crucial in the partitioning of long-chain fatty acids between oxidation and reesterification, increases food intake of fat-fed rats (48).

The results described above suggest that signals controlling food intake are generated by changes in hepatic metabolism. Many of the biochemical decisions to either oxidize or store metabolic fuels are made in the liver. It is possible that the consequences of these decisions are appreciated by the hepatic mechanism that monitors energy metabolism to control food intake. Liver metabolism can be markedly perturbed in obesity. Perhaps these metabolic disturbances contribute to overeating by affecting hepatic signals for satiety and hunger.

ACKNOWLEDGMENTS

The research described in this chapter was supported by National Institutes of Health grants DK-36339, DC-00214, DC-00014, and MH-50363, and from a grant from the Howard Heinz Endowment.

REFERENCES

1. Friedman MI. Making sense out of calories. In: Stricker EM, ed. *Handbook of Behavioral Neurobiology: Food and Water Intake.* New York: Plenum Publishing; 1990:513–529.
2. Friedman MI, Stricker EM. The physiological psychology of hunger: a physiological perspective. *Psychol Rev.* 1976;83:409–431.
3. Russek M. An hypothesis on the participation of hepatic glucoreceptors in the control of food intake. *Nature.* 1963;197:79–80.
4. Russek M. Current status of the hepatostatic theory of food intake control. *Appetite.* 1981;2:137–143.
5. Novin D, VanderWeele DA. Visceral involvement in feeding: there is more to regulation than the hypothalamus. *Prog Psychobiol Physiol Psychol.* 1977;7:193–241.
6. Langhans W, Scharrer E. Metabolic control of eating. *World Rev Nutr Diet.* 1992;70:1–67.
7. Tordoff MG, Friedman MI. Hepatic portal glucose infusions decrease food intake and increase food preference. *Am J Physiol.* 1986; 251:R191–R196.
8. Tordoff MG, Tluczek JP, Friedman MI. Effect of hepatic portal glucose concentration on food intake and metabolism. *Am J Physiol.* 1990;257:R1474–R1480.
9. Friedman MI. Hyperphagia in rats with experimental diabetes mellitus: a response to a decreased supply of utilizable fuels. *J Comp Physiol Psychol.* 1978;92:109–117.
10. Friedman MI, Granneman J. Food intake and peripheral factors after recovery from insulin-induced hypoglycemia. *Am J Physiol.* 1983;244:R374–R382.
11. Tordoff MG, Friedman MI. Hepatic control of feeding: effect of glucose, fructose, and mannitol infusion. *Am J Physiol.* 1988;254:R969–R976.
12. Novin D, VanderWeele DA, Rezek M. Infusions of 2-deoxy-d-glu-

cose into the hepatic portal system causes eating: evidence for peripheral glucoreceptors. *Science.* 1973;181:858–860.

13. Russell PJD, Mogenson GJ. Drinking and feeding induced by jugular and portal infusions of 2-deoxy-D-glucose. *Am J Physiol.* 1976; 229:1014–1018.

14. Miselis R, Epstein AN. Feeding induced by intracerebroventricular 2-deoxy-D-glucose in the rat. *Am J Physiol.* 1975;229:1438–1447.

15. Riquelme PT, Kneer NM, Wernette-Hammond ME, Lardy HS. Inhibition of glycolysis in isolated rat hepatocytes and in Ehrlich ascites cells. *Proc Natl Acad Sci USA.* 1985;82:78–82.

16. Stevens HC, Covey TR, Dills WL. Inhibition of gluconeogenesis by 2,5-anhydro-D-mannitol in isolated rat hepatocytes. *Biochim Biophys Acta.* 1985;845:502–506.

17. Tordoff MG, Rafka R, DiNovi MJ, Friedman MI. 2,-5-Anhydro-D-mannitol: a fructose analogue that increases food intake in rats. *Am J Physiol.* 1988;254:R150–R153.

18. Tordoff MG, Rawson N, Friedman MI. 2,5-Anhydro-D-mannitol acts in liver to initiate feeding. *Am J Physiol.* 1991;261:R283–R288.

19. Mayer J. Regulation of energy intake and the body weight: the glucostatic theory and the lipostatic hypothesis. *Ann NY Acad Sci.* 1955; 63:15–42.

20. Friedman MI, Tordoff MG. Fatty acid oxidation and glucose utilization interact to control food intake in rats. *Am J Physiol.* 1986;251: R840–R845.

21. Friedman MI, Tordoff MG, Ramirez I. Integrated metabolic control of food intake. *Brain Res Bull.* 1986;17:855–859.

22. Scharrer W, Langhans E. Metabolic and hormonal factors controlling food intake. *Int J Vitam Nutr Res.* 1988;58:249–261.

23. Nicolaidis S, Even PC. The ischymetric control of feeding. *Int J Obes.* 1990;14(suppl 3):35–52.

24. Friedman MI. Metabolic control of calorie intake. In: Friedman MI, Tordoff MG, Kare MR, eds. *Appetite and Nutrition.* Vol. 4 of *Chemical Senses.* New York: Marcel Dekker; 1991:19–38.

25. Riquelme PT, Wernette-Hammond ME, Kneer NM, Lardy HA. Regulation of carbohydrate metabolism by 2,5-anhydro-D-mannitol. *Proc Natl Acad Sci USA.* 1983;80:4301–4305.

26. Rawson NE, Blum H, Osbakken MD, Friedman MI. Hepatic phosphate trapping, decreased ATP and increased feeding after 2,5-anhydro-D-mannitol. *Am J Physiol.* 1994;266:R112–R117.

27. Rawson NE, Friedman MI. Phosphate-loading prevents the decrease in ATP and increase in food intake produced by 2,5-anhydro-D-mannitol. *Am J Physiol.* 1994;266:R1792–R1796.

28. Shull KH, McConomy J, Vogt M, Castillo A, Farber E. On the mechanism of induction of hepatic adenosine triphosphate deficiency by ethionine. *J Biol Chem.* 1966;241:5060–5070.

29. Smith LJ, Murphy E, Gabel SA, London RE. In vivo ^{31}P NMR studies of the hepatic response to L-ethionine in anesthetized rats. *Toxicol Appl Pharmacol.* 1987;88:346–353.

30. Russek M. Current hypothesis in the control of feeding behavior. In: Mogenson GJ, Calaresu FR, eds. *Neural Integration of Physiological Mechanisms and Behaviour.* Toronto: University of Toronto Press; 1975:128–147.

31. Langhans W, Scharrer E. Evidence for a role of the sodium pump of hepatocytes in the control of food intake. *J Auton Nerv Syst.* 1987; 20:199–205.

32. Ashcroft FM. Adenosine 5'-triphosphate-sensitive potassium channels. *Annu Rev Neurosci.* 1988;11:97–118.

33. Beavis AD, Lu Y, Garlid KD. On the regulation of K$^+$ uniport in intact mitochondria by adenine nucleotides and nucleotide analogs. *J Biol Chem.* 1993;268:997–1004.

34. Friedman MI, Sawchenko PE. Evidence for hepatic involvement in the control of ad libitum food intake in rats. *Am J Physiol.* 1984;247: R106–R113.

35. Geary N, Smith GP. Selective hepatic vagotomy blocks pancreatic glucagon's satiety effect. *Physiol Behav.* 1983;31:391–394.

36. Langhans W, Egli G, Scharrer E. Selective hepatic vagotomy eliminates the hypophagic effect of different metabolites. *J Auton Nerv Syst.* 1985;13:255–262.

37. Prechtl JC, Powley TL. A light and electron microscopic examination of the vagal hepatic branch of the rat. *Anat Embryol (Berl).* 1987; 176:115–126.

38. Berthoud H-R, Kressel M, Neuhuber WL. An anterograde tracing study of the vagal innervation of rat liver, portal vein and biliary system. *Anat Embryol (Berl).* 1992;186:431–442.

39. Prechtl JC, Powley TL. Organization and distribution of the rat subdiaphramatic vagus and associated paraganglia. *J Comp Neurol.* 1985;235:182–195.

40. Berthoud H-R, Carlson NR, Powley TL. Topography of efferent va-

gal innervation of the rat gastrointestinal tract. *Am J Physiol.* 1991; 260:R200–R207.

41. Prechtl JC, Powley TL. The fiber composition of the abdominal vagus of the rat. *Anat Embryol (Berl).* 1990;181:101–115.

42. Tordoff MG, Friedman MI. Altered hepatic metabolic response to carbohydrate loads in rats with hepatic branch vagotomy or cholinergic blockade. *J Auton Nerv Syst.* 1994;47:255–261.

43. Geary N, Le Sauter J, Noh U. Glucagon acts in liver to control spontaneous meal size in rats. *Am J Physiol.* 1993;264:R116–R122.

44. Ritter S, Dihn TT, Friedman MI. Induction of Fos-like immunoreactivity (Fos-li) and stimulation of feeding by 2,5-anhydro-D-mannitol (2,5-AM) require the vagus nerve. *Brain Res.* 1994;646: 53–64.

45. Grill HJ, Friedman MI, Norgren R, Scalera G, Seeley R. Parabrachial nucleus lesions impair the feeding response elicited by 2,5-anhydro-D-mannitol but not 2-deoxy-D-glucose. *Am J Physiol.* 1995;268: R676–R682.

46. Ritter S, Calingasan NY, Hutton B, Dihn TT. Cooperation of vagal and central neural systems in monitoring metabolic events controlling feeding behavior. In: Ritter S, Ritter RC, Barnes CD, eds. *Neuroanatomy and Physiology of Abdominal Vagal Afferents.* Boca Raton, FL: CRC Press; 1992;249–277.

47. Friedman MI. Body fat and the metabolic control of food intake. *Int J Obes.* 1990;14(suppl 3):53–64.

48. Friedman MI, Ramirez I, Bowden CR, Tordoff MG. Fuel partitioning and food intake: role for mitochondrial fatty acid transport. *Am J Physiol.* 1990;258:R216–R221.

DAVID N. BRINDLEY and CHEUN-NEU WANG

Contribution of Glucocorticoids and Insulin Resistance to Dyslipidemias

ABSTRACT

Insulin resistance is a central feature of android (visceral) obesity, and it is associated with hypertension, high concentrations of very low density lipoproteins (VLDL) plus low density lipoproteins (LDL), and low concentrations of high density lipoproteins (HDL). Cortisol produces insulin resistance in tissues and increases the sensitivity of adipose tissue to lipolytic hormones. This causes an accelerated release of fatty acids from adipose tissue, and delivery to the liver is particularly large because of the high visceral mass of adipose tissue in android obesity. Fatty acids themselves cause further insulin resistance in the liver, and they stimulate gluconeogenesis and triacylglycerol synthesis. Glucocorticoids and insulin also stimulate fatty acid synthesis synergistically. The increased availabilities of fatty acids and glucocorticoids provide strong stimuli for the secretion of VLDL. Dexamethasone (a synthetic glucocorticoid) stimulates triacylglycerol secretion, and particularly apolipoprotein B (apoB) secretion from isolated hepatocytes. These effects are antagonized by insulin. The mechanisms for the increased secretion of apoB involve increased synthesis and decreased degradation of apoB: effects that are opposite to those of insulin. The increase in apoB secretion means that more VLDL particles are produced under the influence of cortisol. This has atherogenic implications, since each VLDL particle is converted to an intermediate-density-lipoprotein, or to LDL. The uptake of these particles is decreased by glucocorticoids through down-regulation of the hepatic apoB/E receptor. Consequently, insulin resistance and high glucocorticoid activity can produce hyperapobetalipoproteinemia. This relationship can partly explain the dyslipidemia associated with android obesity, diabetes, and stress, and why these conditions predispose to premature atherosclerosis.

Introduction

Insulin resistance is a central feature of the "metabolic syndrome" (syndrome X) and it is associated with android (visceral) obesity, type II diabetes, hypertension, hypertriglyceridemia, hyperapobetalipoproteinemia, and low concentrations of high density lipoproteins (HDL) (1). All of these conditions are not necessarily observed in a particular individual with the metabolic syndrome, since the expression of the various pathologies depends upon genetic predisposition and environmental pressures. The pathologies that are associated with android obesity (Fig. 1) represent powerful risk factors for the development of premature atherosclerosis, coronary thrombosis, and stroke. Patients need not have hypercholesterolemia, but they often exhibit high concentrations of dense low density lipoproteins (LDL) in their circulation (2). Each of these particles contains one molecule of apolipoprotein B (apoB), which explains the hyperapobetalipoproteinemia.

This paper will consider some of the metabolic complications of insulin resistance and the role of counterregulatory factors, including cortisol and nonesterified fatty acids (NEFA). It is proposed that the association of hyperinsulinemia and increased regulation of metabolism

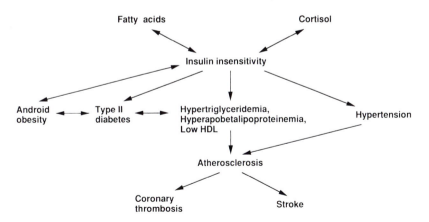

Figure 1. Proposed interactions between cortisol and fatty acids and pathological changes associated with the metabolic syndrome.

by cortisol and NEFA produce a type of metabolism that is potentially atherogenic (3, 4). We observed that this type of metabolism occurs in many of the risk factors associated with atherosclerosis, including stress, diabetes, android obesity, smoking, and the consumption of diets rich in fats and refined sugar but low in vitamin C. This observation not only provides a link between the various risk factors for athero-sclerosis, but also an explanation of why these factors might interact (3). The metabolic interactions of cortisol and fatty acids with insulin are therefore to be discussed in relationship to the production of dys-lipidemias.

Interactions of Insulin, Cortisol, and Nonesterified Fatty Acids

The interactions between insulin and cortisol in regulating metabolism fall into two distinct categories; namely, antagonism and synergism. The antagonistic actions are well known in terms of the control of glu-cose homeostasis. Insulin promotes the uptake of glucose by muscle and adipose tissue and stimulates subsequent glycolysis. By contrast, cortisol produces insulin resistance in tissues within a few hours, thus inhibiting insulin-mediated glucose uptake (3, 5). Cortisol also in-creases the activity of the regulatory enzymes for hepatic gluconeoge-nesis and the production of gluconeogenic precursors. For example, cortisol promotes protein breakdown in muscle and the delivery of amino acids to the liver, whereas insulin has the opposite effect. Simi-larly, insulin inhibits lipolysis in adipose tissue, thus lowering the sup-ply of NEFA and glycerol to the liver. The insulin resistance produced by cortisol decreases the ability of insulin to prevent lipolysis, and thus increased quantities of fatty acids and glycerol are released (Fig. 2). Furthermore, cortisol sensitizes adipose tissue to the lipolytic effects of catecholamines and growth hormone (6). Glycerol is an important glu-coneogenic precursor, and fatty acid oxidation and the formation of acetyl-CoA stimulate hepatic gluconeogenesis acutely. Furthermore, NEFA prevent the binding of insulin to the hepatic receptor, and this is one of the factors leading to insulin resistance and hyperinsulinemia (7–11). As a consequence of the increased fatty acid supply to the liver, hepatic β-oxidation is stimulated, and glucose is diverted to peripheral tissues.

The increased supply of fatty acids to the liver, especially in android obesity, often exceeds the need for β-oxidation, and the excess fatty

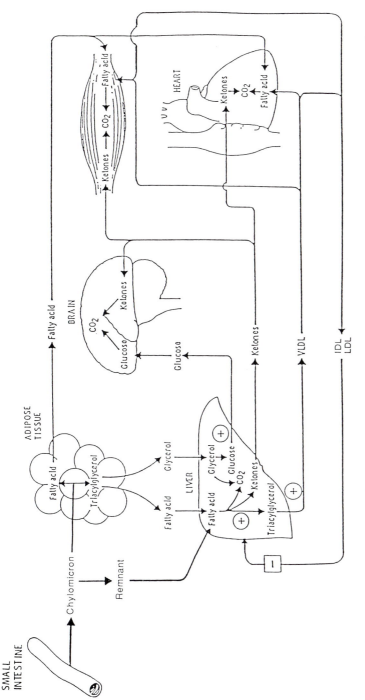

Figure 2. Schematic representation of the changes in lipid and lipoprotein metabolism that can occur in android obesity and type II diabetes. The effects of cortisol on gluconeogenesis, hepatic triacylglcyerol synthesis, VLDL secretion, and the uptake of IDL and LDL are shown: □ = decrease; ⊕ = increase. The hyperphagia and high-fat diet can increase fatty acid supply to the liver via chylomicron remnants. Furthermore, high carbohydrate intake and increased concentrations of insulin and cortisol can stimulate hepatic fatty acid synthesis.

acids are esterified to form triacylglycerols. This effect depends upon an increased availability of fatty acids and glycerol phosphate, which is partly derived from gluconeogenic precursors (Fig. 2). In addition, NEFA are acute activators of phosphatidate phosphohydrolase, which is an important enzyme that facilitates high rates of hepatic triacylglycerol synthesis (12, 13). In the long term, the phosphohydrolase activity is increased by the combined action of cortisol and glucagon on the liver. Such an effect is seen in stress and diabetic conditions. This type of regulation of phosphatidate phosphohydrolase (long-term control by cortisol and glucagon and short-term stimulation by NEFA) is reminiscent of that of the key regulatory enzymes involved in gluconeogenesis (12, 13). Consequently, there appears to be a coordination between the secretion of glucose and very low density lipoproteins (VLDL) triacylglycerol from the liver, both of which are intended to provide peripheral tissues with sources of energy.

The secretion of triacylglycerols from the liver in VLDL is stimulated by substrate availability, especially the supply of NEFA (14, 15). This is increased in android obesity because of the large, abdominal adipose tissue mass and the insulin insensitivity of this tissue. Furthermore, the supply of fatty acids to the liver is also increased through the uptake of chylomicron remnants and the high fat intake associated with android obesity (Fig. 2). The hyperphagia and increased carbohydrate availability can also stimulate hepatic fatty acid synthesis, which is increased by the synergistic actions of cortisol and high insulin concentrations. The increased availability of fatty acids in the liver stimulates the secretion of VLDL, probably by expanding the core of triacylglycerol. In some experimental systems (Hep G2 cells) NEFA also stimulate the secretion of apoB. However, in primary cultures of rat hepatocytes, this effect on apoB secretion is not observed (15).

Cortisol is also an important regulatory factor in controlling VLDL secretion. Glucocorticoids stimulate the secretion of triacylglycerols but have an even more pronounced effect in promoting apoB secretion (14, 16). This has potentially atherogenic implications, since each VLDL particle is metabolized to intermediate density lipoproteins (IDL), or LDL (Fig. 2). The mechanisms for the stimulation of apoB secretion were examined in greater detail using primary cultures of rat hepatocytes. Incubation of rat hepatocytes for 16 hours with 10 nanomolar dexamethasone (a synthetic glucocorticoid) increased the synthesis of apoB100 and apoB48 from [^{35}S]methionine over a 10 minute incubation by about 2- and 1.5-fold, respectively, despite producing a 28% decrease in overall protein synthesis (17). It should be noted that in rat hepatocytes, both apoB100 and apoB48 are produced, whereas in human liver only apoB100 is synthesized. The dexamethasone-induced increases in apoB synthesis occur without a significant increase in the steady-state concentration of mRNA for apoB (17), indicating that glucocorticoids may increase translational efficiency. Pulse-chase studies demonstrated that preincubation of rat hepatocytes with 10 nanomolar dexamethasone for 16 hours decreased the degradation of apoB100 and apoB48 over the first 60 minutes of the chase period. This is indicated by the relative amount of apoB recovered from cells plus medium (Table 1). There was also a significant increase in the relative secretion of apoB100 and apoB48 into the medium. Furthermore, dexamethasone also increased the time required for 50% of the labeled apoB100 and apoB48 in the cells to disappear from the peaks of radioactivities after a 10 minute pulse with [^{35}S]methionine (half-lives of decay) from 77 to 112 minutes and 145 to 250 minutes, respectively (17). The secretion of labeled apoB100 and apoB48 was also increased by dexamethasone in these experiments by 2- and 1.5-fold, respectively, after 180 minutes of chase (17). It was concluded that dexamethasone increased secretion by a combination of increased apoB synthesis and decreased degradation.

Table 1. Effects of Dexamethasone on the Degradation and Secretion of apoB100 and apoB48 in Cultured Rat Hepatocytes

Apolipoprotein	Location	Control	+ 10 nmolar dexamethasone
ApoB100	Cells	42 ± 7	55 ± 11*
	Medium	11 ± 3	28 ± 8**
	Total	53 ± 8	83 ± 13***
ApoB48	Cells	63 ± 5	80 ± 7*
	Medium	9 ± 2	14 ± 4*
	Total	72 ± 5	94 ± 5*

Hepatocytes were incubated for 16 hours in the presence or absence of 10 nmolar dexamethasone. Cells were labeled for 1 hour with [^{35}S]methionine and then washed with medium containing 10 nmolar L-methionine and 3 mmolar L-cystein over 40 minutes. The chase was then begun and it lasted 1 hour. Results are means ± SD from four independent experiments and are presented as percentages of the initial radioactivity in the cells at the beginning of the chase period. Significant differences between control cells and those treated with 10 nmolar dexamethasone are indicated by a paired t test: *$P \leq 0.05$; **$P \leq 0.01$; ***$P < 0.001$.

These effects of glucocorticoids on the synthesis, stability, and secretion of apoB are opposite to those produced by insulin (18, 19). Most current biochemical evidence indicates that insulin decreases the secretion of apoB and VLDL (14, 20), though this is somewhat controversial. Hyperinsulinemia and insulin resistance are commonly associated with hypertriglyceridemia. However, this can be interpreted as an effect of insulin resistance rather than a direct stimulation of VLDL secretion by insulin. In the case of insulin resistance, insulin is unable to suppress lipolysis in adipose tissue and VLDL secretion from the liver (Fig. 2). The high supply of fatty acids to the liver and the stimulating effects of NEFA and glucocorticoids on hepatic VLDL secretion can account for the hypersecretion of VLDL that occurs in stress, type II diabetes, and android obesity. These effects resemble those that explain increased glucose output from the liver in insulin resistance.

This role of insulin in suppressing VLDL secretion can be understood in physiological terms, since insulin is produced after a meal when chylomicrons are available to supply fatty acids to muscle and adipose tissue (16, 20). As the concentrations of chylomicrons and insulin subside, the liver is then able to secrete VLDL to provide an alternative source of fatty acids from triacylglycerols.

Effects of Cortisol and the Uptake of IDL and LDL by the Liver

The hydrolysis of the triacylglycerols in VLDL is catalyzed by lipoprotein lipase and occurs mainly in adipose tissue and muscle. The clearance of VLDL from the circulation may be depressed in the metabolic syndrome (21), thus exaggerating the hypertriglyceridemia that is produced by the increased secretion of VLDL from the liver. The removal of the triacylglycerol core of the VLDL leads to the formation of IDL and LDL, which are cholesterol-rich and still contain apoB. These particles are potentially atherogenic. The clearance of the IDL and LDL from the circulation depends mainly upon the activity of the hepatic LDL receptor (the apoB/E receptor). Expression of this receptor and the degradation of LDL are increased by insulin and decreased by cortisol. Consequently, the increased action of cortisol relative to insulin can produce a hypertriglyceridemia linked to hypercholesterolemia and hyperapobetalipoproteinemia (3, 4, 14). This profile of dyslipidemia is an important risk factor for the development of premature atherosclerosis.

Synergistic Interactions Between Insulin and Cortisol

By contrast to the antagonistic actions of insulin and cortisol on the hepatic production of glucose and VLDL, many of the pathways of energy storage are stimulated synergistically by cortisol and insulin. Cortisol facilitates the action of insulin in stimulating the synthesis of fatty acids (22, 23) and glycogen (24) and in increasing the activity of lipoprotein lipase and adipose tissue (25). However, the expression of lipoprotein lipase may be modulated by other events and this activity may be decreased in android obesity (21). The combination of high cortisol and high insulin concentrations appears to be a signal for energy deposition, and this signal is observed after meals when there is a release of both of these hormones (26–28). The balance between the release of cortisol and insulin is likely to depend upon the composition of the diet. Glucose will release more insulin relative to fructose, alcohol, and fat, which will have little effect on insulin secretion.

Cortisol can also: 1) increase food intake and insulin secretion (29); 2) decrease energy expenditure at least in rodents (30); 3) stimulate adipose tissue development (31); and 4) decrease the production of adipsin (32). Adipsin is a protein that is produced by adipose tissue and its concentration can be decreased in obese animals (32). Adipsin is probably involved in controlling the extent of adipose tissue development, and its secretion may be coordinated with the production of acylation stimulating protein (ASP), which is now known to be identical with C3adesArg (33). C3adesArg is derived by the interaction of three proteins: adipsin, factor B, and factor C3. C3adesArg is derived by the removal of arginine from C3a, which is catalyzed by a peptidase present in the plasma (33). It is postulated that ASP stimulates triacylglycerol synthesis in adipose tissue and that its defective action will make more fatty acids available to stimulate the hepatic secretion of VLDL. This is thought to be an important component leading to hyperapobetalipoproteinemia (34).

Conclusions

The available evidence suggests that excessive sensitivity to the action of cortisol relative to other stimuli such as corticotropin-releasing factor is one of the factors that is involved in the development of upper-body obesity (5, 7, 35–37). This may explain why adrenalectomy (38), or decreasing the effects of glucocorticoids on metabolism by use of antiglucocorticoids (39, 40), or the serotonergic agents dexfenfluramine (41) or benfluorex (42), may arrest the progress of obesity that is observed in many experimental models. It is also significant that impairment of type II glucocorticoid-receptor function in transgenic mice diminished feedback regulation of the hypothalamic-pituitary-adrenal axis (43). This raised the concentrations of corticotropin and corticosterone in the mice and produced obese animals. The authors suggest that the hypothalamic-pituitary-adrenal function of these animals is reminiscent of severe depression, and that the transgenic mice could provide a useful model for studying the relationship between depression and obesity.

The effect of cortisol in producing obesity need not be accompanied by dramatic increases in cortisol concentrations in the blood, since relatively modest increases in total circulating cortisol are accompanied by larger increases in the concentrations of the active, free cortisol. Obesity may also be a result of increased sensitivity of tissues to cortisol action, which in turn may also be related to the production of insulin insensitivity.

This paper emphasizes the role of glucocorticoids and fatty acids in the pathogenesis of obesity and in producing insulin resistance. Cortisol and fatty acids are increased in this condition and many people overeat in response to perceived stressors in their lives (4). This type of hyperphagia is often associated with an increased consumption of fatty foods. Furthermore, the consumption of high-fat diets is associated with an increased sensitivity to stress reactions and an increased release of glucocorticoids (44–46). Thus, we have a potentially vicious cycle that will predispose to obesity and particularly android obesity.

This paper has concentrated upon the role of glucocorticoids and fatty acids in contributing to the dyslipidemia. Cortisol and fatty acids are stimulators of VLDL secretion, and cortisol, together with insulin resistance, leads to a decreased removal of LDL from the circulation. The consequent hypertriglyceridemia, hypercholesterolemia, and hyperapobetalipoproteinemia represent a strong atherogenic risk profile. This is a component in producing the observed increase in coronary thrombosis and stroke that is associated with the metabolic syndrome.

ACKNOWLEDGMENTS

This work was supported by the Heart and Stroke Foundation of Alberta and the Canadian Diabetes Association.

REFERENCES

1. Reaven GM. Role of insulin resistance in human disease. *Diabetes.* 1988;37:1595–1607.
2. Brunzell JD. Overview: Low density Lipoprotein Subclass Phenotype B as a Biochemical Marker for Visceral Obesity and Insulin Resistance. In: Bray GA, Ryan DH, eds. *Molecular and Genetic Aspects of Obesity.* Pennington Center Nutrition Series 5. Baton Rouge, LA: Louisiana State University Press; 1996;5:355–363.
3. Brindley DN, Rolland Y. Possible connections between stress, diabetes, obesity, hypertension and altered lipoprotein metabolism that may result in atherosclerosis. *Clin Sci.* 1989;77:453–461.
4. Brindley DN, McCann BS, Niaura R, Stoney CM, Suarez EC. Stress and lipoprotein metabolism: modulators and mechanisms. *Metabolism.* 1993;9(suppl. 1):3–15.
5. Brindley DN. Neuroendocrine regulation and obesity. *Int J Obes.* 1992;16:S75–S79.
6. Fain JN. Hormonal regulation of lipid mobilization from adipose tissue. In: Litwack G, ed. *Biochemical Actions of Hormones.* New York: Academic Press; 1980;1:119–204.
7. Björntorp P. Classification of obese patients and complications related to the distribution of surplus fat. *Nutrition.* 1990;5:131–137.
8. Randle PJ, Garland PB, Hales CN, Newsholm EA. The glucose fatty acid cycle: its role in insulin sensitivity and the metabolic disturbances of diabetes mellitus. *Lancet.* 1963;1:785–789.
9. Bevilacqua S, Bonadonna R, Buzzigoli G, *et al.* Acute elevation of free fatty acid levels leads to hepatic insulin resistance in obese subjects. *Metabolism.* 1987;36:502–506.
10. Hennes MMI, Shrago E, Kissebah AH. Mechanism of free fatty acid effects on hepatocyte insulin receptor binding and processing. *Obesity Res.* 1993;1:28–33.
11. Després J-P, Moorjani S, Lupien PJ, Trembley A, Nadeau A, Bouchard C. Regional distribution of body fat, plasma lipoproteins, and cardiovascular disease. *Arteriosclerosis.* 1990;10:497–511.

12. Brindley DN. Intracellular translocation of phosphatidate phosphohydrolase and its possible role in the control of glycerolipid synthesis. *Prog Lipid Res.* 1984;23:115–133.

13. Brindley DN. Phosphatidate phosphohydrolase activity in the liver. In: Brindley, PN, ed. *Phosphatidate Phosphohydrolase.* Boca Raton, FL: CRC Press; 1988;1:21–77.

14. Brindley DN, Salter AM. Hormonal regulation of the hepatic low density lipoprotein receptor and the catabolism of low density lipoproteins: relationship with the secretion of very low density lipoproteins. *Prog Lipid Res.* 1991;30:349–360.

15. Dixon JL, Ginsberg HN. Regulation of hepatic secretion of apolipoprotein B-containing lipoproteins: information obtained from cultured liver cells. *J Lipid Res.* 1993;34:167–179.

16. Martin-Sanz P, Vance JE, Brindley DN. Stimulation of apolipoprotein secretion in very-low-density and high-density lipoproteins by dexamethasone. *Biochem J.* 1990;271:575–583.

17. Wang CN, McLeod RS, Yao Z, Brindley DN. Effects of dexamethasone on the synthesis, degradation and secretion of apolipoprotein B in cultured rat hepatocytes. *Vasc Biol.* 1995;15:1481–1491.

18. Sparks JD, Sparks CE. Insulin modulation of hepatic synthesis and secretion of apolipoprotein B by rat-hepatocytes. *J Biol Chem.* 1990; 265:8854–8862.

19. Sparks JD, Zolfaghari RR, Sparks CE, Smith HC, Fisher EA. Impaired hepatic apolipoprotein B and E translation in streptozotocin diabetic rats. *J Clin Invest.* 1992;89:1418–1430.

20. Gibbons GF. Assembly and secretion of hepatic very low density lipoproteins. *Biochem J.* 1990;268:1–13.

21. Eckel R. Role of lipoprotein lipase in the insulin resistant syndrome. *Int J Obes.* 1994. In press.

22. Minshull M, Strong CR. The stimulation of lipogenesis in white adipose tissue from fed rats by corticosterone. *Int J Biochem.* 1985; 17:529–532.

23. Al-Sieni AII, Plested P, Rolland Y, Brindley, DN. Decreased incorporation of glucose into lipids and increased lactate production by adipose tissue after long-term treatment of rats with D-fenfluramine. *Biochem Pharmacol.* 1989;38:3661–3667.

24. Whitton PD, Hems DA. Glycogen synthesis in the perfused liver of adrenalectomized rats. *Biochem J.* 1976;156:585–592.

25. Speake BK, Parkin SM, Robinson DS. Regulation of the synthesis

of lipoprotein lipase in adipose tissue by dexamethasone. *Biochim Biophys Acta.* 1986;881:155–157.

26. Quigley ME, Yen SSC. A mid-day surge in cortisol levels. *J Clin Endocrinol Metab.* 1976;49:945–947.

27. Slag MR, Ahmed M, Gannon MC, Nutall FO. Meal stimulation of cortisol secretion: a protein induced effect. *Metabolism.* 1981;30: 1104–1108.

28. Follenius M, Brandenberger G, Hietter B, Siméoni M, Reinhard B. Diurnal cortisol peaks and their relationships to meals. *J Clin Endocrinol Metab.* 1982;55:757–761.

29. Dallman MF, Darlington DN, Suemaru S, Cascio CS, Levin N. Corticosteroids in homeostasis. *Acta Physiol Scand.* 1989;583:27–34.

30. Holt S, York DA, Fitzsimmons JTR. The effects of corticosterone, cold exposure and overfeeding with sucrose on brown adipose tissue of obese Zucker rats *(fa/fa)*. *Biochem J.* 1983;214:215–223.

31. Hauner H, Entenmann G, Wabitsch M, *et al.* Promoting effect of glucocorticoids on the differentiation of human adipocyte precursor cells cultured in a chemically defined medium. *J Clin Invest.* 1989;84:1663–1670.

32. Spiegelman BM, Lowell B, Napolitano A, *et al.* Adrenal corticoids regulate adipsin gene expression in genetically obese mice. *J Biol Chem.* 1989;264:1811–1815.

33. Baldo A, Sniderman AD, St-Luce S, *et al.* The adipsin-acylation stimulating protein system and regulation of intracellular triglyceride synthesis. *J Clin Invest.* 1993;92:1543–1547.

34. Sniderman A, Baldo A, Cianflone K. The potential role of acylation stimulating protein as a determinant of plasma triglyceride clearance and intracellular triglyceride synthesis. *Curr Opin Lipid.* 1992; 3:202–207.

35. Rivera MP, Svec F. Is cortisol involved in upper body obesity? *Med Hypotheses.* 1989;30:95–100.

36. Langley SC, York DA. Glucocorticoid receptor numbers in the brain and liver of the obese Zucker rat. *Int J Obes.* 1992;16:135–143.

37. York DA. Central regulation of appetite and autonomic activity by CRH, glucocorticoids and stress. *Prog Neuroendocrinol Immunol.* 1992;5:153–165.

38. Bray GA, York DA. Hypothalamic and genetic obesity in experimental animals: an autonomic and endocrine hypothesis. *Physiol Rev.* 1979;59:719–809.

39. Baulieu EE. Contragestion and other clinical applications of RU486, an antiprogesterone, at the receptor. *Science.* 1989;245:1351–1357.

40. Langley SC, York DA. Effects of antiglucocorticoid RU486 on development of obesity in obese *fa/fa* Zuckers rats. *Am J Physiol.* 1990; 259:R539–R544.

41. Brindley DN, Hales P, Al-Sieni AII, Russell JC. Sustained decreases in weight and serum insulin, glucose, triacylglycerol and cholesterol in JCR:LA-corpulent rats treated with D-fenfluramine. *Br J Pharmacol.* 1992;105:679–685.

42. Brindley DN. Mechanisms for the effects of benfluorex in the obese-diabetic-dyslipidemic syndrome. *Diabetes Metab Rev.* 1993;9(suppl 1):515–565.

43. Pepin M-C, Pothier F, Barden N. Impaired type II glucocorticoid-receptor function in mice bearing antisense RNA transgene. *Nature.* 1992;355:725–728.

44. Brindley DN, Cooling J, Glenny HP, Burditt SL, McKechnie IS. Effects of chronic modification of dietary fat and carbohydrate on the insulin, corticosterone and metabolic responses of rats fed acutely with glucose, fructose or ethanol. *Biochem J.* 1981;200:275–283.

45. Tannenbaum BM, Brindley DN, Dallman MF, Meaney MJ. Hypothalamic-pituitary dysregulation associated with a high fat diet. In: Program of annual meeting of the Society for Neuroscience; Annaheim, CA;1992;18:1540.

46. Tannenbaum BM, Francis D, Tannenbaum GS, Brindley DN, Dallman MF, Meaney MJ. High-fat feeding impairs both basal and stress-induced hypothalamic-pituitary-adrenal responsiveness. In: Program of the annual meeting of the Society for Neuroscience; Washington, DC; 1993;19:1188.

PART IV

Adipose Tissue

JOHN D. BRUNZELL, DAVID N. NEVIN,
ROBERT S. SCHWARTZ, MELISSA A. AUSTIN,
and WILFRED Y. FUJIMOTO

Overview: Low Density Lipoprotein Subclass Phenotype B as a Biochemical Marker for Visceral Obesity and Insulin Resistance

ABSTRACT

The insulin resistance syndrome is defined as an accumulation of intraabdominal fat, as identified by computed tomography, resistance to the action of insulin, elevated plasma free fatty acid levels, impaired glucose tolerance, dyslipidemia, hypertension, and premature coronary artery disease. The dyslipidemia consists of hypertriglyceridemia caused by increased very low density lipoproteins, decreased high density lipoprotein cholesterol levels, and the presence of small-dense low density lipoproteins (LDL). The presence of small LDL, identified by gradient gel electrophoresis, has been suggested to be a common trait, with autosomal dominant inheritance, termed LDL subclass phenotype B. It is proposed that LDL subclass phenotype B is a biochemical marker for the insulin resistance–intraabdominal obesity syndrome.

The pathogenesis of obesity-related dyslipidemia is uncertain, in part because of the occurrence of obesity with non–insulin-dependent diabetes mellitus (NIDDM) and familial combined hyperlipidemia (FCHL), both of which are commonly associated with hyperlipidemia. Patients with NIDDM experience an increased risk of coronary heart disease. Many studies have suggested an association of both NIDDM and coronary heart disease as part of a broader syndrome that includes obesity, insulin resistance, hyperinsulinemia, hypertriglyceridemia, and low levels of high density lipoprotein (HDL) (1–11). Obesity (12) as well as other components of this metabolic syndrome (13) has also been reported in FCHL, a common cause of premature coronary artery disease.

The obesity observed in this syndrome is usually centripetal, which has been defined by computed tomography to be intraabdominal or visceral (14–17). Centripetal obesity has been shown to be an important risk factor for NIDDM and cardiovascular disease independent of total body fat mass and is correlated with plasma levels of various lipoproteins and insulin, independent of body mass index (BMI) (1–11, 18).

Elevated fasting plasma insulin levels occur with centripetal obesity and are a marker of insulin resistance (19–25). Fasting insulin is often used as a proxy for insulin resistance, though various techniques are available that provide quantitative assessment of in vivo insulin sensitivity (26, 27). A more recently developed method is the minimal model devised by Bergman *et al.* (28), which has been applied to the study of visceral obesity (29).

Insulin resistance is common in NIDDM (30, 31) and has been associated with hypertriglyceridemia and low HDL (32–35). The often present hypertriglyceridemia of treated NIDDM (36) and FCHL (37) have been attributed to increased production of very low density lipoprotein (VLDL). Hypertriglyceridemia is often accompanied by low HDL levels, a well-recognized risk factor for atherosclerosis (38). Although it is not known if hypertriglyceridemia has a major independent effect on atherosclerosis risk, it is one marker for the other lipoprotein abnormalities that occur (39), including decreased HDL cholesterol. Other important determinants of plasma HDL cholesterol levels are the activity of the triglyceride lipases, lipoprotein lipase and hepatic lipase. Both low plasma lipoprotein lipase activity and high hepatic lipase activity have been associated with reduced HDL levels (40–43).

Although elevated low density lipoprotein (LDL) levels are an important risk factor for coronary heart disease, LDL-cholesterol levels are not consistently abnormal in NIDDM or FCHL. In the presence of hypertriglyceridemia, however, LDL-cholesterol measurements do not accurately reflect the number of plasma LDL particles, since cholesterol content is decreased in LDL particles (26, 44). Moreover, centripetal obesity has been directly related to increased numbers of small and dense particles (8, 11, 29, 45, 46). Most individuals can be classified on the basis of the size and density of their LDL particles into one of two LDL subclass phenotypes: phenotype A, characterized by a predominance of larger and more buoyant LDL; and phenotype B, characterized by smaller, denser LDL particles. Phenotype B has been postulated to be a more atherogenic lipoprotein profile (47). Recently, LDL size, buoyancy, and composition have been shown to be a function of post-heparin plasma hepatic lipase activity in men with or without premature coronary disease (48), which implies that hepatic lipase mediates changes in LDL size and density. Phenotype B has been proposed to be caused by a major gene in population-based studies of families (49) and in FCHL (50), interacting with an independent gene that affects apolipoprotein B levels (51). It is possible that one of these putative genes may have an effect on insulin action and, in the presence of another gene affecting insulin secretion, causes NIDDM.

A recent study has been performed to examine in greater detail the interaction between visceral body fat and these metabolic processes in normal-weight men (29). This study examined the associations between fasting plasma levels of lipoproteins, plasma free fatty acid levels, LDL subclass phenotype, post-heparin plasma lipolytic activity, insulin sensitivity, and visceral body fat assessed by computed tomography (Fig. 1).

Intraabdominal fat was significantly correlated with insulin sensitivity ($r = -0.559$), plasma free fatty acid ($r = 0.677$), plasma triglyceride ($r = 0.541$), LDL density (relative flotation rate, $r = -0.803$), and plasma HDL cholesterol ($r = -0.717$). Insulin sensitivity was inversely correlated with plasma free fatty acids ($r = -0.546$) and also tended to be inversely related to hepatic lipase activity ($r = -0.512$). Although associations do not prove cause and effect, some potential mechanisms

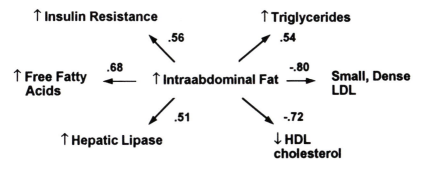

Figure 1. Correlation of area of intraabdominal fat by computed tomographic scan with variables measured in the visceral obesity–insulin resistance syndrome. Numbers are correlation coefficients.

From reference 29.

through which these factors might interrelate can be determined from studies that perturb individual components of this visceral obesity–insulin resistance syndrome.

One possible model for this syndrome is that an unknown primary defect causes intraabdominal fat accumulation resulting in insulin resistance. This is then followed by elevated plasma free fatty acids and finally dyslipidemia (Fig. 2). Perturbations at any point in this model are postulated to cause changes in variables occurring downstream, but variables upstream from the point of perturbation would be unaffected. Treatment of the dyslipidemia seen in NIDDM (52) and FCHL (26, 53) with fibric acid derivatives lowers the plasma triglyceride level and raises the HDL cholesterol level without changing upstream events. Treatment with pharmacologic doses of nicotinic acid causes insulin resistance (54) but lowers free fatty acid levels and corrects all components of the dyslipidemia. Preliminary studies of the effect of weight loss due to caloric restriction demonstrate that all components of the syndrome from accumulation of intraabdominal fat through the dyslipidemia correct after stabilization at a new lower weight (55). These stepwise perturbations strongly suggest that the primary event in the cascade is the accumulation of abdominal fat followed sequentially by the other steps (Fig. 2). The mechanisms responsible for the accumulation of intraabdominal fat remain unexplained.

Treatment directed at the components of this visceral obesity–insulin resistance syndrome would be expected to delay the onset of coronary artery disease in this syndrome. The ideal drug would be one that corrects the defect causing intraabdominal fat accumulation, or possibly one that can increase insulin sensitivity directly.

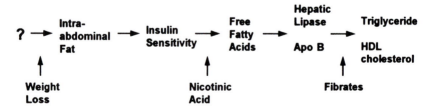

Figure 2. Proposed cascade to relate visceral obesity and insulin resistance to dyslipidemia. Perturbations in system indicated by vertical arrows.

ACKNOWLEDGMENTS

Research was supported in part by National Institutes of Health grant
DK02456. A portion of this study was performed in the University of
Washington Medical Center Clinical Research Center (NIH RR37). Aus-
tin was an established investigator at the American Heart Association.

REFERENCES

1. Després J-P, Moorjani S, Ferland M, *et al.* Adipose tissue distribution and plasma lipoprotein levels in obese women: importance of
intra-abdominal fat. *Arterioscler Thromb.* 1989;9:203–210.
2. Kaplan NM. The deadly quartet: upper-body obesity, glucose intolerance, hypertriglyceridemia, and hypertension. *Arch Intern
Med.* 1989;149:1514–1520.
3. Kissebah AH, Vydelingum N, Murray R, *et al.* Relation of body fat
distribution to metabolic complications of obesity. *J Clin Endocrinol
Metab.* 1982;54:254–260.
4. Krotkiewski M, Bjorntorp P, Sjostrom L, Smith U. Impact of obesity
on metabolism in men and women—importance of regional adipose tissue distribution. *J Clin Invest.* 1983;72:1150–1162.
5. Lapidus L, Bengtsson C, Larsson B, Pennert K, Rybo E, Sjostrom L.
Distribution of adipose tissue and risk of cardiovascular disease
and death: a 12-year follow-up of participants in the population
study of women in Gothenburg, Sweden. *Br Med J.* 1984;289:1257–
1261.
6. Larsson B, Svardsudd K, Welin L, Wilhelmsen L, Bjorntorp P, Tibblin G. Abdominal adipose tissue distribution, obesity, and risk of
cardiovascular disease and death: 13-year follow-up of participants
in the study of men born in 1913. *Br Med J.* 1984;288:1401–1404.
7. Ohlson L-O, Larsson B, Svardsudd K, *et al.* The influence of body
fat distribution on the incidence of diabetes mellitus: 13.5 years of
follow-up of the participants in the study of men born in 1913.
Diabetes. 1985;34:1055–1058.
8. Peeples LH, Carpenter JW, Israel RG, Barakat HA. Alterations in
low-density lipoproteins in subjects with abdominal obesity. *Metabolism.* 1989;38:1029–1036.
9. Reaven GM. Role of insulin resistance in human disease. *Diabetes.*
1988;37:1595–1607.

360   JOHN D. BRUNZELL *et al.*

10. Stern MP, Haffner SM. Body fat distribution and hyperinsulinemia as risk factors for diabetes and cardiovascular disease. *Arterioscler Thromb.* 1986;6:123–130.

11. Terry RB, Wood PD, Haskell WL, Stefanick ML, Krauss RM. Regional adiposity patterns in relation to lipids, lipoprotein cholesterol, and lipoprotein subfraction mass in men. *J Clin Endocrinol Metab.* 1989;68:191–199.

12. Brunzell J. Obesity and risk for cardiovascular disease. In: Greenwood MRC, ed. *Contemporary Issues in Clinical Nutrition, Obesity.* New York: Churchill Livingston, Inc; 1983;4:3–16.

13. Cabezas MC, de Bruin TWA, de Valk HW, Shoulders CC, Jansen H, Erkelens DW. Impaired fatty acid metabolism in familial combined hyperlipidemia: a mechanism associating hepatic apolipoprotein B overproduction and insulin resistance. *J Clin Invest.* 1993;92:160–168.

14. Ashwell M, Cole TJ, Dixon AK. Obesity: new insight into the anthropometric classification of fat distribution shown by computed tomography. *Br Med J.* 1985;290:1692–1694.

15. Fujioka S, Matsuzawa Y, Tokunaga K, Tarui S. Contribution of intraabdominal fat accumulation to the impairment of glucose and lipid metabolism in human obesity. *Metabolism.* 1987;36:54–59.

16. Shuman WP, Newell Morris LL, Leonetti DL, *et al.* Abnormal body fat distribution detected by computed tomography in diabetic men. *Invest Radiol.* 1986;21:483–487.

17. Sparrow D, Borkan GA, Gerzof SG, Wisniewski C, Silbert CK. Relationship of fat distribution to glucose tolerance: results of computed tomography in male participants of the normative aging study. *Diabetes.* 1986;35:411–415.

18. Després J-P, Moorjani S, Lupien PJ, Tremblay A, Nadeau A, Bouchard C. Regional distribution of body fat, plasma lipoproteins, and cardiovascular disease. *Arterioscler Thromb.* 1990;10:497–511.

19. Bagdade JD, Bierman EL, Porte D Jr. The significance of basal insulin levels in the evaluation of the insulin response to glucose in diabetic and nondiabetic subjects. *J Clin Invest.* 1967;46:1549–1557.

20. Barakat HA, Carpenter JW, McLendon VD, *et al.* Influence of obesity, impaired glucose tolerance, and NIDDM on LDL structure and composition: a possible link between hyperinsulinemia and atherosclerosis. *Diabetes.* 1990;39:1527–1533.

21. Garg A, Helderman H, Koffler M, Ayuso R, Rosenstock J, Raskin

P. Relationship between lipoprotein levels and in vivo insulin action in normal young white men. *Metabolism.* 1988;37:982–987.

22. Kahn SE, Beard JC, Schwartz MW, *et al.* Increased beta-cell secretory capacity as mechanism for islet adaptation to nicotinic acid-induced insulin resistance. *Diabetes.* 1989;38:562–568.

23. Laakso M. How good a marker is insulin level for insulin resistance? *Am J Epidemiol.* 1993;137:959–965.

24. Lillioja S, Mott DM, Zawadzki JK, *et al.* In vivo insulin action is familial characteristic in nondiabetic Pima Indians. *Diabetes.* 1987; 36:1329–1335.

25. Olefsky J, Farquhar JW, Reaven G. Relationship between fasting plasma insulin level and resistance to insulin-mediated glucose uptake in normal and diabetic subjects. *Diabetes.* 1973;22:507–513.

26. Hokanson JE, Austin MA, Zambon A, Brunzell JD. Plasma triglyceride and LDL heterogeneity in familial combined hyperlipidemia. *Arterioscler Thromb.* 1993;13:427–434.

27. Shen S-W, Reaven GM, Farquhar JW. Comparison of impedance to insulin-mediated glucose uptake in normal subjects and in subjects with latent diabetes. *J Clin Invest.* 1970;49:2151–2160.

28. Bergman RN, Ider YZ, Bowden CR, Cobelli C. Quantitative estimation of insulin sensitivity. *Am J Physiol.* 1979;236:E667–E677.

29. Fujimoto WY, Abbate SL, Kahn SE, Hokanson JE, Brunzell JD. The visceral adiposity syndrome in Japanese-American men. *Obesity Res.* 1994;2:364–371.

30. Ginsberg H, Kimmerling G, Olefsky JM, Reaven GM. Demonstration of insulin resistance in untreated adult-onset diabetic subjects with fasting hyperglycemia. *J Clin Invest.* 1975;55:454–461.

31. Reaven GM, Silvers A, Farquhar JW. Study of the relationship between plasma insulin concentration and efficiency of glucose uptake in normal and mildly diabetic subjects. *Diabetes.* 1970;19:571–578.

32. Golay A, Felber JP, Jequier E, DeFronzo RA, Ferrannini E. Metabolic basis of obesity and non-insulin dependent diabetes mellitus. *Diabetes Metab Rev.* 1988;4:727–747.

33. Orchard TJ, Becker DJ, Bates M. Plasma insulin and lipoprotein cholesterol concentrations: an atherogenic association? *Am J Epidemiol.* 1983;118:326–337.

34. Sims EAH, Danford E, Horton ES, Bray GA, Glennon JA, Salans

LB. Endocrine and metabolic effects of experimental obesity in man. *Recent Prog Horm Res.* 1973;29:457–496.

35. Stewart MW, Laker MF, Dyer RG, *et al.* Body fat distribution and hyperinsulinemia as risk factors for diabetes and cardiovascular disease. *Arterioscler Thromb.* 1986;6:123–130.

36. Brunzell JD, Chait A. Lipoprotein pathophysiology and treatment. In: Rifkin H, Porte D Jr, eds. *Ellenberg and Rifkin's Diabetes Mellitus.* New York: Elsevier; 1990;756–767.

37. Chait A, Albers JJ, Brunzell JD. Very low density lipoprotein over-production in genetic forms of hypertriglyceridemia. *Eur J Clin Invest.* 1980;10:17–22.

38. Castelli WP, Doyle JR, Gordon TR, *et al.* HDL cholesterol and other lipids in coronary heart disease: the cooperative lipoprotein phenotyping study. *Circulation.* 1977;55:767–772.

39. Austin MA. Plasma triglyceride as a risk factor for coronary heart disease. *Arterioscler Thromb.* 1991;11:2–14.

40. Babirak SP, Iverius P-H, Fujimoto WY, Brunzell JD. Detection and characterization of the heterozygote state for lipoprotein lipase deficiency. *Arterioscler Thromb.* 1989;9:326–334.

41. Magill P, Rao SN, Miller NE, *et al.* Relationships between the metabolism of high density and very low density lipoproteins in man: studies of apolipoprotein kinetics and adipose tissue lipoprotein lipase activity. *Eur J Clin Invest.* 1982;12:113–120.

42. Nikkila EA, Taskinen M-R, Sane T. Plasma high-density lipoprotein concentration and subfraction distribution in relation to triglyceride metabolism. *Am Heart J.* 1987;113:543–548.

43. Patsch JR, Prasad S, Gotto AM Jr, Patsch W. High density lipoprotein$_2$: relationship of the plasma level of this lipoprotein species to its composition, to the magnitude of postprandial lipemia, and to the activities of lipoprotein lipase and hepatic lipase. *J Clin Invest.* 1987;80:341–347.

44. Deckelbaum RJ, Granot E, Oschry Y, Rose L, Eisenberg S. Plasma triglyceride determines structure-composition in low and high density lipoproteins. *Arterioscler Thromb.* 1984;4:225–231.

45. Houmard JA, Wheeler WS, McCammon MR, *et al.* An evaluation of waist to hip ratio measurement methods in relation to lipid and carbohydrate metabolism in men. *Int J Obesity.* 1991;15:181–188.

46. Selby JV, Austin MA, Newman B, *et al.* LDL subclass phenotypes and the insulin resistance syndrome. *Circulation.* 1993;88:381–387.

47. Austin MA, Breslow JL, Hennekens CH, Buring JE, Willett WC, Krauss RM. Low-density lipoprotein subclass patterns and risk of myocardial infarction. *JAMA*. 1988;260:1917–1921.
48. Zambon A, Austin MA, Brown BG, Hokanson JE, Brunzell JD. Effect of hepatic lipase on LDL in normal men and those with coronary artery disease. *Arterioscler Thromb*. 1993;13:147–153.
49. Austin MA, King M-C, Vranizan KM, Krauss RM. Artherogenic lipoprotein phenotype: a proposed genetic marker for coronary heart disease risk. *Circulation*. 1990;82:495–506.
50. Austin MA, Brunzell JD, Fitch WL, Krauss RM. Inheritance of low density lipoprotein subclass patterns in familial combined hyperlipidemia. *Arterioscler Thromb*. 1990;10:520–530.
51. Jarvik GP, Brunzell JD, Austin MA, Krauss RM, Motulsky AG, Wijsman E. Genetic predictors of FCHL in four large pedigrees. Influence of apo B level major locus predicted genotype and LDL subclass phenotype. *Arterioscler Thromb*. 1994;14:1687–1694.
52. Garg A, Grundy SM. Management of dyslipidemia in NIDDM. *Diabetes Care*. 1990;13:153–169.
53. Bruckert E, Dejager S, Chapman MJ. Ciprofibrate therapy normalises the atherogenic low-density lipoprotein subspecies profile in combined hyperlipidemia. *Atherosclerosis*. 1993;100:91–102.
54. Kahn SE, Beard JC, Schwartz MW, *et al.* Increased β-cell secretory capacity as mechanism for islet adaptation to nicotinic acid-induced insulin resistance. *Diabetes*. 1989;38:562–568.
55. Nevin DN, Schwartz RS, Kahn SE, Brunzell JD. Metabolic associations in insulin resistance syndrome: effect of weight perturbation. *Circulation*. 1993;88:I–455.

GÉRARD AILHAUD, RAYMOND NEGREL, and PAUL
GRIMALDI

Adipogenic Hormones, Fatty Acids, and Adipose Cell Differentiation

ABSTRACT

The process of adipose cell differentiation is a multistep phenomenon. Commitment of adipoblasts to preadipose cells expressing early markers does not require adipogenic factors, in contrast to terminal differentiation of preadipose to adipose cells expressing late and very late markers as well as accumulating triacylglycerol. Terminal differentiation of Ob1771 preadipose cells requires a combination of circulating and locally produced hormones. Recent results indicate that, in addition to hormones, fatty acids can play the role of transcriptional regulators of lipid-related genes, favoring subsequent events which lead in vitro to the formation of adipose cells. The action of fatty acids appears to be mediated through nuclear trans-acting factors recently cloned and sequenced. The relevance of these findings is discussed with respect to adipose tissue hyperplasia observed in vivo in response to high-carbohydrate or high-fat diet.

Numerous investigations have been performed during the last decade with respect to the process of adipose cell differentiation. Adipose precursor cells from clonal lines (3T3-L1, 3T3-F442A, and Ob17 among the most frequently used) or isolated from the stromal-vascular fraction of white or brown adipose tissue of various species (from mouse to human) have been used extensively. In the case of the various "preadipocyte" clonal lines, the process of adipose cell differentiation, which can be analyzed in vitro, corresponds to the following phenotypic changes: adipoblast $\xrightarrow{\text{commitment}}$ preadipose cell (usually termed preadipocyte) $\xrightarrow{\text{terminal differentiation (start)}}$ immature adipose cell $\xrightarrow{\text{terminal differentiation (end)}}$ mature adipose cell or adipocyte. In the case of adipose precursor cells isolated from fat tissue, though the presence of adipoblasts cannot be excluded, this process corresponds primarily to the sequence: preadipose cell $\rightarrow$ immature adipose cell $\rightarrow$ mature adipose cell. This tentative conclusion is based upon the fact that mouse, rat, and human stromal-vascular cells contain the bulk of clone 9 mRNA (a member of the pentaxin family) and that of A2COL6/pOb24 mRNA (encoding for the α2-chain of collagen VI), and that these cells express lipoprotein lipase (LPL) and insulin-like growth factor-1 (IGF-1) mRNAs which are markers characterizing the preadipose state of cells from clonal lines. Other early markers include clone 5 (encoding for AP27) (1), clone 154 (encoding for an adipose differentiation-related protein) (2), and clone FAT (encoding for a protein involved in fatty acid uptake) (3). Growth arrest at the G1/S of the cell cycle, rather than contact among arrested cells, is necessary to trigger the process of cell commitment. The process of terminal differentiation is characterized by the induction of late and very late markers. The enzymatic machinery required for lipogenesis, triacylglycerol synthesis, and hydrolysis is then turned on and is responsible for lipid accumulation and mobilization. The acquisition in rodent cells of a β-adrenoreceptor–mediated lipolytic response by means of β2- and β3-adrenoreceptors is also observed, followed by that of an α2-adrenoreceptor–mediated antilipolytic response at the end of the differentiation process (for review see 4). It should be pointed out that dormant preadipocytes are present in old rodents and elderly people (5). Consequently, a fair knowledge of the adipogenic and antiadipogenic factors constitutes a requisite to gain some insights into the process of terminal differentiation.

Control of Terminal Differentiation of Preadipose Cells by Adipogenic and Antiadipogenic Factors

The critical role played by various hormones in regard to differentiating cells should not be confused with the role of the same hormones in regard to differentiated cells. A combination of hormonal factors is able to trigger terminal differentiation acting via cell surface receptors and nuclear receptors.

Involvement of Cell Surface Receptors

Insulin-like growth factor-I and insulin act by means of receptors having intrinsic tyrosine-kinase activity, whereas growth hormone acts by

means of a receptor that activates a phospholipase C activity hydro-
lyzing phosphatidylcholine to diacylglycerol and phosphocholine (6)
and a tyrosine-kinase associated activity (7). An important role appears
to be played by prostacyclin (PGI_2) which is, with prostaglandin E_2
(PGE_2), the major prostaglandin locally produced in adipose tissue both
in rodents and man (8). As shown in Figure 1, PGI_2 exerts a specific
adipogenic role on the terminal differentiation of Ob1771 cells and that
of preadipocytes from rat and human. It activates adenylate cyclase
and induces, in addition to a cAMP production, a rapid and transient
increase in intracellular free calcium. Both phenomena are required to
trigger terminal differentiation. Once differentiated, cells do not respond any longer to PGI_2, as no receptor appears to be present in adipose cells (9). In contrast, PGE_2 shows no effect on preadipose cells and
affects exclusively adipose cells, behaving as an antilipolytic-hypertrophic effector (10). The results indicate that PGI_2 has a critical window
of action with respect to terminal differentiation. As predicted, antibodies directed against a stable analogue of PGI_2-carbaprostacyclin is
able to block the terminal differentiation of Ob1771 cells (8). Altogether,
these results strongly suggest also that PGI_2 and PGE_2 have separate
target cells in adipose tissue and appear to act in concert rather than in
an opposite manner, controlling its hyperplastic and hypertrophic development, respectively. A similar situation takes place in regard to

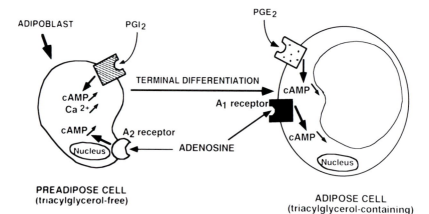

Figure 1. Shift in receptor composition during terminal differentiation of
preadipose to adipose cells. This model is based upon various results obtained
in Ob1771 preadipose cells and rat preadipocytes.

adenosine action and adenosine receptors: in rat preadipocytes, the A_2 receptor subtype is coupled positively to adenylate cyclase, whereas in rat adipocytes, adenosine induces a negative modulation of adenylate cyclase via the A_1 receptor subtype (11). Similar results have been obtained with respect to the differentiation of Ob1771 preadipose cells to adipose cells (J. Börglum et al., unpublished work).

Involvement of Nuclear Receptors

Triiodothyronine appears to be essential for the differentiation of Ob17 preadipose cells both in serum-supplemented and serum-free medium (12, 13). Similar observations have been made in 3T3-F442A cells (14). Triiodothyronine is active within a physiological range of concentrations ($EC_{50} = 0.1$ nmol) close to the dissociation constant value of the receptor for its natural ligand (15). Glucocorticoids stimulate terminal differentiation of 3T3-L1, TA-1, and Ob1771 cells as well as that of adipose precursor cells derived from rat, rabbit, and human adipose tissues (for review see 4). According to the order of potency and the range of concentration of various steroids, the glucocorticoid receptor appears to be involved. The effect of glucocorticoids may be mediated, at least in part, by an increase in the production of PGI_2 (Fig. 2) from arachidonic acid of exogenous or endogenous origin. Sex steroids such as β-estradiol, testosterone, and progesterone fail to enhance adipose cell differentiation, and only steroids with glucocorticoid activity are effective (16). Quite recently, retinoids have been shown to enhance the terminal differentiation of Ob1771 preadipose cells both in serum-supplemented and serum-free medium as well as that of rat preadipocytes in serum-free medium. This positive effect involves in particular the retinoic acid receptor α (RARα) subtype. When present at concentrations below or close to the dissociation constant value of the retinoic acid receptors, all-trans retinoic acid behaves also as a potent adipogenic hormone, in contrast to earlier reports (17).

Fatty Acids and Nuclear Receptors

We have recently shown that fatty acids play a central role in the control of the expression of genes involved in their own metabolism, both in Ob1771 preadipose and adipose cells. The effects of fatty acids from exogenous origin or originating from glucose by de novo synthesis take

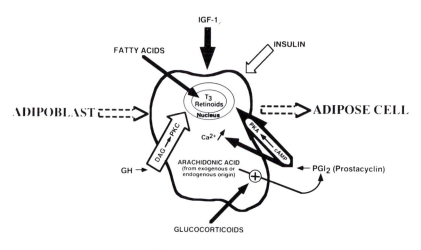

PREADIPOSE CELL

Figure 2. Hormonal factors and nutrients involved in the terminal differentiation of preadipose to adipose cells. This model is based upon various results
obtained in Ob1771 preadipose cells, 3T3-F442A preadipose cells, and rat and
human preadipocytes.

place primarily at a transcriptional level; they are fully reversible upon
fatty acid or glucose removal (18, 19). In this process, fatty acids per se
are actually the inducers of gene expression, since 2-bromopalmitate,
which is neither activated into acyl-CoA nor incorporated into lipids
in preadipose cells, is fully active in inducing the expression of various
lipid-related genes that include genes encoding for a fatty acid transporter (FAT) (3 and P. Grimaldi *et al.*, unpublished work), lipoprotein
lipase (LPL) (E. Amri *et al.*, unpublished work), adipocyte-lipid binding
protein (ALBP), and acyl-CoA synthetase (ACS) (18). More recently, it
has been observed that the critical role of fatty acids occurs during the
first three days following the commitment of adipoblasts to preadipose
cells. After fatty acid removal, this leads to overexpression of terminal
differentiation–related genes (20). Altogether, these observations suggest that fatty acids exert their adipogenic effects by acting at early steps
of the differentiation process. If one recalls that high-carbohydrate or
high-fat diet induces, in adult rodents, adipose tissue hyperplasia independently of sex, strain, or depot (21), and if we assume that under
these conditions an increased flux of fatty acids entering preadipose
and adipose cells from chylomicrons or very low density lipoproteins,

these results provide at the molecular level a potential link between high-carbohydrate or high-fat diet and the hyperplastic development of adipose tissue. The effects of fatty acids raise the question of their mechanism(s) of action. Fatty acids, like retinoic acid and fibrates, are amphipathic carboxylates. All-*trans* retinoic acid, 9-*cis* retinoic acid, and fibrates are recognized by receptors that belong to the superfamily of hormone steroid receptors, which includes retinoic acid receptors (RARα, β, and γ), retinoic X receptors (RXRα, β, and γ), and the peroxisome proliferator activated receptor (PPAR and related receptors), respectively (22). Quite recently, we have cloned and sequenced from fatty acid–treated Ob1771 cells a new member of this family showing strong homologies with human NUC-1 (23).

This receptor is a fatty acid–activated receptor (FAAR). In vitro, it is of interest to note that no expression of the FAAR gene occurs in adipoblasts; it becomes activated at the time of commitment to preadipose cells. In fibroblast cells stably transfected by FAAR, a fatty acid responsiveness is observed where they become adipose cells, strongly suggesting a critical role of FAAR in the initial events leading to the formation of adipocytes.

Conclusions

So far, in regard to terminal differentiation of preadipose cells, no unique adipogenic hormone appears critical, but rather a combination of hormonal factors above threshold concentrations appears involved (Fig. 2). It is worth pointing out that all these factors have to be present at the same time to trigger terminal differentiation. It is assumed that frequent ill-timed hormone secretion induced by diets or stress, as well as a diet-related increase in the flux of fatty acids entering adipose tissue, will increase the probability that threshold levels are attained, leading to hyperplasia of adipose tissue. Clearly, in vivo, the actual concentrations of adipogenic hormones and fatty acids in the vicinity of preadipose cells, in particular according to diets, are not precisely known. Nevertheless, in the case of low-molecular weight hormones such as PGI_2, in situ microdialysis has been used successfully to get information on this point. Our results show that its concentration in the nanomolar range is compatible with a physiological effect on differentiation (24). However, our results do not exclude the possibility that (specific?) inhibitory factors are preventing terminal differentiation of preadipose cells in vivo unless this inhibition is removed. No such factor or factors have been described so far, though, in vitro, the transforming growth factor-β (TGF-β) appears rather unique among growth factors, since after exposure of preadipose cells to this effector, no subsequent differentiation is observed following TGF-β removal (25).

REFERENCES

1. Wenz HM, Hinck L, Cannon P, Navre M, Ringold GM. Reduced expression of AP27 protein, the product of a growth factor-repressible gene, is associated with diminished adipocyte differentiation. *Proc Natl Acad Sci USA.* 1992;89:1065–1069.
2. Jiang HP, Serrero G. Isolation and characterization of a full-length cDNA coding for an adipose differentiation-related protein. *Proc Natl Acad Sci USA.* 1992;89:7856–7860.
3. Abumrad NA, El-Maghrabi MR, Amri EZ, Lopez E, Grimaldi PA. Cloning of a rat adipocyte membrane protein implicated in binding or transport of long-chain fatty acids that is induced during preadipocyte differentiation: homology with human CD36. *J Biol Chem.* 1993;268:17665–17668.
4. Ailhaud G, Grimaldi P, Négrel R. Cellular and molecular aspects of adipose tissue development. *Annu Rev Nutr.* 12:207–233.
5. Ailhaud G, Amri E, Bertand B, *et al.* Cellular and molecular aspects of adipose tissue growth. In: Bray G, Ricquier D, Spiegelman B, eds. *Obesity: Towards a Molecular Approach.* New York: Liss; 1990: 219–236.
6. Catalioto RM, Ailhaud G, Négrel R. Diacylglycerol production induced by growth hormone in Ob1771 preadipocytes arises from phosphatidylcholine breakdown. *Biochem Biophys Res Commun.* 1990;173:840–848.
7. Argetsinger LS, Campbell GS, Yang X, *et al.* Identification of JAK2 as a growth hormone receptor-associated tyrosine kinase. *Cell.* 1993; 74:237–244.
8. Catalioto RM, Gaillard D, Maclouf J, Ailhaud G, Négrel R. Autocrine control of adipose cell differentiation by prostacyclin and PGF$_{2\alpha}$. *Biochim Biophys Acta.* 1991;1091:364–369.
9. Vassaux G, Gaillard D, Ailhaud G, Négrel R. Prostacyclin is a specific effector of adipose cell differentiation: its dual role as a cAMP- and Ca^{2+}-elevating agent. *J Biol Chem.* 1992;267:11092–11097.

10. Vassaux G, Gaillard D, Darimont C, Ailhaud G, Négrel R. Differential response of preadipocytes and adipocytes to PGI$_2$ and PGE$_2$: physiological implications. *Endocrinology.* 1992;131:2393–2398.

11. Vassaux G, Gaillard D, Mari B, Ailhaud G, Négrel R. Differential expression of adenosine A$_1$ and A$_2$ receptors in preadipocytes and adipocytes. *Biochem Biophys Res Commun.* 1993;193:1123–1130.

12. Grimaldi P, Djian P, Négrel R, Ailhaud G. Differentiation of Ob17 preadipocytes to adipocytes: requirement of adipose conversion factor(s) for fat cell cluster formation. *EMBO J.* 1982;1:687–692.

13. Darimont C, Gaillard D, Ailhaud G, Négrel R. Terminal differentiation of mouse preadipocyte cells: adipogenic and antimitogenic role of triiodothyronine. *Mol Cell Endocrinol.* 1993;98:67–73.

14. Flores-Delgado G, Marsh-Moreno M, Kuri-Harcuch W. Thyroid hormone stimulates adipocyte differentiation of 3T3 cells. *Mol Cell Biochem.* 1987;76:35–43.

15. Gharbi-Chihi J, Grimaldi P, Torresani J, Ailhaud G. Triiodothyronine and adipose conversion of Ob17 preadipocytes: binding to high affinity sites and effects on fatty acid synthetizing and esterifying enzymes. *J Recept Res.* 1981;2:153–173.

16. Gaillard D, Wabitsch M, Pipy B, Négrel R. Control of terminal differentiation of adipose precursor cells by glucocorticoids. *J Lipid Res.* 1991;32:569–579.

17. Safonova I, Darimont C, Amri EZ, *et al.* Retinoids are positive effectors of adipose cell differentiation. *Mol Cell Endocrinol.* 1994;104:201–211.

18. Amri E, Bertrand B, Ailhaud G, Grimaldi P. Regulation of adipose cell differentiation, I: Fatty acids are inducers of the aP2 gene expression. *J Lipid Res.* 1991;32:1449–1456.

19. Amri E, Ailhaud G, Grimaldi P. Regulation of adipose cell differentiation, II: kinetics of induction of the aP2 gene by fatty acids and modulation by dexamethasone. *J Lipid Res.* 1991;32:1457–1463.

20. Amri E, Ailhaud G, Grimaldi P. Fatty acids as signal transducing molecules: involvement in the differentiation of preadipose to adipose cells. *J Lipid Res.* 1994;35:930–937.

21. Faust IM, Miller WH Jr. Hyperplastic growth of adipose tissue in obesity. In: Angel A, Hollenberg CH, Roncari DAK, eds. *The Adipocyte and Obesity: Cellular and Molecular Mechanisms.* New York: Raven; 1983:41–51.

22. Green S. Promiscuous liaisons. *Nature.* 1993;361:590–591.

23. Amri EZ, Bonino F, Ailhaud G, Abumard NA, Grimaldi P. Cloning of a protein that mediates transcriptional effects of fatty acids in preadipocytes. Homology to peroxisome proliferator-activated receptors. *J Biol Chem.* 1995;270:2367–2371.

24. Darimont C, Vassaux G, Ailhaud G, Négrel R. In situ microdialysis of prostaglandins in adipose tissue: stimulation of prostacyclin release by angiotensin II. *Int J Obes.* 1994;18:783–788.

25. Vassaux G, Négrel R, Ailhaud G, Gaillard D. Removal of anti-andipogenic agents leads to distinct effects on the resumption of rat preadipocyte differentiation. *J Cell Physiol.* 1994;161:249–256.

TIMOTHY G. RAMSAY

Insulin-like Growth Factors and Adipose Tissue

ABSTRACT

Insulin-like growth factors (IGFs) I and II are adipogenic when supplemented to cell lines or preadipocytes in primary culture. In addition, these cell lines and primary cultures express IGF mRNA and protein. Thus, the cells of adipose tissue generate an adipogenic factor. Use of various media treatments can induce differential expression of IGF-I between the adipocyte and stromal-vascular cell population of adipose tissue. This suggests differential regulation of IGF-I production by the various cell types. The paracrine actions of IGF-I on cell cultures derived from adipose tissue is complicated by the production of a variety of IGF binding proteins (IGFBP) by these cells. These IGFBPs may have beneficial or inhibitory actions on adipose tissue; their role has yet to be defined. These in vitro data recently have been confirmed in vivo. Expression of IGF-I, IGF-II, and IGFBPs within adipose tissue can respond to external stimuli, with the levels of IGF protein in adipose tissue exceeding the levels in liver. Thus, the insulin-like growth factors and their binding proteins may be considered to be important factors in the prenatal and postnatal development of adipose tissue.

Introduction

The insulin-like growth factors (IGF-I and IGF-II) are members of the insulin family, sharing structural homology to proinsulin. They are small polypeptides with molecular weights of approximately 7500. The IGFs can be readily detected in serum and are present in concentrations that exceed other known growth factors (EGF, FGF, etc.). The liver was originally considered to be the major site of synthesis, but many peripheral tissues are now known to synthesize the insulin-like growth factors. These growth factors have potent mitogenic and metabolic actions during cell and tissue development (for review, see 1). This discussion will focus on a review of in vitro and in vivo studies that support a role for insulin-like growth factors in the growth and development of adipose tissue.

In Vitro Assessment of IGF Action

Research into the potential function of IGFs in adipocyte development began during the period when IGFs were first discovered. Use of insulin antibodies demonstrated that inactivation of insulin in a serum sample did not eliminate all insulin-like activity of that serum when assessed by monitoring glucose metabolism of isolated adipocytes (nonsuppressible insulin-like activity) (2). Since that time, numerous studies have evaluated the metabolic actions of IGF-I and IGF-II on glucose metabolism by adipocytes. The IGFs have a limited but significant ability to induce glucose transport, oxidation, and lipogenesis in adipocytes. This ability has been ascribed to binding to the insulin receptor because of the high concentrations of IGFs necessary to elicit a response.

Assessment of other functions for IGFs in adipose tissue began by a more indirect route. Growth hormone was demonstrated to be an adipogenic factor for 3T3 preadipocytes by Howard Green's laboratory in a series of elegant experiments (3, 4, 5). The last of this series demonstrated that growth hormone exposure was necessary for IGF-I to induce mitogenesis during clonal expansion (6). However, use of growth hormone in primary cultures derived from rodents or swine could not produce an adipogenic effect at physiological concentrations (7, 8; for review, see 9).

The observation of growth hormone induction of IGF-I secretion in various cell types led to assessment of IGF-I action on primary cultures containing preadipocytes. Supplementation of IGF-I to either serum-containing or serum-free medium demonstrated that IGF-I is adipogenic within the physiological range (20–500 ng/mL) to primary cultures containing rat or pig preadipocytes (8, 10, 11, 12). This effect is not limited to IGF-I, but can also be induced by IGF-II at physiological concentrations (Fig. 1a). The IGFs induce both a mitogenic and differentiation response in preadipocytes (9, 11, 13). The mitogenic response is not specific to the preadipocyte population but also occurs in other cells within the stromal-vascular cell population (Fig. 1b). This is not

Differentiation Response by Primary Cultures to IGF-I or -II Supplementation

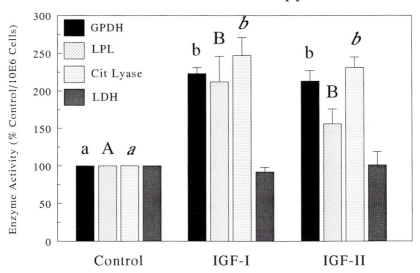

Figure 1a. Differentiation response by primary cultures to IGF-I or -II supplementation. Primary cultures containing porcine preadipocytes were exposed to IGF-I (50 ng/mL medium) or IGF-II (50 ng/mL medium) at confluency. Cultures were harvested 9 days later for analysis of enzyme activities as a monitor for differentiation. Values are expressed as percent activity of cultures exposed to basal medium per 10^6 cells. Means not sharing a common superscript for each enzyme are significantly different ($P < .01$). GPDH = sn-glycerol-3-phosphate dehydrogenase; LPL = lipoprotein lipase; Cit Lyase = citrate lyase; LDH = lactate dehydrogenase.

Derived from ref. 23 by permission of the American Institute of Nutrition.

surprising, as numerous cell types (including fibroblasts and endothelial cells) have been reported to demonstrate a mitogenic response to IGFs (for review, see 1).

The adipogenic cell lines have permitted examination of a variety of responses that are specific to preadipocyte cells, since they are clonal in origin, thus eliminating the confounding influences or interactions with other cell types present in the stromal-vascular fraction of adipose tissue during primary culture. Supplementation of IGF-I to the cell culture media of the Ob17 adipogenic cell line results in cell proliferation (14). Direct effects of IGF-I on differentiation in Ob17 cells have not

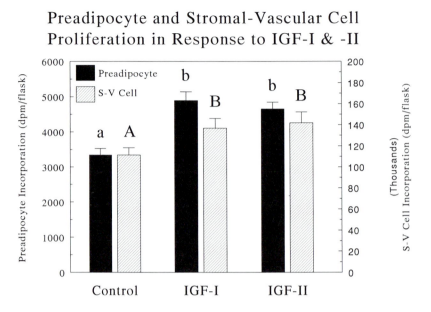

Figure 1b. Preadipocyte and stromal-vascular cell proliferation in response to IGF-I and -II. Primary cultures containing porcine preadipocytes were exposed to IGF-I (50 ng/mL medium) or IGF-II (50 ng/mL medium) on days 1–5 of culture, prior to confluency. Cells were pulse-labeled with ^{3}H-thymidine (0.05 μCi/25 cm^2 flask) on day 4 of culture. Following confluency and differentiation, cell populations were separated on percoll density gradients (see ref. 11 for details of method). Data are expressed as dpm incorporated per flask for each cell population. Means not sharing a common superscript for each cell population are significantly different ($P < .05$).

been reported. In contrast, genes associated with both early and late events of differentiation in 3T3 preadipocyte cell lines have been evaluated in response to IGF-I supplementation to the medium. Differentiation of the 3T3-L1 preadipocyte can be augmented with the supplementation of IGF-I to culture medium with or without serum (15, 16, 17). The initial action of IGF-I may occur very early during differentiation, since c-fos transcription and c-fos expression have been reported to increase rapidly following exposure of 3T3-442A cells to IGF-I (18). This action is through the IGF-I receptor and not the insulin receptor, since Weiland *et al.* (19) showed induction of c-fos mRNA by IGF-I parallels its receptor occupancy during acute experiments in 3T3-L1 cells.

The various lines of evidence from supplemental IGF additions to in vitro culture systems indicate that IGF-I at physiological concentrations is a potent inducer of differentiation of preadipocytes. Attempts to develop extensive dose response curves for IGF-I and IGF-II by preadipocytes in primary cultures met with limited success and often revealed great variability (unpublished observations). At the time, the causative factors for this variability were unknown. Then, Doglio *et al.* (20) reported that Ob17 cells generate mRNA for IGF-I when exposed to growth hormone (GH). Insulin-like growth factor-I gene expression was rapid in response to GH, reaching a maximum within two hours of GH exposure and returning to baseline within twenty-four hours of withdrawal. The autocrine/paracrine production of IGFs could account for the apparent inability to generate extensive dose response curves with IGFs in primary cultures containing preadipocytes. This report with Ob17 cells resulted in several experiments to examine the regulation of IGF-I expression in primary cultures containing porcine preadipocytes.

Utilization of human growth hormone (1 nmol) in primary cultures resulted in an increase in IGF-I mRNA steady state levels within one and one-half hours of exposure, and these levels were still elevated following twenty-four hours of incubation (21). The estimated ED_{50} for this mRNA response is 0.25 nmol to 0.5 nmol GH when assessed using rat stromal cells (22). The changes in level of mRNA abundance correlated with changes in IGF-I protein concentration in the medium; IGF-I was detectable in the medium by radioimmunoassay within three hours of exposure to GH (21). Immunofluorescent localization demonstrated that IGF-I was associated with both adipocytes and stromal elements in the primary culture, suggesting no cell specificity in the response. However, this experiment could not determine if differential regulation of IGF-I abundance occurs between the adipocyte versus stromal-vascular cell fractions.

Use of Percoll density gradients permits separation of adipocytes from stromal cells for use in mRNA analysis (23). Exposure of primary cultures containing porcine preadipocytes to porcine GH (pGH, 4.54 nmol) results in a coordinated increase in IGF-I mRNA abundance in both the adipocyte and stromal cell fractions of primary cultures (Fig. 2). This increase in mRNA abundance is accompanied by a similar proportional increase in IGF-I protein secreted into the culture medium, in agreement with the report of Gaskins *et al.* (21). Thus, growth hormone

Relative IGF-I mRNA and Protein Response by Primary Cultures to Growth Hormone

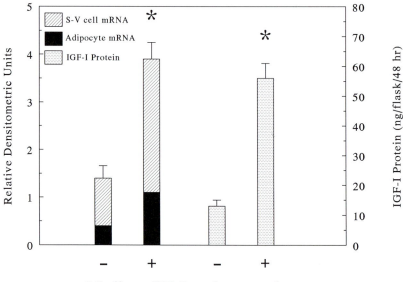

Medium GH Supplementation

Figure 2. Relative IGF-I mRNA and protein response by primary cultures to growth hormone. Primary cultures derived from porcine adipose tissue were exposed to a basal medium supplemented without ($-$) or with ($+$) porcine growth hormone (100 ng/mL medium) for 48 hours. The medium was then collected for analysis of IGF-I content by radioimmunoassay. Adipocytes and stromal-vascular cells were harvested from the flasks and separated on percoll density gradients. Total RNA was isolated from each cell population and screened for IGF-I mRNA by Northern analysis. * = different from basal medium ($P < .001$).

Derived from ref. 23 by permission of the American Institute of Nutrition.

is a nonspecific inducer of IGF-I gene expression in adipose tissue, affecting both adipocytes and stromal cells in a similar manner. Adipocyte synthesis is confirmed by the data of Vikman *et al.* (24) that demonstrated that isolated adipocytes in short-term culture (2–3 days) synthesize and secrete IGF-I in response to growth hormone exposure (1–100 ng/mL).

Exposure of primary cultures to hypophysectomized pig serum and use of these Percoll gradients has permitted identification of differential regulation of IGF-I between adipocytes and stromal cells (Fig. 3). Abundance of IGF-I mRNA is significantly reduced in the adipocyte fraction of the total cell population, whereas expression is increased in the stromal cells. The result is that IGF-I protein levels are significantly elevated in the medium in comparison to medium from cultures incubated with sera from pituitary-intact pigs. This elevation in IGF-I in the medium may account for the reported excessive proliferation of

Relative IGF-I mRNA and Protein Levels in Primary Cultures

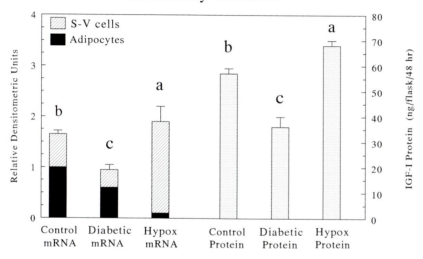

Figure 3.   Relative IGF-I mRNA and protein levels in primary cultures. Primary cultures derived from porcine adipose tissue were exposed to a basal medium supplemented with 2% porcine serum derived from intact (control), diabetic, or hypophysectomized (hypox) pigs following differentiation of preadipocytes. The medium was collected after 48 hours of incubation for analysis of IGF-I content by radioimmunoassay. The IGF-I protein content of the medium was corrected for the amount of protein derived from the serum supplements. Adipocytes and stromal-vascular cells were harvested from the flasks and separated on percoll density gradients. Total RNA was isolated from each cell population and screened for IGF-I mRNA by Northern analysis. Means not sharing a common superscript within each assay are significantly different ($P < .05$).

stromal cells in primary cultures exposed to sera from hypophysectomized animals (8).

Growth hormone is not the only regulator of IGF-I gene expression
(for review see 1 and 25). Glucocorticoids are commonly included in
differentiation medium to induce adipocyte formation in cell line or
primary culture. Nougues *et al.* (26) reported that dexamethasone (100
nmol) can alter the quantity of IGF-I secreted by primary cultures of
stromal-vascular cells from rabbit adipose tissue.

In addition, exposure of primary cultures to sera from diabetic animals results in a reduction in IGF-I mRNA abundance and protein
secretion (Fig. 3). This also indicates that GH is not the only regulator
of IGF-I gene expression, since diabetic serum contains elevated levels
of growth hormone in comparison to serum from normal animals. Insulin has been shown to stimulate IGF-I gene expression in tissues from
diabetic rats and pigs, whereas growth hormone could not induce IGF-
I in diabetic animals (27, 28). These data might suggest that the routine
use of high concentrations of insulin (10 nmol to 1 μmol) in differentiation media for preadipocytes in many culture systems may function
by inducing paracrine IGF-I expression, especially in serum-free systems in which no growth hormone is present. Further research is necessary to elucidate this hypothesis, but if true, reevaluation of many
studies from the past will be necessary.

Measurement of mRNA abundance and protein secretion into cell
culture medium does not conclusively demonstrate that a factor is a
paracrine adipogenic factor. The secreted protein must be functional
and be able to induce an adipogenic response. Recently, Nougues *et al.*
(26) performed this essential experiment by supplementing a monoclonal IGF-I antibody to primary cultures of rabbit stromal-vascular cells
containing preadipocytes. Addition of the antibody resulted in approximately a 25% reduction in ^{3}H-thymidine incorporation and a 50% decrease in differentiation as assessed by sn-glycerol-3-phosphate dehydrogenase activity. Thus, IGF-I can be considered an autocrine/
paracrine adipogenic factor in vitro.

Recent evidence suggests that physiological concentrations of IGF
are functioning through specific IGF receptors rather than cross-reacting with the insulin receptor to induce differentiation. Two types of IGF
receptors have been detected on adipocytes or stromal-vascular cells
from adipose tissue or preadipocyte cell lines (29, 30, 31, 32, 33). The
type I receptor demonstrates highest affinity for IGF-I, and the type II

receptor demonstrates highest affinity to IGF-II and is structurally dis-similar to the type I receptor or the insulin receptor (for review see 34). Physiological concentrations of IGF-I that bind to the IGF type I recep-tor result in proliferation and differentiation of preadipocytes (26). Also, IGF-I can induce glucose transport and changes in GLUT4 levels in 3T3 adipocytes by binding to the type I receptor (19). This response cannot be duplicated with human adipocytes; pharmacological concen-trations of IGF-I are required to induce glucose transport (31). The re-sponse to specific binding at the type II receptor is currently unknown, but physiological concentrations of IGF-II can induce differentiation as previously mentioned (Fig. 1a). IGF-II is not cross-reacting with the insulin receptor to generate a response, since the affinity of the insulin receptor for IGF-II is several orders of magnitude lower than for the IGF type II receptor, but IGF-II binding to the IGF type I receptor cannot be excluded. Irrespective of the IGF-II mechanism of action, the IGFs affect preadipocyte proliferation and differentiation at physiological concentrations in vitro through binding to the IGF receptors and not to insulin receptors.

These in vitro experiments have permitted identification of the IGFs as potential autocrine/paracrine adipogenic factors. Second, these in vitro experiments have been important in characterizing components of the IGF system that may be of functional significance to adipose tissue in vivo. However, in vitro experiments are not a replacement for in vivo experiments to assess the overall biological significance of IGF physiology.

In Vivo Assessment of IGF Action

Only a very few experiments have examined IGF status in adipose tissue in vivo. Historically, the liver was believed to be the major site of synthesis, but this has changed as more and more tissues have been discovered to express these proteins. The evaluation of the potential role of IGFs in adipose tissue development must begin during fetal development when adipose tissue undergoes extensive development by proliferation and differentiation of preadipocytes, but limited hy-pertrophy (35). Few animal models develop adequate adipose tissue during prenatal development to permit extensive experimentation. The fetal pig contains limited adipose tissue stores, but the large size of the fetus permits a relatively easy dissection in comparison to the fetal rat or mouse.

The pig fetus accumulates most of its adipocyte population during the second half of gestation by the process of preadipocyte proliferation and differentiation. Levels of IGF-I mRNA within developing fetal adipose tissue also increase during this time (Fig. 4). Assessment of IGF mRNA levels during this period has shown that fetal adipose tissue has greater abundance of this mRNA than liver or skeletal muscle (Fig. 5). Both perirenal and subcutaneous adipose express higher levels of IGF-I mRNA than liver or muscle throughout the second half of gestation. Additional research is necessary to determine: 1) if these transcripts are translated into immunologically reactive protein; and 2) if

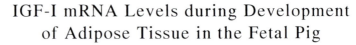

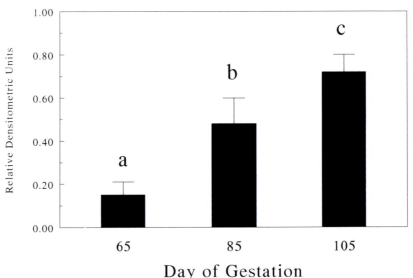

Figure 4. IGF-I mRNA levels during development of adipose tissue in the fetal pig. Subcutaneous adipose tissue was obtained by dissection following cesarean section at 65 or 85 or 105 days of a 114-day gestation. Total RNA was extracted and probed for IGF-I mRNA by Northern analysis. Data are expressed as relative densitometric units. Means not sharing a common superscript are significantly different ($P < .05$).

Relative IGF-I mRNA Levels in Tissues from the Late Gestation Fetal Pig

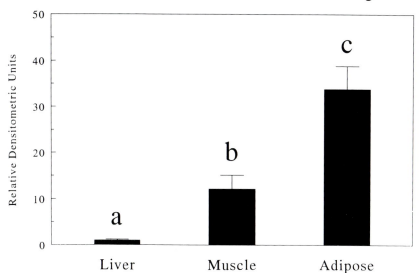

Figure 5.   Relative IGF-I mRNA levels in tissues from the late gestation fetal pig. Liver, subcutaneous adipose tissue, and semitendinosus were obtained by dissection following cesarean section at day 105 of gestation. Total RNA was extracted and probed for IGF-I mRNA by Northern analysis. Data are expressed as relative densitometric units. Means not sharing a common superscript are significantly different ($P < .01$).

the changes in IGF-I mRNA abundance regulate the development of adipose tissue or are a consequence of the development of adipose tissue. The in vitro data delineated above would suggest that protein production does occur in these cells and that IGFs can induce preadipocyte proliferation and differentiation, but in vivo analysis would strengthen the argument.

The IGF genes in fetal adipose tissue can respond to changes in the environment, which suggests that expression is regulated and not intrinsic. For example, diabetes has been used as a model to evaluate IGF physiology in the postnatal animal (for review, see 36). Induction of maternal diabetes during the third trimester (day 70 of a 114-day gestation) results in an alteration in IGF-I mRNA abundance when sampled during late gestation at day 105 (Fig. 6). Thus a chronic alteration

Relative IGF-I mRNA Levels in Adipose Tissue from Fetuses of Diabetic Pigs

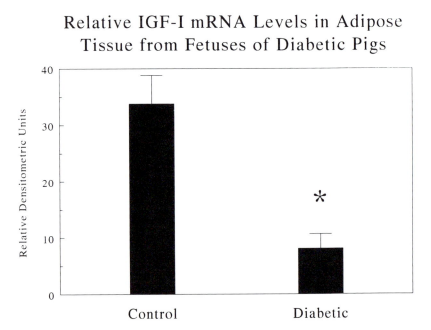

Figure 6. Relative IGF-I mRNA levels in adipose tissue from fetuses of diabetic pigs. Pregnant pigs were rendered diabetic on day 75 of a 114-day gestation with alloxan (50 mg/kg bwt). Subcutaneous adipose tissue was obtained from fetuses by dissection following cesarean section at day 105 of gestation. Total RNA was extracted and probed for IGF-I mRNA using a RNase protection assay. Data are expressed as relative densitometric units. * = different from control fetal tissue ($P < .01$).

in maternal metabolic/endocrine status can affect IGF-I gene expression within adipose tissue of the fetal animal. Maternal diabetes is a severe perturbation of the maternal and fetal physiology. An acute perturbation of the maternal metabolic/endocrine status can produce a similar response in IGF-I mRNA abundance in fetal adipose tissue. Fasting of a pregnant animal for 72 hours during late gestation also results in a reduction in IGF-I mRNA abundance within adipose tissue of the fetal pig (Fig. 7). These studies demonstrate that either chronic or acute alterations in maternal metabolic/endocrine status and the subsequent changes in the fetal environment affect adipose tissue gene expression. Unfortunately, neither experiment was directly designed to examine adipose tissue development, so additional measurements of tissue composition, metabolism, etcetera, were not performed. The abil-

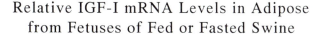

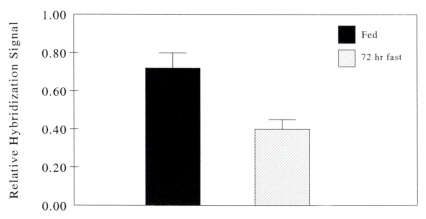

Figure 7. Relative IGF-I mRNA levels in adipose from fetuses of fed or fasted swine. Pregnant pigs were fasted for 72 hours prior to cesarean section on day 105 of a 114-day gestation. Fetal subcutaneous adipose tissue was obtained by dissection. Total RNA was extracted and probed for IGF-I mRNA by Northern analysis. Data are expressed as relative densitometric units. * = different from control fetal tissue ($P < .01$).

ity to alter the mRNA abundance suggests that IGF-I mRNAs are produced in response to some mechanism of regulation. Currently, the mechanisms that regulate prenatal IGF expression are not clearly understood, though growth hormone and nutrition can impact on serum levels of IGFs (for review, see 37).

Postnatally, growth hormone, insulin, and nutrition are the known regulators of IGF-I (1). Injection of growth hormone for four weeks in swine results in a significant elevation in IGF-I mRNA abundance (Fig. 8). The level of all transcripts is increased, but the 7.4 kilobase transcript comprises greater than 90% of all IGF-I mRNA. Peter *et al.* (22) and Vikman *et al.* (24) have demonstrated the same phenomenon in hypophysectomized rats using chronic treatment with GH. The hypophysectomized rat studies demonstrated that adipocytes and stromal cells both respond in vivo with increases in IGF-I mRNA abundance. Insulin-like growth factor-I protein concentrations in tissue extracts increased in response to GH injection in association with these chronic changes in IGF-I mRNA levels (22). However, chronic treatment with

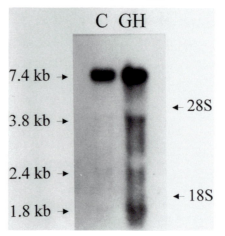

Figure 8. Northern analysis of IGF-I mRNA in porcine adipose tissue obtained from swine following injection of a buffer or growth hormone (60 ug/kg bwt) for 4 weeks. 40 µg of total RNA was separated by electrophoresis and transferred to nylon membrane. The membrane was hybridized with a ^{32}P-labeled pIGF-I cDNA fragment. Sizes of mRNA were estimated based on relative migration distance of 18 and 28S ribosomal bands.

growth hormone has a variety of effects in vivo that result in alterations in endocrinology, protein metabolism, and lipid metabolism. Thus, it could be argued that growth hormone may not be directly acting on the adipose tissue to produce these changes in IGF-I mRNA abundance.

Therefore, the response to a single injection of growth hormone was evaluated to preclude most adaptive responses. Vikman *et al.* (24) reported that epididymal adipose tissue in rats responded to GH by two hours post-injection. In swine, GH (200µg/kg) induced a maximal increase in IGF-I mRNA concentration in subcutaneous and perirenal adipose by eight hours following injection (Fig. 9). This was the same time frame as the response by hepatic tissue, and the level of response was similar to liver. The rapid change in IGF-I mRNA level in swine and rats suggests that this phenomenon in adipose tissue is directly responsive to growth hormone status.

Changes in the level of IGF-I protein require a longer period of time (unpublished observation); however, extraction of immunologically reactive IGF-I demonstrated that the concentrations in perirenal and subcutaneous adipose tissue exceed the concentration of liver (Fig. 10). Adipose tissue contains relatively small quantities of protein because

Relative IGF-I mRNA Levels in Tissues following a Single GH Injection

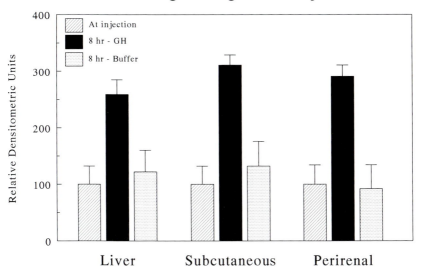

Figure 9.   Relative IGF-I mRNA levels in tissue following a single GH injection. Swine (45 kg) were given a single injection of either a buffer or growth hormone (200 μg/kg bwt). Animals were euthanized at various time points following injection. Tissues were then collected by dissection. Data are presented for the 0- and 8-hour time points, representing the basal and peak responses. Total RNA was extracted and probed for IGF-I mRNA using a RNase protection assay. Data are expressed as relative densitometric units.

the cell volume is primarily lipid. Thus, data expressed on a protein basis can be skewed by this method of interpretation. However, it does indicate that IGF-I may be an important cell product in the adipocyte. Peter *et al.* (22) recently reported that rat adipose tissue also expresses high levels of IGF-I protein, though a direct comparison of IGF-I concentration between liver and adipose tissue was not performed in that study. The liver has been considered to be the major site of IGF-I protein production in rodent species based on analysis of the effluent from perfused liver (38). However, the present data suggest that liver may not be the only major site of IGF-I production. Secretion of these high levels of IGF-I has not been demonstrated using perfusion techniques, but this protein may be secreted by the tissue, since primary cultures

Immunoreactive IGF-I Concentrations in Tissues of the Pig

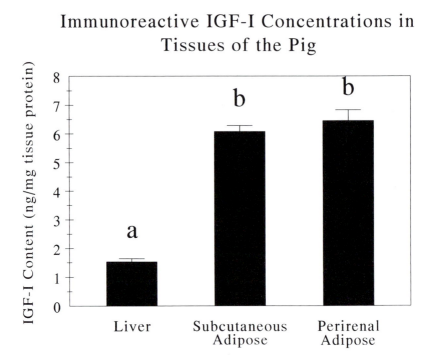

Figure 10. Immunoreactive IGF-I concentrations in tissues of the pig. Tissues from 45 kg swine were extracted for IGF-I protein using the procedures of D'Ercole and Underwood (67). Samples were corrected for blood contamination according to the procedures of D'Ercole and Underwood (67). IGF-I protein concentrations were determined by radioimmunoassay and are expressed as ng/mg tissue protein. Means not sharing a common superscript are significantly different ($P < .001$).

from porcine adipose tissue can be induced to secrete IGF-I in response to GH stimulation (21, 23). Interestingly, human adipose tissue contains a greater abundance of IGF-I mRNA than liver (39); thus this phenomenon may also exist in the human.

The most direct method to evaluate the response of adipose tissue to changes in IGF-I status is to inject the protein into the animal. Unfortunately, the expense has limited the number of these experiments and only a very few have examined the adipose tissue or lipid component of the animals. Infusion of IGF-I into rats during an acute euglycemic clamp resulted in a stimulation of lipogenesis within the epididymal adipose tissue at a concentration of approximately 50 nmol

(40). This concentration is outside the normal physiological range for the rat and may be affecting lipogenesis as a consequence of binding to the insulin receptor. Chronic infusion of IGF-I into broiler chickens was reported to induce a reduction in abdominal fat, but this effect also may have been the consequence of a change in thyroid hormone status (41). Similar changes in adiposity were observed in children with Laron-type dwarfism (low serum IGF-I) receiving daily injection of IGF-I for three to ten months; chronic IGF-I injection in children resulted in a rapid increase in linear growth with a reduction in subcutaneous adipose tissue (42).

Injection of growth hormone into growth hormone–deficient humans results in a reduction in subscapular skinfold thickness and mean adipose tissue volume of the thigh, as determined by computerized tomography analysis, and an elevation of serum GH by 112% and IGF-I levels by 130% (43). This effect may be specific to certain regions of adipose deposition in humans, since Rosenbaum et al. (44) reported an increase in serum IGF-I and a decrease in abdominal subcutaneous adipocyte volume (µg lipid/cell) as a result of chronic injection of growth hormone (100 µg/kg/day) into children of short stature, but no effect on gluteal adipocyte volume. These studies suggest that serum IGF-I elevation as a response to GH administration is associated with a reduction in adipose tissue accretion. Research with swine has shown a similar effect; chronic GH injection (60 µg/kg/day) results in a reduction in adipose tissue accretion and inhibition of lipid metabolism by subcutaneous adipose while increasing serum IGF-I and the abundance of IGF-I mRNA in adipose tissue (45).

Thus a paradigm exists:

1. IGF-I is a paracrine/autocrine adipogenic factor in vitro.
2. IGF-I is present in high concentrations within adipose tissue in vivo.
3. GH induces the secretion of endocrine IGF-I in vivo and paracrine/autocrine IGF-I in vitro.
4. Growth hormone treatment induces IGF-I, yet there is a reduction in adipose tissue accretion.

A portion of this paradigm can be explained by the known action of growth hormone to inhibit lipid metabolism by adipose tissue (45, 46, 47, 48). However, the inability of the putative paracrine IGF-I to demonstrate an adipogenic effect may be a consequence of another action of growth hormone: the induction of insulin-like growth factor binding proteins (IGFBPs).

Insulin-like Growth Factor Binding Proteins

The IGFBPs are currently a family of six proteins: IGFBP-1, -2, -3, -4, -5, and -6. The overall function of these proteins is the point of some controversy as they do not demonstrate a uniform response to stimuli, but appear to be independently regulated (for review, see 49). These proteins bind IGF-I and IGF-II with high affinity. In general, IGFBPs have been proposed to regulate the transfer of IGFs through the extracellular compartment and the interaction of the IGFs with their receptors. They can either stimulate or inhibit this interaction of IGFs with the receptors. For example, supplementation of a purified serum fraction enriched for IGF binding activity to incubation medium inhibits IGF-I induction of glucose oxidation and lipogenesis by adipose tissue fragments (50). This experiment was repeated utilizing a more purified serum fraction enriched for IGFBP-3 with the same inhibitory results (51). This IGFBP-3 is the major IGFBP in serum and forms a complex of 150 kilodaltons that binds approximately 90% of the IGF-I (52).

Growth hormone and IGF-I induce an increase in the serum level of IGFBP-3 (53). Thus, increases in IGFBPs as a result of GH injection may result in an inhibition of the potential adipogenic actions of endocrine IGF-I. Second, the activity of paracrine IGF-I induced by systemic GH may be blocked under some circumstances by paracrine IGFBPs. Gaskins *et al.* (21) were the first to report that GH induces IGFBP secretion by primary cultures derived from adipose tissue. The types of IGFBPs induced were not identified because of the nature of the binding assay used.

Western ligand blot analysis was utilized in a recent study to characterize the binding proteins secreted by primary cultures containing preadipocytes. Cultures derived from rabbit adipose tissue secrete three binding proteins with M_r = 40 000, 30 000, and 24 000 (26). The cells appear to secrete higher levels of IGFBPs prior to confluency than after confluency and subsequent differentiation. In addition, dexamethasone was able to inhibit the secretion of the predominant M_r = 30 000 form of binding protein (BP-2 or 4?) while promoting IGF-I secretion. Dexamethasone has commonly been included in differentiation medium for preadipocyte cell lines and primary cultures. Thus, one of the mechanisms by which glucocorticoids may function to promote differentiation is to increase the availability of IGF-I in the paracrine environment by promoting IGF-I secretion and inhibiting IGFBP release. This paracrine IGF-I can then perform its adipogenic function by inducing post-confluent mitosis and differentiation.

In vivo analysis of IGFBPs in adipose tissue was recently reported (22). Rat adipose tissue was reported to contain BP-2, -3, -4, -5, and -6, according to Western ligand blot analysis. These binding proteins were differentially expressed as suggested by comparing extracts of adipose tissue from control and hypophysectomized rats. Chronic infusion of GH into hypophysectomized rats using osmotic pumps resulted in an increase in mRNA abundance for BP-2, -3, -5, and -6 according to Northern analysis (Table 1). Interestingly, this phenomenon could not be replicated in vitro by supplementing GH to cells isolated from the adipose tissue of hypophysectomized rats. This suggests an even more complex regulation of paracrine IGF physiology, but this experiment must be replicated prior to comment.

Collagenase digestion of the adipose tissue from these hypophysectomized and pituitary-intact rats permitted assessment of the contribution of adipocytes versus the stromal-vascular cells to the total abundance of mRNA for IGFBPs (22). This experiment demonstrated a differential expression of mRNA for the IGFBPs between the cell types (Fig. 11). Adipocytes expressed only a limited abundance of IGFBP-5 (approximately 30% of the level in stromal-vascular cells) and no other binding proteins in this experiment. Stromal-vascular cells contained mRNA for IGFBP-2, -3, -5. No mention was made of the absence of

Table 1. IGF-I and IGFBP mRNA Levels in Rat Adipose Tissue In Vivo[1]

	Normal	Hypox	Hypox + GH
IGF-I	100	4.6 ± 2.5	80 ± 25
IGFBP-3	100	127 ± 9	483 ± 32
IGFBP-4	100	104 ± 23	115 ± 22
IGFBP-5	100	53 ± 16	128 ± 22
IGFBP-6	100	16 ± 5	41 ± 10

[1]Values are derived from analysis of epididymal adipose tissue from 3–5 rats by densitometry. Values in adipose tissue from pituitary intact (normal) animals were defined as 100%. Data are expressed as percent of the normal value.
Derived from ref. 22 and used by permission of the Endocrine Society.

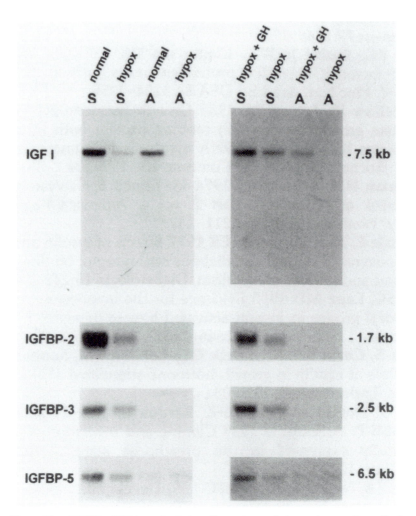

Figure 11. IGFBP mRNA analysis in adipocytes and stromal-vascular cells derived from adipose tissue of hypophysectomized and pituitary-intact rats following collagenase digestion. Epididymal adipose tissue was digested with collagenase and the adipocytes were separated from the stromal-vascular cells by centrifugation. Total RNA of adipocytes (A) and stromal vascular cells (S) from normal, hypox, and GH-treated hypox rats (two sc GH injections) was hybridized with cDNA probes specific for IGF-I, IGFBP-2, -3, and -5.

Derived from ref. 22 and reproduced by permission of the Endocrine Society.

BP-4 and -6 from the isolated cells versus the intact tissue, but this suggests some problems with the analysis. Incubation with collagenase may have had an adverse effect on mRNA stability in the adipocytes, though this has not been demonstrated. Irrespective of this anomaly, the data do indicate that some differences exist between regulation of IGFBPs in adipocytes and the surrounding stromal elements of adipose tissue. Pretreatment of hypophysectomized animals with GH prior to cell isolation resulted in changes in transcript abundance only within the stromal-vascular cells and not in the adipocytes; IGFBP-5 mRNA levels were unaffected by GH in adipocytes but were increased in stromal-vascular cells. Peter *et al.* (22) proposed that these paracrine IGFBPs in adipose tissue may function to inhibit any lipogenic activity of paracrine IGFs, since IGF-I is present in very high concentrations in rat adipose tissue. Otherwise, insulin regulation of glucose oxidation and lipogenesis would be superseded by paracrine IGFs in vivo, and thus insulin would not be integral to systemic glucose regulation. This would be an even greater consideration in the human, where IGF mRNA abundance is greater in adipose tissue than in liver, but the converse is true in the rat (39).

The synthesis and secretion of high concentrations of IGF-I within the paracrine environment of adipose tissue and the additional paracrine production and release of IGFBPs is illogical if the IGFBPs are inhibitory. The most logical hypothesis would be that the stromal cells synthesize an inhibitory group of binding proteins and the adipocytes synthesize facilitatory binding proteins (or the converse) to produce a very strict modulation of this very high IGF activity within adipose tissue. The data of Peter *et al.* (22) suggest stromal cell specific production of IGFBP-2 and BP-3. However, there are limited data to support a specific mode of action for any IGFBP; some evidence suggests that under specific conditions some IGFBPs facilitate the binding of IGFs to their receptors, but it is exceeded by the evidence supporting an inhibitory function (for review, see 49).

More likely, binding proteins are produced by all cells within adipose tissue, but the relative amounts of binding proteins vary between the cell types. The data of Peter *et al.* (22) indicate that adipocytes contain limited amounts of IGFBP mRNA, suggestive of limited amounts of protein in comparison to the stromal-vascular cells. However, accurate assessment must await the development of radioimmunoassays for the various binding proteins, since Western ligand blotting is not truly a quantifiable procedure.

The data collected from the various in vivo and in vitro studies suggest that consideration of the activity of the IGFs requires consideration of the IGFBPs. Thus, it may be more accurate to conceptualize the relationship and its consequences as the result of the ratio of IGF to IGFBP, similar to evaluating insulin/glucagon during assessment of gluconeogenesis or the analysis of T_3/thyroid binding globulin for determination of thyroid status. A ratio greater than one would permit an adipogenic response, and a ratio of less than one would result in an inhibition of adipogenic activity. It may be hypothesized that expression of IGFBP by the stromal-vascular cells functions to modulate the adipogenic stimulus of IGF-I (and possibly IGF-II). Thus the stimulus for adipocyte formation or recruitment is continually present, and the production and release of IGFBPs serves to modulate this stimulus.

IGFs and Obesity

In men, IGF-I concentrations in sera from moderately obese individuals are depressed in comparison to the concentrations in sera from nonobese individuals (54, 55, 56). This may be a consequence of the depressed GH levels often observed in these individuals (57). However, IGF-I levels are not reduced in obese, adult women (55, 58, 59), despite GH levels that are depressed by approximately 66% (59). This sex difference suggests that IGF-I regulation in obese women may differ from that in men. The potential contribution of this difference in IGF-I status to the regional differences in adiposity between the sexes has not been explored.

Correlation analysis of IGF-I to the obese state has been somewhat confusing. The concentration of serum IGF-I was negatively correlated to triceps skinfold thickness in men (54). However, serum IGF-I concentration has not been correlated to the degree of adiposity, whether male or female (56, 59); although Marin *et al.* (56) reported that depressed serum IGF-I was inversely related to visceral adipose mass but not to subcutaneous or total fat mass in men. These studies evaluated as a group do not suggest that serum IGF-I is directly associated with the obese state or to the severity of the obesity.

None of these studies evaluated the IGFBP status of the obese and nonobese subjects. The reported depression in serum GH levels in the obese would probably cause a reduction in IGFBP-3 levels, since it has been demonstrated to be GH dependent (49). Also, Conover *et al.* (58) have reported that serum IGFBP-1 is severely depressed in obese women but the IGF-I concentration remains normal (Fig. 12). Thus, the relative IGF/IGFBP ratio may be altered in the obese such that the amount of free IGF relative to the amount of IGFBP is increased, despite the depression in total concentration of IGF in the obese state. Further analysis of the IGFBP status in the obese versus nonobese may indicate

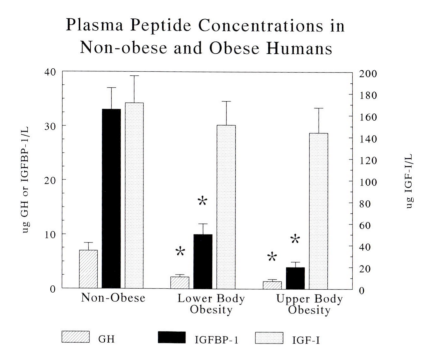

Figure 12.   Plasma GH, IGFBP-1, and IGF-I concentrations in non-obese humans and humans with lower body obesity or upper body obesity. Regional obesity was defined by waist:hip ratio; upper body obese individuals had ratios greater than 0.85, whereas lower body obese individuals had ratios less than 0.76. Controls had a body mass index of 22 ± 0.4 kg/m², and the obese had a body mass index of 30–36 kg/m². IGF-I and GH values are the means of blood samples collected during the last 30 minutes of a 90-minute saline infusion, and the IGFBP-1 values were measured on samples collected at the end point of the infusion period. All peptides were measured using specific radioimmunoassays. * = different from non-obese ($P < .05$).

Derived from ref. 58 and reproduced by permission of the Endocrine Society.

a defective IGFBP regulation in the obese, thus removing the inhibition on IGF-I to function as an adipogenic factor in the adipose tissue.

Another potential reason for a lack of correlation of IGF-I serum levels with adiposity is that all of these studies were performed on adults with existing obesity rather than during the development of obesity. The IGFs and IGFBPs may have a functional role during the recruitment of new adipocytes for hyperplastic development of the adipose tissue. Assessment of serum IGF-I in children with obesity has demonstrated elevated IGF-I serum levels (60, 61, 62), the opposite of the observations in adults. Childhood obesity is often a consequence of hyperplasia and hypertrophic development of adipocytes, whereas adult onset obesity is often hypertrophic, except in extreme obesity in which some hyperplasia does occur (for review, see 63). Insulin-like growth factor-I is a potent stimulator of mitogenesis and differentiation as reviewed above; thus it would be a likely candidate for stimulation of hyperplastic development of adipose tissue in children during the development of obesity. The source of this IGF-I may be both endocrine and paracrine in nature, since IGF-I mRNA abundance is greater in adipose tissue than in liver or skeletal muscle of the human (39). The status of the binding proteins is unknown in obese children, but the data of Conover *et al.* (58) that demonstrate reduced IGFBP-1 concentrations in obese adults suggests that binding protein analysis should be performed in these children. The consequences of an absolute increase in IGF-I concentration and a potential decrease in IGFBP concentration would be a potent adipogenic stimulus, since the relative IGF/IGFBP would be very large.

Conclusions

All of the studies that have evaluated IGF or IGFBP status in the obese versus nonobese have examined blood samples rather than samples directly from the adipose tissue. The data presented in this review indicate that the paracrine IGFs are effective adipogenic factors. The IGFBPs are also produced in the paracrine environment and may mediate this potent adipogenic signal to limit the recruitment of new adipocytes from the stromal-vascular environment. Growth hormone administration results in a large increase in IGF-I in the paracrine environment, which is counteracted by an increase in IGFBPs. In contrast, the tight paracrine regulation of IGF action by IGFBPs within adipose tissue may become disturbed during the development of obesity. Thus, a higher effective concentration of IGF may be present within adipose tissue to stimulate proliferation and differentiation of preadipocytes in hyperplastic obesity. This concept may also be worth examining in the excessively obese when hyperplastic obesity develops subsequent to hypertrophic obesity. Hyperplastic obesity has been proposed to be the consequence of a recruitment of new adipocytes from the preadipocyte pool caused by a release of a putative adipogenic factor from the very large adipocytes (64, 65, 66). The IGFs may be these adipogenic signals, but again their efficacy may be dependent upon the IGFBP response. Reexamination of a potential role for IGFs may be necessary, since only systemic IGF has been examined, whereas paracrine IGFs and IGFBPs have not been critically evaluated during the development of obesity.

REFERENCES

1. Daughaday WH, Rotwein P. Insulin-like growth factors I and II: peptide messenger ribonucleic acid and gene structures, serum, and tissue concentrations. *Endocr Rev.* 1989;10:68–91.

2. Froesch ER, Burgi H, Ramseier EB, Bally P, Labhart A. Antibody suppressible and non-suppressible insulin-like activities in human serum and their physiological significance. *J Clin Invest.* 1963;42: 1816–1834.

3. Morikawa M, Nixon T, Green H. Growth hormone and the adipose conversion of 3T3 cells. *Cell.* 1982;29:783–789.

4. Morikawa M, Green H, Lewis UJ. Activity of human growth hormone and related polypeptides on the adipose conversion of 3T3 cells. *Mol Cell Biol.* 1984;4:228–231.

5. Nixon T, Green H. Contribution of growth hormone to the adipogenic activity of serum. *Endocrinology.* 1984;114:527–532.

6. Zezulak KM, Green H. The generation of insulin-like growth factor-1 sensitive cells by growth hormone action. *Science.* 1986;233:551–553.

7. Wiederer O, Loffler G. Hormonal regulation of the differentiation of rat adipocyte precursor cells in primary culture. *J Lipid Res.* 1987; 28:649–658.

8. Ramsay TG, Wolverton CK, Hausman GJ, Kraeling RR, Martin RJ. Alterations in adipogenic and mitogenic activity of porcine serum

in response to hypophysectomy. *Endocrinology.* 1989;124:2268–2276.

9. Hausman GJ, Wright JT. Genetic, endocrine and paracrine/autocrine aspects of porcine adipocyte differentiation. *Proc Recip Meats Conf.* 1990;43:73.

10. Deslex S, Negrel R, Ailhaud G. Development of a chemically defined serum-free medium for differentiation of rat adipose precursor cells. *Exp Cell Res.* 1987;168:15–30.

11. Ramsay TG, White ME, Wolverton CK. Insulin-like growth factor 1 induction of differentiation of porcine preadipocytes. *J Anim Sci.* 1989;67:2452–2459.

12. Hausman GJ. The influence of insulin, triiodothyronine (T₃) and insulin-like growth factor-I (IGF-I) on the differentiation of preadipocytes in serum-free cultures of pig stromal-vascular cells. *J Anim Sci.* 1989;67:3136–3143.

13. Butterwith SC, Goddard C. Regulation of DNA synthesis in chicken adipocyte precursor cells by insulin-like growth factors, platelet-derived growth factor and transforming growth factor-beta. *J Endocrinol.* 1991;131:203–209.

14. Grimaldi P, Djian P, Forest C, Poli P, Negrel R, Ailhaud G. Lipogenic and mitogenic effects of insulin during conversion of ob17 cells to adipose-like cells. *Mol Cell Endocrinol.* 1983;29:271–285.

15. Blake WL, Clarke SD. Induction of adipose fatty acid binding protein by insulin-like growth factor-I in 3T3-L1 preadipocytes. *Biochem Biophys Res Commun.* 1990;173:87–91.

16. Schmidt W, Jordan GP, Loffler G. Adipose conversion of 3T3-L1 cells in a serum free culture system depends on epidermal growth factor, insulin-like growth factor I, corticosterone, and cyclic AMP. *J Biol Chem.* 1990;265:15489–15495.

17. Smith PJ, Wise LS, Berkowitz R, Wan C, Rubin CS. Insulin-like growth factor-I is an essential regulator of the differentiation of 3T3-L1 adipocytes. *J Biol Chem.* 1988;263:9402–9408.

18. Ashcom G, Gurland G, Schwartz J. Growth hormone synergizes with serum growth factors in inducing c-fos transcription in 3T3-442A cells. *Endocrinology.* 1992;131:1915–1921.

19. Weiland M, Bahr F, Hohne M, Schurmann A, Ziehm D, Joost HG. The signaling potential of the receptors for insulin and insulin-like growth factor I (IGF-I) in 3T3-L1 adipocytes: comparison of glucose

transport activity, induction of oncogene c-fos, glucose transporter mRNA, and DNA synthesis. *J Cell Physiol.* 1991;149:428–435.

20. Doglio A, Dani C, Fredrikson G, Grimaldi P, Ailhaud G. Acute regulation of insulin-like growth factor-I gene expression by growth hormone during adipose cell differentiation. *EMBO J.* 1987;13: 4011–4016.

21. Gaskins HR, Kim J-W, Wright JT, Rund LA, Hausman GJ. Regulation of insulin-like growth factor-I ribonucleic acid expression, polypeptide secretion, and binding protein activity by growth hormone in porcine preadipocytes cultures. *Endocrinology.* 1990;126: 622–630.

22. Peter MA, Winterhalter KH, Boni-Schnetzler M, Froesch ER, Zapf J. Regulation of insulin-like growth factor-I (IGF-I) and IGF-binding proteins by growth hormone in rat white adipose tissue. *Endocrinology.* 1993;133:2624–2631.

23. Ramsay TG, Rao SV, Wolverton CK. In vitro systems for the analysis of the development of adipose tissue in domestic animals. *J Nutr.* 1992;122:806–817.

24. Vikman K, Isgaard J, Eden S. Growth hormone regulation of insulin-like growth factor-I mRNA in rat adipose tissue and isolated rat adipocytes. *J Endocrinol.* 1991;131:139–145.

25. Chatelain P, Naville D, Avallet O, *et al.* Paracrine and autocrine regulation of insulin-like growth factor I. *Acta Paediatr Scand.* 1991; 372(suppl):92–95.

26. Nougues J, Reyne Y, Barenton B, Chery T, Garandel V, Soriano J. Differentiation of adipocyte precursors in a serum-free medium is influenced by glucocorticoids and endogenously produced insulin-like growth factor-1. *Int J Obes.* 1993;17:159–167.

27. Fagin JA, Roberts CT Jr, Leroith D, Brown AT. Coordinate decrease of tissue insulinlike growth factor I posttranscriptional alternative mRNA transcripts in diabetes mellitus. *Diabetes.* 1989;38:428–433.

28. Leaman DW, White ME, Ramsay TG, Simmen FA. Expression of insulin-like growth factor-I and II mRNA in muscle, heart and liver tissues of streptozotocin-diabetic swine. *Endocrinology.* 1990;126: 2850–2857.

29. Burguera B, Frank BH, DiMarchi R, Long S, Caro JF. The interaction of proinsulin with the insulin-like growth factor-I receptor in human liver, muscle, and adipose tissue. *J Clin Endocrinol Metab.* 1991; 72:1238–1241.

30. Eriksson J, Gause-Nilsson I, Lonnroth P, Smith U. The insulin-like effect of growth hormone on insulin-like growth factor II receptors is opposed by cyclic AMP: evidence for a common post-receptor pathway for growth hormone and insulin action. *Biochem J.* 1990; 268:353–357.

31. Sinha MK, Buchanan C, Leggett N, *et al.* Mechanism of IGF-I stimulated glucose transport in human adipocytes. Demonstration of specific IGF-I receptors not involved in stimulation of glucose transport. *Diabetes.* 1989;38:1217–1225.

32. Sinha MK, Buchanan C, Raineri-Maldonado C, *et al.* IGF-II receptors and IGF-II stimulated glucose transport in human fat cells. *Am J Physiol.* 1990;258:E534–E542.

33. Tanti JF, Gremeaux T, Cormont M, Van Obberghen E. Okadaic acid stimulates IGF-II receptor translocation and inhibits insulin action in adipocytes. *Am J Physiol.* 1993;264:E868–E873.

34. Nissley P, Lopaczynski W. Insulin-like growth factor receptors. *Growth Factors.* 1991;5:29–43.

35. Hausman GJ. The comparative anatomy of adipose tissue. In: Cryer A, Van RLR, eds. *New Perspectives in Adipose Tissue: Structure, Function and Development.* London: Butterworths; 1985:1–21.

36. Bach LA, Rechler MM. Insulin-like growth factors and diabetes. *Diabetes Metab Rev.* 1992;8:229–257.

37. D'Ercole AJ. The insulin-like growth factors and fetal growth. In: Spencer EM, ed. *Modern Concepts of Insulin-like Growth Factors.* New York: Elsevier; 1991:9–23.

38. Schwander J, Hauri C, Zapf J, Froesch ER. Synthesis and secretion of insulin-like growth factor and its binding protein by the perfused rat liver: dependence on growth hormone status. *Endocrinology.* 1983;113:297–305.

39. Möller C, Arner P, Sonnenfeld T, Norstedt G. Quantitative comparison of insulin-like growth factor mRNA levels in human and rat tissues analysed by a solution hybridization assay. *J Endocrinol.* 1991;7:213–222.

40. Schmitz F, Hartmann H, Stumpel F, Creutzfeldt W. In vivo metabolic action of insulin-like growth factor I in adult rats. *Diabetologia.* 1991;34:144–149.

41. Huybrechts LM, Decuypere E, Buyse J, Kuhn ER, Tixier-Boichard M. Effect of recombinant human insulin-like growth factor-I on

weight gain, fat content, and hormonal parameters in broiler chickens. *Poult Sci.* 1992;71:181–187.

42. Laron Z, Anin S, Kliper-Aurbach Y, Klinger B. Effects of insulin-like growth factor on linear growth, head circumference and body fat in patients with Laron-type dwarfism. *Lancet.* 1992;339:1258–1261.

43. Jorgensen JO, Pedersen SA, Thuesen L, *et al.* Beneficial effects of growth hormone treatment in GH-deficient adults. *Lancet.* 1989;1:1221–1225.

44. Rosenbaum M, Gertner JM, Gidfar N, Hirsch J, Leibel RL. Effects of systemic growth hormone (GH) administration on regional adipose tissue in children with non-GH-deficient short stature. *J Clin Endocrinol Metab.* 1992;75:151–156.

45. Wolverton CK, Azain MJ, Duffy JY, White ME, Ramsay TG. The influence of somatotropin on lipid metabolism and IGF gene expression in porcine adipose tissue. *Am J Physiol.* 1992;263:E637–E645.

46. Glenn KC, Shieh JJ, Laird DM. Characterization of 3T3-L1 storage lipid metabolism: effect of somatotropin and insulin on specific pathways. *Endocrinology.* 1992;131:1115–1124.

47. Goodman HM. Biological activity of bacterial derived human growth hormone in adipose tissue of hypophysectomized rats. *Endocrinology.* 1984;114:131–137.

48. Magri KA, Adamo M, Leroith D, Etherton TD. The inhibition of insulin action and glucose metabolism by porcine growth hormone in porcine adipocytes is not the result of any decrease in insulin binding or insulin receptor kinase activity. *Biochem J.* 1990;266:107–113.

49. Baxter RC. Physiological roles of IGF binding proteins. In: Spencer EM, ed. *Modern Concepts of Insulin-like Growth Factors.* New York: Elsevier;1991:371–380.

50. Zapf J, Schoenle E, Jagars G, Sand I, Grunwald J, Froesch ER. Inhibition of the action of nonsuppressible insulin-like activity on isolated rat fat cells by binding to its carrier protein. *J Clin Invest.* 1979;63:1077–1084.

51. Walton PE, Gopinath R, Etherton TD. Porcine insulin-like growth factor (IGF) binding protein blocks IGF-I action on porcine adipose tissue. *Proc Soc Exp Biol Med.* 1989;190:315–319.

52. Baxter RC. Insulin-like growth factor (IGF) binding proteins: the

role of serum IGFBPs in regulating IGF availability. *Acta Paediatr Scand.* 1991;372(suppl):107–14.

53. Clemmons DR, Thissen JP, Maes M, Ketelslegers JM, Underwood LE. Insulin-like growth factor-I (IGF-I) infusion into hypophysectomized or protein-deprived rats induces specific IGF binding proteins in serum. *Endocrinology.* 1989;125:2967–2972.

54. Colletti RB, Copeland KC, Devlin JT, Roberts JD, McAuliffe TL. Effect of obesity on plasma insulin-like growth factor-I in cancer patients. *Int J Obes.* 1991;15:523–527.

55. Copeland KC, Colletti RB, Devlin JT, McAuliffe TL. The relationship between insulin-like growth factor-I, adiposity, and aging. *Metabolism.* 1990;39:584–587.

56. Marin P, Kvist H, Lindstedt G, Sjöstrom L, Björntorp P. Low concentrations of insulin-like growth factor-I in abdominal obesity. *Int J Obes.* 1993;17:83–89.

57. Veldhuis JD, Iranmanesh A, Ho KKY, Waters MJ, Johnson ML, Lizarralde G. Dual defects in pulsatile growth hormone secretion and clearance subserve the hyposomatotropism of obesity in man. *J Clin Endocrinol Metab.* 1991;72:51–59.

58. Conover CA, Lee PDK, Kanaley JA, Clarkson JT, Jensen MD. Insulin regulation of insulin-like growth factor binding protein-1 in obese and nonobese humans. *J Clin Endocrinol Metab.* 1992;74:1355–1360.

59. Cordido F, Casanueva FF, Vidal JI, Dieguez C. Study of insulin-like growth factor I in human obesity. *Horm Res.* 1991;36:187–191.

60. Van Vliet G, Bosson D, Rummens E, Robyn C, Water R. Evidence against growth hormone releasing factor deficiency in children with idiopathic obesity. *Acta Endocrinol Suppl.* 1986;279:403–408.

61. Loche S, Cappa M, Borrelli P, *et al.* Reduced GH response to GHRH in children with simple obesity: evidence for somatomedin-C mediated inhibition. *Clin Endocrinol Oxf.* 1987;27:145–153.

62. Rosskamp R, Becker M, Soetadji S. Circulating somatomedin C levels and the effect of growth hormone-releasing factor on plasma level growth hormone and somatostatin-like immunoreactivity in obese children. *Eur J Pediatr.* 1987;146:48–52.

63. Björntorp P, Sjöstrom L. Adipose tissue dysfunction and its consequences. In: Cryer A, Van RLR, eds. *New Perspectives in Adipose Tissue: Structure, Function and Development.* London: Butterworths; 1985:447–458.

64. Allen CE. Cellularity of adipose tissue in meat animals. *Fed Proc.* 1976;35:2302–2307.

65. Björntorp P, Karlsson M, Pettersson P. Expansion of adipose tissue storage capacity at different ages in rats. *Metabolism.* 1982;31:366–373.

66. Faust IM, Johnson PR, Stern JS, Hirsch J. Diet induced adipocyte number increase in adult rats: a new model of obesity. *Am J Physiol.* 1978;235:E279–E286.

A. DONNY STROSBERG

Structure, Function, and Regulation of the β3-Adrenergic Receptors

ABSTRACT

Adipocytes express three subtypes of β-adrenergic catecholamine receptors: β_1, β_2, and β_3. Their relative proportion varies widely from species to species. Quantitative analysis of mRNA content by polymerase chain reaction suggests that in mice and rats, the β_3 subtype is much more abundant than the β_1, and that the β_2 is almost undetectable. In man, both semiquantitative polymerase chain reaction and lipolytic activity measurement using a β_3 selective agonist suggest that the β_3 adrenergic receptor albeit functional is less abundant than β_1 and β_2 expressed at almost equivalent levels. Using model systems such as the adipocyte-like 3T3-F442A, or β_3-transfected Chinese hamster ovary, Chinese hamster fibroblast, or L-cells, we performed an in-depth analysis of the ligand-binding and adenylyl cyclase activating properties of the available β_3 adrenergic agonists. The regulation of the expression of the murine and human β_3 receptors was studied in the presence of a variety of compounds including β_3 agonists, dexamethasone, butyrate, and insulin. Using β_2/β_3 chimeras we started to define regions responsible for differential regulation of subtype expression.

Introduction

It has long been known that lipolysis and thermogenesis in fat tissues can not be blocked by potent β-adrenergic antagonists such as propranolol or alprenolol, though these physiologic effects are induced by compounds that appear as weak agonists in β_1- and β_2-adrenergic model systems (1, 2, 3). These observations led us (4) to clone the human gene coding for a third β-adrenergic receptor subtype, which was designated as β_3AR and which we showed to be responsible for the atypical β-adrenergic effects observed earlier. The subsequent cloning of the murine (5) and rat β_3AR (6, 7) confirmed these similarities between the atypical and the newly cloned receptors (8).

The β_3AR is essentially expressed in fat tissues and in part of the gut, including the gall bladder and colon (9), and is obviously involved in the metabolic effects of noradrenaline. Its expression is narrowly regulated and varies with time, location, and concentration of cyclic adenosine monophosphate (cAMP), glucocorticoids, butyrate, or insulin. In contrast to the β_1 and β_2 subtypes, the β_3 is resistant to short-term desensitization induced by agonists but does, as do the other subtypes, become down-regulated when studied over several hours to several days. Metabolic effects of β_3 agonists in animals clearly suggest that these types of compounds, which are often antagonists toward the β_1-adrenergic receptor (β_1AR) and β_2-adrenergic receptor (β_2AR), may play an important role in future approaches to treat diabetes and obesity.

Structure

The β_3ARs have now been cloned from a variety of species and all display the major characteristics of receptors coupled to guanosine-triphosphate–binding proteins from the R_7G family (10). They possess an extracellular glycosylated N-terminus, an intracellular C-terminus, and seven hydrophobic transmembrane domains, separated from each other by three extra- and intracellular loops, as represented in Figure 1. The β_3AR from mouse, rat, and man are highly homologous (85% to 98%) and share with β_1 and β_2 subtypes up to 51% of the amino acid residues mainly located in the seven transmembrane regions and in the portion of the intracellular loops that are most proximal to the membrane (Fig. 1). These localized homologies may be explained by the fact that the three β-adrenergic receptors (βAR) bind the same natural ligands noradrenaline and adrenaline, couple to the same trimeric G_s protein, and activate the same effector: adenylyl cyclase (10).

Characterization of the β_2AR ligand binding site by affinity labeling and site-directed mutagenesis has helped define the amino acid residues likely to be involved in the interaction with agonists and antagonists. Most of these residues, represented in Figure 2, are conserved in the three βAR subtypes, but some differences may explain why a variety of β_1 and β_2 antagonists are β_3 agonists (10, 11). Site-directed

Human ß3AR

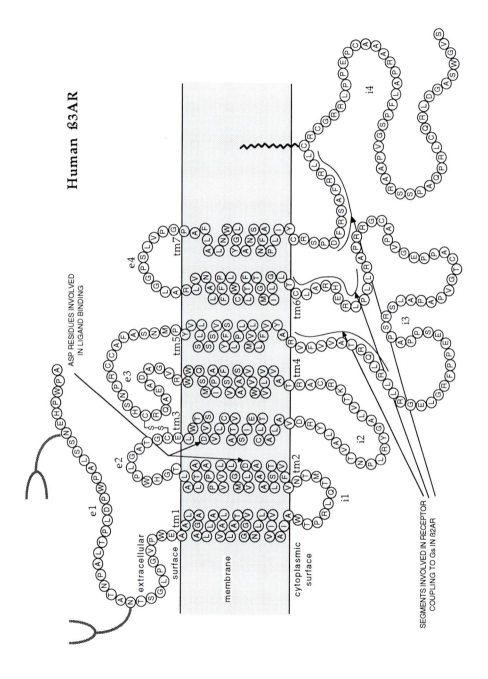

ASP RESIDUES INVOLVED IN LIGAND BINDING

SEGMENTS INVOLVED IN RECEPTOR COUPLING TO Gs IN ß2AR

extracellular surface

membrane

cytoplasmic surface

e1

e2

e3

e4

tm1

tm2

tm3

tm4

tm5

tm6

tm7

i1

i2

i3

i4

mutagenesis of the β_3AR has so far confirmed predictions made on the basis of the β_2AR studies (Manning, unpublished data).

Pharmacology

Numerous β-adrenergic agonists and antagonists have been used to characterize the pharmacologic properties of the β_1 and β_2 subtypes, and a large variety of drugs are currently used to treat cardiovascular disease by antagonizing the β_1 subtype, the main receptor expressed in the heart, or to work as agonists toward the β_2 receptor, the main receptor expressed in the lung, for instance to treat asthma. To analyze the ligand binding and adenylyl cyclase activating properties of the three subtypes in the same conditions, each receptor was expressed separately in Chinese hamster ovary cells (CHO) normally devoid of β-adrenergic receptors (12).

Five characteristics distinguish β_3 from β_1 and β_2 (11): 1) atypically low affinity for conventional β antagonists, including reference radioligands; 2) atypically low stereoselectivity index for agonist and antagonist enantiomers; 3) atypically low potencies of reference agonists; 4) high potency of a novel class of compounds, the phenylethanolamines, initially described as potent activators of lipolysis and thermogenesis in white and brown adipose tissues of rodents; and 5) partial agonistic activities of several β_1/β_2-antagonists (oxprenolol, pindolol, alprenolol), reflecting intrinsic sympathomimetic activities in tissues. In particular, CGP-12177 and ICI-201651 increase cyclic adenosine monophosphate (cAMP) accumulation in CHO-β_3 and decrease cAMP in CHO-β_1 and CHO-β_2. The first of these compounds stimulates lipolysis in human omental fat (13).

When comparing human to rodent β_3AR, a few differences were observed: propranolol, a leading β_1/β_2 blocker, is a weak agonist toward the human β_3 but an antagonist toward the murine β_3AR (5).

Figure 1. Primary structure of the human β_3AR. The sequences are represented in the one-letter code for amino acids. The single polypeptide chain is arranged according to the model for rhodopsin. The disulfide bond essential for activity linking Cys[111] and Cys[190] is represented by -S-S-. The two N-glycosylation sites in the amino-terminal portion of the protein are indicated by Y. The palmitoylated Cys[360] residue in the N-terminus of the i_4 loop is indicated by a ⧘.

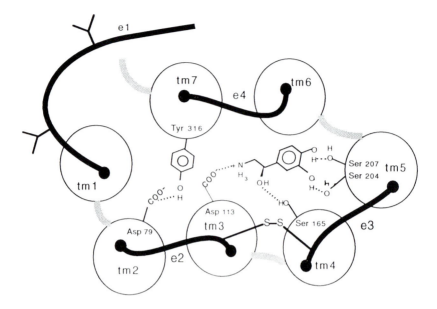

Figure 2. Schematic view of the chemical interactions of noradrenaline with various residues of the β2-adrenergic receptor binding site. A composite image of the β_2AR ligand-binding region. Proposed interactions in the ligand-binding area of the βAR viewed from the outside of the cell. All seven tm domains are essential for ligand binding. The ligand noradrenaline is shown surrounded by several of the amino acid chains that are speculated to be involved in agonist binding. These are Asp[113] in tm3, Ser[165] in tm5, Ser[204], and Ser[207] in tm5. The movement of Tyr[316] after agonist binding toward Asp[79] may be important for signal transmission to Gs. Whether all the interactions with the ligand occur simultaneously or sequentially is not known (10).

Several other β_3 agonists are more potent at the rodent than at the human receptor, possibly because they were developed using rodent in vivo models (8). Occasionally, however, opposite effects have been noted.

Regulation

SHORT-TERM HOMOLOGOUS DESENSITIZATION

β_1-adrenergic receptor and β_2AR are regulated through several mechanisms that have been well described. Short-term (minutes) regulation usually referred to as desensitization may be homologous, through treatment with agonists, or heterologous, through treatment with a variety of other compounds. Several steps in homologous desensitization have been identified. The first of these, following binding of agonist to β_1AR or β_2AR, leads to phosphorylation of the receptor by protein kinase A, acting on well-identified R-R-S-S (β_2AR) or R-R-P-S (β_1AR) sequences. The absence of these sequences from the β_3AR explains the resistance of this subtype to short-term desensitization. This resistance could be partially transferred to β_2/β_3AR chimeras in which the incriminated β_2 sequences were substituted by the β_3 stretches (14).

LONG-TERM DESENSITIZATION

AGONIST

Long-term treatment (hours to several days) with agonists (Table 1) induces down-regulation of all three βAR subtypes, probably through accelerated degradation of mRNA and, possibly, additional mecha-

Table 1.   Agonist-Induced Regulation of β_3 Adrenergic Receptors

Agonist-treated Cells	mRNA	Receptor sites	References
Rat WAT, BAT	↓	↓	(15) (16) (20)
Murine L Huβ_3 AR	↓	→	(20)
Murine 3T3 F442A	↑	↑	(17) (19)
Hamster CHW-Huβ_3	→*	→	(20)
Agonist-treated Animals			
6-day perfusion of hamsters	No change in β_3AR modulated lipolysis while down-regulation of β_1 and β_2AR		(18)
Long-term treatment of dogs	Strong increase of BAT expressing β_3AR		(23)
Cold-treated Animals			
Exposure of hamsters to cold	Decrease of β_3AR responsiveness		(25) (26)

*A transient down-regulation was observed by Nantel *et al.* (1994).

nisms including, from the Gs protein, increased activity of phospho-diesterase, etcetera.

In rat white and brown adipose tissues, hours-long agonist treatment resulted in a reduction in both β_3AR binding sites (15) and mRNA levels (15, 16). On the other hand, studies with murine adipocyte-like 3T3-F442A cells (17) and hamster adipocytes (18) or β_3-transfected Chinese hamster fibroblast (CHW) cells (19) showed almost complete resistance to long-term desensitization.

A detailed study of murine L cells and hamster CHW cells transfected with the human β_3AR gene confirmed that sustained agonist-promoted down-regulation of β_3AR may be a cell-specific phenomenon that could be observed in the L cells but not in the CHW cells (20).

TREATMENT WITH OTHER COMPOUNDS

Treatment with other compounds induces strikingly different patterns of down-regulation (Table 2): exposure of 3T3-F442A cells to dexamethasone leads to an increase in β_2-mediated adenylyl cyclase and a decrease in β_1 and β_3 effector activity, best explained by reduced levels of transcription of the β_1AR and β_3AR genes.

Treatment of these cells with n-butyrate, a dietary factor produced from colonic fermentation, increased β_1AR and β_2AR while sharply decreasing β_3AR as detected by direct ligand binding and competition studies. The mRNA levels and gene transcription rates paralleled the protein variations (21). Exposure of the same type of cells to insulin for four days caused a 3.5-fold decrease in the density of the β_3AR, whereas β_1AR remained unchanged and β_2AR became undetectable. Reverse transcriptase–polymerase chain reaction (RT-PCR) analysis confirmed unchanged levels of β_1, but also β_2AR mRNA and sharp decrease of β_3AR mRNA. Nuclear run-on assays showed that insulin actually in-

Table 2. Differential Up- and Down-Regulation of the Three β Subtypes

	β_1	β_2	β_3	References
Adipose differentiation	↓	↓	↑	(27, 28)
cAMP	↓	↓	↑	(17)
Dexamethasone	↓	↑	↓	(27, 28)
Butyrate	↑	↑	↓	(21)
Insulin	→	→	↓	(22)

hibited the β_3AR transcription rate by 90% (22). These findings provide a convincing demonstration of the interplay between insulin and β_3AR expression.

LONG-TERM REGULATION IN ANIMALS

Long-term treatment of mice or dogs with ICI D77114 or mice with BRL 37344, two potent β_3AR agonists, increases the amount of brown adipose tissue and reduces body fat (23).

Physiopathology

In an adult man, mRNA for β_3AR is detected in most white fat tissue depots as well as in isolated brown adipocytes, identified by the expression of uncoupling protein (UCP) mRNA. Pheochromocytoma patients who accumulate organized brown adipose tissue around the adrenal tumor express abundant mRNA in that location (a). In addition, β_3 mRNA was also detected in the gall bladder and in various parts of the colon.

Available data thus suggest that β_3AR is involved in the modulation by catecholamines of storage and usage of fat. In rodents, thermogenesis of brown adipose fat is controlled by sympathetic innervation and may be induced by lowering temperature (cold-induced thermogenesis) or increasing food intake (diet-induced thermogenesis).

The presence of β_3AR in the gall bladder and the gastrointestinal tract suggests an additional level of control regulating fat intake and degradation. This hypothesis is in line with the frequent dysfunction of gall bladder (hypomobility, lithiasis) in obese patients. After a fat-rich meal, jejunal absorption of lipids is thus faster and more efficient in obese than in lean individuals (24). These observations thus confirm that the β_3AR may participate in the control of energetic balance by acting on intestinal assimilation of lipids and their storage, their mobilization or dissipation in adipose tissue. Actors in such control may be free fatty acids or their metabolic products (ketones, volatile fatty acids), acting locally or through the sympathic nervous system on the expression or activity of the β_3AR. A noncontrolled assimilation caused by the failure of one of these steps could induce a dysregulation of insulin function, thus favoring a type II diabetes associated with obesity.

Perspectives

Long-term treatment of obese animals (rodents, dogs) with lipolytic-selective agents induces weight loss and restores insulin sensitivity. These effects appear to be mediated by the β_3-adrenergic receptor expressed in adipose tissues and in the digestive tract. The first β_3 agonists, developed using animal models, appear in short-term clinical studies to be much less efficient in man than in rodents. New compounds selective for their activity on the cloned human β_3AR expressed in model cells should be more efficacious in man, in whom they may help treat some forms of obesity and diabetes.

ACKNOWLEDGMENTS

Support for this work comes mostly from the Centre National de la Recherche Scientifique, the Institut National de la Santé et de la Recherche Médicale, University Paris VII, the Ministry for Research, and the Bristol-Myers-Squibb Company. I am also grateful for help from the Ligue Nationale Contre le Cancer, the Foundation pour la Recherche Médicale Française, and the Association pour la Recherche sur le Cancer.

REFERENCES

1. Arch JRS, Bywater RJ, Coney KA, et al. Influence on body composition and mechanism of action of the β-adrenoceptor agonist BRL26830A. In: Lardy F, Stratman F, eds. Hormones, Thermogenesis and Obesity. Amsterdam: Elsevier; 1989:465–476.
2. Arch JR, Coney KA, Gusterson BA, et al. β-adrenoceptor-mediated control of thermogenesis, body composition and glucose homeostasisin obesity and cachexia. In: Rothwell NJ, Stock MJ, eds. Obesity and Cachexia. London: J. Willey & Sons; 1991:241–268.
3. Zaagsma J, Nahorski SR. Is the adipocyte β-adrenoceptor a prototype for the recently cloned atypical β$_3$-adrenoceptor? Trends Pharmacol Sci. 1990;11:3–7.
4. Emorine LJ, Marullo S, Briend-Sutren MM, et al. Molecular characterization of the human β$_3$-adrenergic receptor. Science. 1989;245: 1118–1121.
5. Nahmias C, Blin N, Elalouf JM, Mattei MG, Strosberg AD, Emorine

LJ. Molecular characterization of the mouse β_3-adrenergic receptor: relationship with the atypical receptor of adipocytes. *EMBO J.* 1991; 10:3721–3727.

6. Granneman JG, Lahners KN, Chaudhry A. Molecular cloning and expression of the rat β_3-adrenergic receptor. *Mol Pharmacol.* 1991;40: 895–899.

7. Muzzin P, Revelli JP, Kuhne F, *et al.* An adipose tissue-specific β-adrenergic receptor: molecular cloning and down-regulation in obesity. *J Biol Chem.* 1991;266:24053–24058.

8. Blin N, Nahmias C, Drumare MF, Strosberg AD. The β_3-adrenergic receptor: a single subtype responsible for atypical β-mediated effects. *Br J Pharmacol.* 1996;112:911–919.

9. Krief S, Lönnqvist F, Raimbault S, *et al.* Tissue distribution of β_3-adrenergic receptor mRNA in man. *J Clin Invest.* 1993;91:344–349.

10. Strosberg AD. Structure, function and regulation of adrenergic receptors. *Protein Sci.* 1993;12:1198–1209.

11. Blin N, Camoin L, Maigret B, Strosberg AD. Structural and conformational features determining selective signal transduction in the β_3-adrenergic receptor. *Mol Pharmacol.* 1993;44:1094–1104.

12. Tate KM, Briend-Sutren MM, Emorine LJ, Delavier-Klutchko C, Marullo S, Strosberg AD. Expression of 3 human β-adrenergic receptor subtypes in transfected Chinese Hamster Ovary cells. *Eur J Biochem.* 1991;196:357–361.

13. Lönnqvist F, Krief S, Strosberg AD, Nyberg B, Emorine LJ, Arner P. Evidence for a functional β_3-adrenergic receptor in man. *Br J Pharmacol.* 1993;110:929–936.

14. Nantel F, Bonin H, Emorine LJ, *et al.* The human β_3-adrenergic receptor is resistant to short-term agonist-promoted desensitization. *Mol Pharmacol.* 1993;43:548–555.

15. Revelli JP, Muzzin P. Modulation in vivo of β-adrenergic receptor subtypes in rat brown adipose tissue by the thermogenic agonist Ro 16 8714. *Biochem J.* 1992;286:743–746.

16. Granneman JG, Lahners KN. Differential regulation of β_1 and β_3 adrenoceptor messenger ribonucleic acids in adipose tissues. *Endocrinology.* 1992;130:109–114.

17. Thomas RF, Holt BD, Schwinn DA, Liggett SB. Long-term agonist exposure induces up-regulation of β_3AR exposure via multiple cAMP response elements. *Proc Natl Acad Sci USA.* 1992;89:4490–4494.

18. Carpéné C, Galitzky J, Collon P, Escalpez F, Dauzats M, Lafontan M. Desensitization of β_1 and β_2 but not β_3-adrenoceptor-mediated lipolytic responses of adipocytes after long-term norepinephrine infusion. *J Pharmacol Exp Ther.* 1993;265:237–247.

19. Liggett SB, Freedman NJ, Schwinn DA, Lefkowitz RJ. Structural basis for receptor subtype-specific regulation revealed by a chimeric β_2/β_3 adrenergic receptor. *Proc Natl Acad Sci USA.* 1993;90: 3665–3669.

20. Nantel F, Marullo S, Krief S, Strosberg AD, Bouvier M. Cell-specific down-regulation of the β_3-adrenergic receptor. *J Biol Chem.* 1994; 269:13148–13155.

21. Krief S, Fève B, Baude B, *et al.* Transcriptional modulation by n-butyric acid of β_1-, β_2-, and β_3- adrenergic receptor balance in 3T3-F442A adipocytes. *J Biol Chem.* 1994;269:6664–6670.

22. Fève B, Elhadri K. Quignard-Boulangé A, Pairault J. Transcriptional down-regulation by insulin of the β_3-adrenergic receptor expression in 3T3-F442A adipocytes: a novel mechanism for repressing the cAMP signalling pathway. *Proc Natl Acad Sci USA.* 1994;91:5677–5681.

23. Champigny O, Ricquier D, Blondel O, Mayers RM, Briscoe MG, Holloway B. β_3-Adrenergic receptor stimulation restores message and expression of brown-fat mitochondrial uncoupling protein in adult dogs. *Proc Natl Acad Sci USA.* 1991;88:10774–10777.

24. Wisén O, Johansson C. Gastrointestinal function in obesity: mobility, secretion and absorption following a liquid test meal. *Metabolism.* 1992;41:390–395.

25. Svoboda P, Unelius L, Cannon B, Nedergaard J. Attenuation of $G_{s\alpha}$ coupling efficiency in brown-adipose-tissue plasma membranes from cold-acclimated hamsters. *Biochem J.* 1993;295:655–661.

26. Unelius L, Bronnikov G, Mohell N, Nedergaard J. Physiological desensitization of β_3-adrenergic responsiveness in brown fat cells. Involvement of a post-receptor mechanism. *Am J Physiol.* 1993;265: 1340–1348.

27. Fève B, Emorine LJ, Lasnier F, *et al.* Atypical β-adrenergic receptor in 3T3-F442A adipocytes: pharmacological and molecular relationship with the human β_3-adrenergic receptor. *J Biol Chem.* 1991;266: 20329–20336.

28. Fève B, Baude B, Krief S, Strosberg AD, Pairault J, Emorine, LJ.

Dexamethasone down-regulates β_3-adrenergic receptors in 3T3-F442A adipocytes. *J Biol Chem.* 1992;267:15909–15915.

29. Liggett SB. Functional properties of the rat and human β_3-adrenergic receptors: differential agonist activation of recombinant receptors in Chinese Hamster Ovary cells. *Mol Pharmacol.* 1992;42:634–637.

MAX LAFONTAN, ANNE BOULOUMIÉ,
ISABELLE CASTAN, DOMINIQUE LARROUY,
PHILIPPE VALET, CHRISTIAN CARPÉNÉ,
and JEAN-SEBASTIEN SAULNIER-BLACHE

Adipocyte Receptors Involved in the Control of Lipolysis: Role of Antilipolytic Mechanisms

ABSTRACT

The lipolytic response of the fat cell depends on the balanced action of the stimulatory and inhibitory pathways involved in the control of lipolysis. The role played by inhibitory modulators of lipolysis will be considered more specifically. In addition to catecholamines (acting via α_2-adrenoceptors) and insulin, which have marked effects on lipolysis, three different antilipolytic agents are involved in the control of antilipolysis: adenosine A1-receptors, EP3-prostaglandin receptors, and neuropeptide Y/peptide YY receptors. Inhibitory regulation of lipolysis seems to involve two major systems: a constitutive system that is related to paracrine mediators (adenosine and prostaglandins) and a regulatory one involving neuroendocrine messengers such as norepinephrine, epinephrine, and NPY/PYY; inhibitory responses to neurotransmitters and hormones such as epinephrine or PYY are only facultative. The differential recruitment, regulation, and coupling to G_i-proteins of the various receptors will also be reviewed. Considering fat cell adrenoceptors, the balance between the various inhibitory and stimulatory subtypes is the point of regulation that determines the final effect of catecholamines. The differences in recruitment of β_1-, β_2-, β_3-, and α_2-adrenoceptors occur on the basis of their relative affinity for the physiological amines. Regarding the coupling of inhibitory receptors to G_i proteins, the adenosine A1-receptor is more strongly coupled than the α_2-adrenoceptor with the G_i protein in adipocyte membranes. Concerning heterologous regulations of receptors inhibiting adenylyl cyclase, androgens have been shown to control the expression of fat cell α_2-adrenoceptor but less is known for the other types.

Adipose tissue is a heterogeneous metabolic organ exhibiting noticeable differences in its regional distribution in laboratory mammals and humans. Although nutritional and neuroendocrine mechanisms play a major role in adipose tissue abundance, it is difficult to delineate their direct contribution to the development of the relative size of the different fat depots. The role of the intrinsic properties of the actual adipose tissue from various deposits is not easy to delineate from other neuroendocrine mechanisms.

Studies of the site-specific properties of adipose tissue have increased since the early eighties. Adipose tissues from different anatomical locations (*e.g.*, intraabdominal and subcutaneous) are relatively easy to analyze after fat cell isolation in laboratory mammals. Tissue-specific differences in fat cell properties have been reported by a large number of laboratories. The major unresolved question concerns the relevance of the results obtained in fat cells of various animal models for the understanding of the human fat cell function and dysfunction.

Unfortunately in humans, it is essentially the adipose tissue, the most convenient and abundant for biopsies (*i.e.*, subcutaneous), that has been chosen most frequently for the study of fat cell function in healthy patients, whereas intraabdominal depots are less easily investigated and generally obtained from patients suffering various kinds of illness and undergoing surgery.

In this paper, the regulation of the lipolytic response of the fat cell will be considered. It depends on the balanced action of stimulatory and inhibitory pathways involved in the control of lipolysis. The normal regulation of antilipolysis will be discussed after a brief review of the biochemical mechanisms that can explain antilipolytic actions. The physiological differences between antilipolytic systems and the major physiological and pathological alterations of lipolytic effects will be considered in laboratory mammals and humans. Special attention will be paid to regional variations in antilipolysis and possible factors modifying the extent of antilipolytic responsiveness. In addition, the physiological and pathophysiological relevance of such local variations will also be discussed in humans.

Antilipolysis in Fat Cells and Its Molecular Mechanisms

Cyclic adenosine monophosphate (cAMP)–dependent pathways play a key role in the control of the lipolytic activity in the fat cell of all species investigated so far (1, 2). The receptor-controlled increment of intracellular cAMP levels promotes activation of cAMP-dependent protein kinase A (PKA) that phosphorylates a serine residue of the hormone sensitive lipase and promotes its activation (2). It is easily understandable that activators and inhibitors of the adenylyl cyclase system and cAMP production are direct regulators of lipolysis. In addition, cyclic guanosine monophosphate (cGMP)–inhibited low-Km phosphodiesterase (cGI-PDE), which hydrolyses cAMP, plays an important role, since it is activated by insulin and also PKA. Although there have been controversies with regard to the ability of insulin to lower the intracellular cAMP, more recent studies have demonstrated that the insulin effect is, to a large extent, exerted through antagonism of the elevation of cAMP promoted by lipolytic hormones (3, 4). Antilipolysis is linked to the lowering of intracellular cAMP levels. Cyclic AMP may be reduced through inhibition of adenylyl cyclase or stimulation of cGI-PDE.

In human fat cells, in addition to insulin, there are at least four different antilipolytic receptors that are negatively coupled to adenylyl cyclase: α_2-adrenoceptors, adenosine A1-receptors, EP3-prostaglandin E2 receptors, and neuropeptide Y/peptide YY (NPY/PYY) receptors. The existence of nicotinic acid receptors is proposed to explain the antilipolytic action of nicotinic acid; but as yet, there is no demonstration that such receptors actually exist.

The in vitro demonstration, on isolated fat cells, of a clear antilipolytic response to an agonist inhibiting lipolysis generally requires the preliminary inhibition of the action of adenosine via the inclusion of adenosine deaminase and/or of an adenosine antagonist in the incubation medium of the fat cells. Methylxanthines (theophylline, isobutylmethylxanthine) have also been used by various investigators. They act as adenosine A1-receptor antagonists and cGI-PDE inhibitors when used in the millimole concentration range. The adenosine concentrations in isolated adipocyte incubations may be abnormally elevated as a consequence of the isolation procedure. Endogenously released adenosine derived from adenine nucleotides extruded by broken and damaged cells provides a permanent inhibition of lipolysis in isolated adipocytes. Addition of adenosine deaminase to the incubation is often followed by an increment of the basal rate of lipolysis, which can reach maximum levels in certain conditions. It results in the "ligand free" state previously described (5) that is accompanied by maximal rates of lipolysis (avoiding any noticeable increment of lipolysis by stimulatory agents). It is clear that any study of the hormonal regulation of the adenylyl cyclase and lipolysis must check the adenosine level in the incubation medium. This point is particularly important for the study of inhibitory mechanisms. Inhibitory antilipolytic effects cannot be demonstrated in fat cells that are inhibited by endogenous adenosine in standard assay conditions. Moreover, inhibitory effects are also weakly operative when higher doses of adenylyl cyclase agonists are used to preactivate fat cells before testing inhibition. Saturating concentrations of lipolytic agents completely abolish the antilipolytic effects of most adenylyl cyclase inhibitors but also those of insulin (4). It is particularly difficult to find the most suitable conditions to investigate inhibition of lipolysis by insulin and adenylyl cyclase–linked inhibiting receptors.

The basal mechanisms underlying the mediation of adenylyl cyclase inhibition and antilipolytic effects via inhibitory receptors seems to be identical for all the receptor classes. When an antilipolytic agonist interacts with an inhibitory receptor, the plasma-membrane–bound receptor acts on a trimeric inhibitory guanosine-triphosphate (GTP)–binding protein (*e.g.*, composed of three subunits named αi, β, and γ), the αi-protein subunit dissociates from the $\beta \gamma$ dimer. It is still unclear whether the GTP-bound αi protein, the $\beta \gamma$ complex, or both inhibit adenylyl cyclase and what mechanism they really operate to lead to inhibition of the catalytic moiety of the enzyme. However, it has now been convincingly demonstrated that both kinds of G protein subunits interact with effectors and receptors and play an active role in signal transduction. Direct inhibition of adenylyl cyclase by activated $G_{\alpha i}$ protein has recently been demonstrated in vitro (6). The inhibitory effect of αi is dependent on the type of adenylyl cyclase and on the nature of the activator of the enzyme. Newer evidence also indicates that the $\beta \gamma$-dimers released by trimeric G protein activation could play a major part in signal transmission (7). However, for the moment, no specific studies have been made in fat cells.

Rat epididymal fat cells and human adipocytes contain the short and long forms of $G_{\alpha s}$ (largely the long isoform), and three forms of $G_{\alpha i}$

protein (αi1, αi2, and αi3), which are detectable by adenosine diphos-phate (ADP)–ribosylation and immunodetection. Both β_{35} and β_{36} sub-units have also been identified (8). Although seven different sorts of G_γ subunits are known and are considered to be more heterogeneous than the G_β subunits, the forms existing in fat cells have not been deter-mined. Adipocyte membranes are devoid of Gαo, whereas its presence is suspected in 3T3-L1 preadipocytes (8). Concerning the catalyst of adenylyl cyclase, six types of mammalian adenylyl cyclase have been cloned (types I–VI); the isoform of the fat cell, which is probably insen-sitive to calmodulin, has not been fully characterized.

Species-Specific–Dependent and Differentiation-Dependent Differences in the Action of Inhibiting Antilipolytic Receptors

SPECIES-SPECIFIC DIFFERENCES IN INHIBITING MECHANISMS

When comparative studies were performed to test the efficiency of four different antilipolytic mechanisms operating in mature fat cells (*e.g.*, α_2-adrenergic-, PGE1-, adenosine-, and NPY/PYY-dependent), important differences were revealed. The inhibitory regulation of lipolysis in white adipocytes seems to involve two kinds of systems: 1) a major constitutive one, found in all the adipocytes, that involves paracrine/autocrine effectors that exert potent inhibiting effects (adenosine, pros-taglandins); 2) a regulatory one, which involves neuro-endocrine agents such as catecholamines, NPY, and PYY, the efficiency of which exhibits striking species-specific differences in normal mature fat cells. Prostaglandin E1– and E2–, and phenylisopropyl adenosine (PIA)–dependent antilipolytic responses are fully developed, whatever the fat cells of the various species (from rodents, hibernating mammals, pri-mates, and humans). The efficiency of the α_2-adrenergic and NPY-ergic systems varies partly according to the level of expression of the re-spective receptors in fat cells (9). These receptors, and specifically the α_2-adrenoceptors, can be submitted to a number of heterologous reg-ulations of its expression (2). In other words, antilipolysis induced by paracrine/autocrine agents such as prostaglandins and adenosine is compulsory, whereas inhibitory responses to hormones and neuro-transmitters are only facultative in white adipocytes and variable under a number of pathophysiological situations. These results show how careful we must be in the future when animal fat cells are chosen as representative models for human adipocytes.

DIFFERENTIATION-DEPENDENT EXPRESSION OF INHIBITING RECEPTORS OF THE FAT CELL

Prostaglandins (PGs) and adenosine are paracrine regulators that are released in adipose tissue and originate from the concerted contribution of different cell types including adipocytes, preadipocytes, and endothelial cells (10). These paracrine/autocrine effectors are involved in the control of lipolysis but also contribute essentially to the control of adipose tissue blood flow. Prostaglandin E2 (PGE2) and prostacyclin (prostaglandin I2, [PGI2]) are the major PGs identified in adipose tissue. Prostaglandin E2 and PGE1 are potent antilipolytic agents that bind to an EP3 receptor and operate through inhibition of adenylyl cyclase in the adipocytes (11). Specific binding of PGE2 has been demonstrated in human and rat fat cells. The EP3 subtype of the PGE2 receptor belongs to the seven-transmembrane domain receptor family. It mediates the diverse physiological actions of PGE2 and probably acts through its coupling to G_i proteins and adenylyl cyclase inhibition. The EP3-receptors exist under at least four isoforms that are produced by alternative splicing (12, 13).

Prostaglandin I2 behaves as a potent and specific adipogenic agent that allows preadipocytes to enter terminal differentiation (14, 15). Conversely, PGE2 exclusively acts on mature adipocytes on which it exerts its well-known antilipolytic action. Since PGI2 retains some lipolytic effect in mature rat cells (16), PGE1, which has an affinity for PGI2 receptors, is less appropriate than PGE2 to investigate antilipolytic mechanisms.

Concerning the other well-known autacoid identified in adipose tissue, adenosine, molecular, and pharmacological approaches have demonstrated the presence of adenosine A2-receptor in preadipocytes, the stimulation of which promotes cAMP production and allows preadipocytes to enter differentiation. Absent from preadipocytes, the adenosine A1-receptor is only expressed in mature adipocytes where its stimulation promotes adenylyl-cyclase inhibition and antilipolysis (17). As for PGs, it is clear that adenosine could have a bimodal action on the fat cell depending on the state of differentiation. The PGI2 and adenosine A2-receptors coupled positively to adenylyl cyclase, mainly expressed and operative in preadipocytes, probably play an important role in the formation of new fat cells and in the control of adipose cell differentiation in vivo.

When considering catecholamine receptors, β-adrenoceptors (β_1, β_2, and β_3) are expressed early in murine cell lines and preadipocytes, but α_2-adrenoceptors have never been identified in various murine cell lines (3T3-L1, 3T3-F442A, and ob17 cells) and under standard conditions of culture. It is noticeable that most of the preadipocyte models were established from rat or mouse, in which the α_2-adrenergic control of lipolysis in mature adipocytes is poorly efficient when compared to man, dog, and rabbit, or hamster. When differentiating cultured hamster preadipocytes were studied in a serum-free medium supplemented with insulin and thyroxine, α_2-adrenergic responsiveness was not found in eight-day post-confluent differentiating preadipocytes though G_i proteins and inhibitory effects of adenosine and PGE2 were. Functional α_2-adrenoceptors, having pharmacological properties identical to those found in mature adipocytes, were identified in differentiated adipocytes (20 days of culture). Apparently and unlike the β-adrenoceptors, the α_2-adrenoceptor seems to be a late marker of preadipose cell differentiation (18).

It is noticeable that all the inhibiting receptors investigated so far appear in differentiated adipocytes, whereas the activating forms of the receptors of the various agents are predominant in preadipocytes. The convergence of all these inhibiting mechanisms activated by various agents could contribute synergistically and/or separately to the development of the adipose mass by the negative control of mobilization of triacylglycerol reserves through modulation of the lipolytic processes under various pathophysiological conditions (Fig. 1).

Physiological and Pathological Variations of Antilipolytic Responses and Antilipolytic Receptors in Various Fat Deposits

From a physiological point of view, insulin is the most important antilipolytic agent, but the situation is less clear for autacoids, catecholamines, NPY, and PYY. The antilipolytic effect of insulin differs between various fat cell deposits in rat and human fat cells. Sensitivity and responsiveness of the antilipolytic effects of insulin are more pronounced in subcutaneous than in omental human fat cells in humans, but the nature of these differences are not fully explained (19).

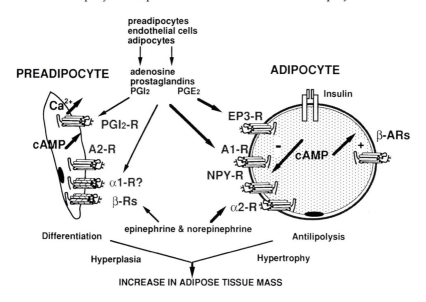

Figure 1. Differentiation-dependent differences in the expression of inhibitory (EP3-R, A_1-R, α_2-R, NPY-R) and stimulatory (PGI2-R, A_2-R, β and α_1-R) receptors for prostaglandins (PGI2 and PGE2), adenosine, catecholamines, and NPY, respectively. Prostaglandin I2 and adenosine A_2-receptors could act in concert locally in the formation of new fat cells and in the control of adipose cell differentiation (15). A putative contribution of the α_1-adrenoceptor is still unsolved. All the inhibitory receptors for paracrine/autocrine agents, neurotransmitters, and hormones (insulin and epinephrine) expressed in the mature fat cell could act in concert to promote and/or sustain hypertrophy of fat cells.

Concerning adenosine and prostaglandins, these compounds are probably metabolized very rapidly in vivo. However, substantial amounts of adenosine were found in the interstitial fluid of adipose tissue using a microdialysis technique (20). The various mechanisms involved in PGs effect have been analyzed in detail and recently reviewed (10).

Adenosine A1-receptors have been characterized in the rat adipocyte by various groups using different kinds of radioligands. The antagonist [3H]DPCPX and the agonist [3H]PIA are the most suitable ones and have allowed characterization of human, rat, and hamster fat cell adenosine A1-receptors. The binding properties of A1-receptors are very different from those of another G_i-coupled receptor, the α_2-adrenoceptor (21). The results obtained in hamster fat cells indicate that adenosine A1-receptors and α_2-adrenoceptors could be differentially coupled with G_i proteins (22).

All the more recent studies have confirmed the diversity and the abundance (number of binding sites) of inhibiting receptors coupled to adenylyl cyclase by comparison with the stimulating receptors. They indicate that endogenous inhibitory agents may have more important effects on triglyceride hydrolysis than previously suspected. Various arguments based on in vitro but also in vivo studies can be reconsidered to support the idea that inhibitory systems (inhibitory receptors and G_i proteins) of the adipocyte could be more important than supposed by a number of investigators. First, it is unquestionable that the addition of adenosine deaminase to adipocyte suspensions always removes the tonic inhibition exerted by adenosine released in fat cell suspensions and increases basal lipolysis (spontaneous glycerol release by isolated fat cells). The extent of the stimulation of lipolysis initiated by adenylyl cyclase stimulators is reduced under such conditions. It is for this reason that the effects of various antilipolytic agents on cAMP production and lipolysis are dependent on the experimental conditions (*e.g.*, the adipocyte number, the incubation time, and the use of stimulators). These parameters should always be defined in order to make comparisons among the different studies. Second, in vitro treatment of adipocytes with pertussis toxin, which inactivates all the G_i proteins and blocks the inhibitory action of all the adenylyl cyclase–linked inhibitory receptors, promotes maximal rates of spontaneous lipolysis and no other lipolytic ligand brings any further noticeable increase. This action could be interpreted as if G_i proteins per se or in the presence of inhibitory ligands exert a tonic action in fat cells. Although rather drastic, in vivo effects of pertussis toxin largely fitted with in vitro observations; reduction or suppression of G_i protein promoted lipid mobilization in vivo. A recent investigation into the role of GTP-binding protein subunit $G_{i\alpha2}$, using transgenic mice in which the αi2-subunit expression of $G_{i\alpha2}$ was suppressed by antisense RNA, has brought positive new arguments concerning the physiological significance of G_i protein levels and at the same time of inhibiting ligands. Basal levels of cAMP are raised in the adipocytes of these transgenic mice in the absence of stimulatory ligands and, moreover, as expected, PIA-induced inhibition of cAMP levels (raised by epinephrine) was strongly attenuated. This study demonstrated that $G_{i\alpha2}$ is a major transducer of the inhibitory response in adipose tissue and that $G_{i\alpha2}$ provides tonic suppression of the basal adenylyl cyclase activity. Nearly total elimination of $G_{i\alpha2}$ subunit largely de-represses the inhibitory control of intracellular accumulation of cAMP; this protein probably plays a major role in fat cells, when compared with $G_{i\alpha1}$ and $G_{i\alpha3}$, in the control of adenylyl cyclase function (23, 24) (Fig. 2).

It is reasonable to propose that under in vivo conditions, in the presence of endogenous ligands, the $G_{i\alpha2}$-dependent inhibitory pathways are under sustained and permanent tonic inhibition. Inhibitory receptors are activated at low levels of their endogenous ligands (prostaglandins, catecholamines, adenosine). When the action (inhibition versus stimulation of adenylyl cyclase) of these agents having dual effects are carefully reconsidered in vitro, it is always the inhibitory pathway that is activated at the lowest concentration of the agent having the dualistic action as shown for prostaglandins (25, 26), adenosine (27), and even catecholamines in human fat cells (28). It is clear that inhib-

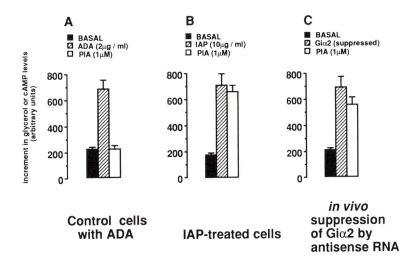

Figure 2. Diagram representing the influence of various fat cell treatments on lipolysis (*A, B*) and cAMP production (*C*). Effects of adenosine deaminase (ADA) (*A*) and pertussis toxin (IAP) treatment (*B*) on glycerol release in human fat cells in vitro. Both treatments promote submaximal glycerol release by the fat cells. Inhibitory effects of PIA are suppressed after IAP treatment. The experiments were repeated five times (unpublished results). Part *C* is interpreted from original results describing attenuation of inhibitory adenylyl cyclase response and increment of basal cAMP production by suppression of $G_{i\alpha2}$ in vivo, published by Moxham *et al.* (24).

itory α_2-adrenoceptors have a higher affinity for catecholamines than β-adrenoceptors and are recruited before β-adrenoceptors (29, 30).

Functionally, the fact that unrestrained fat cell adenylyl cyclase proceeds at increased rates suggests that a certain degree of inhibition might be necessary for fat cell adenylyl cyclase to be susceptible to stimulation. In vivo pertussis-toxin treatments that are known to promote lipid mobilization, probably by the relief of the action of inhibitory ligands (31), and the far more selective "knock out" of the specific $G_{i\alpha2}$-protein subunit by antisense RNA expression in vivo offer a convincing demonstration of the importance of inhibitory pathways in contributing to the setting of adenylyl cyclase and in the ambient levels of cAMP that control basal lipolysis. Increments of lipolysis can be considered to operate by a modulation of inhibitory pathways; these pathways are overcome in the presence of high concentrations of stimulating ligands. As suggested previously from in vitro studies a certain level of tonic inhibition of lipolysis might be necessary for fat cell lipolysis to be susceptible to stimulation (32).

Although it is unequivocal that adenylyl cyclase–linked inhibitory systems involving PGs, adenosine, catecholamines, and NPY/PYY and controlling antilipolysis are operative in vitro, more research is needed to evaluate the possible physiological role of such systems in in vivo conditions using more physiological approaches such as in situ microdialysis. It is obvious that reducing endogenous production of PGs in adipose tissue by chronic indomethacin treatment results in enhanced EP3-receptor binding, enhanced antilipolytic sensitivity to exogenous PGE2, and increased ADA-stimulated lipolysis. A dynamic equilibrium between adenosine and PG production and action might exist at the adipose tissue level (33). The activation state of adenylyl cyclase is determined by such a complex equilibrium; the various steps involved in the setting up of such an equilibrium are difficult to investigate. Concerning the adrenergic system, a basal tonic activity always exists (34); local denervation of retroperitoneal fat deposits in rats is followed by a large increment of α_2-adrenoceptors and smaller changes in β-adrenoceptors (35).

Concerning catecholamine action, in vitro studies have clearly established that catecholamines stimulate their various adrenoceptors on the basis of their relative affinities for each kind. The existence of a differential recruitment of the various adrenoceptors, in the order $\alpha_2 > \beta_1 > \beta_2 > \beta_3$ depending on the relative affinity of catecholamines for each adrenoceptor type, has been demonstrated in various fat cells and recently discussed (2). The physiological relevance of the results obtained in vitro were assessed using in situ microdialysis methods. The studies have shown, using the α_1/α_2-adrenoceptor antagonist phentolamine, that α_2-adrenoceptors could be involved in the modulation of lipolysis at rest (36). Although further studies are required using more selective α_2-antagonists and defining catecholamine levels and putative changes in blood flow in situ, it is suggested that a certain degree of tonic inhibition of lipolysis could occur at low levels of catecholamines through α_2-adrenoceptor stimulation. This view agrees with previous studies of the group demonstrating the high affinity of catecholamines for fat cell α_2-adrenoceptors (29).

The role of fat cell α_2-adrenoceptors, which largely outnumber β-adrenoceptors in human fat cells, has never been clearly understood. In fact, they could play a major role in the regulation of lipolysis at low levels of sympathetic nervous system (SNS) activation (at rest or under very weak SNS activity). In addition, contribution of the vascular β-, α_1-, and α_2-adrenoceptors involved in the control of adipose tissue blood flow also requires extended investigations. A recent study using in situ microdialysis approaches has revealed the importance of this component (37).

Alpha$_2$-Adrenoceptors and Adipose Tissue Dysfunction: Regulatory Considerations

Involvement of the various antilipolytic systems can be suspected whenever alterations of the lipolytic processes are described. A large number of reports, sometimes contradictory, exist in animal models and humans; an exhaustive review will not be performed here, since some aspects have recently been reviewed (2, 10, 38). Some points concerning recent results on α_2-adrenoceptor regulation will be treated more specifically.

Obesity and Aging

When comparisons of omental and subcutaneous deposits were made to test the efficiency of the antilipolytic systems in standard animals and normal patients, the adenylyl cyclase regulation differed noticeably between the various deposits; intraabdominal fat is far less sensitive to inhibition by α_2-agonists, PYY, and adenosine than subcutaneous fat in humans (39, 40) and laboratory mammals (41, 42, 43). Regional differences in the lipolytic responsiveness agree with the adenylyl cyclase assays. In humans, among the antilipolytic compounds tested so far, UK14304, clonidine, epinephrine, PYY, and insulin have reduced antilipolytic properties in omental adipocytes as compared with subcutaneous adipocytes (19, 40, 44). Prostaglandin E2 has similar antilipolytic properties in the adipocytes from the various depots, whereas adenosine exhibits intersite differences in its antilipolytic action (38, 44).

Enhanced basal lipolysis was reported in the adipocytes of obese subjects. It was considered to be due in part to an impaired antilipolytic action of PGE2 and adenosine (45, 46). The reduced antilipolytic effect of PGE2 and adenosine does not seem to involve a more general impairment of the antilipolytic pathways (insulin, α_2-adrenergic). Conversely, it is an increment of α_2-adrenergic responsiveness that is observed in subcutaneous adipocytes of obese men and women (47, 48).

In humans, it is clearly demonstrated that regional differences in catecholamine-induced lipolysis are regulated at the adrenoceptor level. When lipolysis is stimulated at the distal part of the "lipolytic cascade" at the level of the PKA-lipase complex, the lipolytic differences between site and sex are completely abolished (49). Omental and pericolonic adipocytes have a considerably higher lipolytic response to physiological amines than subcutaneous fat cells. The regional differences involve changes in β_1/β_2- and α_2-adrenoceptor number. The highest number of β_1/β_2-adrenoceptors is found in the highly responsive fat deposits (omental, pericolonic), and conversely, an increased α_2-adrenoceptor number is found in tissues characterized by a weak responsiveness to norepinephrine and other antilipolytic agents (adenosine, insulin, NPY) (30, 40, 49, 50). Nevertheless, when considering site heterogeneity more precisely it is not excluded that the α_2-adrenergic effects of catecholamines in fat cells may be governed by undefined sex factors, since differences between catecholamine-induced lipolysis and α_2-adrenergic effects exist between fat cells of men and women. Influence of sex-steroid–dependent regulation of the various elements of the adenylyl cyclase system requires further investigations (49, 51).

FAT CELL SIZE CHANGES AND FASTING

It has been reported in humans and laboratory animals that differences in the hormonal sensitivity of adipocytes could be due to differences in cell size with the idea that if large cells were less sensitive to inhi-bition of lipolysis they would release stored fat more easily than smaller fat cells. This suggestion is supported by the finding that large fat cells of obese individuals or young infants (52, 53) have a weaker sensitivity to inhibition and a higher rate of basal lipolysis. Nevertheless, a number of observations in humans and numerous animal models are in contra-diction with such a view. In humans under normal conditions omental fat cells are smaller than subcutaneous fat cells and they have a lower sensitivity to various inhibiting ligands (α_2-agonists, adenosine, NPY/PYY). The larger adipocytes of the gluteal region of women are those that exhibit the highest α_2-adrenergic responsiveness and the highest number of α_2-adrenoceptors (30, 49). In different species (rat, dog, hamster) fattening, which is associated with cell size enlargement, is associated with a specific increase of α_2-adrenoceptor expression and improvement of α_2-adrenoceptor–mediated effects (54, 55, 56, 57) as-sociated with a concomitant decrease in $\beta1/\beta2$-adrenoceptor number in some of them and no changes in adenosine and prostaglandins ef-fects (Fig. 3). A striking fall of α_2-adrenoceptor–mediated effects ap-pears on cell size reduction after a long period of fasting. The phenom-enon is also observed whether or not the experimental strategy is used to promote emaciation of the animals (41, 58, and unpublished results).

HETEROLOGOUS REGULATION OF THE EXPRESSION OF THE INHIBITORY RECEPTORS BY SEX STEROIDS IN THE FAT CELL

Previous studies from our group revealed that a physiological modu-lation of the expression of fat cell α_2-adrenoceptors and α_2-mediated antilipolytic effects existed in hamster fat cells over the year, with a weaker effect in winter (short-day photoperiod) (59). Surgical castration also decreases α_2-adrenoceptor number and efficiency in the hamsters (60). In fact, in male hamster fat cells, the expression of the adipocyte α_2-adrenoceptor is under the control of photoperiod by a testosterone-dependent mechanism mediated by the hypothalamic-pituitary axis (59). Moreover, the androgenic regulation of the adipocyte α_2-adreno-ceptor is not limited to males and to photoperiodic manipulations. Tes-tosterone and dihydrotestosterone administration also induce a large up-regulation of the adipocyte α_2-adrenoceptor in female hamster fat cells and in young hamsters. Testosterone also increases α_2-adrenocep-tors in fat cells of male and female rats (unpublished results). Adeno-

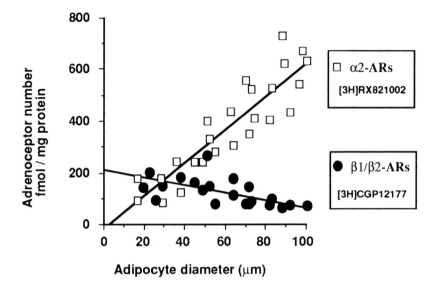

Figure 3. Changes in α₂- and β₁/β₂-adrenoceptor number in hamster white fat cells are correlated with development of fat cell hypertrophy. Alpha₂- and β₁/β₂-adrenoceptor numbers were determined using saturation binding studies on the same batch of fat cell membranes.

sine A1-receptors are not affected by testoterone administration (61), β-adrenergic responsiveness and β-adrenoceptor number are unchanged. The up-regulating effect of testosterone was also found in the α₂-adrenoceptor mRNA levels; a transcriptional mechanism can be hypothesized. In order to verify if the regulation in vivo can be attributed to a direct effect of androgens on the adipocyte, adipose precursor cells from male hamsters were exposed to testosterone in primary culture. The effect was exclusively androgen-specific; among the various steroids tested (estradiol, progesterone, androstenedione, and dexamethasone) only testosterone, dihydrotestosterone, and the synthetic androgen agonist R-1881 enhanced α₂-adrenoceptor expression (Fig. 4). To conclude, androgens promote up-regulation of fat cell α₂-adrenoceptors in vivo and in vitro. The effect is adipose-tissue specific; the hamster α₂A adrenoceptor isotype expressed in human fat cells and existing in various other tissues such as kidney, brain, and colocytes exhibits a strong tissue-specific regulation limited to the white fat cell (Bouloumié *et al.*, unpublished results). Considering the noticeable role played by

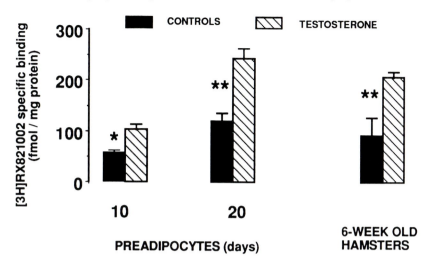

Figure 4. Kinetics of the up-regulating effect of testosterone on preadipocyte α_2 adrenoceptors during adipose conversion. Confluent adipocytes from male hamsters were treated with 1 µmol testosterone or maintained in a defined medium (controls). The medium was changed every two days. Alpha$_2$-adrenoceptor density was determined 10 and 20 days post-confluence. Binding parameters determined in isolated fat cell membranes of 6-week-old male hamsters treated with testosterone are given for comparison. * $P < 0.05$, ** $P < 0.01$ (student t test).

α_2-adrenoceptors in the control of human fat cell function, it is important to demonstrate if such a mechanism could exist in human fat cells and if testosterone sensitivity is an intrinsic property of the α_2A-adrenoceptor gene. Experiments are currently being performed in the laboratory to determine whether the promoter of the human α_2A-adrenoceptor gene linked to a CAT reporter gene and transfected in 3T3-F442A cells exhibits testosterone responsiveness.

Conclusions and Future Trends

Apart from insulin, which could be considered the major antilipolytic agent, adenylyl cyclase–coupled inhibitory receptors of the fat cell, though diverse and numerous, represent the neglected part of fat cell function for a number of fat cell biologists. The inhibitory arm of the fat cell adenylyl cyclase probably acts to counterregulate the stimulatory arm. Lipolysis is the result of increased stimulation without change in inhibition or of reduction in inhibition without changes in stimulation or is a mixture of both events. The most suitable conditions to explore involvement of both systems under balanced conditions is not reached in vitro. Depending on the intention of the authors, one arm of the regulatory system is always privileged with respect to its counterpart.

Numerous differences reported in humans and animals between intraabdominal and subcutaneous depots and even within the various subcutaneous depots show that each adipose tissue deposit has its own specificity in terms of its lipolytic and antilipolytic system. These systems permit triacylglycerol to be hydrolyzed at different rates from fat cells of the different regions. Regional differences in fat cell stimulators and inhibitors of adenylyl cyclase may explain why fat tends to accumulate more specifically in particular adipose tissue sites. Moreover, the diversity and the site differences reported in antilipolytic pathways suggest that the antilipolytic-hypertrophic pathways, involving numerous effectors produced in highly variable physiological or pathological conditions, represent an important part of the lipolytic system. It is expected that the development of in vivo approaches using in situ microdialysis will facilitate the analysis of the agents released in the vicinity of the fat cells. The study of their direct action on fat cells and the vascular bed will also be considerably facilitated. Moreover, genetic techniques should enable the cell-targeted "knock out" of various genes coding for the numerous elements of the inhibitory pathways and open new perspectives for the delineation of the physiological relevance of these inhibitory pathways of lipolysis.

REFERENCES

1. Fain JN, Garcia-Sainz JA. Adrenergic regulation of adipocyte metabolism. *J Lipid Res.* 1983;24:945–966.
2. Lafontan M, Berlan M. Fat cell adrenergic receptors and the control of white and brown fat cell function. *J Lipid Res.* 1993;34:1057–1091.
3. Manganiello VC, Degerman E, Smith CJ, Vasta V, Tornqvist H, Belfrage P. Mechanisms for activation of the rat adipocyte particulate cyclic-GMP-inhibited cyclic AMP phosphodiesterase and its importance in the antilipolytic action of insulin. In: Strada SJ, Hidaka H, eds. *Advances in Second Messenger and Phosphoprotein Research.* New York: Raven Press Ltd; 1992;25:147–164.

4. Wesslau C, Eriksson JW, Smith U. Cellular cyclic AMP levels modulate insulin sensitivity and responsiveness: evidence against a significant role of G_i in insulin signal transduction. *Biochem Biophys Res Commun.* 1993;196:287–293.

5. Honnor RC, Dhillon GS, Londos C. cAMP-dependent protein kinase and lipolysis in rat adipocytes, II: definition of steady-state relationship with lipolytic and antilipolytic modulators. *J Biol Chem.* 1985;260:15130–15138.

6. Taussig R, Iniguez-Lluhi JA, Gilman AG. Inhibition of adenylyl cyclase by G_i alpha. *Science.* 1993;261:218–221.

7. Clapham DE, Neer EJ. New roles for G-protein beta/gamma-dimers in transmembrane signalling. *Nature.* 1993;365:403–406.

8. Begin-Heick N, McFarlane-Anderson N. G-proteins in obesity. In: Milligan G, Wakelam M, eds. *G-Proteins.* London: Academic Press Ltd; 1992;129–156.

9. Castan I, Valet P, Quideau N, *et al.* Antilipolytic effects of alpha$_2$-adrenergic agonists, neuropeptide Y, adenosine and PGE1 in mammal adipocytes. *Am J Physiol.* 1994;266:R1141–R1147.

10. Richelsen B. Prostaglandins in adipose tissue. *Dan Med Bull.* 1991; 38:228–244.

11. Strong P, Coleman RA, Humphrey PP. Prostanoid-induced inhibition of lipolysis in rat isolated adipocytes: probable involvement of EP3-receptors. *Prostaglandins.* 1992;43:559–566.

12. Sugimoto Y, Negishi M, Hayashi Y, *et al.* Two isoforms of the EP3 receptor with different carboxyl-terminal domains: identical ligand binding properties and different coupling properties with G_i proteins. *J Biol Chem.* 1993;268:2712–2718.

13. Namba T, Sugimoto Y, Negishi M, *et al.* Alternative splicing of C-terminal tail of prostaglandin E receptor subtype EP3 determines G-protein specificity. *Nature.* 1993;365:166–170.

14. Vassaux G, Gaillard D, Ailhaud G, Négrel R. Prostacyclin is a specific effector of adipose cell differentiation: its dual role as cAMP and Ca^{2+} elevating agent. *J Biol Chem.* 1992;267:11092–11097.

15. Vassaux G, Gaillard D, Darimont C, Ailhaud G, Négrel R. Differential response of preadipocytes and adipocytes to prostacyclin and prostaglandin E2: physiological implications. *Endocrinology.* 1992; 131:2393–2398.

16. Chatzipantelli K, Rudolph S, Axelrod L. Coordinate control of li-

polysis by prostaglandin E2 and prostacyclin in rat adipose tissue. *Diabetes.* 1992;41:927–935.

17. Vassaux G, Gaillard D, Mari B, Ailhaud G, Négrel R. Differential expression of adenosine A_1 and A_2 receptors in preadipocytes and adipocytes. *Biochem Biophys Res Commun.* 1993;193:1123–1130.

18. Saulnier-Blache J-S, Dauzats M, Daviaud D, *et al.* Late expression of alpha$_2$-adrenergic-mediated antilipolysis during differentiation of hamster preadipocytes. *J Lipid Res.* 1991;32:1489–1499.

19. Bolinder J, Kager L, Ostman J, Arner P. Differences at the receptor and post-receptor level between human omental and subcutaneous adipose tissue in the action of insulin on lipolysis. *Diabetes.* 1983; 32:117–123.

20. Lönnroth P, Jansson P-A, Fredholm BB, Smith U. Microdialysis of intercellular adenosine concentration in subcutaneous tissue in humans. *Am J Physiol.* 1989;256:E250–E255.

21. Larrouy D, Galitzky J, Lafontan M. A1 adenosine receptors in the human fat cell: tissue distribution and regulation of radioligand binding. *Eur J Pharmacol.* 1991;206:139–147.

22. Larrouy D, Remaury A, Daviaud D, Lafontan M. Coupling of inhibitory receptors with G_i-proteins in hamster adipocytes: comparison between adenosine A_1 receptor and alpha$_2$-adrenoceptor. *Eur J Pharmacol.* (Mol Pharmacol Sect) 1994;267:225–232.

23. Moxham CM, Hod Y, Malbon CC. Induction of Gα2i-specific antisense RNA in vivo inhibits neonatal growth. *Science.* 1993;260:991–995.

24. Moxham CM, Hod Y, Malbon CC. $G_{i\alpha2}$ mediates the inhibitory regulation of adenylyl cyclase in vivo: analysis in transgenic mice with $G_{i\alpha2}$ suppressed by inducible antisense RNA. *Dev Genet.* 1993;14:266–273.

25. Kather H, Simon B. Biphasic effects of prostaglandin E2 on the human fat cell adenylate cyclase. *J Clin Invest.* 1979;64:609–612.

26. Cohen-Luria R, Rimon G. Prostaglandin E2 can bimodally inhibit and stimulate the epididymal adipocyte adenylyl cyclase. *Cell Signal.* 1992;4:331–335.

27. Garcia-Sainz JA, Torner ML. Rat fat cells have three types of adenosine receptors (Ri, Ra and P): differential effects of pertussis toxin. *Biochem J.* 1985;232:439–443.

28. Lafontan M, Berlan M. Characterization of physiological agonist selectivity of human fat cell alpha$_2$-adrenoceptors: adrenaline is the

major stimulant of the alpha$_2$-adrenoceptor. *Eur J Pharmacol.* 1982; 82:107–111.

29. Berlan M, Lafontan M. Evidence that epinephrine acts preferentially as an antilipolytic agent in abdominal human subcutaneous fat cells: assessment by analysis of beta- and alpha$_2$-adrenoceptors properties. *Eur J Clin Invest.* 1985;15:341–346.

30. Mauriège P, Galitzky J, Berlan M, Lafontan M. Heterogeneous distribution of beta- and alpha$_2$-adrenoceptor binding sites in human fat cells from various fat deposits: functional consequences. *Eur J Clin Invest.* 1987;17:156–165.

31. Garcia-Sainz AJ. Decreased sensitivity to alpha$_2$-adrenergic amines, adenosine and prostaglandins in white fat cells from hamsters treated with pertussis vaccine. *FEBS Lett.* 1981;126:306–308.

32. Kather H, Bieger W, Michel G, Aktories K, Jakobs KH. Human fat cell lipolysis is primarily regulated by inhibitory modulators acting through distinct mechanisms. *J Clin Invest.* 1985;76:1559–1565.

33. Thompson GE, Vernon RG. Prostaglandin E2 in adipose tissue extracellular fluid of sheep. *Exp Physiol.* 1992;77:363–367.

34. Berlan M, Montastruc J-L, Lafontan M. Pharmacological prospect for alpha$_2$-adrenoceptor antagonist therapy. *Trends Pharmacol Sci.* 1992;13:277–282.

35. Cousin B, Casteilla L, Lafontan M, et al. Local sympathetic denervation of white adipose tissue in rats induces preadipocyte proliferation without noticeable changes in metabolism. *Endocrinology.* 1993;133:2255–2262.

36. Arner P, Kriegholm E, Engfeldt P, Bolinder J. Adrenergic regulation of lipolysis in situ at rest and during exercise. *J Clin Invest.* 1990;85: 893–898.

37. Galitzky J, Lafontan M, Nordenström J, Arner P. Role of vascular alpha$_2$-adrenoceptors in regulating lipid mobilization from human adipose tissue. *J Clin Invest.* 1993;91:1997–2003.

38. Ohisalo JJ. Regulatory functions of adenosine. *Med Biol.* 1987;65: 181–191.

39. Richelsen B. Prostaglandin E2 action and binding in human adipocytes: effect of sex, age and obesity. *Metabolism.* 1988;37:268–275.

40. Castan I, Valet P, Larrouy D, et al. Distribution of PYY receptors in human fat cells: an antilipolytic system alongside the alpha$_2$-adrenergic one. *Am J Physiol.* 1993;265:E74–E80.

41. Carpéné C, Galitzky J, Saulnier-Blache J-S, Lafontan M. Selective

reduction of alpha$_2$-adrenergic responsiveness in hamster adipose tissue during prolonged starvation. *Am J Physiol.* 1990;259:E80–E88.

42. Dieudonné M-N, Pecquery R, Giudicelli Y. Characteristics of the alpha$_2$/beta-adrenoceptor-coupled adenylate cyclase system and their relationship with adrenergic responsiveness in hamster fat cells from different anatomical sites. *Eur J Biochem.* 1992;205:867–873.

43. Vanucci SJ, Klim CM, Martin LF, LaNoue KF. A1-adenosine receptor-mediated inhibition of adipocyte adenylate cyclase and lipolysis in Zucker rats. *Am J Physiol.* 1989;257:E871–E878.

44. Richelsen B, Pedersen SB, Moller-Pedersen T, Bak JF. Regional differences in triglyceride breakdown in human adipose tissue: effects of catecholamines, insulin and prostaglandin E2. *Metabolism.* 1991; 40:990–996.

45. Vikman H-L, Ohisalo JJ. Regulation of adenylate cyclase in plasma membranes of human intraabdominal and abdominal subcutaneous adipocytes. *Metabolism.* 1993;42:739–742.

46. Martin LF, Klim CM, Vannuci SJ, Dixon LB, Landis JR, LaNoue KF. Alterations in adipocyte adenylate cyclase activity in morbidly obese and formerly morbidly obese humans. *Surgery.* 1990;108:228–235.

47. Mauriège P, Després JP, Prudhomme D, *et al.* Regional variation in adipose tissue lipolysis in lean and obese men. *J Lipid Res.* 1991;32: 1625–1633.

48. Mauriège P, Després J-P, Moorjani S, *et al.* Abdominal and femoral adipose tissue lipolysis and cardiovascular disease risk factors in men. *Eur J Clin Invest.* 1993;23:729–740.

49. Wahrenberg H, Lönnqvist F, Arner P. Mechanisms underlying regional differences in lipolysis in human adipose tissue. *J Clin Invest.* 1989;84:458–467.

50. Richelsen B. Increased alpha$_2$- but similar beta-adrenergic receptor activities in subcutaneous gluteal adipocytes from females compared with males. *Eur J Clin Invest.* 1986;16:302–309.

51. Leibel RL, Hirsch J. Site and sex-related differences in adrenoceptor status in human adipose tissue. *J Clin Endocrinol Metab.* 1987;64: 1205–1210.

52. Arner P, Marcus C, Karpe B, Sonnenfeld T, Bolme P. Role of alpha-adrenoceptors for adipocyte size in man. *Eur J Clin Invest.* 1987;17: 58–62.

53. Marcus C, Karpe B, Bolme P, Sonnenfeld T, Arner P. Changes in catecholamine-induced lipolysis in isolated human fat cells during the first year of life. *J Clin Invest.* 1987;79:1812–1818.
54. Pecquery R, Giudicelli Y. Ontogenic development of alpha-adrenergic receptors and responsiveness in white adipocytes. *Biochem J.* 1980;192:947–950.
55. Lafontan M. Alpha-adrenergic responses in rabbit white fat cells: the influence of obesity and food restriction. *J Lipid Res.* 1981;22:1084–1093.
56. Berlan M, Carpéné C, Lafontan M, Dang-Tran L. Alpha$_2$-adrenergic antilipolytic effect on dog fat cells: incidence of obesity and adipose tissue localization. *Horm Metab Res.* 1982;14:257–260.
57. Carpéné C, Rebourcet M-C, Guichard C, Lafontan M. Increased alpha$_2$-adrenergic binding sites and antilipolytic effect in adipocytes from genetically obese rats. *J Lipid Res.* 1990;31:811–819.
58. Carpéné C, Berlan M, Lafontan M. Influence of development and reduction of fat stores on the antilipolytic alpha$_2$-adrenoceptor in hamster adipocytes: comparison with adenosine and beta-adrenergic lipolytic responses. *J Lipid Res.* 1983;24:766–774.
59. Saulnier-Blache J-S, Larrouy D, Carpene C, Quideau N, Dauzats M, Lafontan M. Photoperiodic control of adipocyte alpha$_2$-adrenoceptors in Syrian hamsters: role of testosterone. *Endocrinology.* 1990;127:1245–1253.
60. Pecquery R, Leneveu M-C, Giudicelli Y. Influence of androgenic status on the alpha$_2$/beta-adrenergic control of lipolysis in white fat cells: predominant alpha$_2$-antilipolytic response in testosterone-treated castrated hamsters. *Endocrinology.* 1988;122:2590–2596.
61. Saulnier-Blache J-S, Bouloumie A, Valet P, Devedjian J-C, Lafontan M. Androgenic regulation of adipocyte alpha$_2$-adrenoceptor expression in male and female Syrian hamsters: proposed transcriptional mechanism. *Endocrinology.* 1992;130:316–327.

PETER ARNER

Regulation of Lipolysis in Obesity

ABSTRACT

The regulation of lipolysis in human obesity is examined in this paper. There is an overall increase in the rate of lipolysis in adipose tissue of obese subjects when examined at rest after an overnight fast. This may explain in part the increase in the circulating levels of free fatty acids in the obese state and can be caused by a combination of increased fat cell size plus increased total mass of adipose tissue. Impaired function of antilipolytic adipocyte receptors for adenosine and prostaglandins might also be involved. Resistance to catecholamines, which are the major lipolytic hormones, is present in obesity and appears to counteract the overall increase in the rate of lipolysis. Insensitivity to the effect of lipolytic catecholamine may be of importance for excessive weight gain during caloric excess and for insufficient weight loss during caloric deprivation in subjects who are prone to develop obesity. The molecular basis of catecholamine resistance in fat cells seems to reside at multiple levels in the lipolytic cascade involving decreased function of β_2-adrenergic receptors, increased function of α_2-adrenergic receptors, and decreased ability of cyclic adenosine monophosphate to activate hormone sensitive lipase. These defects appear to be related to age, gender, and severity of the obesity. It is unclear whether resistance to the antilipolytic action of insulin is present also in obese subjects. Some data suggest that lipolytic resistance to insulin and catecholamines is more marked in upper-body obesity than in lower-body obesity. So far abnormalities in lipolysis regulation have been demonstrated only in the peripheral (*i.e.*, subcutaneous) fat depots. Lipolytic defects in the more active visceral fat region remain to be established in obese subjects. Furthermore, it is not known if abnormal regulation of lipolysis is primarily or secondarily associated with the obese state.

Introduction

It is an intriguing possibility that disturbances in lipid metabolism of obese subjects could be related to changes in turnover of triglycerides in white adipose tissue. Adipocytes in this tissue are the body's largest reservoir of triglycerides, which are synthesized through esterification of free fatty acids and hydrolyzed to glycerol and free fatty acids through the lipolytic process. Since the discovery, about forty years ago, that adipose tissue is a metabolically active organ, there has been a continuous search for a defect in the turnover of triglycerides in white fat cells, which could be linked to obesity. These studies have focused on lipolysis, which is relatively easy to measure, since the end products—free fatty acids and glycerol—can be quantified. The synthesis of triglycerides, on the other hand, has received less attention perhaps because the synthesis can not be directly quantified.

The regulation of lipolysis has been studied in obese humans and in several animal models of obesity. Although multiple defects have been demonstrated in dogs (1), mice (2, 3) and rats (4), earlier studies of lipolysis in human obesity have yielded conflicting results. In a review published in 1988 it was concluded that there were no apparent defects in lipolytic regulation in humans (5). However, new methods have been developed since then to study lipolysis in vivo and in vitro in humans. The results of these studies will be reviewed in some detail in order to re-evaluate the possibility that lipolytic regulation might be altered in the adipose tissue of obese human subjects.

Regulation of Lipolysis in Humans

The regulation of lipolysis in human fat cells is in many ways different from that in laboratory animals. There is a marked in vitro lipolytic activity of human fat cells when they are incubated in the absence of lipolytic agents. This is in contrast to fat cells of most other species, which show very low basal rates of lipolysis. Numerous studies have shown that the basal lipolytic rate of human fat cells strongly depends on fat cell size (5). Large cells have a higher rate than small ones. The mechanisms responsible for basal lipolysis are unknown. On the other hand, this lipolytic activity may just be an artifact. The basal rate is much lower in isolated fat cells than in fragments of adipose tissue (6). This can be caused by altered metabolism of cyclic adenosine monophosphate (cAMP) (6) and purines (7) during the collagenase isolation procedure, which may cause artificial changes in the spontaneous lipolytic activity of fat cells. Large cells may be more sensitive to these alterations than small cells.

Another important species difference is that catecholamines are the only hormones with a pronounced lipolytic activity in adult human fat cells (5). In most other species a number of additional hormones have marked lipolytic effects. Catecholamines regulate lipolysis through four different receptor subtypes, which are the stimulatory β_1, β_2, and β_3 and the inhibitory α_2. As reviewed (8), the activity of α_2 receptors is very strong in human fat cells so that the lipolytic action of the naturally occurring catecholamines (noradrenaline and adrenaline) is much less in man than in several other species. As regards the β receptors it is well established that human fat cells possess fully functional β_1- and β_2-adrenoceptors, but it is unclear at present if these two receptors have different or equal importance for lipolytic regulation (8). It is a matter of debate if the recently cloned β_3 receptor is of importance for human lipolysis since no (9, 10), small (11), or marked (12) lipolytic effects of β_3 receptor agonists have been demonstrated in human fat cells.

Quite in contrast to lipolytic stimulation, a number of hormones and parahormones can inhibit lipolysis in human fat cells. These include insulin, prostaglandins, adenosine, insulin-like growth factors, and neuropeptide Y. Because of the existence of few lipolytic but many antilipolytic regulatory systems it has been suggested that lipolysis in human fat cells is under chronic tonic inhibition and is above all stimulated by relief of endogenous inhibition (13).

Basal Lipolysis in Obesity

Numerous studies have shown that after an overnight fast the turnover rates of free fatty acids and glycerol in vivo as well as the basal release of glycerol from fat cells in vitro are increased in obese subjects (5). These effects of obesity on basal lipolysis, however, may be more apparent than real. When the influence of fat cell size, which is increased in obesity, is taken into account, most of the differences in the in vitro rate of basal lipolysis between lean and obese subjects disappear (5). The same is true in vivo. Thus, the influx of glycerol and free fatty acids to the circulation after an overnight fast is increased by total body mass in obese subjects but normal or even decreased when expressed per kilogram of fat mass (14–16). A recent attempt was made to directly estimate the rate of basal lipolysis in vivo in subcutaneous adipose tissue by combining a microdialysis technique to determine the extra-cellular concentration of glycerol with a Xenon washout technique to determine blood flow (17). It was demonstrated that the rate of glycerol release was increased when expressed per fat cell but normal when expressed per adipose tissue weight in obesity.

Thus, when earlier and recent data are considered together it appears that the basal rate of lipolysis, whether determined in vivo or in vitro, is increased in obesity because of a mass effect. Thus, the rate is accelerated mainly because fat cell size is enlarged and the total fat mass is expanded in obese subjects. When these differences between lean and obese are taken into account there appear to be none, or minor, differences in the basal rates of lipolysis. It should, however, be borne in mind that additional defects in the utilization of lipids (not dealt with in this review) might cause a further elevation of circulating free fatty acids in the basal state in obesity.

Antilipolytic Mechanisms in Obesity

The effect of insulin, which is the major antilipolytic hormone, has been intensively examined in obese subjects in the past (5). Those earlier investigations have shown conflicting results. Evidence for increased, decreased, or normal antilipolytic effect has been presented in vivo and in vitro. Even recent in vivo data are conflicting. In one study insulin was infused in graded doses under euglycemic conditions and free fatty acid production rate was determined (15). A normal sensitivity to the antilipolytic of insulin was observed in obese subjects. In two other investigations it was observed that, during infusion of a constant insulin dose as well as postprandially (when there is insulin excess), free fatty acid production rates were elevated in upper-body obese subjects as compared to lean subjects (18, 19). There may be many reasons for the conflicting results. The optimal conditions for investigating the antilipolytic effect of insulin are not yet established. Insulin has complex interactions with catecholamines in human fat cells, and the antilipolytic sensitivity depends on the prevailing catecholamine concentration (20). These interactions between the two major counteracting hormone systems have not been considered in previous lipolytic studies in obesity. Furthermore, the antilipolytic effect of insulin in human fat cells is governed by the availability of glucose, and different results are obtained when fat cells are obtained before as compared with after glucose ingestion in obese and normal subjects (21). Finally, there might be regional variations in the antilipolytic effect of insulin as discussed below. It should be noted, however, that the results with antilipolysis and obesity are quite different from those concerning glucose transport and obesity. As discussed in detail (22) the latter results uniformly show decreased ability of insulin to stimulate glucose transport in fat cells of obese subjects.

Other antilipolytic effects besides those of insulin have also been investigated in obesity. The antilipolytic actions of prostaglandins and adenosine are decreased in vitro in obese subjects (23, 24). However, these data must be interpreted with caution because prostaglandins and adenosine, as well as insulin, have complex interactions with the counteracting catecholamines (25). This cross talk between lipolytic and antilipolytic pathways has not been evaluated in obesity.

Thus, it is still an open question whether or not the antilipolytic effect of insulin is altered in obesity. Although the antilipolytic effects of prostaglandins and adenosine might be impaired in obese subjects, the pathophysiological meaning of those defects are unclear at present, as discussed in detail recently (26). The clinical use of drugs that interact with prostaglandins and adenosine, such as methylxanthines and salicylic acid, seems to have little or no effect on body weight regulation. In theory, however, impaired function of receptors for prostaglandins and adenosine might play a role in the overall (basal) increase in lipolysis after an overnight fast.

Catecholamine Action

Until recently surprisingly little has been known about the catecholamine-induced lipolysis in obese subjects (5). During the last few years three independent in vivo studies have been published showing decreased lipolytic response to catecholamine infusions in obese as compared with lean subjects (14, 27, 28). One study also presented data regarding the lipolytic response to short-term fasting, which is a state of sympathetic activation. In normal subjects the in vivo production of lipolytic markers rose markedly with 87 hours of fasting, whereas the increase was modest in obese subjects (27).

There is also new information about catecholamine action in vitro in subcutaneous abdominal fat cells of obese subjects. In adipocytes of women with uncomplicated upper-body obesity, decreased lipolytic sensitivity to noradrenaline was observed, which was attributed to a posttranscriptional decrease in the β_2-adrenoceptor expression (29). Other adrenoceptors and postadrenoceptor activation of lipolysis were normal in these cells. When elderly men with so-called metabolic syndrome (upper-body obesity, glucose intolerance, insulin resistance, and hyperinsulinemia) were investigated, multiple defects in catecholamine-induced lipolysis were observed in the fat cells (30). The lipolytic noradrenaline resistance was almost complete. It was due to the same β_2-receptor defect as described above in combination with decreased ability of cAMP to activate hormone-sensitive lipase. Finally, lipolytic adrenaline resistance in adipocytes from young men with uncomplicated obesity also has been demonstrated (31). This defect was solely ascribed to an increased α_2-adrenergic response. Beta receptors were reported to be normal in the obese subjects. The observed defects of adrenoceptor function in these studies correlated with body-mass index (29, 31). The different lipolytic abnormalities in adipocytes of obese subjects might be related to gender and age. As discussed in detail (32) catecholamine-induced lipolysis differs between men and women. These sex-related variations are localized at the level of adrenoceptor function in fat cells. In addition, lipolytic catecholamine resistance due to the inability of cAMP to activate hormone-sensitive lipase is observed in abdominal fat cells of elderly healthy nonobese male subjects as compared with young ones (33).

In summary, when recent in vivo and in vitro data are considered together it is clear that lipolytic catecholamine resistance is present in abdominal subcutaneous adipocytes of obese subjects. This defect might be involved in the development of overweight and resistance to sliming in certain individuals. The mechanisms appear above all to involve the function of adrenoceptors (decreased β_2, increased α_2) and can be gender related. However, additional defects, which are located at the final step in lipolysis activation (hormone-sensitive lipase) also might be present in more severe cases of obesity, at least in elderly male subjects.

Heterogeneity of Obesity and Adipose Tissue Metabolism

It is well known that not all human obesity is the same. Upper body obesity, which is more frequent among men than women, has a strong association with the metabolic and cardiovascular complications of overweight. Lower-body obesity, which is more often observed in women than in men, is less harmful regarding these complications. So far, only a few studies have compared lipolytic regulation in different types of obesity. Greater in vivo resistance to the antilipolytic effect of insulin and to the lipolytic effect of catecholamines is found in upper-body obesity as compared with lower-body obesity (19, 28). The basal rate of free fatty acid release was higher in upper-body obese subjects than in normal or lower-body obese subjects (19). These data may suggest that abnormalities in lipolytic regulation are more apparent in upper-body-obese subjects than in lower-body-obese subjects.

Another important aspect in the regulation of lipolysis in obesity is the existence of regional differences in lipolytic activity, which has recently been reviewed in detail (34). The lipolytic activity is low in peripheral subcutaneous adipose tissue, intermediate in the subcutaneous abdominal site, and high in the visceral adipose regions. The site differences can be attributed to regional variations in the function of insulin receptors and adrenoceptors of fat cells. As far as I know, only one study has been published so far dealing with regional aspects of lipolysis in obese versus nonobese subjects (31). Normal catecholamine-induced lipolysis in femoral subcutaneous fat cells but decreased hormone response in subcutaneous abdominal fat cells was found in young obese men. Regarding regional aspects of lipolysis, it would be of greater interest to study the visceral region than to compare various subcutaneous sites. It is increasingly apparent that release of free fatty acids to the portal system through lipolysis in visceral fat cells is of major importance for several of the metabolic complications to upper-body obesity as reviewed in detail (35).

Are Lipolytic Defects Primary or Secondary to Obesity?

In order to understand the pathophysiology of obesity it is essential to find out whether metabolic abnormalities precede the disease or develop as secondary phenomenon. So far, little is known about this aspect of lipolytic regulation in obesity. In three studies, subcutaneous adipose tissue was obtained from obese subjects before and after their weight was partly normalized (but stabilized) following dieting or gastrointestinal anti-obesity surgery (36–38). Basal- and noradrenaline-induced rates of lipolysis were reduced, the antilipolytic effect of adenosine was improved, but the antilipolytic effect of insulin was unchanged in vitro after body weight reduction. In another study, the in vivo lipolytic response to catecholamines was increased in formerly obese subjects as compared with never-obese subjects (39).

It is hard to draw any firm conclusions regarding primary and secondary events in lipolytic regulation in obese subjects on the basis of the data discussed above. Obviously more investigations are needed. This might include family studies, longitudinal studies, and investigations on obese subjects before and after complete normalization of body weight.

Conclusions

The results of several recent studies suggest that at least two abnormalities are observed in the regulation of lipolysis in obese subjects. These lipolytic defects are probably more common in upper-body obesity than in lower-body obesity. First, there is an increased rate of lipolysis in the resting state (*i.e.*, after an overnight fast). This is largely due to a mass effect, because fat cell volume and total fat mass are increased in obesity. Resistance to the antilipolytic effects of prostaglandins and adenosine might also play a role in this acceleration of the rate of lipolysis. The increase of circulating free fatty acids, which often is observed in obese subjects, could partly be explained by an overall enhancement of the lipolysis in the resting state.

The second defect involves catecholamine action and is so far established only in the abdominal subcutaneous region. Lipolytic catecholamine resistance is present in obese subjects. This is above all due to abnormalities in adipocyte adrenoceptor function, which may be gender related. Beta$_2$ receptor function is decreased in obese women. Alpha$_2$ receptor function is increased in young obese men. These adrenoceptor-related abnormalities of catecholamine function can be of importance for the development of overweight and may cause resistance to slimming in some obese subjects. In elderly upper-body-obese subjects with complications to obesity (*i.e.*, the so-called metabolic or insulin-resistance syndrome), the lipolytic resistance to catecholamines is even more marked, which presumably is caused by additional defects in hormone sensitive lipase.

Whether abnormalities in lipolysis regulation are present also in visceral adipose tissue in obese subjects is unclear yet. In addition, the question of whether the antilipolytic effect of insulin is altered in obesity is not settled. Another open question is whether the abnormalities in lipolytic regulation are primary or secondary to the obese state.

ACKNOWLEDGMENTS

This study was supported by grants from the Swedish Medical Research Council and by Medicus Bromma Company.

REFERENCES

1. Taosis M, Valet P, Estan L, Lafontan M, Montastruc P, Berlan M. Obesity modifies the adrenergic status of dog adipose tissue. *J Pharmacol Exp Ther.* 1989;250:1061–1066.

2. Shepherd RE, Malbon CC, Smith CJ, Fain JN. Lipolysis and adenosine 3′, 5′-monophosphate metabolism in isolated white fat cells from genetically obese hyperglycaemic mice (*ob/ob*). *J Biol Chem.* 1977;252:7243–7248.

3. Bégin-Heick N. The response of adenylate cyclase to ACTH in adipocyte membranes of lean and obese mice. *Mol Cell Endocrinol.* 1987;53:1–8.

4. Muzzin P, Revelli JP, Kuhne F, *et al.* An adipose tissue-specific β-adrenergic receptor: molecular cloning and down-regulation in obesity. *J Biol Chem.* 1991;266:24053–24058.

5. Arner P. Control of lipolysis and its relevance to development of obesity in man. *Diabetes Metab Rev.* 1988;4:507–515.

6. Engfeldt P, Arner P, Ostman J. Influence of adipocyte isolation by collagenase on phosphodiesterase activity and lipolysis in man. *J Lipid Res.* 1980;21:443–448.

7. Kather H. Purine accumulation in human fat cell suspensions. *J Biol Chem.* 1988;263:8803–8809.

8. Lafontan M, Berlan M. Fat cell adrenergic receptors and the control of white and brown fat cell function. *J Lipid Res.* 1993;34:1057–1092.

9. Langin D, Portillo MP, Saulnier-Blache J-S, Lafontan M. Coexistence of three β-adrenoceptor subtypes in white fat cells of various mammalian species. *Eur J Pharmacol.* 1991;199:291–301.

10. Rosenbaum M, Malbon CC, Hirsch J, Leibel RL. Lack of β$_3$-adrenergic effect on lipolysis in human subcutaneous adipose tissue. *J Clin Endocrinol Metab.* 1993;77:352–355.

11. Hollenga C, Brouwer F, Zaagsma J. Differences in functional cyclic AMP compartments mediating lipolysis by isoprenaline and BRL 37344 in four adipocyte types. *Eur J Pharmacol.* 1991;200:325–330.

12. Lönnqvist F, Krief S, Strosberg AD, Nyberg B, Emorine LJ, Arner P. Evidence for a functional β_3-adrenergic receptor in man. *Br J Pharmacol.* 1993;110:929–936.

13. Kather H, Bieger W, Michel G, Aktories K, Jakobs KH. Human fat cell lipolysis is primarly regulated by inhibitory modulators acting through distinct mechanisms. *J Clin Invest.* 1985;76:1559–1565.

14. Connacher AA, Bennet WM, Jung RT, *et al.* Effect of adrenaline infusion on fatty acid and glucose turnover in lean and obese human subjects in post-absorptive and fed states. *Clin Sci.* 1991;81: 635–644.

15. Groop LC, Saloranta C, Shank M, Bonadonna RC, Ferrannini E, DeFronzo RA. The role of free fatty acid metabolism in the pathogenesis of insulin resistance in obesity and noninsulin-dependent diabetes mellitus. *J Clin Endocrinol Metab.* 1991;72:96–107.

16. Le Stunff C, Bougnères PF. Glycerol production and utilization during the early phase of human obesity. *Diabetes.* 1992;41:444–450.

17. Jansson P-A, Larsson A, Smith U, Lönnroth P. Glycerol production in subcutaneous adipose tissue in lean and obese humans. *J Clin Invest.* 1992;89:1610–1617.

18. Jensen MD. Regulation of forearm lipolysis in different types of obesity. *J Clin Invest.* 1991;87:187–193.

19. Roust LR, Jensen MD. Postprandial free fatty acid kinetics are abnormal in upper body obesity. *Diabetes.* 1993;42:1567–1573.

20. Engfeldt P, Hellmér J, Wahrenberg H, Arner P. Effects of insulin adrenoceptor binding and the rate of catecholamine-induced lipolysis in isolated human fat cells. *J Biol Chem.* 1988;263:15553–15560.

21. Arner P, Bolinder J, Engfeldt P, Hellmér J, Ostman J. Influence of obesity on the antilipolytic effect of insulin in isolated human fat cells obtained before and after glucose ingestion. *J Clin Invest.* 1984; 73:673–680.

22. Foley JE. Mechanisms of impaired insulin action in isolated adipocytes from obese and diabetic subjects. *Diabetes Metab Rev.* 1988; 4:487–505.

23. Richelsen B. Prostaglandin E_2 action and binding in human adipocytes: effects of sex, age and obesity. *Metabolism.* 1988;37:268–275.

24. Ohisalo JJ, Ranta S, Huhtaniemi IT. Attenuated adenosine R-site effect in adipocytes in obesity. *Metabolism.* 1988;35:143–146.

25. Lönnqvist F, Arner P. Interactions between adenylate cyclase inhibitors and beta-adrenoceptors in isolated human fat cells. *Biochem Biophys Res Commun.* 1989;161:654–660.

26. Arner P. Adenosine, prostaglandins and phosphodiesterase as targets for obesity pharmacotherapy. *Int J Obes.* 1993;17:S57–S59.

27. Wolfe RR, Peters EJ, Klein S, Holland OB, Rosenblatt J, Gary H. Effect of short-term fasting on lipolytic responsiveness in normal and obese human subjects. *Am J Physiol.* 1987;2523:E189–E196.

28. Jensen MD, Haymond MW, Rizza RA, Cryer PE, Miles JM. Influence of body fat distribution on free fatty acid metabolism in obesity. *J Clin Invest.* 1989;83:1168–1173.

29. Reynisdottir S, Wahrenberg H, Carlström K, Rössner S, Arner P. Catecholamine resistance in fat cells of women with upper-body obesity due to decreased expression of beta$_2$-adrenoceptors. *Diabetologia.* 1994;37:428–435.

30. Reynisdottir S, Ellerfeldt K, Wahrenberg H, Lithell H, Arner P. Multiple lipolysis defects in the insulin resistance (metabolic) syndrome. *J Clin Invest.* 1994;93:2590–2599.

31. Mauriège P, Després JP, Prud'homme D, *et al.* Regional variation in adipose tissue lipolysis in lean and obese men. *J Lipid Res.* 1991;32: 1625–1633.

32. Bouchard C, Després J-P, Mauriége P. Genetic and nongenetic determinants of regional fat distribution. *Endocr Rev.* 1993;14:72–93.

33. Lönnqvist F, Nyberg B, Wahrenberg H, Arner P. Catecholamine-induced lipolysis in adipose tissue of the elderly. *J Clin Invest.* 1990; 85:1614–1621.

34. Leibel RL, Edens NK, Fried SK. Physiologic basis for the control of body fat distribution in humans. *Annu Rev Nutr.* 1989;9:417–443.

35. Björntorp P. Metabolic implications of body fat distribution. *Diabetes Care.* 1991;14:1132–1143.

36. Smith U, Hammersten J, Björntorp P, Kral JG. Regional differences and effect of weight reduction on human fat cell metabolism. *Eur J Clin Invest.* 1979;9:327–332.

37. Sörbris R, Petersson B-G, Nilsson-Ehle P. Effects of weight reduction on plasma lipoproteins and adipose tissue metabolism in obese subjects. *Eur J Clin Invest.* 1981;11:491–498.

38. Ohisalo JJ, Kaartinen JM, Ranta S, *et al.* Weight loss normalizes the

inhibitory effect of N^6-(phenylisopropyl)adenosine on lipolysis in fat cells of massively obese human subjects. *Clin Sci.* 1992;83:589–592.

39. Leibel R, Berry EM, Hirsch J. Metabolic and hemodynamic response to endogenous and exogenous catecholamines in formerly obese subjects. *Am J Physiol.* 1991;29:R785–R791.

PART V

Genetics of Human Obesity

R. ARLEN PRICE

Obesity Genes in Human Populations

ABSTRACT

Previous research suggests that there are several relatively rare genes that have significant effects in particular families. Common genes are likely to have less pronounced effects, and the inherited polygenic background against which single obesity genes segregate will be made up of many genes with smaller quantitative effects. Animal studies suggest that most human variation in obesity could be accounted for by as few as six to ten of these genes. Studies aimed at identifying obesity-predisposing genes should adopt strategies that take into account genetic heterogeneity, varying gene-effect sizes, and environmentally mediated gene penetrance and expression. One design that appears to be robust in the face of such complexities requires the sampling of families with at least two extremely obese siblings and at least one normal-weight parent and a normal-weight adult sibling. Simulation studies indicate this combination of phenotypes maximizes gene segregation and thus information for linkage under a wide range of models of inheritance. Power calculations are presented indicating that African-American families show particular promise for identifying obesity genes. Candidate gene approaches will be most promising if a homologous gene or region has been identified in an animal model.

Genetics of Human Obesity

Genes play a major role in determining proneness to obesity (1). Family, twin, and adoption studies indicate that genes also play a role in determining levels of fatness or thinness in the normal range (2–5). In adults, environmental influences appear to originate outside the family (4–5), and genes mediate response to the environment (6). Obesity associated with single-gene mutations in animals and chromosome abnormalities in humans indicate that disruption or deletion of single genes or several contiguous genes can result in obesity, even in the absence of special obesity-promoting diets (1, 7–8). Multigene models of obesity depend on both genotype and exposure to high-fat diets (9). These studies indicate that genes influence proneness to obesity across a broad range of fat and thin phenotypes and possess a range of susceptibility to the environmental influences of diet and exercise.

Single-gene effects are apparent for certain animal obesity mutants and are suggested even for some human syndromes (1). Moreover, several segregation studies suggest a recessive mode of inheritance for normal variation in obesity (1–2). The recessive pattern could be due in part to temporal increases in prevalence and level of obesity between generations in Pima Indians (10–11). However, new segregation analyses show that the recessive pattern, whether due to single or multiple genes, cannot be explained completely by obesity increases following World War II, as appears to be the case for Pima Indians (11). The recessive pattern is particularly strong in African-Americans, and the major gene accounted for more variance. We may even speculate that there could be common recessive genes for obesity in humans, for example, homologous to the *ob* and other obesity mutations in the mouse. It would be fortunate indeed if this were true, for the power to detect linkage is greatest under the recessive model. In any case, no single model can explain the inheritance of obesity in all families, and it is likely that several different genes are needed to account for most human variation (1).

Gene locus and allele effect sizes are likely to vary considerably. In rare cases of extreme obesity that is independent of diet, there may well be genes with large effects that account for most of the risk for obesity in the families in which they are segregating. This is a heterogeneity model. These genes would be analogous to obesity mutants such as *ob* and *fa* or chromosome abnormalities such as the Prader-Willi syndrome. More common genes may have relatively smaller effects and are likely to be diet dependent and act in combination with other genes in either an additive (oligogenic model) or interactive (epistatic model) manner. These genes could be causes of diet-sensitive obesity in animals (9) and may account for cases of extreme obesity in human families. Genes accounting for variation of body fatness within the normal range are likely to be more numerous and to have smaller individual effects (polygenic model). On the other hand, mapping studies of quantitative traits in plants and animals suggest that even for obesity that is polygenic in origin only a few genes (say, six to ten) could account for most variation (12).

Obesity genes causing common forms of obesity appear to depend on diet for expression. The rationale for this assertion comes in part from the high prevalence of obesity and in part from the parallel temporal changes in obesity, diet, and exercise (1, 10) over the last half century. Together, these observations suggest common obesity genes that have become increasingly penetrant with modern living conditions (1, 10). Currently, it is impossible to know just how many genes with each magnitude of effect are present, but as noted, several single-gene obesities have been identified already in animals, and additional genes probably contribute significantly to common human obesities and to normal variation in levels and distribution of body fat.

Previous research has not been able to resolve the number and type of genes involved in common forms of obesity. However, the studies do suggest hypotheses that are necessary to guide linkage, biochemical, and molecular genetic studies. Genetic linkage studies of obesity should exercise care that the sampling and analytic methods selected are compatible and the approaches chosen maximize the efficiency of the search for human obesity genes that differ in patterns of inheritance and expression.

Optimal Selection Strategies for Linkage Studies

One possible sampling design is as follows. Selecting families with extreme obesity (for example, at least 80% overweight in one individual and 50% overweight in another) and some normal-weight individuals (for example, at least one parent and one adult sibling who never have been more than 20% overweight) will optimize the probability of genetic differences *between families* as well as maximize gene segregation *within families* under a range of modes of inheritance. Focusing only on the obese siblings within such families will avoid problems associated with reduced gene penetrance and expression due to genetic background and environmental conditions. However, our simulation studies have shown that inclusion of a normal-weight adult sibling also increases gene segregation and thus information for linkage analyses. Utilizing a sibling design also makes it feasible to use analytic methods that do not require genetic homogeneity among families. This family sampling design should be useful for identifying genes with a wide range of effect sizes from major genes to quantitative trait loci, since power will depend on sample size and not on idiosyncrasies of specific family structures.

GENDER AND ETHNICITY

Obesity is more prevalent in women than in men (13, 14). Whereas obesity is a problem for women in virtually all Western and developing countries, it particularly affects certain groups. The prevalence and extent of obesity are higher in African-American women and in American Indians. African-Americans have a high admixture (15) (about 26%) with American whites and a large difference in prevalence of obesity. The high level and prevalence of obesity in the ascertained families assure that they have both the genetic and dietary factors needed for obesity (necessary and sufficient genetic and environmental factors). An increased variance in African-American women, the extremely obese phenotypes in ascertained families, the high level of genetic admixture, and the requirement that at least one parent and one adult sibling never were even moderately overweight (lifetime body mass index [BMI] $< 27\text{kg}/\text{m}^2$) all maximize the segregation of genes that vary *within and between populations.* There are also ethnic differences in inheritance patterns. Based on our recent studies, recessive major-gene inheritance appears stronger (accounts for more variance) and polygenic inheritance weaker (accounts for less variance) in the African-American families compared with whites. Onset appears to be later and bimodal in African-American families and earlier and unimodal in whites.

POWER

Forty-one African-American families who meet the selection criteria described above have been identified. Simulations have been completed on those family structures expanded to a total sample of 165 families. For the nonparametric sibling pair analyses, a qualitative classification (fat vs normal) and use only "affected" sibling pairs were used. Using a threshold BMI of 33, and a total sample size of 165 sibships, 559 affected siblings were projected. By controlling for nonindependence of pairs in sibships with 3 or more affected (16), these families provided 409 sibling pair-equivalents. The overall best-fitting model (recessive) from segregation analyses of African-American families (17, and new analyses within birth cohort) applied to transformed data was used to estimate gene frequency and penetrances for each genotype (calculated as the proportion of each theoretical genotypic distribution above the chosen BMI threshold). The number of sibling pairs needed to detect linkage was estimated using equations published by Suarez and others (18) with fully informative markers. Power was estimated under two sets of assumptions: Level 1, screening, alpha 0.01 (similar to a logarithm of odds [LOD] score of 2), 80% power, distance 5 centimorgans (cM) (5% recombination); Level 2, confirmation, alpha 0.001 (similar to a LOD score of 3), 80% power, distance 1 cM (1% recombination). In all cases, linkage was detected, even if only a portion of the families are linked (about 7% for recessive genes and 20% for dominant or additive genes). These results confirm observations of Lander and Botstein (11) and Carey and Williamson (19), who reported that sample size may be dramatically reduced by sampling only the distribution tails of a quantitative trait in segregating F1 backcross and F2 progeny. It appears that the high values were achieved in these simulations because the method of sampling and model parameters used give a high probability of parental segregation. This level of power should allow investigators to detect obesity predisposing genes at the boundary between major genes and quantitative trait loci (QTL) determining polygenic variation in overall fatness. By using all the information available in the quantitative phenotypes and highly polymorphic markers, it should be possible to detect linkage with random markers, even in the presence of substantial heterogeneity.

Whenever there is genetic heterogeneity, the central question for parametric (LOD score) analyses is whether there is sufficient power to detect the heterogeneity (see 20). This is because all LOD scores may sum across families to equal zero or a negative number, even when a subset of the families is closely linked to the marker. For the parametric analyses, SIMLINK (21) was used to simulate four allele markers linked at a distance of 1 cM or 5 cM to a gene influencing BMI. For the multiplex nuclear families, three models were assumed: the genetic model supported in a sample of African-Americans (17, and previously unpublished analyses within birth cohort), and dominant and additive models that were devised to account for the uppermost component group in analyses of the same samples [*i.e.,* q^2(recessive) = 2pq(dominant) = 2pq(additive)].

Since the most reasonable hypothesis for a random marker is that it is not linked to an obesity gene, power to detect heterogeneity was examined assuming a recombination value of 50% for the majority of families, that is, in which the maximum LOD score would be near zero in the combined sample of all families (about .11 at 44–49 cM). Thus, evidence for linkage will come only from a positive test of heterogeneity. Here again power was calculated under two sets of assumptions: Level 1, screening, alpha 0.01 (similar to a LOD score of 2), 80% power, distance 5 cM (5% recombination); Level 2, confirmation, alpha 0.001 (similar to a LOD score of 3), 80% power, distance 1 cM (1% recombination). In all cases, heterogeneity was detected even with only 3% of the families being linked to the marker. As with the sibling analyses, the high power in analyses of nuclear families appears to have been achieved because the sampling design assures both extreme genotypes and gene segregation.

Finally, under a heterogeneity model segregation of a single gene should be apparent in at least some individual families. If instead gene effects are summed to generate the phenotype, sibling phenotypes will be affected by segregation at multiple gene loci. Simulations by Carey and Williamson (19) indicate that one should be able to detect linkage to such an additive gene if it accounts for as much as 20% to 25% of the variance. All these power calculations assumed no interaction of loci. If this assumption is violated, then power is greatly reduced. The main loss of information, however, should be from the unaffected individuals, just as with the heterogeneity model.

Overall, the results of simulations are encouraging. Existing samples or those currently being collected by several investigators should provide power to detect genes segregating in as few as 3% of families under a heterogeneity model or accounting for as little as 20% to 25% of the total variance under a polygenic (QTL) model.

Mapping Strategies

Genome searches aimed at finding linkage between obesity and random genetic markers offer the best strategy for mapping obesity genes. More biologically based "candidate gene" approaches have intuitive appeal, but in most cases they will be inefficient because of the complexity of the "candidate" biological systems (1). The best candidates for mapping obesity genes in humans will be homologous genes or chromosome regions linked to obesity in animals (see 7–9).

Conclusions

Overall, previous research suggests that there are several relatively rare genes that have significant effects in particular families. Common genes are likely to have less pronounced effects, and the inherited polygenic background against which single obesity genes segregate will be made up of many genes with smaller quantitative effects. Studies aimed at identifying obesity-predisposing genes should adopt strategies that take into account genetic heterogeneity, varying gene-effect sizes, and environmentally mediated gene penetrance and expression. One design that appears to be robust in the face of such complexities requires the sampling of families with at least two extremely obese siblings with one normal-weight parent and a normal-weight adult sibling. Power calculations are presented indicating that African-American families show particular promise for identifying obesity genes. Finally, random gene mapping approaches to identifying obesity-predisposing genes appear to have greater efficiency than more biologically intuitive candidate gene approaches. Candidate gene approaches can work if a homologous gene or region has been identified in an animal model.

ACKNOWLEDGMENTS

The research for this paper was supported in part by National Institutes of Health Grant number RO1-DK44073. Thanks to Dr. Danielle Reed for useful comments on an earlier draft.

REFERENCES

1. Price RA. The case for single gene effects on human obesity. In: Bouchard C, ed. *The Genetics of Obesity.* Boca Raton, Florida: CRC Press; 1994. In press.
2. Price RA, Ness R, Laskarzewski P. Common major gene inheritance of extreme overweight. *Hum Biol.* 1990;62:747–765.
3. Price RA, Gottesman II. Body fat in Shields' cohort of identical twins reared apart. *Behav Genet.* 1991;21:1–7.

4. Price RA, Cadoret RJ, Stunkard AJ, Troughton E. Genetic contributions to human fatness: an adoption study. *Am J Psychol.* 1987; 144:1003–1008.

5. Sørensen TIA, Price RA, Stunkard AJ, Schulsinger F. Genetics of obesity in adult adoptees and their biological siblings. *Br Med J.* 1989;298:87–90.

6. Bouchard C, Tremblay A, Després J-P, *et al.* The response to long-term overfeeding in identical twins. *N Engl J Med.* 1990;322:1477–1482.

7. Friedman JM, Leibel RL, Bahary N. Molecular mapping of the mouse ob mutation. *Mammalian Genome.* 1991;1:130–144.

8. Johnson PR, Greenwood MRC, Horwitz BA, Stern JS. Animal models of obesity: genetic aspects. *Annu Rev Nutr.* 1991;11:325–353.

9. West DB, Waguespack J, Price RA. A genetic model for the control of dietary obesity in AKR/J and SWR/J mice. *Mammalian Genome.* 1994;4: under revision following peer review.

10. Price RA, Charles MA, Pettitt DJ, Knowler WC. Obesity in Pima Indians: large increases among post-World War II birth cohorts. *Am J Phys Anthropol.* 1993;92:473–479.

11. Price RA, Charles MA, Pettitt DJ, Knowler WC. Obesity in Pima Indians: genetic segregation analysis of human obesity complicated by temporal increases in obesity. *Hum Biol.* 1994;66:249–272.

12. Lander ES, Botstein D. Mapping Mendelian factors underlying quantitative traits using RFLP linkage maps. *Genetics.* 1989;121:185–199.

13. Dawson DA. Ethnic differences in female overweight: data from the 1985 National Health Interview Survey. *Am J Public Health.* 1988; 78:1326–1329.

14. Pi-Sunyer FX. Obesity in black Americans. *Diabetes Care.* 1990;13:1144–1149.

15. Chakraborty R, Kamboh MI, Ferrell RE. "Unique" alleles in admixed populations: a strategy for determining "heredity" population differences of disease frequencies. *Ethnic Dis.* 1991;1:245–256.

16. Hodge SE. The information contained in multiple sib pairs. *Genet Epidemiol.* 1984;1:109–122.

17. Ness R, Laskarzewski P, Price RA. Inheritance of extreme overweight in black families. *Hum Biol.* 1991;63:39–52.

18. Suarez BK, Rice J, Reich T. The generalized sib pair IBD distribu-

tion: its use in the detection of linkage. *Ann Hum Genet.* 1978;42: 87–94.

19. Carey G, Williamson J. Linkage analysis of quantitative traits: increased power by using selected samples. *Am J Hum Genet.* 1991; 49:786–796.

20. Cavalli-Sforza LL, King MC. Detecting linkage for genetically heterogeneous diseases and detecting heterogeneity with linkage data. *Am J Hum Genet.* 1986;38:599–616.

21. Ploughman LM, Boehnke M. Estimating the power of a proposed linkage study for a complex genetic trait. *Am J Hum Genet.* 1989;44: 543–551.

THORKILD IA SØRENSEN

Adoption Studies of Obesity

ABSTRACT

Adoption studies have been among the most useful methods of assessing the genetic and environmental influences on human obesity. Resemblance of the adoptee and the members of the adoptive family reflects the effects of the shared family environment, and resemblance of the adoptee and the biological family is due to shared genes (assuming no effect of the shared preadoptive environment). Six partial adoption studies, in which there is no information from the biological relatives of the adoptees, have been carried out: genetic influence is estimated by the difference in the resemblance of the adoptees and the members of the adoptive family and the resemblance of members of natural families (different families or biologically related members of the adoptive families). These studies, all addressing obesity in childhood or adolescence, have produced conflicting results. One Danish and one American study using the complete adoption method agree that there is a strong genetic influence on adult obesity, which fully explains the familial resemblance. The Danish and another American study both showed a similar strong genetic influence in childhood, but only the Danish one suggested in addition that the rearing environment has a weak influence on childhood obesity. In view of the methodological properties of the partial versus the complete adoption studies, it may be concluded that there is strong evidence for a genetic influence that accounts for most, if not all, familial resemblance in human obesity.

The interest in the genetic aspects of obesity must be viewed on the background of the obvious strong environmental influence. The evidence for this stems from the observed spontaneous changes in the occurrence of obesity both within populations and within individuals over time as well as the changes induced by environmental manipulation in populations, clinical settings, and laboratories (1). On the other hand, many studies in different populations have shown a remarkable stability of familial resemblance in various obesity measures (1). The parent-offspring correlations are in the range of 0.15 to 0.25, the full sibling correlations between 0.25 and 0.35. Such familial resemblance may be due to genes shared by relationship, but shared exposure to environmental factors, or a combination of shared genes and shared exposure to environmental factors, may be operating as well.

The observation of a familial resemblance usually raises the question about the heritability, which is assumed to be a measure of the strength or importance of the genetic influence. Strictly speaking, the heritability, h^2, as estimated statistically is a measure of the proportion of the interindividual within-population variance of the phenotype, here the measure of obesity, that can be ascribed to the variance between individuals in the effect of their genes. There are several theoretical problems with the use of heritability as a measure of the genetic influence (2). Therefore, this paper will not address this question, but rather will aim at answering the following more straightforward questions.

To what extent can the familial correlations be attributed to the shared genes or shared exposure of environmental factors? Does shared exposure to environmental factors contribute to the familial correlations after the rearing family environment is left? The answers do not rely on the same assumptions as the heritability estimate. The questions may be addressed by several different methods with different strengths and weaknesses.

The classical strategy is the twin method, which has been used in several studies (1). The correlations in obesity measures between monozygotic twins range from 0.70 to 0.90, and between dizygotic twins from 0.35 to 0.45. The finding that the monozygotic correlations are about double the size of the dizygotic correlations strongly suggests that genes are fully responsible for the twin resemblance. However, the greater correlations between dizygotic twins than between nontwin full siblings suggests that nongenetic influences are at work as well. Thus, age differences between nontwin siblings or less similarity of the shared environment of these siblings may be responsible for the smaller correlations. If such shared sibling environment is important, it is conceivable that it may contribute to an even greater correlation between monozygotic twins, and hence inflate the estimated genetic influence. One approach to solve the difficulties may be to study twins reared apart (3), but they are very rare, and there is often doubt about the degree of separation of their rearing environments.

An alternative to the twin method is the adoption method, which separately estimates the genetic and familial environmental influences. By this method, subjects adopted away from their biological family to an unrelated family early in life are compared to their biological and adoptive relatives. Some studies have used foster children or stepchildren, but they are not as appropriate because of the remaining admixture of shared genetic and shared environmental influences.

In the so-called complete adoption method, there is access to both the adoptive and biological family, whereas in the partial adoption method information is available only on the members of the adoptive family. We assume that resemblance of the adoptee and the members of the biological family—parents and siblings—is due to shared genes. Similarly, resemblance of the adoptee and the members of the adoptive family—parents and siblings—is due to shared environment. Resemblance may be measured by the phenotypic correlations, and the statistical test for genetic and for familial environmental effects is the test of whether the correlations differ significantly from zero.

The partial adoption method provides the same estimate of the influence of the shared family environment as the complete adoption method, namely, the phenotypic correlations between the adoptees and the adoptive family members. The partial adoption method may be used to estimate the genetic influence as well. This requires a comparison of these correlations with the phenotypic correlations observed between members of natural families, in which biologically related family members also share the family environment. These correlations may be generated from the biologically related members of the adoptive family as well as from other natural families. The difference in the correlations between the adoptee and the adoptive family members and the correlations between the members of the natural family may then be interpreted as a measure of the genetic influence. This difference between the correlations should then be statistically tested for departure from zero.

There are a number of assumptions built into the adoption method. The separation of the adoptee and the biological family should be early and maintained until the study. The adoptee should not be selectively placed in an adoptive family similar to the biological family with respect to the phenotype in question or related aspects. There should be no sustained influences of the shared preadoptive (prenatal or postnatal) environment. The biological and adoptive families should be representative with respect to familial resemblance of the phenotype. There should be no assortative mating of the biological parents, and the paternity should be correctly assigned. The partial adoption method for assessment of the genetic influences relies on the additional asumptions that the shared environmental influences in the adoptive family are equal to those in the natural family and that they act additively upon the genetic effects.

Six partial and three complete adoption studies have been carried out (4–17) (Table 1). The results of these studies are most easy to summarize and interpret if they are grouped according to whether they estimated parent-offspring correlations or sibling correlations, and whether they dealt with correlations for the adoptee in childhood and adolescence or with correlations in adulthood. The results are presented in Table 2 with regard to the extent to which they indicate a genetic or a familial environmental influence on the familial resemblance, using a semiquantitative scale with $+ + + +$ representing the entire familial resemblance.

Table 2 shows the results of parent-offspring analysis for childhood and adolescence. The partial adoption studies provide a rather confusing picture with some studies indicating major genetic influences and others indicating little genetic influence. The two complete adoption studies both support a major genetic influence as being responsible for the parent-offspring resemblance. The Danish study, but not the Colorado study, suggests a little effect of the shared environment.

Except for a single partial adoption study, all partial and the only complete adoption study using sibling correlations showed that the genetic influence is the major reason for sibling resemblance in childhood or adolescence (Table 3).

There are no partial adoption studies addressing parent-offspring or sibling correlations in adulthood. The only two complete adoption studies of parent-offspring correlations and the single study of sibling correlations all indicated a major genetic influence on familial resemblance (Table 4). This means that the shared rearing environment seems to have no sustained effect into adulthood.

Most, if not all, the discrepancies between the results of the various adoption studies may be attributed to methodological problems, par-

Table 1. Description of Adoption Studies of Human Obesity

Author(s)	Year of Publication of First Report	Reference No.	Study Name	Number of Adoptees	Measure of Obesity
Partial adoption studies					
Withers	1964	4	London Study	142	Percentage overweight
Garn et al.	1979	5	Tecumseh Study	160	Skinfold thickness
Hartz et al.	1977	6	TOPS Study	254	Percentage overweight
Biron et al.	1977	7–8	Montreal Study	374	Several BMIs, W for H
Bouchard et al.	1985	9–10	Québec City Study*	409	BMI, skinfolds, fat mass
Cardon et al.	In press	11	Colorado Study*	245	BMI, W for H
Complete adoption studies					
Stunkard et al.	1986	12–16	Danish Study	3651	BMI, silhouette
Price et al.	1987	17	Iowa Study	357	BMI
Cardon et al.	In press	11	Colorado Study*	245	BMI, W for H

*Partial adoption study of siblings and complete adoption study of parent-offspring relations.

Table 2. Genetic and Familial Environmental Influences on Obesity in Parents Versus Offspring in Childhood or Adolescence as Estimated in Partial and Complete Adoption Studies

Study	Genetic Influence	Familial Environmental Influence
Partial		
London	+	+ + +
Tecumseh	+ +	+ +
TOPS	+ +	+ +
Montreal	+ + +	+
Québec	+	+ + +
Complete		
Danish	+ + +	+
Colorado	+ + + +	0

+ + + + Extent of familial resemblance.

Table 3. Genetic and Familial Environmental Influences on Obesity in Siblings in Childhood or Adolescence as Estimated in Partial and Complete Adoption Studies

Study	Genetic Influence	Familial Environmental Influence
Partial		
TOPS	+	+ + +
Montreal	+ + + +	0
Québec	+ + + +	0
Colorado	+ + + +	0
Complete		
Danish	+ + +	+

+ + + + Extent of familial resemblance.

ticularly in the partial adoption studies. For example, the selection of adoptive families for study may be quite critical. If the recruitment procedure in some way selects for families in which the parent and the young adopted child each tends to be obese, or just similar to each other in degree of obesity, then the parent-offspring correlations on the adoptive side will be inflated and the generated estimate of genetic influence will be spuriously reduced.

In conclusion, all the complete adoption and some of the partial

Table 4.   Genetic and Familial Environmental Influences on Obesity in
Parents Versus Offspring and in Siblings in Adulthood as Estimated in Partial
and Complete Adoption Studies

Study	Genetic Influence	Familial Environmental Influence
Partial		
None		
Complete		
Parent-offspring		
Danish	+ + + +	0
Iowa	+ + +	+
Siblings		
Danish	+ + + +	0

+ + + + Extent of familial resemblance.

adoption studies indicate that the familial resemblance in obesity from
childhood through adulthood is mainly due to shared genes. All the
complete and some of the partial adoption studies found little or no
influence of the shared family environment, particularly after the adoptee had left the home. The principles and design of the complete adoption studies suggest that their results are more valid than those of the
partial adoption studies (1).

The adoption studies performed so far encourage future studies that
use more accurate measures of the size and distribution of the fat mass,
that assess gender- and age-related effects, nonadditive genetic effects,
components of the familial environmental influences, gene-environment interactions, and behavioral, physiological, and biochemical mediators of genetic and environmental effects.

REFERENCES

1. Bouchard C, ed. *The Genetics of Obesity.* Boca Raton, Fla: CRC Press;
   1994.
2. Feldman MW, Lewontin RC. The heritability hang-up. *Science.* 1975;
   190:1163–1168.
3. Stunkard AJ, Harris JR, Pedersen NL, McClearn GE. The body-mass
   index of twins who have been reared apart. *N Engl J Med.* 1990;322:
   1483–1487.

4. Withers RFJ. Problems in the genetics of human obesity. *Eugen Rev.* 1964;56:81–90.

5. Garn SM, Cole PE, Bailey SM. Living together as a factor in family-line resemblance. *Hum Biol.* 1979;51:565–587.

6. Hartz A, Giefer E, Rimm AA. Relative importance of the effects of family environment and heredity on obesity. *Ann Hum Genet.* 1977; 41:185–193.

7. Biron P, Mongeau JG, Bertrand D. Familial resemblance of body weight and height in 374 homes with adopted children. *J Pediatr.* 1977;91:555–558.

8. Annest JL, Sing CF, Biron P, *et al.* Family aggregation of blood pressure and weight in adoptive families, III: analysis of the role of shared genes and shared household environment in explaining family resemblance for height, weight and selected height/weight indices. *Am J Epidemiol.* 1983;117:492–506.

9. Bouchard C, Savard R, Després J-P, Tremblay A, Leblanc C. Body composition in adopted and biological siblings. *Hum Biol.* 1985;57: 61–75.

10. Bouchard C, Perusse L, Leblanc C, Tremblay A, Theriault G. Inheritance of the amount and distribution of human body fat. *Int J Obes.* 1988;12:205–215.

11. Cardon LR, Fulker DW. Genetic influences on body fat from birth to age 9. *Genet Epidemiol.* 1992.

12. Stunkard AJ, Sørensen TIA, Hanis C, *et al.* An adoption study of human obesity. *N Engl J Med.* 1986;314:193–198.

13. Sørensen TIA, Price RA, Stunkard AJ, Schulsinger F. Genetics of obesity in adult adoptees and their biological siblings. *BMJ.* 1989; 298:87–90.

14. Sørensen TIA, Holst C, Stunkard AJ, Skovgaard LT. Correlations of body mass index of adult adoptees and their biological and adoptive relatives. *Int J Obes.* 1992;16:227–236.

15. Sørensen TIA, Holst C, Stunkard AJ. Childhood body mass index— genetic and familial environmental influences assessed in a longitudinal study. *Int J Obes.* 1992;16:705–714.

16. Sørensen TIA, Stunkard AJ. Does obesity run in families because of genes? Danish adoption study using silhouettes as measure of obesity. *Acta Psychiatr Scand.* 1993;S370:67–72.

17. Price RA, Cadoret RJ, Stunkard AJ, Troughton E. Genetic contributions to human fatness: an adoption study. *Am J Psychiatry.* 1987; 144:1003–1008.

CLAUDE BOUCHARD

Genetic Epidemiology, Association, and Sib-Pair Linkage: Results from the Québec Family Study

ABSTRACT

The Québec Family Study has been in progress for about fifteen years. It was initially based on a panel of 375 families, which included several types of relatives by descent or adoption (Phase 1). A subsample of about 100 families from Phase 1 plus a panel of 40 families with obese probands are incorporated in Phase 2. Those families will be remeasured every five years for a panel of body-fat, regional fat distribution, and metabolic phenotypes. The results from several genetic epidemiology studies reveal that heritability of body-fat content attains about 25%. Studies have also indicated that an autosomal recessive gene could potentially contribute to variation in body fat in the Québec Family Study Phase 1 cohort. Association and linkage studies with candidate genes and other markers reveal that it is useful to take into account both total body fat and fat distribution phenotypes. The first few reports suggest that a good number of genes and chromosomal regions need to be considered in the investigation of the genetic architecture of body-fat content and subcutaneous fat distribution.

Introduction

Systematic attempts to define the genetic basis of obesity began with the study of Davenport reported in 1923 (1). More than seventy years after the publication of the monograph by Davenport, progress has been made in the understanding of the genetic basis of human obesity, particularly from the genetic epidemiology perspective. The understanding of the genetic and molecular basis of obesity and of various fat distribution phenotypes has now moved to the top of the agenda of the obesity research community. There is a consensus to the effect that some or all of the genes determining the predisposition to become obese or to exhibit android obesity or to have a large amount of abdominal visceral fat can be identified through a variety of research methods applied to animal and human studies.

The tools of genetic epidemiology can tell whether the phenotype is inherited and to what extent in a given population. They also allow testing of the hypotheses about the segregation of major genes and their mode of inheritance. Association studies and sib-pair linkage studies are also part of the approaches that can be used to investigate complex multifactorial phenotypes such as those commonly assessed in human obesities.

This paper provides an overview of the results published so far on the genetic epidemiology characteristics of body-fat content and regional fat distribution phenotypes based on the Québec Family Study cohort. It also summarizes the association and sib-pair linkage data with candidate genes that have been reported up to now with the same cohort.

The Québec Family Study

We initiated the Québec Family Study in 1978. The preliminary results of relevance to obesity were presented in 1980 (2), and the first paper dealing with familial characteristics and body fat was published in 1983 (3). The Québec Family Study monitors a wide range of phenotypes. So far, about seventy papers have been published based on the data generated on this cohort, and 60% of these papers deal with body fat, fat distribution, or the influence of these phenotypes on the metabolic profile.

There are three phases in the Québec Family Study (Fig. 1). The first phase includes the data collection that took place from 1979 to 1981 on 375 families and a total of 1650 individuals. Members of the parental generation ranged in age from 30 to 59 years. Ages of the offspring generation were from 8 to 26 years. These families were all of French descent (as ascertained from an interview conducted during the preliminary home visit) and were living within 80 kilometers of Québec City. These families were recruited through the media (*i.e.,* local and regional newspapers, radio, television, and flyers distributed in churches and schools). The socioeconomic status (SES) of the families was rated on

THE QUÉBEC FAMILY STUDY

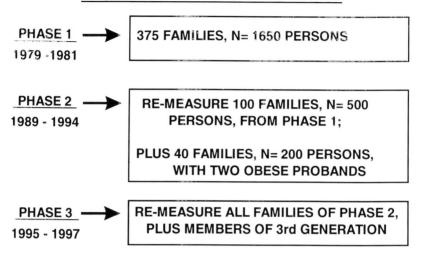

Figure 1. The three phases of the Québec Family Study with number of families and sample sizes.

the basis of occupation using the Blishen and McRoberts (4) index. The average SES rating for the fathers in this study was 54 (range 23 to 75), which was comparable to the general French-Canadian population (5).

The second phase of the Québec Family Study is currently in progress (1989–1994). In this phase, about 100 families from Phase 1 are remeasured and an additional 40 families with a minimum of three adult offspring are recruited and incorporated in the cohort. For the latter panel of families, one of the parents and at least one of the offspring must have a body mass index (BMI) greater than or equal to 32. Phase 2 will therefore incorporate data on 140 families with a minimum of 700 persons. Finally, during Phase 3 (1995–1997), members of the Phase 2 cohort will be remeasured and the children (third generation) of the adult offspring will be recruited when they reach 10 years of age. Permanent lymphoblastoid cell lines are established for all members of the Phases 2 and 3 cohorts. For these individuals, percent body fat (underwater weighing assessment of body density), subcutaneous fat distribution (eight skinfolds and girths), and abdominal visceral fat (computed tomographic [CT] scan) are obtained along with a large number of metabolic, physiological, and behavioral variables.

Table 1 summarizes the nature of the samples available in the Québec Family Study to address various types of research questions along with the approximate sample sizes. In addition, a maximum of 100 families with about 500 subjects, 200 unrelated adults and about 150 pairs of siblings, are part of the prospective design with data over the three phases of the study. We plan to follow all members of Phase 3 plus the additional children of the third generation when they reach 10 years of age in Phase 4, which we intend to undertake from 1998 to 2000.

Overview of Heritability and Segregation Analysis

Of interest here are the results of the Québec Family Study pertaining to heritability levels, commingling of score distributions, and complex segregation analysis for body-fat content and indicators of regional fat distribution. All the results published so far on these issues are based on the Phase 1 data base. Thus they do not deal with abdominal visceral fat, as the CT assessment of this phenotype became part of the protocol in Phase 2.

Table 2 provides an overview of the findings reported to date, which were derived from the tools of genetic epidemiology. The information is presented separately for body-fat content and for regional fat distribution phenotypes. Let us review briefly these findings for each class of phenotypes.

Table 1. Sample Sizes in the Québec Family Study for Various Types of Research Questions

	Phase 1 (1979–1981)	Phase 2 (1989–1994)
Heritability and related issues	375 families; 9 types of relatives	140 families
Segregation analysis	301 families	140 families
Association with markers	727 unrelated adults; 393 unrelated offspring	280 unrelated adults; 140 unrelated offspring
Sib-pair linkage	About 400 pairs	About 250 pairs

Table 2. A Summary of the Québec Family Study Results (Phase 1 data)

	Body Fat*	Fat Distribution**
Total transmission (%)	35 to 55	30 to 70
Heritability (%)	25	30 to 50
Maternal effect	No	No
Commingling of distributions	Yes, in adults	Yes
Major effect	Yes	Yes
Major gene effect	Yes, about 45%	Yes, about 35%
Model	Autosomal recessive	Autosomal recessive
Gene frequency	0.2 to 0.3	0.3

*From % fat, FM, sum of 6 skinfolds or BMI.
**From trunk to limb skinfolds ratio, principal component of skinfolds, or sum of skinfolds to FM ratio.

BODY-FAT CONTENT

Total body fat is assessed here by a variety of standard measures, such as percent body fat or total fat mass derived from underwater weighing, sum of six skinfolds, or body mass index. Based on the data available in Phase 1 of the Québec Family Study, studies have revealed that the total transmission effect across generations ranged from 35% to 55% with genetic heritability reaching approximately 25% of the age- and gender-adjusted phenotype variance (3, 6). No specific maternal or paternal effect was detected in the genetic heritability of body-fat content (6).

Commingling of distributions was consistently observed in the adults (parents) of the study for the body-fat content phenotypes, but skewness alone characterized the distribution of scores in the offspring (7). Complex segregation analysis applied to a subset of 176 families, for which body composition data derived from underwater weighing were available, revealed that a major effect could be inferred, that it accounted for about 45% of the age- and gender-adjusted percent body fat variance, and that it was compatible with a single autosomal recessive gene effect (8). The gene frequency was of the order of 0.2 to 0.3 in that particular study. In a separate study, the major gene effect hypothesis for the BMI was not accepted (9) unless the segregation model allowed the contribution of genotype-specific age and gender effects (10). The results suggested that the individuals with the high recessive genotype showed the greatest degree of heaviness early in life, with a subsequent trend toward lower values of the BMI throughout life. In addition, the high genotype conferred a greater degree of heaviness in women than in men. The results suggested a higher penetrance of the heavy genotype in the young (10).

FAT DISTRIBUTION

We have also considered in the Québec Family Study Phase 1 several anthropometric indicators of regional fat distribution. They include the trunk (sum of suprailiac + subscapular + abdominal skinfolds) to limb (sum of biceps + triceps + medial calf skinfolds) skinfolds ratio, the sum of six skinfolds to fat mass ratio, and the second principal component of a principal component analysis of the six skinfold measurements. In the latter case, the first component describes a general fatness component and the second component describes a trunk to limb fatness profile.

The multifactorial transmission of the regional fat distribution phenotypes in the Québec Family Study cohort ranged from 40% to 70% of the age- and gender-adjusted phenotype variance with a genetic heritability level of about 30% to 50% (11–14). There was no evidence of a specific maternal or paternal effect in the regional fat distribution phenotypes transmission or genetic heritability.

Commingling analysis of regional fat distribution measures revealed that significant distributional heterogeneity was observed for most phenotypes, but adjusting them for total fat mass tended to eliminate the heterogeneity (15). More recently, complex segregation analysis was performed for the same phenotypes (16). Results indicated that a major locus may govern the tendency to store fat in subcutaneous versus visceral and deep fat depots. In addition, a significant major gene effect could also be inferred for the relative distribution of subcutaneous fat on the trunk versus the limbs without and with adjustment for total body fat. For these two important indicators of fat distribution, namely, the sum of skinfolds to total fat mass ratio and the trunk to limb skinfolds ratio, evidence for the segregation of a major gene was quite consistent. The best model was for an autosomal recessive gene accounting for about 35% of the age-, gender-, and fat mass–adjusted phenotype variance, with a gene frequency of about 0.3 (16).

Results from Association and Linkage Studies

A large number of association studies with candidate genes and of linkage studies with candidate genes and other markers are being undertaken on the subjects of Phase 1 and Phase 2 of the Québec Family Study. Only those that have been published or are currently in press will be reviewed here.

Association Studies

The first report dealt with the A, B, and C loci of the HLA system and their relations with several phenotypes of body-fat content and regional fat distribution (17). The analyses were performed on a maximum of 348 adult males, 357 adult females, 468 boys and male adolescents, and 405 girls and female adolescents. No consistent pattern of association emerged for any of the phenotypes. The observation made by others that allelic variation at the class 1 loci of the HLA system (chromosomal assignment: 6p21.3) was associated with the BMI could not be confirmed in the Québec Family Study.

We also investigated the relation between allelic variation at the alpha 1, alpha 2, and beta genes of the Na,K-ATPase and percent body fat, resting metabolic rate, and respiratory quotient in 261 subjects from 58 families from Phase 2 of the Québec Family Study (18). Five restriction fragment length polymorphisms (RFLP) were determined: one at the alpha 1 locus with the restriction enzyme *Bgl II*, two at the alpha 2 locus with *Bgl II*, and two at the beta locus with *MspI* and *PvuII*. There was a consistent trend for percent body fat to be related to the RFLP generated in exons 21–22 of the alpha 2 gene in both males ($P = 0.06$) and females ($P = 0.05$). The respiratory quotient was associated with the alpha 2 exon 1 *Bgl II* RFLP with data adjusted for age, fat mass, and fat-free mass ($P = 0.02$). The respiratory quotient was also associated with the alpha 2 exon 1 and exons 21–22 haplotype ($P = 0.04$). None of the markers of the Na,K-ATPase genes was associated with variation in resting metabolic rate adjusted for age, fat mass, and fat-free mass. The alpha 2 locus has been mapped to 1cen-q32.

The association between DNA sequence variation in the brown adipose tissue uncoupling protein gene and body-fat content was investigated in 261 individuals from 64 families of Phase 2 (19). DNA samples were digested with nine restriction enzymes, but only *Bcl I* generated a RFLP with a 4.5 kb fragment (frequency = 0.72) and a 8.3 kb fragment (frequency = 0.28). No difference was observed in percent body fat, the sum of six skinfolds, and resting metabolic rate among the three UCP *Bcl I* genotypes when data were analyzed cross-sectionally. However, those who gained more than 7% body fat over twelve years were more frequently carriers of the 8.3 kb minor allele (62%) than those who gained less percent body fat (32%). The UCP gene has been mapped to 4q31.

Finally, an association study dealing with the relationship between a RFLP generated by *Bgl II* in the 3 beta-hydroxysteroid dehydrogenase locus (mapped to chromosome 1) and body-fat content and regional adipose tissue distribution phenotypes was completed with 132 unrelated subjects from the Québec Family Study (20). No association was found for BMI, percent body fat, sum of six skinfolds, and several fat distribution phenotypes in either sex when data were analyzed cross-sectionally. However, significant relationships were observed between genotypes for the 11.3-year changes in the sum of six skinfolds (P = 0.04), abdominal skinfold (P = 0.01), and abdominal skinfold adjusted for the sum of six skinfolds (P = 0.03) at entry in the study. The relations were observed only in women who gained considerably more fat than men over the 11.3-year span. Homozygotes for the polymerase chain reaction (PCR) generated 371 bp allele had the largest body fat and abdominal fat gain over time, whereas the homozygotes for the 575 bp allele gained the least.

Linkage Studies

The only linkage data reported thus far from the Québec Family Study are based on the sib-pair linkage method (21, 22). It is a useful method to screen for potential linkage between obesity phenotypes and genetic or molecular markers. The method assumes that pairs of siblings who share a greater proportion of alleles at a linked gene by descent will also tend to share alleles at the phenotype locus of interest. These pairs of siblings should therefore have a more similar phenotype than pairs who share fewer or no marker alleles. The slope of the regression of the squared sib-pair differences for the phenotype on the proportion of genes identical by descent is expected to be negative if there is a linkage. A one-sided *t*-test is used to assess whether the slope is significantly negative. Sib-pair linkage analysis on the Québec Family Study data is carried out using the program SIBPAL from SAGE 2.1 (18, 23).

The first study was conducted with about 400 pairs of siblings from Phase 1 of the Québec Family Study on red blood cell antigenic groups and enzyme polymorphic markers that we originally used to verify biological relationships and twin zygosity (24). Several potential linkage relationships were found involving the adenosine deaminase locus (20q13) with BMI ($P < 0.001$) and sum of six skinfolds ($P < 0.02$), the Kell blood group (7q33) with BMI ($P < 0.0001$) and sum of six skinfolds ($P < 0.0001$) as well as the trunk to limb skinfolds ratio adjusted for body fat ($P < 0.04$), and the esterase D enzyme marker (13q14) with percent body fat ($P < 0.04$) and the sum of six skinfolds adjusted for body fat ($P < 0.05$). Other marginal linkages were observed with markers on the short arm of chromosome 1 (1p22 to 1p36) including the Rh alleles and the phosphoglucomutase-1 locus.

The sib-pair linkage approach was also used by Dériaz *et al.* (18) in their study of the alpha 1, alpha 2, and beta genes of the Na,K-ATPase. They reported that the polymorphic markers did not reveal any evidence for potential linkage with either percent body fat or resting metabolic rate. However, they found that the respiratory quotient seemed to be linked to the beta gene *Msp*l and *Pvu*ll haplotype ($P = 0.008$). The beta locus is located on 1q.

Finally, Oppert *et al.* (19) also used the sib-pair linkage approach to test whether there was any evidence of potential linkage between the *Bcl I* polymorphic site of the uncoupling protein gene and body fat and resting metabolic rate. The results were consistently negative. They also applied the same procedure to the twelve-year changes in body fat. Again, all results were negative.

Conclusions

Several studies are currently in progress using Phase 1 and/or Phase 2 of the Québec Family Study data base. They cover a wide range of issues and involve genetic epidemiology, association, and linkage topics. An important area of work at present is the problem of the cross-phenotype familial resemblance incorporating body-fat or regional fat distribution phenotypes with health-related phenotypes such as blood pressures, blood lipids and lipoproteins, and others. We also remain very active on the candidate gene front, the present investigations covering about forty such genes. Finally, all members of Phase 2 of the study are being typed for a large number of anonymous markers, including di-, tri-, and tetra-nucleotide repeats, variable number of tandem repeats, and others. Our goal is to obtain a dense set of markers covering the whole genome, including mitochondrial DNA, on all members of the Québec Family Study Phase 2.

The results already available from the Québec Family Study and others that we reviewed recently (25, 26) strongly suggest that a large number of genes may be involved in the determination of the susceptibility to obesity. All the accumulated evidence seems to indicate that human obesity will be associated with complex multigenic systems and an intricate network of gene-gene and gene-environment interaction effects. Genetic heterogeneity will undoubtedly be a major issue as progress is made in the definition of the genetic architecture of human excessive body-fat content, upper-body obesity, and visceral obesity.

ACKNOWLEDGMENTS

The Québec Family Study was initiated in 1978 with funding from the Fonds pour la formation de chercheurs et l'action concertée du Québec (FCAC), Conseil pour la recherche en santé du Québec (CRSQ), Ministère du loisir, de la chasse et de la pêche du Québec (MLCP), and from Health and Welfare Canada. From 1989 to 1992, the Québec Family Study was funded by an operating grant from the Medical Research Council of Canada (MRC) (MA-10499). The study is now funded by a program grant from MRC (PG-11811).

The author would like to express his gratitude to Drs. D. C. Rao, F. T. Dionne, L. Pérusse, and M. C. Thibault, coprincipal investigators for the genetic component of the MRC Program Grant; A. Tremblay, principal investigator for the energy metabolism component; and J. P. Després, principal investigator for the lipid-lipoprotein component. Thanks are also expressed to Drs. C. Allard, G. Thériault, A. Nadeau, P. J. Lupien, S. Moorjani, M. Province, T. Rice, and I. Borecki for their contribution to the study and to G. Fournier, L. Allard, C. Leblanc, M. Chagnon, G. Bouchard, and others who have been involved in the data collection, laboratory work, and data analysis over the years.

REFERENCES

1. Davenport CB. *Body build and its inheritance.* Washington, DC: Carnegie Institution of Washington; 1923:329.
2. Bouchard C, Tremblay A, Leblanc C, Savard R, Lortie G, Després JP. Familiarity in subcutaneous fat: genetic or cultural. *Med Sci Sports Exerc.* 1980;12:97. Abstract.
3. Savard R, Bouchard C, Leblanc C, Tremblay A. Familial resemblance in fatness indicators. *Ann Hum Biol.* 1983;10:111–118.
4. Blishen BR, McRoberts HA. A revised index for occupations in Canada. *Can Rev Soc Anthropol.* 1976;13:71–79.
5. Blishen BR. Social class and opportunity in Canada. *Can Rev Soc Anthropol.* 1970;7:110–127.
6. Bouchard C, Pérusse L, Leblanc C, Tremblay A, Thériault G. Inheritance of the amount and distribution of human body fat. *Int J Obes.* 1988;12:205–215.
7. Borecki IB, Rice T, Bouchard C, Rao DC. Commingling analysis of generalized body mass and composition measures: the Québec Family Study. *Int J Obes.* 1991;15:763–773.
8. Rice T, Borecki IB, Bouchard C, Rao DC. Segregation analysis of fat mass and other body composition measures derived from underwater weighing. *Am J Hum Genet.* 1993;52:967–973.
9. Rice T, Borecki IB, Bouchard C, Rao DC. Segregation analysis of body mass index in an unselected French-Canadian sample: the Québec Family Study. *Obesity Res.* 1993;1:288–294.
10. Borecki IB, Bonney GE, Rice T, Bouchard C, Rao DC. Influence of genotype-dependent effects of covariates on the outcome of segregation analysis of the body mass index. *Am J Hum Genet.* 1993; 53:676–687.
11. Bouchard C. Inheritance of human fat distribution. In: Bouchard C, Johnston FE, eds. *Fat Distribution During Growth and Later Health Outcomes. Current Topics in Nutrition and Disease.* New York: Alan R. Liss Inc.; 1988;17:103–125.
12. Bouchard C. Genetic factors in the regulation of adipose tissue distribution. *Acta Med Scand.* 1988;723:135–141.
13. Bouchard C. Genetic and environmental influences on regional fat distribution. In: Oomura Y, Tarui S, Inoue S, Shimazu T, eds. *Progress in Obesity Research 1990.* London: Libbey; 1991:303–308.
14. Bouchard C, Després JP, Mauriège P. Genetic and nongenetic determinants of regional fat distribution. *Endocr Rev.* 1993;14:72–93.

15. Rice T, Borecki IB, Bouchard C, Rao DC. Commingling analysis of regional fat distribution measures: the Québec Family Study. *Int J Obes.* 1992;16:831–844.

16. Borecki IB, Rice T, Pérusse L, Bouchard C, Rao DC. Major gene influence on the propensity to store fat in trunk versus extremity depots: evidence from the Québec Family Study. *Obesity Res.* 1995; 3:1–8.

17. Bouchard C, Pérusse L, Rivest J, *et al.* HLA system, body fat and fat distribution in children and adults. *Int J Obes.* 1985;9:411–422.

18. Dériaz O, Dionne FT, Pérusse L, Tremblay A, Vohl MC, Côté G, Bouchard C. DNA variation in the genes of the Na,K-Adenosine Triphosphatase and its relation with resting metabolic rate, respiratory quotient, and body fat. *J Clin Invest.* 1994;93:838–843.

19. Oppert JM, Vohl MC, Chagnon M, *et al.* DNA polymorphism in the uncoupling protein (UCP) gene and human body fat. *Int J Obes.* 1994;18:526–531.

20. Vohl MC, Dionne FT, Pérusse L, Dériaz O, Chagnon M, Bouchard C. Relation between Bgl II polymorphism in 3β-hydroxysteroid dehydrogenase gene and adipose tissue distribution in human. *Obesity Res.* 1994;2:444–449.

21. Haseman JK, Elston RC. The investigation of linkage between a quantitative trait and a marker locus. *Behav Genet.* 1972;2:3–19.

22. Amos CI, Elston RC, Wilson AF, Bailey-Wilson JE. A more powerful test of linkage for quantitative traits. *Genet Epidemiol.* 1989;6:435–449.

23. Statistical Analysis for Genetic Epidemiology Rel. 2.1. (SAGE) Department of Biometry and Genetics, LSU Medical Center, New Orleans. 1992.

24. Borecki IB, Rice T, Pérusse L, Bouchard C, Rao DC. An exploratory investigation of genetic linkage with body composition and fatness phenotypes: the Québec Family Study. *Obesity Res.* 1994;2:213–219.

25. Bouchard C, Pérusse L. Genetics of obesity. *Ann Rev Nutr.* 1993;13: 337–354.

26. Bouchard C. Genetics of obesity: overview and research directions. In: Bouchard C, ed. *Genetics of Obesity.* Boca Raton: CRC Press Inc.; 1994.

TRUDY L. BURNS, PATRICIA PEYSER MOLL,
and RONALD M. LAUER

The Muscatine Ponderosity Family Study

ABSTRACT

A family study was conducted in Muscatine, Iowa, to examine the risk of cardiovascular disease in adult relatives of children with different patterns of ponderosity (body weight relative to height), and to estimate the genetic contribution to familial clustering of levels of ponderosity. Four groups of probands were selected from students who participated in three consecutive biennial school surveys: a random group (n = 70); a lean group (n = 72); a gain group (n = 70); and a heavy group (n = 72). The parents, siblings, a related aunt or uncle, and a first cousin of these probands were examined. Death certificates were obtained for deceased adult relatives. The relative risk of dying from cardiovascular disease for the heavy group versus the random group relatives was 1.41 (95% confidence interval 1.01, 1.98). Complex segregation analysis indicated strong support for a single recessive locus with a major effect that accounted for almost 35% of the age-gender–adjusted variability in body mass index. Genotypic probabilities were assigned to family members, and the effect of the recessive major locus on other measures of body habitus and cardiovascular risk factors was examined. This analysis suggested that individuals whose obesity may be caused by a gene at a single genetic locus are at higher cardiovascular risk because of mechanisms associated with their risk factor profile. We are currently searching for genetic factors responsible for the variability in body mass index. This may lead to early identification of individuals and families at high risk for the development of the chronic diseases associated with obesity.

482

Introduction

In adult population studies, obesity has been shown to be related to abnormal cardiovascular risk factor levels and to have adverse effects on morbidity and mortality from cardiovascular disease (1, 2, 3, 4). Whether this relationship is directly causal or whether obesity acts indirectly through its effects on other cardiovascular risk factor levels is not clear. Several studies have shown that obesity acquired in childhood is highly predictive of adult obesity (5) and that the prevalence of obesity in the United States is increasing, particularly among children and adolescents (6, 7).

Individual differences in ponderosity (body weight relative to height) are important determinants of health status. We conducted a family study in Muscatine, Iowa, to evaluate the relationship between ponderosity in children and cardiovascular risk factor levels in the children and in their family members, to estimate the genetic contribution to familial clustering of levels of ponderosity, and to examine the risk of cardiovascular disease in adult relatives of children with different patterns of ponderosity.

Identification and Examination of Families

A total of 284 families in four study groups were ascertained on the basis of the relative weight quintile pattern of a family member (proband) who had participated as a child in three consecutive Muscatine school surveys conducted in 1977, 1979, and 1981. For each survey year, the relative weight (weight/median weight for the appropriate age, height, and gender group × 100) was determined for every participating student. Use of relative weight allowed us to consider the weight of each student in relation not only to his or her age and gender but also to height-matched peers. The relative weights were rank ordered and grouped into quintiles, and the quintile pattern from each of the three surveys was used to identify four study groups: 1) 70 families ascertained through a child with a random quintile pattern over the three survey periods (random group); 2) 72 families ascertained through a child who was in the lowest quintile of relative weight on all three surveys (lean group); 3) 70 families ascertained through a child who gained at least two quintiles of relative weight from the first or second survey to the second or third survey (gain group); and 4) 72 families ascertained through a child who was in the highest quintile of relative weight on all three surveys (heavy group) (8).

For each family, a complete pedigree was constructed that included age, gender, and vital status information for every first-, second-, and third-degree relative of the proband. In each family, the proband, parents, siblings, a related aunt or uncle, and a first cousin were targeted for examination. Among these persons, several genetic and environmental contrasts are represented in terms of genetically related persons living together and apart and nonrelated persons living together and apart. These family members, along with the proband, were asked to come to our clinic in the Hotel Muscatine where the following were obtained: 1) a fasting venous blood sample that was used to measure total cholesterol, total triglycerides, and high density lipoprotein (HDL) cholesterol levels and to calculate low density lipoprotein (LDL) cholesterol levels in the Lipid Laboratory at the University of Iowa; 2) three right-arm blood pressures using a random zero sphygmomanometer with the subject seated comfortably for at least five minutes; 3) heart rate; 4) height, weight, skinfolds (triceps, subscapular, and abdominal), and circumferences (chest, abdominal, hip, and upper arm); and 5) a medical history questionnaire (8). In addition, copies of death certificates were obtained for first- and second-degree relatives who were 30 years of age or older at the time of death. All of the participating families were of white European descent.

Probands

An individual with a relative weight of 100% is exactly at the median for his or her age, height, and gender group. The mean relative weight for random group probands was close to 100% in each of the three school surveys. Lean group probands had a mean relative weight that was approximately 15% below the median weight in each survey, whereas the mean for heavy group probands was approximately 30% above the median weight. At the first survey, the mean relative weight for gain group probands was 6% below the median weight, by the second survey the mean was 2% above the median, and at the time of the third survey it was 7% above the age-gender-height-survey-specific median weight. At the time of each school survey, the heavy group probands had significantly higher age-gender–adjusted mean body mass index and triceps skinfold thickness ($P < 0.0001$), indicating that they persistently had a greater degree of ponderosity and adiposity than the probands in the other three study groups.

Of the 284 probands, 280 were reexamined along with their family members, at which time they ranged in age from 12 to 22 years. At the time of the family study examination, the heavy group probands had significantly higher age-gender–adjusted mean weight, body mass index (= weight in kg / height^2 in m^2), skinfolds, and circumferences (8). They also had significantly higher age-gender–adjusted systolic blood pressure and triglyceride levels and significantly lower HDL-cholesterol levels. When these risk factor levels were adjusted for body mass index in addition to age and gender, the group differences in systolic blood pressure, triglycerides, and HDL-cholesterol were no longer significant, which suggests that the differences were associated with differences in ponderosity.

Cardiovascular Disease Mortality

The pedigrees for the 214 lean, random, and heavy group families contained a total of 2567 mothers, fathers, aunts, uncles, grandmothers, and grandfathers. Copies of death certificates were obtained for 387 of the 399 first- and second-degree relatives in these families who were 30 years of age or older at the time of death (9). The gain group families were not included in the mortality analyses. A certified nosologist, "blind" to the study groups, assigned codes for every condition listed on the death certificates using the *International Classification of Diseases,* ninth edition. Cardiovascular disease, the most frequently listed cause of death for relatives in each of the study groups, was listed more frequently for heavy group relatives (60%) than for random (43%) or lean (48%) group relatives. Ischemic heart disease and cerebrovascular disease were the two major causes of death from cardiovascular disease, and the higher proportion of cardiovascular disease deaths in heavy group relatives appeared to be due to ischemic heart disease (30% lean, 27% random, 42% heavy; $P < 0.05$) rather than to cerebrovascular disease (15% lean, 16% random, 16% heavy).

Twenty of the heavy group probands had systolic blood pressures above the age-gender survey-specific ninetieth percentile for at least two of the three school surveys. The families of these 20 probands were classified as the hypertensive-heavy group and the remaining 52 heavy group families were classified as the nonhypertensive-heavy group.

Probands in the hypertensive-heavy group had a mean relative weight more than 10% higher than probands in the nonhypertensive-heavy group. Cardiovascular disease was listed as a cause of death on 76% of the death certificates for hypertensive-heavy group relatives in contrast to 51% for nonhypertensive-heavy group relatives ($P < 0.01$). This increased cardiovascular mortality was seen in both the male and female relatives of the hypertensive-heavy group probands.

Estimates of the relative risk of death from cardiovascular disease that accounted for person-years at risk for each relative, using the experience of relatives in the random group as reference, were obtained using proportional hazards analysis. The risk of death from cardiovascular disease for lean group relatives was not significantly different from that for random group relatives (relative risk = 0.94; 95% confidence interval 0.65, 1.36); however, the risk of death for heavy group relatives was significantly increased (1.41; 1.01, 1.98). When the heavy group was divided on the basis of the blood pressure pattern of the probands, the risk of death from cardiovascular disease for nonhypertensive-heavy group relatives was not significantly different from the risk for random group relatives (1.11; 0.75, 1.65); however, the risk for relatives in the hypertensive-heavy group compared with the random group was more than doubled (2.20; 1.43, 3.37). This magnitude of increased risk persisted when grandfathers and grandmothers were analyzed separately (9). Thus, although there appeared to be an increased risk of death from cardiovascular disease in relatives of obese children, it was most remarkable in both male and female relatives of the children whose obesity was accompanied by elevated blood pressure.

Examined Family Members

A total of 1607 probands and relatives from the 284 families were examined. In nearly one-half of the families (n = 130) the proband, mother, father, at least one sibling, a related aunt or uncle, and a first cousin were examined; 69% (n = 197) included the proband, mother, father, and at least one sibling.

The levels of body mass index in the probands for this family study clustered with the levels of body mass index in their relatives (8). Overweight relatives had consistently higher blood pressure, total cholesterol, LDL-cholesterol, and total triglyceride levels, and lower HDL-cholesterol levels. When these levels were adjusted for body mass index in addition to age and gender, the differences between overweight and nonoverweight groups disappeared.

The distribution of age-gender–adjusted body mass index in the relatives was examined using commingling analysis to determine whether it could best be explained by a mixture of normal distributions rather than a single normal distribution. We found that a mixture of two component distributions fit the data as well as a mixture of three component distributions, and fit significantly better than a single component distribution (10). The maximum likelihood parameter estimates from fitting the two-component model suggest that 7.5% of the population from which these relatives were recruited falls in the upper component distribution with a body mass index mean of 34.6 kg/m^2, and 92.5% of the population falls in the lower component with a body mass index mean of 23.4 kg/m^2. Several factors, both genetic and environmental, could lead to the rejection of a single normal distribution in favor of a mixture of distributions.

Complex Segregation Analysis

A possible genetic basis for the aggregation of age-gender–adjusted body mass index in these families was investigated using complex segregation analysis (11, 12) to test a specific series of models that represented combinations of genetic and environmental factors that might explain the evidence that we found for a mixture of two normal distributions for adjusted body mass index. We assumed that the observed distribution of body mass index was a consequence of the independent contributions of a single genetic or nontransmitted environmental factor with a major effect on body mass index, the additive allelic effects of a large number of independent polygenic loci each with a small effect, the effects of shared environments, and individual-specific environmental influences. The major factor was modeled as having two alternatives, L (leaner) and H (heavier), that might be of either genetic or nontransmitted environmental origin. Based on the model comparisons, there was evidence that the distribution of adjusted body mass index is influenced to a small extent by environmental factors shared by siblings living in the same house and shared by spouses living together (10). However, more than 75% of the variability in adjusted body mass index is influenced by genetic factors that include a single recessive major locus (35% of the variability) in addition to polygenic loci

(42% of the variability). The mean body mass index for homozygous HH individuals was estimated to be 34.8 kg/m^2 and the mean for LL and LH individuals was estimated to be 23.8 kg/m^2. Approximately 6% of the individuals in the population from which these pedigrees were ascertained are predicted to have two copies of the recessive gene (genotype HH), and 37% of the individuals are predicted to have one copy of the gene (genotype LH).

Assignment of Major Locus Genotype Probabilities and Calculation of Genotypic Probability Estimators

Because the existence of a major locus was inferred from complex segregation analysis, genotypic probabilities for each major locus genotype were estimated for each participating family member (12, 13). For example, the genotypic probabilities for one 17-year-old female participant with a body mass index of 29.3 kg/m^2 were as follows: Pr(LL) = 0.12, Pr(LH) = 0.60, and Pr(HH) = 0.28. The genotypic probabilities for a 23-year-old male participant with a body mass index of 31.8 kg/m^2 were 0.03, 0.13, and 0.84, respectively. There were 58 families (four lean group, eight random group, 18 gain group, and 28 heavy group) that contained at least two members who were classified as either LH or HH using a Pr $\geq$ 0.60 criterion. One such pedigree is displayed in Figure 1. For this pedigree Pr(LH) = 0.99 for both of the parents, individuals 111 and 112. Two of their children, including the proband, have a very high body mass index for their age with Pr(HH) = 0.98 for the proband and Pr(HH) = 0.99 for her brother.

Major locus genotype frequencies, quantitative trait genotypic means, and the percent of the variability in traits that could be attributed to the recessive major locus were estimated using the genotypic probability estimator approach (13). With this approach, our first example individual with major locus genotype probabilities of 0.12, 0.60, and 0.28 would contribute 12% of her quantitative trait level to genotype LL, 60% to genotype LH, and 28% to genotype HH.

The estimated major locus genotype frequencies are displayed in Table 1 for all family study participants by study group and gender, and by age and gender. Also displayed are the estimated genotype frequencies for probands by study group. The estimated frequency of HH individuals increases from 2% in lean group families to 5% to 7% in random and gain group families and to 12% to 14% in heavy group

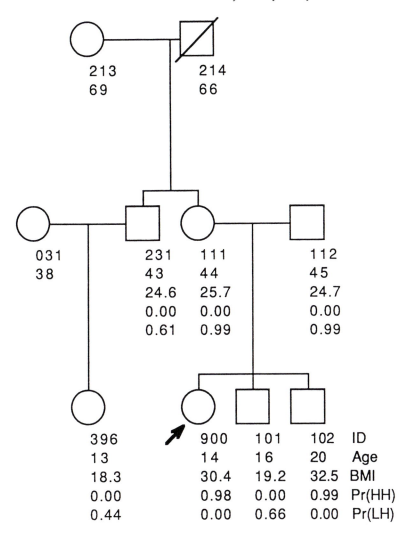

Figure 1. Muscatine Ponderosity Family Study pedigree number 214 200, including age, body mass index, and the unmeasured genotypic probabilities that the examined individuals have the HH and the LH genotypes.

families. Across the age groups, there is no indication of a major difference in the frequency of LH or HH individuals. The frequency of the HH genotype was very low among lean, random, and gain group probands; however, we estimate that 21% of the probands identified be-

Table 1. Body Mass Index Genotype Frequencies by Study Group and Gender, and by Age and Gender for All Family Study Participants (n = 1573), and by Study Group for Probands (n = 277)

	Males			Females			Probands		
	N	LH	HH	N	LH	HH	N	LH	HH
Study Group									
Lean	200	0.34	0.02	220	0.35	0.02	69	0.34	0.01
Random	190	0.36	0.05	202	0.35	0.05	69	0.37	0.02
Gain	181	0.39	0.06	205	0.38	0.07	67	0.41	0.03
Heavy	183	0.41	0.12	192	0.42	0.14	72	0.35	0.21
Age (years)									
<20	298	0.38	0.06	295	0.37	0.06			
20 to 39	214	0.38	0.07	293	0.37	0.08			
≥40	242	0.36	0.05	231	0.39	0.06			
	754	0.37	0.06	819	0.37	0.06	277	0.37	0.07

Frequencies were estimated using genotypic probability estimators (13).

cause of a persistent pattern of increased relative weight have the HH genotype.

Tables 2 and 3 show the estimated body habitus means by body mass index major locus genotype and the estimated percent of the phenotypic variance due to the major locus for all family study participants (Table 2) and for study participants younger than 20 years of age (Table 3). With the exception of height, the HH genotype is associated with significantly increased ($P < 0.0001$) age-gender–adjusted levels for each of these body habitus measures and indices. The percent of the variance in these traits that may be attributable to this purported major locus for body mass index is significant ($P < 0.0001$) for each of the measures except height, but it is considerably higher for the body habitus measures than it is for the indices.

Tables 4 and 5 show the estimated cardiovascular risk factor means by body mass index major locus genotype and the estimated percent of the phenotypic variance caused by the major locus for all family study participants (Table 4) and for study participants younger than 20 years of age (Table 5). The HH genotype is also associated with significantly higher ($P < 0.005$) estimated mean levels of blood pressure, total

Table 2.   Body Habitus Means by Body Mass Index Major Locus Genotype and Percent of the Phenotypic Variance Due to the Major Locus for All Family Study Participants (n = 1573)

	LL	LH	HH*	%VAR**
Weight (kg)	67	67	97	30.2
Height (cm)	167	167	166	0.3
Triceps skinfold (mm)	17	17	31	18.7
Subscapular skinfold (mm)	17	17	34	19.0
Waist circumference (cm)	76	77	101	26.7
Hip circumference (cm)	95	95	116	26.5
Waist-to-hip ratio	0.80	0.81	0.87	6.0
Conicity index (from ref. 14)	1.12	1.12	1.22	7.1

Means are adjusted for age and gender and were estimated using genotypic probability estimators. Genotypes were permuted 1000 times among family study participants, and the genotypic probability estimators were recomputed each time to test for significance (13).
*For each trait, HH is significantly different from LL or LH ($P < 0.0001$), except for height, which is not significant.
**For each trait $P < 0.0001$, except for height, in which $P < 0.01$.

Table 3.   Body Habitus Means by Body Mass Index Major Locus Genotype and Percent of the Phenotypic Variance Due to the Major Locus for Family Study Participants < 20 Years of Age (n = 593)

	LL	LH	HH*	%VAR**
Weight (kg)	56	57	84	28.6
Height (cm)	162	163	163	0.1
Triceps skinfold (mm)	14	14	28	21.6
Subscapular skinfold (mm)	12	13	29	22.0
Waist circumference (cm)	69	69	90	23.0
Hip circumference (cm)	88	89	106	21.3
Waist-to-hip ratio	0.78	0.78	0.85	6.7
Conicity index (from ref. 14)	1.09	1.09	1.17	4.8

Means are adjusted for age and gender and were estimated using genotypic probability estimators. Genotypes were permuted 1000 times among family study participants and the genotypic probability estimators were recomputed each time to test for significance (13).
*For each trait, HH is significantly different from LL or LH ($P < 0.0001$), except for height, which is not significant.
**For each trait $P < 0.0001$, except for height, which is not significant.

cholesterol and triglycerides, and LDL-cholesterol, and significantly lower estimated mean levels of HDL-cholesterol when all family study participants are included in the analysis (Table 4). Although the esti-

Table 4. Coronary Risk Factor Means by Body Mass Index Major Locus Genotype and Percent of the Phenotypic Variance Due to the Major Locus for All Family Study Participants (n = 1573)

	LL	LH	HH*	%VAR**
Systolic BP (mmHg)	113	114	122	3.7
Diastolic BP (mmHg)	74	74	80	2.2
Total cholesterol (mg/dL)	176	177	184	0.4
HDL-cholesterol (mg/dL)	49	49	42	2.3
LDL-cholesterol (mg/dL)	108	108	116	0.5
Total triglycerides (mg/dL)	106	108	147	2.7

Means are adjusted for age and gender and were estimated using genotypic probability estimators. Genotypes were permuted 1000 times among family study participants, and the genotypic probability estimators were recomputed each time to test for significance (13).
*For each trait, HH is significantly different from LL or LH (*P* < 0.0001), except for total cholesterol and LDL-cholesterol, in which *P* < 0.005.
**For each trait *P* < 0.0001, except for total cholesterol and LDL-cholesterol, in which *P* < 0.005.

Table 5. Coronary Risk Factor Means by Body Mass Index Major Locus Genotype and Percent of the Phenotypic Variance Due to the Major Locus for Family Study Participants < 20 Years of Age (n = 593)

	LL	LH	HH*	%VAR**
Systolic BP (mmHg)	107	108	119	6.4
Diastolic BP (mmHg)	69	70	77	3.5
Total cholesterol (mg/dL)	156	156	160	0.1
HDL-cholesterol (mg/dL)	49	49	40	4.7
LDL-cholesterol (mg/dL)	92	92	97	0.3
Total triglycerides (mg/dL)	77	78	118	5.4

Means are adjusted for age and gender and were estimated using genotypic probability estimators. Genotypes were permuted 1000 times among family study participants, and the genotypic probability estimators were recomputed each time to test for significance (13).
*For each trait, HH is significantly different from LL or LH (*P* < 0.0001), except for total cholesterol and LDL-cholesterol, which are not significant.
**For each trait *P* < 0.0001, except for total cholesterol and LDL-cholesterol, which are not significant.

mated percent of the phenotypic variance attributable to the major locus is much smaller for these risk factors, it is nonetheless significant (*P* < 0.005). The estimated mean total cholesterol and LDL-cholesterol levels for HH family study participants younger than 20 years of age was not significantly different from the mean for LL or LH individuals (Table 5), nor was the percent of the variance significant. However, the mean blood pressures and HDL-cholesterol and triglyceride levels for HH individuals differed from LL and LH participants ($P < 0.0001$), and the percent of the variance was also significant for these traits ($P < 0.0001$). The results of the analyses summarized in Tables 2 through 5 suggest that individuals whose obesity may be due in part to a gene at a single locus are at higher cardiovascular risk because of mechanisms associated with their risk factor profile.

Discussion

The role of genetic and environmental factors in determining variability in indices of body size has been investigated using complex segregation analysis in several different populations employing a variety of sampling designs and with quite consistent results (10, 15–20). A major unanswered question from these investigations is, What inherited factors carry an associated risk for excess ponderosity? There are probably multiple mechanisms, and the specific mechanisms and specific genes may vary among families. A number of possible factors exist, including genes associated with basal metabolism, dietary thermogenesis, appetite, satiety, endocrine function, and fat storage, and many of these factors are described in the other papers from this symposium. There are several rodent models of obesity that have been extensively characterized. For example, in the Zucker fatty rat (*fa/fa*), the diabetic mouse (*db/db*), and the obese mouse (*ob/ob*), obesity is inherited as an autosomal recessive trait. In each of these rodent models, metabolic abnormalities that may be responsible for the obesity have been identified and the genes have been localized as detailed in other contributions from this symposium.

In humans, excess ponderosity is associated with increased cardiovascular risk. Among the participants in the Muscatine Ponderosity Family Study, those with the HH genotype had higher blood pressure and triglyceride levels and lower HDL-cholesterol levels than those with the LL or LH genotype. This suggests that individuals whose obesity is caused by a gene at a single genetic locus with a major effect are at increased cardiovascular risk because of mechanisms associated with their cardiovascular risk factor profile. When the genes with major effects on the determination of body habitus in humans are located, we will have the potential to identify individuals with a genetic predisposition to developing obesity, as well as those at risk for the development of hypertension and atherosclerosis.

ACKNOWLEDGMENTS

This research was supported by the Iowa Specialized Center of Research Grant in Atherosclerosis (HL 14320) from the National Heart, Lung, and Blood Institute, and by HD 29569 from the National Institute of Child Health and Human Development. We recognize the efforts of our field team coordinator, Catherine Rost; our genealogist, Kathleen Schreiber; the Muscatine field team of Verna Mae Wilson, Elizabeth Fletcher, Carol Bendle, and Ann Shopa; and the data management skills of John Witt and Richard Paulos. We thank the children of Muscatine and their families for their participation in this study.

REFERENCES

1. Bray GA. Complications of obesity. *Ann Intern Med.* 1985;103:1052–1062.
2. Hubert HB, Feinleib M, McNamara PM, *et al.* Obesity as an independent risk factor for cardiovascular disease: a 26-year follow-up of participants in the Framingham heart study. *Circulation.* 1983;67:968–977.
3. Hartz AJ, Rupley DC, Rimm AA. The association of girth measurements with disease in 32 856 women. *Am J Epidemiol.* 1984;119:71–80.
4. Van Itallie TB. Health implications of overweight and obesity in the United States. *Ann Intern Med.* 1985;103:983–988.
5. Johnston FE. Health implications of childhood obesity. *Ann Intern Med.* 1985;103:1068–1072.
6. Bray GA, ed. *Obesity in America.* Bethesda, MD: National Institutes of Health, Publications Unit, Fogerty International Center; November, 1979. NIH Publication No. 79-359.
7. Kolata G. Obese children: a growing problem. *Science.* 1986;232:20–21.
8. Burns TL, Moll PP, Lauer RM. The relation between ponderosity and coronary risk factors in children and their relatives: the Muscatine Ponderosity Family Study. *Am J Epidemiol.* 1989;129:973–987.
9. Burns TL, Moll PP, Lauer RM. Increased familial cardiovascular

mortality in obese school children: the Muscatine Ponderosity Family Study. *Pediatrics.* 1992;89:262–268.

10. Moll PP, Burns TL, Lauer RM. The genetic and environmental sources of body mass index variability: the Muscatine Ponderosity Family Study. *Am J Hum Genet.* 1991;49:1243–1255.

11. Elston RC, Stewart J. A general model for the genetic analysis of pedigree data. *Hum Hered.* 1971;21:523–542.

12. Hasstedt SJ. *PAP: Pedigree Analysis Package, Rev 3.* Salt Lake City, Utah: Department of Human Genetics, University of Utah; 1989.

13. Hasstedt SJ, Moll PP. Estimation of genetic model parameters: variables correlated with a quantitative phenotype exhibiting major locus inheritance. *Genet Epidemiol.* 1989;6:319–332.

14. Valdez R, Seidell JC, Ahn YI, Weiss KM. A new index of abdominal adiposity as an indicator of risk for cardiovascular disease: a cross-population study. *Int J Obes.* 1993;17:77–82.

15. Hasstedt SJ, Ramirez ME, Kuida H, Williams RR. Recessive inheritance of a relative fat pattern. *Am J Hum Genet.* 1989;45:917–925.

16. Price RA, Ness R, Laskarzewski P. Common major gene inheritance of extreme overweight. *Hum Biol.* 1990;62:747–765.

17. Province MA, Arnqvist P, Keller J, Higgins M. Strong evidence for a major gene for obesity in the large unselected total community health study of Tecumseh. *Am J Hum Genet.* 1990;45:A143.

18. Ness R, Laskarzewski P, Price RA. Inheritance of extreme overweight in black families. *Hum Biol.* 1991;63:39–52.

19. Rice T, Borecki IB, Bouchard C, Rao DC. Segregation analysis of fat mass and other body composition measures derived from underwater weighing. *Am J Hum Genet.* 1993;52:967–973.

20. Borecki IB, Bonney GE, Rice T, Bouchard C, Rao DC. Influence of genotype-dependent effects of covariates on the outcome of segregation analysis of the body mass index. *Am J Hum Genet.* 1993; 53:676–687.

LAURA E. MITCHELL and D. C. RAO

Genetic Epidemiology of Obesity

ABSTRACT

There is little doubt that familial factors play an important role in the development of obesity and influence the distribution of fat on the human body. Twin, adoption, and traditional family studies strongly suggest that the familial nature of such traits is determined, at least partially, by genetic factors. Identification of the specific genetic factors involved in the development of these traits and characterization of their effects is, however, a complex task. Recent developments in both statistical genetic modeling and molecular genetics offer opportunities to gain new insights into the genetic epidemiology of complex traits such as obesity. Multivariate extensions of the traditional segregation analysis models provide an opportunity to explore the interrelationships among correlated phenotypes and their covariates. Moreover, the identification of polymorphic DNA markers throughout the human genome dramatically increases the prospects of identifying specific genetic factors involved in the development of obesity.

Introduction

Significant familial correlations have been documented for many of the phenotypes that characterize the amount and distribution of fat on the human body (1–5). Since these aspects of the human physique are clearly influenced by a familial component, it is believed that their development is determined, at least in part, by genetic factors. Although nongenetic factors may also contribute to the familial nature of these phenotypes, several lines of evidence support the view that genes are involved in the development of obesity and influence the distribution of fat on the human body.

The existence of several rodent models of obesity, in which specific patterns of fat accumulation are attributable to the effects of a single

gene or to polygenic influences, illustrates that genes can and do influence the development of obesity in mammals. Interestingly, the mouse
obesity genes all appear to fall within highly conserved syntenic groups
between human and mouse (6). The highly conserved nature of these
genes suggests that the human homologues may also influence the development of obesity, and provides several candidate genes for human
obesity.

Several human syndromes of known genetic etiology are also associated with specific obesity-related phenotypes. The Prader-Willi
syndrome, which is associated with a deletion of the paternally derived
chromosome 15 (15q11-13) in over 50% of cases, and characterized by
hypotonia in infancy, moderate developmental delay, hypogonadism,
and obesity with hyperphagia beginning in early childhood (7), is perhaps the most widely recognized of these disorders. However, Smith
(8) lists five additional syndromes that are known to be or are suspected
of being inherited in a Mendelian fashion (e.g., Carpenter, Cohen,
Grebe, Laurence-Moon-Biedl, Albright hereditary osteodystrophy),
and four chromosomal syndromes (e.g., Down's syndrome, XO, XXY,
XXXY) that are also characterized by an excess of body fat. Although
individuals with obesity as part of a recognized genetic syndrome account for only a small percentage of the obese population, they clearly
illustrate the effect that genetic variation can have on both the absolute
amount and distribution of fat on the body.

Statistical analyses of family data also provide evidence that genetic
factors contribute to the familial nature of at least some obesity-related
phenotypes. For example, heritability analyses have quite consistently
supported the involvement of genetic factors in the determination of
the body mass index (BMI) (9–12). Although genetic and cultural
sources of familiality may be difficult to untangle in such analyses, the
convergence of conclusions from twin, adoption, and traditional family
studies (each of which has its own set of strengths and weaknesses with
regard to resolving genetic and cultural heritability) strongly supports
a genetic role in the determination of the BMI. Moreover, segregation
analyses have shown that the familial patterns exhibited by several
obesity-related phenotypes are consistent with the involvement of a
major gene (13–19).

The use of molecular genetic techniques to identify genes that may
be involved in the development of human obesity is a relatively new
area of endeavor. Such analyses, however, have already led to the iden-

tification of genes that appear to be associated with, or in strong linkage disequilibrium with genes that are associated with, specific obesity phenotypes (20, 21). In addition, sib-pair linkage analyses have identified several blood group antigens and enzyme polymorphisms that appear to be associated with (or in strong linkage disequilibrium with genes that are associated with) specific obesity phenotypes (22, 23).

Considering the level of evidence supporting the role of genetic factors in the development of human obesity, we have relatively few clues regarding the specific factors (*i.e.,* the number of genes involved, the magnitude of their effect, their location within the human genome) that are involved in determining the obesity-related phenotypes. The characterization of the genetic contribution to individual obesity-related phenotypes has been, and is likely to continue to be, a complex undertaking. The complexity of this task is influenced by the lack of a clear biologic basis for defining the relevant phenotype(s), as well as the potential for genetic heterogeneity, developmental effects, temporal trends, phenotypic covariates that may themselves be under genetic control, and interactions among phenotypic determinants.

Genetic Epidemiology of Human Obesity

Genetic epidemiology is a relative newcomer to the multidisciplinary efforts aimed at expanding our understanding of the etiology and natural history of human fatness. Despite a relatively short history in the arena of human obesity research (the majority of genetic epidemiologic analyses of human obesity date only as far back as the early 1980s), findings based on the genetic epidemiologic approach have radically altered our view of the primary determinants of obesity. Once considered to be strongly determined by behavioral characteristics, obesity is increasingly viewed as a condition with strong genetic underpinnings.

The genetic epidemiology of the BMI (weight in kilograms/[height in meters]^2) has been more thoroughly evaluated than that of any other obesity-related phenotype. Although the BMI is actually a composite measure of heaviness (24), it exhibits substantial correlations with fat mass (25) and is relatively simple to measure. Hence, the BMI provides an attractive proxy measure for fatness. Because the BMI can be reliably measured in even the most remote field study and can often be reconstructed from historical data, it has been studied in a number of populations in which data on other obesity-related phenotypes are unavailable, unreliable, or difficult to obtain. Past and ongoing efforts to delineate the genetic epidemiology of the BMI, therefore, largely define our current understanding of the genetic epidemiology of obesity and provide a paradigm for the study of other obesity-related phenotypes.

Genetic Epidemiology of the Body Mass Index

Studies of Genetic Heritability

Estimates of the genetic heritability of a trait (*i.e.*, the proportion of the overall variance exhibited by a trait that is attributable to genetic factors) can be obtained from twin, adoption, and traditional family data. Each of these study designs has its own set of strengths and weaknesses with regard to the resolution of genetic and environmental sources of phenotypic variance. Adoption studies that include information on both biologic and adoptive relatives of the adoptee (*i.e.*, the complete adoption design) and studies of monozygotic (MZ) twins reared together and apart are, however, two of the more powerful approaches for resolving the relative impact of genetic and environmental influences on a trait.

In a recent study of Danish adoptees, their biologic parents, siblings and half-siblings, and their adoptive parents, approximately 34% of the variance in adult BMI levels was attributable to genetic effects. The shared family environment had no significant impact on adult BMI levels in this population, whereas the nonshared environment accounted for approximately 66% of the variance in this phenotype (10, 12). Similar conclusions regarding the relative impact of genetic, family environment and the nonshared environment on the BMI have been drawn from analyses of traditional (*i.e.*, nonadoptive) families in Utah (9) and Gubbio, Italy (11).

Comparison of MZ twins reared together and apart also supports the view that familial resemblance for the BMI is largely, if not entirely, attributable to genetic effects. In general, the MZ twin correlation for the BMI has been found to be independent of whether or not the twins were reared together (26–28). However, estimates of the genetic heritability of the BMI obtained from twin studies tend to be substantially higher than those from nontwin studies.

The discrepancy in the estimates of genetic heritability of the BMI from twin and family studies is not easily reconciled. The involvement of nonadditive genetic factors in the determination of the BMI could contribute to the higher estimates of genetic heritability obtained in twin data. Factors, such as age, that make co-twins (even those reared apart) more similar than other types of relatives may also account for some of this discrepancy.

COMMINGLING ANALYSES

Commingling in the population distribution of a phenotype is consistent with major gene involvement in the determination of the trait. It does not, however, establish a genetic etiology for a phenotype, since nongenetic factors may also give rise to commingling. The distribution of the BMI has been assessed in several diverse populations, including Caucasians (14, 25, 29–32), African Americans (33), Pima Indians (34), and members of the Reddy caste in Andhra Pradesh, India (35). With few exceptions, the BMI has been best described by a mixture of two or three component distributions (Table 1) and, therefore, is compatible with the expectations for a trait that is influenced by a major gene.

The presence of heterogeneity in the distribution of a phenotype between subgroups of the population may also provide clues regarding the determinants or covariates of the phenotype. If a trait is determined by a major gene, such heterogeneity suggests that the effect of the gene is modified by, or interacts with, the characteristic(s) that define the relevant subgroups of the population. Evidence of significant heterogeneity in the distribution of the BMI has been reported between population subgroups defined by age (25) and sex (30, 35). Hence, when evaluating the potential causes of familial resemblance for the BMI, the possibility that age and/or sex effects may obscure the evidence for a major gene should be considered.

SEGREGATION ANALYSES

The primary goal of segregation analysis is to determine if the familial patterns exhibited by a phenotype are consistent with the expectations for a trait that is at least partially determined by a major gene. Several studies have evaluated the segregation patterns of the BMI using the parametric mixed model. Under this model, a phenotype may be determined by the effects of a biallelic major gene, multifactorial trans-

Table 1. Summary of Commingling Analyses[a] for the BMI

Population	Data Adjusted for:	Subgroups	#	E	u	d	t	q	p
Andhra Pradesh, India (34)	age, sex	males (≥ 30y) females (≥ 30y)	2S 1S	0.59 0.94	-0.05 -0.11	[0] [0]	1.46 [0]	0.81 [0]	-0.03 -0.91
	age, sex, energy intake, and expenditure	males + females (≥ 30y)	2N	0.76	0.11	[0]	1.76	0.34	[1]
Pima Indians, S. Arizona (33)	age, sex, birth year, residence (on/off reservation)	males + females (15–65y)	3N or 1S	0.48 0.96	0.00 -0.11	0.43 [0]	3.49 [0]	0.12 [0]	[1] -0.37
Québec Family Study (25)	age, sex	adults (30–60y) offspring (8–26y)	3N 1S	0.58 0.97	0.03 -0.12	0.36 [0]	5.33 [0]	0.07 [0]	[1] -0.42
Danish Draft Board (31)	age, IQ, education, region, birth cohort (males only)	Copenhagen, 1939–58 S. Denmark, 1947–58	2S 2S	0.75 0.71	-0.07 -0.08	[0] [0]	2.45 2.20	0.17 0.20	0.17 -0.02
Tecumseh Comm. Health Study (32)	age, sex	males + females (<80y)	2S	0.68	-0.10	[0]	1.74	0.26	-0.36
LRC Family Study (14)	age, sex, social class, clinic	males + females (8–74y)	3S	0.63	-0.06	0.47	4.80	0.03	0.19
NAS-NRC Twin Registry (29)	age (males only)	at induction ($\overline{X} = 20y$) at follow-up ($\overline{X} = 44y$)	3S 3S	0.65 0.72	-0.05 0.01	0.41 0.35	4.03 4.48	0.06 0.05	0.42 1.10
Danish Adoption Registry (30)	age, sex	adult males + females	3S	0.48	-0.02	0.42	3.88	0.09	0.83

[a]Parsimonious model for the distribution of the BMI, as specified by the authors. #, number of component distributions and whether normal (N) or skewed (S); E, the within-component variance which is assumed to be equal for all component distributions; u, the overall mean; d, the displacement of the intermediate mean of the lowest component; t, the displacement between the means of the two extreme components; q, the square root of the relative proportion of the component distribution with the highest mean; p, the power transformation to eliminate skewness in the component distributions.

mission, and a unique, residual effect. With only one exception (a small study of African-American families [33]), such studies have concluded that a model including both a major effect and multifactorial transmission provides the best fit to the familial patterns exhibited by the BMI (14–16, 36). In each of these studies, the best Mendelian model for the BMI included a major autosomal recessive gene (with approximately 2% to 6% of the population having the high risk genotype), acting against a multifactorial background.

GENOTYPE-DEPENDENT COVARIATE EFFECTS:
THE QUÉBEC FAMILY STUDY

Two segregation analyses of the BMI have been undertaken, using data from 375 French-Canadian families enrolled in the Québec Family Study (17, 36). These data were initially analyzed, after adjusting the BMI for the effects of age within sex and generation, using the parametric mixed model. Under this model, the null hypotheses of no major effect and no multifactorial transmission were rejected. However, Mendelian transmission of the major effect was not confirmed (36).

To determine if genotype-dependent effects of age and/or sex may have obscured the evidence for Mendelian transmission of the BMI in the Québec Family Study data, the data were reevaluated using a model that allows for genotype-dependent covariate effects. Under this model, there was evidence that both age and sex exert significant genotype-dependent effects on the BMI. After accounting for these genotype-dependent effects, the hypothesis of no major effect was again rejected. Moreover, in contrast to the earlier analyses, the hypothesis of Mendelian transmission of the major effect could not be rejected (17).

GENOTYPE-DEPENDENT COVARIATE EFFECTS:
THE ANDHRA PRADESH FAMILY STUDY

Variation in individual levels of energy intake and energy expenditure has been shown to significantly influence the familial correlations and transmission of the BMI (5, 37). To further delineate the effects of these energy variables on familial resemblance for the BMI, data from the Andhra Pradesh Family Study were analyzed using an extension of the mixed (segregation analysis) model that allows for genotype-dependent covariate effects (38).

The data employed in these analyses are drawn from a family study of arterial blood pressure conducted among members of the Reddy caste, residing in the Chittoor district of Andhra Pradesh, India. The study sample includes 1441 individuals, ranging in age from 5 to 80 years, from 395 nuclear families (details regarding study design and data adjustment procedures are provided in references 5, 34, and 36). The present analyses are based on the BMI adjusted for the significant effects ($P < 0.05$) of age, age^2, age^3, energy intake, and energy expenditure on both the mean and the variance. These adjustments were performed separately in males and females, and the effects of both the absolute and weight-adjusted (kcal/kg) measures of energy intake and expenditure were considered. The adjusted phenotype was standardized, within sex, to mean zero and unit variance.

The mixed model used in these analyses includes six basic parameters: p, the frequency of the allele (A) that is associated with low values of the BMI; three genotype-specific means (μ_{AA}, μ_{Aa}, μ_{aa}); the within-genotype standard deviation (SD), which is assumed to be homogeneous across genotypes; and multifactorial heritability (h^2). In addition, the model includes three regression coefficients (β), one for each of the three genotypes, for each genotype-dependent covariate. The transmission probabilities were set to their Mendelian expectations (*i.e.*, τ_1 = 1.0, τ_2 = 0.5, τ_3 = 0.0), unless otherwise noted, since the assumption of Mendelian transmission is implicit in the evaluation of genotype-dependent covariate effects.

The genotype-dependent covariate effects of age, sex, energy intake per kilogram of body weight (EI) and energy expenditure per kilogram of body weight (EE) were considered (Table 2). Prior adjustment for the effects of these variables on the overall mean and variance of the BMI is expected to have removed effects of these covariates that are common across all genotypes. Hence, these analyses focus specifically on evaluation of the evidence for genotype-dependent effects of the four covariates. Since failure to account for such effects may result in erroneous conclusions regarding the genetic contribution to a trait, hypotheses regarding the significance of the genotype-dependent covariate effects were assessed relative to an unrestricted Mendelian mixed model. Parameter estimation was carried out using an extension of Hasstedt's mixed model likelihood approximation (39), which allows for genotype-dependent covariate effects (38). Hypotheses were evaluated by the likelihood ratio test.

The significance of the genotype-dependent effects of each covariate was assessed by comparing the likelihood of the basic six-parameter

Table 2. Segregation Analysis of the BMI with Genotype-Dependent Covariate Effects

Model	Covariate	−2 log Likelihood	Likelihood Ratio Test (3df)	P-value
Base[a]		3985.60	—	—
Base plus[b]	Age	3971.81	13.79	0.0032
	Sex	3977.30	8.30	0.0402
	EI	3977.28	8.32	0.0398
	EE	3979.09	6.51	0.0893
Base + age, plus[c]	Sex	3961.47	10.34	0.0159
	EI[e]	3958.14	13.67	0.0034
	EE	3965.82	5.99	0.1121
Base + age + EI, plus[d]	Sex	3950.76	7.38	0.0607
	EE	3956.54	1.60	0.6594

[a]Parameters of base model: p, μ_{AA}, μ_{Aa}, μ_{aa}, SD, h^2.
[b]Assessed relative to base model.
[c]Assessed relative to base model + Age.
[d]Assessed relative to base model + Age + EI.
[e]Comparison of likelihood for (base model + Age + EI) vs (base model + Age): $X_3^2 = 19.14$, $P = 0.0003$, indicates that the genotype by age effects are significant, even when genotype by EI effects are included in the model.

mixed model and the model containing the six basic parameters plus the three genotype-dependent regression coefficients for that covariate. In all cases, the three genotype-dependent regression coefficients were considered as a unit (*i.e.*, either all three or none of the coefficients were included in the model). The covariate associated with the most significant ($P < 0.05$) improvement in the fit of the model (as judged by the likelihood ratio test, with 3 degrees of freedom) was added to the model, and the process was repeated. After the addition of each covariate, all other covariates in the model were reevaluated and removed from the model if they were no longer statistically significant ($P \geq 0.05$). This process was repeated until all significant covariates were included in the model, and all covariates in the model were significant, given the other covariates in the model.

Using this approach there was evidence that age and energy intake (but not sex or energy expenditure) exert significant genotype-dependent effects on the BMI. (The same results were obtained by starting with a model that included all four covariates and removing the non-significant, genotype-dependent effects in a stepwise manner.) Hypotheses regarding the significance of the multifactorial and major gene components were evaluated within the context of models that included the genotype-dependent effects of both age and energy intake. The hypotheses of no multifactorial transmission ($\chi_1^2 = 62.68$, $P < 0.0001$), and no major gene ($\chi_7^2 = 109.73$, $P < 0.0001$) were clearly rejected. Autosomal recessive ($\chi_3^2 = 15.03$, $P = 0.0018$) and autosomal dominant ($\chi_3^2 = 58.69$, $P < 0.0001$) models of inheritance were also rejected.

The Mendelian model that provides the best fit to these family data, therefore, includes the six parameters of the basic mixed model, three genotype-dependent regression coefficients for age, and three genotype-dependent regression coefficients for energy intake (Table 3, unrestricted model). Under this model, the mean value for heterozygous individuals (Aa) is, however, less than that of the low risk homozygotes (AA). In the absence of prior evidence for an overdominance effect, this relationship is difficult to explain under a genetic hypothesis. Consequently, the analyses were repeated under the constraint that the major gene acts in a recessive fashion. Conclusions regarding the significance of the genotype-dependent covariate effects were identical to those obtained using the unconstrained model, and the hypotheses of no multifactorial inheritance and no major gene were again rejected.

The autosomal recessive model (Table 3) predicts that the BMI is

Table 3. Segregation Analysis of the BMI: Parameter Estimates and Standard Errors

Parameter	Unrestricted Model	Autosomal Recessive Model
$p(A)$	0.74 ± 0.03	0.75 ± 0.03
μ_{AA}	-0.07 ± 0.26	-0.49 ± 0.15
μ_{Aa}	-0.99 ± 0.31	-0.49^a
μ_{aa}	4.05 ± 0.79	4.11 ± 0.81
SD	0.83 ± 0.02	0.86 ± 0.02
h^2	0.55 ± 0.06	0.48 ± 0.06
$\beta_{age(AA)}$	-0.010 ± 0.003	0.006 ± 0.002
$\beta_{age(Aa)}$	-0.0006 ± 0.004	0.006^a
$\beta_{age(aa)}$	-0.015 ± 0.009	-0.015 ± 0.009
$\beta_{EI(AA)}$	-0.003 ± 0.004	0.003 ± 0.002
$\beta_{EI(Aa)}$	0.011 ± 0.005	0.003^a
$\beta_{EI(aa)}$	-0.030 ± 0.010	-0.031 ± 0.011

[a]Parameters constrained to be equal to the parameter directly above them in the table.

directly related to age and energy intake in low risk homozygous (AA) and heterozygous (Aa) individuals (Fig. 1), but indirectly related to these covariates in the high risk homozygous (aa) individuals (Fig. 2). The inverse association between energy intake and BMI levels, among individuals with the high risk genotype, may be attributable either to the proportional nature of the measure of energy intake used in these analyses (*e.g.,* if the absolute level of energy intake is homogeneous among individuals with the high risk genotype, the relative energy intake [intake/kg] would tend to decrease as BMI increased), or to a systematic tendency for heavier individuals to underreport energy intake.

The genotype-dependent effects of age detected in this population are similar to those reported in the Québec Family Study data (17). As suggested by Borecki *et al.* (17), a decline in BMI values with increasing age, among individuals with the high risk genotype, may be attributable to the adoption of a more prudent life-style by individuals who are genetically predisposed to heaviness, or to a secular increase in factors that produce a higher penetrance among individuals with the

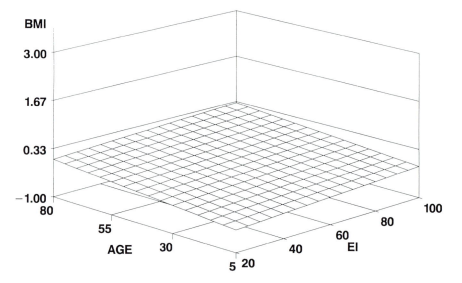

Figure 1. Expected effects of age and energy intake (EI) on the BMI, among AA and Aa individuals, under the autosomal recessive, mixed segregation analysis model.

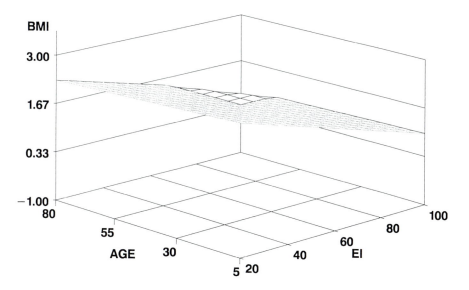

Figure 2. Expected effects of age and energy intake (EI) on the BMI, among aa individuals, under the autosomal recessive, mixed segregation analysis model.

high risk genotype. It is also possible that the simple linear effects considered in these analyses do not fully account for the relationship between age and the BMI.

Summary and Future Directions

Genetic analyses provide ample support for the involvement of genes in the development of the BMI. The BMI is, however, a composite measure of heaviness, reflecting not only fat mass but also body build, proportions, and lean body mass, and it is unclear which of these aspects are under genetic control. Hence, evaluation of more direct measures of obesity and intermediate phenotypes, which are likely to be more closely related to the effects of an individual gene, is a critical aspect of efforts to increase our understanding of the genetic epidemiology of obesity.

The Québec Family Study includes data on what is perhaps the largest battery of obesity-related measurements to be obtained in a study of its magnitude (*i.e.*, 1630 individuals in 375 families). Underwater weighing, from which some of the most direct measures of obesity (*i.e.*, percent body fat and fat mass) are derived, was performed on approximately one-half of the participants in this study. Commingling analyses of the percent body fat and fat mass data from the Québec Family Study indicate that there is significant heterogeneity in the distribution of both phenotypes between the parental and offspring generations (25). Hence, if major genes are involved in the determination of these phenotypes, their effects may be age dependent. Segregation analyses have indicated that the family data for both the percent body fat and fat mass are best described by a model that includes a major autosomal recessive gene plus multifactorial transmission (18).

Analyses of the BMI and other obesity-related phenotypes strongly suggest that the effects of obesity genes are modified by age and sex, and may also be influenced by factors such as energy intake. Identification of additional covariates that exert genotype-dependent effects should help to further elucidate the genetic contribution to many obesity-related phenotypes and, ultimately, may aid in the identification of individuals at high risk of developing patterns of obesity associated with adverse health consequences.

Characterization and identification of genes that contribute to the observed correlations between obesity and other anthropomorphic, physiologic, and biochemical measures also represents a major challenge for future research. Our understanding of the genetic basis for such associations is likely to be aided by developments in statistical modeling that allow for explicit tests regarding pleiotropic genetic effects. Preliminary analyses of pleiotropic effects on the BMI indicate that only a small portion (e.g., 1%–3%) of the additive genetic variance for this phenotype can be attributed to the effects of individual pleiotropic genes (11). The potential for pleiotropic effects of major genes on the BMI and other obesity-related phenotypes is currently being evaluated using data from the Québec Family Study.

Past research supports the view that genes contribute to the development of obesity and confirms what has long been suspected: the genetic contribution to obesity is unlikely to be straightforward. Ongoing and future research efforts, directed by our current understanding of the genetic epidemiology of obesity, are likely to focus on the analysis of obesity-related phenotypes that provide relatively direct measures of obesity and intermediate phenotypes, on genotype-dependent covariate effects, and on the genetic basis for the associations between obesity and other phenotypes. In addition, due to the availability of polymorphic DNA markers throughout the human genome, ongoing and future research efforts will, undoubtedly, be aimed at identifying and mapping individual genetic loci involved in the development of human obesity.

ACKNOWLEDGMENTS

This work was partly supported by grants from the National Institutes of Health (GM28719) and the Medical Research Council of Canada (GM 28719).

REFERENCES

1. Savard R, Bouchard C, Leblanc C, Tremblay A. Familial resemblance in fatness indicators. *Ann Hum Biol.* 1983;2:111–118.
2. Bouchard C, Savard R, Després J-P, Tremblay A, Leblanc C. Body composition in adopted and biological siblings. *Hum Biol.* 1985;57: 61–75.
3. Bouchard C, Perusse L, Leblanc C, Tremblay A, Thériault G. Inheritance of the amount and distribution of human body fat. *Int J Obes.* 1988;12:205–215.
4. Friedlander Y, Kark JD, Kaufmann NA, Berry EM, Stein Y. Familial aggregation of body mass index in ethnically diverse families in Jerusalem: the Jerusalem Lipid Research Clinic. *Int J Obes.* 1988;12: 237–247.
5. Nirmala A, Mitchell LE, Reddy PC, Rao DC. Assessment of adiposity in an Indian population: familial correlations. *Genet Epidemiol.* 1993;10:133–143.
6. Friedman JM, Leibel RL, Bahary N. Molecular mapping of obesity genes. *Mammalian Genome.* 1991;1:130–144.
7. Hall JG. How imprinting is relevant to human disease. *Development.* 1990;Suppl:141–148.
8. Smith DW. *Recognizable Patterns of Human Malformation.* Philadelphia: WB Saunders Company;1982:642.
9. Hunt SC, Hasstedt SJ, Kuida H, Stults BM, Hopkins PN, Williams RR. Genetic heritability and common environmental components of resting and stressed blood pressures, lipids, and body mass index in Utah pedigrees and twins. *Am J Epidemiol.* 1989;129:625–638.
10. Vogler GP, Srinivasan MR, Stunkard AJ, Sørensen TIA, Rao DC.

The significance of genetic and nonshared environmental influences on human obesity. *Am J Hum Genet.* 1990;47:A81.

11. Schork NJ, Weder AB, Trevisan M, Laurenzi M. The contribution
of pleiotropy to blood pressure and body-mass index variation: the
Gubbio Study. *Am J Hum Genet.* 1994;54:361–373.

12. Vogler GP, Sørensen TIA, Stunkard AJ, Srinivasan MR, Rao DC.
Influences of genes and shared family environment on adult body
mass index assessed in an adoption study by a comprehensive path
model in adoption studies. *Relat Metab Disord.* 1995;19:40–45.

13. Hasstedt SJ, Ramirez ME, Kuida H, Williams RR. Recessive inheritance of a relative fat pattern. *Am J Hum Genet.* 1989;45:917–925.

14. Price RA, Ness R, Laskarzewski P. Common major gene inheritance
of extreme overweight. *Hum Biol.* 1990;14:747–765.

15. Province MA, Arnqvist P, Keller J, Higgins M, Rao DC. Strong ev-
idence for a major gene for obesity in the large, unselected total
Community Health Study of Tecumseh. *Am J Hum Genet.* 1990;47:
A143.

16. Moll PP, Burns TL, Lauer RM. The genetic and environmental
sources of body mass index variability: the Muscatine Ponderosity
Family Study. *Am J Hum Genet.* 1991;40:1243–1255.

17. Borecki IB, Bonney GE, Rice T, Bouchard C, Rao DC. Influence of
genotype-dependent effects of covariates on the outcome of segregation analysis of the body mass index. *Am J Hum Genet.* 1993;
53:676–687.

18. Rice T, Borecki IB, Bouchard C, Rao DC. Segregation analysis of fat
mass and other body composition measures derived from underwater weighing. *Am J Hum Genet.* 1993;52:967–973.

19. Borecki IB, Rice T, Perusse L, Bouchard C. Major gene influence on
the propensity to store fat in trunk versus extremity depots: evidence from the Québec Family Study. *Obes Res.* 1995;3:1–8.

20. Beales P, Kopelman P, Vijayaraghavan S, Hitman G. The molecular
genetics of obesity. In: Bray GA, Ryan DH, eds. *Molecular and Genetic Aspects of Obesity.* Pennington Center Nutrition Series, 5. Baton
Rouge, LA: Louisiana State University Press; 1995:534–545.

21. Oppert J-M, Tourville J, Chagnon M, Mauriège P, Dionne FT, Bouchard C. Adrenoceptor genes and regional fat distribution in humans: an association study. In: Abstract booklet of Pennington Biomedical Research Center Symposium on Molecular and Genetic

Aspects of Obesity. Baton Rouge: Pennington Biomedical Research Center; 1994.

22. Wilson AF, Elston RC, Siervogel RM. Possible evidence of linkage for a relative fat pattern index (RFPI) and other anthropomorphic traits using the robust sib-pair method. *Am J Hum Genet.* 1990;47: A149.

23. Borecki IB, Rice T, Pérusse L, Bouchard C, Rao DC. An exploratory investigation of genetic linkage with body composition and fatness phenotypes: the Québec Family Study. In press.

24. Garn SM, Leonard WR, Hawthorne VM. Three limitations of the body mass index. *Am J Clin Nutr.* 1986;44:996–997.

25. Borecki IB, Rice T, Bouchard C, Rao DC. Commingling analysis of generalized body mass and composition measures: the Québec Family Study. *Int J Obes.* 1991;15:763–773.

26. Macdonald A, Stunkard AJ. Body mass indexes of British separated twins. *N Engl J Med.* 1990;322:1530.

27. Stunkard AJ, Harris JR, Pedersen NL, McClearn GE. The body-mass index of twins who have been reared apart. *N Engl J Med.* 1990;322: 1483–1487.

28. Price RA, Gottesman II. Body fat in identical twins reared apart: roles for genes and environment. *Behav Genet.* 1991;21:1–7.

29. Price RA, Stunkard AJ. Commingling analysis of obesity in twins. *Hum Hered.* 1989;39:121–135.

30. Price RA, Sørensen TIA, Stunkard AJ. Component distributions of body mass index defining moderate and extreme overweight in Danish women and men. *Am J Epidemiol.* 1998;130:193–201.

31. Price RA, Ness R, Sørensen TIA. Changes in commingled body mass index distributions associated with secular trends in overweight among Danish young men. *Am J Epidemiol.* 1991;133:501–510.

32. Province MA, Keller J, Higgins M, Rao DC. A commingling analysis of obesity in the Tecumseh Community Health Study. *Am J Hum Biol.* 1991;3:435–445.

33. Ness R, Laskarzewski P, Price RA. Inheritance of extreme overweight in black families. *Hum Biol.* 1991;63:39–52.

34. Price RA, Lunetta K, Ness R, *et al.* Obesity in Pima Indians: distribution characteristics and possible thresholds for genetic studies. *Int J Obes.* 1992;16:851–857.

35. Mitchell LE, Nirmala A, Rice T, Reddy PC, Rao DC. Commingling

analysis of adiposity in an Indian population. *Int J Obes.* 1994;18: 1–8.

36. Rice T, Borecki IB, Bouchard C, Rao DC. Segregation analysis of body mass index in an unselected French-Canadian sample: the Québec Family Study. *Obesity Res.* 1993;1:288–294.

37. Mitchell LE, Nirmala A, Rice T, Reddy PC, Rao DC. The impact of energy intake and energy expenditure of activity on the familial transmission of adiposity in an Indian population. *Am J Hum Biol.* 1993;5:331–339.

38. Konigsberg LW, Blangero J, Kammerer CM, Mott GE. Mixed model segregation analysis of LDL-C concentration with genotype-covariate interaction. *Genet Epidemiol.* 1991;8:69–80.

39. Hasstedt SJ. A mixed-model likelihood approximation on large pedigrees. *Comput Biomed Res.* 1982;15:295–307.

PART VI

Molecular Markers in Human Obesity

PER BJÖRNTORP

Overview: Biology of Regional Fat Distribution

ABSTRACT

Visceral obesity predicts non–insulin-dependent diabetes mellitus, cardiovascular disease, and stroke and is associated statistically with the established metabolic risk factors of these diseases. The condition shows several endocrine abnormalities in which a hypersensitive hypothalamo-adrenal axis seems to be a prominent feature. This axis responds to challenges at central, pituitary, and adrenal levels with elevated, protracted cortisol secretion, but it is not necessarily abnormally active in steady-state conditions, suggesting consequences of central, depressive responses to perceived stress with diminished feed-forward inhibition of cortisol secretion. There is suggestive evidence for serotonergic involvement including regulation of both corticotropin-releasing factor and appetite. Other hormonal abnormalities in the hypothalamo-gonadal and growth hormone axes might be secondary consequences.

The multiple hormonal abnormalities provide possible explanations for both cardinal symptoms of the condition: insulin resistance and disproportional visceral accumulation of depot fat. Insulin resistance is a well-known consequence of hypercortisolemia but may also be caused by low sex steroid hormone secretions, and is probably amplified by free fatty acids from lipolytically active central depots. Visceral fat accumulation seems to be a result of the hormonal abnormalities via combined effects of elevated cortisol and insulin to accumulate triglycerides, whereas testosterone and growth hormone have opposite effects. Consequently low levels of the latter hormones will facilitate triglyceride accumulation. These events are probably more pronounced in visceral than other fat depots because of combined effects of high densities of adipocytes, specific steroid hormone receptors, and innervation as well as a high blood flow, resulting in a depot with a rapid turnover.

515

The hyperactivity of the hypothalamo-adrenal axis suggests influence of perceived stress on susceptible personalities, a supposition supported by findings of associated psychosomatic and psychiatric disease, with depressive traits. There is also evidence for psychosocial and socioeconomic handicaps, and influence of smoking and alcohol consumption, which might provide background factors.

Introduction

A number of cross-sectional and recent epidemiological studies have demonstrated that abdominal or visceral obesity is associated with the metabolic risk factors for cardiovascular disease, non–insulin-dependent diabetes mellitus, and stroke, as well as an increased incidence of these diseases (1). Although prospective studies are rare (2), it seems that it is actually the visceral adipose tissue that is the critical subcompartment because numerous studies have now shown closer relationships between the metabolic risk factors and visceral adipose tissue mass (1) and function (3) than other fractions of adipose tissue.

Visceral Adipose Tissue

In cross-sectional and epidemiological studies, visceral obesity is indicated to be the entity that is associated with the major hazards for development of disease. Visceral obesity consists of two components: a mass factor in terms of total adipose tissue mass and a distribution factor, the fraction of total adipose triglycerides localized to the visceral subcompartment. The question then arises, which of these two factors is the most important. In prospective epidemiological studies, the distribution factor, measured as the surrogate waist/hip circumference ratio (WHR), has been found to be a stronger predictor for disease than a measurement of general obesity, the body mass index (BMI) (4, 5). Also in cross-sectional studies, the WHR seems to be more closely connected with the metabolic risk factors and elevated blood pressure than the BMI (6). This seems to be particularly true for smoking and coagulation variables (1). These analyses thus indicate that the distribution factor is more important than the total body fat mass.

Another more complicated question is whether the absolute mass of visceral adipose tissue is important, or just the proportion of depot fat in this region. To take an example, is a man with a total of 15 kg body fat, of which 30% (4.5 kg) is in the visceral depots, at a higher risk than a man with 30 kg body fat with 20% (6 kg) in the same depots? Statistical studies employing absolute mass measurements of visceral fat by computed tomographic (CT)-scans, related statistically to the risk factor pattern, have suggested that the absolute mass is the critical factor. Consequently the man above with a lower proportion (20%) but higher absolute mass (6 kg) would be expected to show more tight coupling between visceral fat mass and the risk factors. This kind of quantitative "dose-response" result is suggestive of a cause-effect relationship, and explanatory mechanisms have been put forward, indicating that free fatty acids, released from the lipolytically very active visceral adipose tissues, may in fact generate metabolic risk factors (7). On the other hand, other studies have consistently shown that the proportion of visceral fat in relation to total fat or subcutaneous fat is the most important factor (8, 9). If this is correct, it may mean that visceral fat distribution is an indicator of mechanisms that direct depot fat disproportionally to visceral adipose tissue. In other words, there may be common factors underlying visceral fat accumulation and generating the metabolic risk factors. This point then might give indications of whether visceral adipose tissue is the villain or an innocent bystander, or with a combination of both alternatives, a participating bystander. There is actually evidence for all these alternatives, as will be seen in the following.

Endocrine and Neuroendocrine Disturbances

Clinicians have long noted that some obese subjects are Cushing-like in appearance as far as fat distribution, hirsutism, elevated blood pressure, and so on. Such cases sometimes require rather elaborate work-ups with hormonal tests to exclude excessive hypercortisolism of pituitary origin or from cortisol-producing adenomas or tumors. It was shown many years ago that cortisol turnover rate is elevated in obesity in general, but that plasma concentrations of cortisol may be normal or even lower than normal. However, in these subjects the diurnal secretory rhythm, as well as suppression tests, is normal, distinguishing such patients from Cushing's disease or syndrome (10–12). Unfortunately these studies did not take into consideration the subgroups of human obesity.

Vague has noted already that patients with android obesity secreted more cortisol after adrenocorticotrophic hormone (ACTH) challenge than gynoid obese patients did (13). This phenomenon has recently attracted considerable attention. We confirmed Vague's finding and showed in addition that physical and mental stressors in centrally obese women caused more cortisol response than in peripherally obese women (14). The stress-response was elevated and protracted, as recently confirmed in an elegant study by Rebuffé-Scrive *et al.* (15). Furthermore, Pasquali *et al.* have recently shown that, in addition to ACTH challenge, the administration of corticotropin-releasing factor (CRF) was followed by elevated ACTH and cortisol release in abdominally obese subjects (16). These studies then show that the hypothalamo-adrenal axis of abdominally obese subjects is sensitive to challenge at the levels of the adrenals, pituitary, and central nervous system. This does not necessarily mean that urinary cortisol levels are elevated, and midday serum cortisol levels actually tend to be low (14). These observations indicate that in resting, steady-state conditions the hypothalamo-adrenal axis may actually show a low activity. This supposition is supported not only by findings of low midday serum cortisol, but also by normal urinary cortisol output under steady-state conditions, as well as by low CRF levels in the cerebrospinal fluid (CSF) (unpublished observations). During stressful conditions, however, such as during "field-conditions," environmental challenges would probably trigger large, prolonged activity along the CRF-ACTH-cortisol axis, as has also been observed (14).

The CRF or ACTH tests (13, 14, 16) indicate that this axis is sensitized to stimuli. This might be due either to sensitive pituitary or adrenal targets, or to a diminished central feed-forward regulation of CRF secretion. In animals subjected to repeated stress the glucocorticoid receptors in the hippocampal area are down-regulated or even disappearing irreversibly. These receptors regulate the secretion of CRF to balance the CRF-adrenal axis (17, 18). It may therefore be considered that a hyperactivity of the CRF-adrenal axis in abdominal obesity may in fact be due to such a diminution of glucocorticoid receptors and their feed-forward inhibition of CRF secretion. This has also been considered to be part of the aging process (17). Recent studies suggest that the feed-forward inhibition of cortisol secretion is indeed diminished (Ljung *et al.*, unpublished).

This condition might, in analogy with the animal studies (17, 18), be triggered by repeated physical and mental stressors, causing an increased activity along the CRF-adrenal axis. Smoking and alcohol abuse are also followed by similar activity increases (19, 20). Interestingly, there is evidence that all these factors are active in abdominally obese subjects, as will be considered in a later section. It is thus possible to consider that the "functional" hypercortisolism in abdominal obesity is actually primarily induced by centrally acting triggers (stress, alcohol, smoking), which when repeated frequently may lead to a down-regulation of central glucocorticoid receptor density, diminishing the feed-forward inhibition of the CRF-adrenal axis with the consequence that this axis becomes sensitive to stimuli at the central nervous system, pituitary, and adrenal levels. Currently available evidence is entirely compatible with this explanation. Evidence for the presence of this mechanism in humans, and not only in rodents, is found in results of studies of Cushing's syndrome (21). Such patients seem to be subjected to cerebral atrophy in the appropriate regions, proportional to their hypercortisolemia, followed by mental handicaps.

Serotonergic neurons are apparently involved in this chain of events. First, 5-hydroxytryptamin (5-HT, serotonin) is regulating the secretion of CRF (22). The 5-HT metabolite 5-hydrox-3-indole acetic acid (5-HIAA) is tightly correlated with CRF concentrations in the CSF in centrally but not peripherally obese women, and both are inversely related to the WHR, again only in the former subgroup (unpublished data). This then suggests that 5-HT and associated CRF are particularly low in the CSF of abdominally obese women, strongly supported by tentative comparisons with normal subjects (unpublished data). This is followed by associations with appetite regulation, including energy in general and carbohydrate in particular, sometimes leading to voracious eating (unpublished data). These observations then strongly suggest that serotonergic neurons are also involved in human eating behavior, as shown repeatedly in previous animal research (23). This is further supported by the effects of serotonin agonists to decrease appetite and food intake in obese humans (23). These observations indicate that such drugs would be particularly efficient in abdominal obesity, but this has not been extensively studied.

In experiments in animals with repeated stress, leading to a low density of glucocorticoid receptors in the hippocampus, the serotonergic system is also participating. The 5-HT1A receptors become down-regulated, but the 5-HT_2 receptors seem to increase in density (18). The exact consequences of these perturbations, as well as a potential involvement of 5-HT secretion, do not seem to be possible to evaluate at present. The observations referred to above demonstrate, however, that serotonergic neurons and receptors are involved in this vicious cycle, and are interesting targets for further studies.

Measurements in CSF of neuropeptides and catecholamine metabolites have resulted in other potentially interesting findings. Some of the correlations between the factors analyzed are found only in abdominal obesity and not in women with peripheral obesity. The interrelations between 5-HIAA and CRF were mentioned above. Tight correlations were also found between 5-HIAA and endorphins as well as homovanillic acid (HVA), a metabolite of dopamine. It is known from animal experiments that 5-HT regulates the secretion of CRF, endorphins, and dopamine from the hypothalamic nuclei (24). The observations mentioned might mean that these couplings are closer in abdominal than peripheral obesity, and that low 5-HT is followed by such phenomena. Whatever the correct interpretation here will turn out to be, there is clearly a difference between abdominal and peripheral obesity in their interrelationships between neuropeptides and catecholamine metabolites in the CSF, as well as with the regulated functions of these factors in terms of eating behavior and the CRF-adrenal axis. These observations indicate that central nervous system regulation of neuroendocrine factors are different in abdominal than in peripheral obesity. As will be reviewed in the following, it seems likely that these perturbations may in fact be at least partially responsible for the endocrine as well as metabolic and anthropometric perturbations in visceral obesity.

The sensitivity of the hypothalamo-adrenal axis is not the only endocrine perturbation in visceral obesity. Sex steroid hormone secretions are blunted. Testosterone secretion is diminished in men (25–28), and women are frequently oligomenorrhoic or amenorrhoic (29). In addition, women tend to be hyperandrogenic (13). Furthermore, recent studies have shown that growth hormone secretion is particularly blunted in visceral obesity (30). There is a possibility that these endocrine abnormalities may be secondary to the increased activity of the CRF-axis, because CRF inhibits the gonadotropin-releasing hormone as well as growth hormone–releasing hormone (GHRH) secretion centrally (31). This possibility then indicates the potential primary importance of the disturbances in the hypothalamo-adrenal axis and its putative central origin.

It should be pointed out, however, that hyperandrogenicity of women does not seem to fit into this attempt to find a common denominator. There are, however, interesting recent observations that may be informative from this particular aspect. CSF concentrations of 5-HIAA are negatively correlated to free testosterone concentrations in serum women (unpublished observations). Furthermore, a recent study has shown that in women with premenstrual syndrome, serotonergic mechanisms might be involved, in connection with hyperandrogenicity. Serotonergic agonists are helpful in this condition (32). These observations suggest some connection between central serotonergic neurons and hyperandrogenicity in women. There is also the possibility that the hyperandrogenicity is an additional consequence of the hyperactive hypothalamic pituitary-adrenal axis, because this abnormality is amplified by HCTH administration (13). This is perhaps the most simple and probable explanation.

Consequences of the Endocrine Perturbations for Insulin Sensitivity

Elevated cortisol, low testosterone concentrations in men, and elevated testosterone in women, as well as a blunted growth hormone secretion, are the endocrine abnormalities now described repeatedly in visceral obesity (see above, and review in 33). Cortisol's ability to induce insulin resistance is well established. Recently it has also been shown that a lower than normal testosterone concentration in men, as well as hyperandrogenicity in women, may well be at least contributing to muscular insulin resistance (for review, see 34). In addition, subjects with total growth hormone deficiency are also insulin resistant (Bengtsson, personal communication). It is thus apparent that the entire set of observed endocrine abnormalities may indeed contribute to establish an insulin resistant condition. In addition, free fatty acids from enlarged visceral and other adipose tissues may well contribute as an additional powerful mechanism (7). Taken together, the observed endocrine perturbations, most likely induced by central mechanisms, may well be causative factors for the insulin resistance characteristic of visceral obesity. Insulin resistance with ensuing hyperinsulinemia has been considered to be a major background factor for other metabolic perturbations as well as elevated blood pressure constituting a cluster of risk factors and diseases called Syndrome X (35) or the Metabolic Syndrome. Visceral distribution of depot fat is most likely a part of this syndrome (6).

Consequences of the Endocrine Perturbations for Body Fat Distribution

As will be briefly reviewed in the following section, there is now considerable evidence to suggest that a concerted action of the multiple endocrine perturbation in visceral obesity with the Metabolic Syndrome may in fact also cause a distribution of body fat with a preponderance to visceral depots. This is based on the following observations.

First, Cushing's syndrome is a dramatic, clinical example demonstrating that hypercortisolemia is followed by visceral fat accumulation. This is further emphasized by the observation that after successful treatment, visceral fat accumulation is vanishing, as shown with detailed CT-scan measurements (Sjöström, personal communication). The effects of cortisol on adipose tissue, in concert with insulin, is to increase the expression of lipoprotein lipase (LPL) via the glucocorticoid receptor and gene interactions as well as enzyme stabilization (36, 37). Furthermore, this combination of hormonal abnormalities decreases the activity of the lipolytic machinery (Ottosson, unpublished). The effects of testosterone are largely opposite, inhibiting LPL activity and stimulating the lipolytic cascade at several levels. These effects are mediated via a specific receptor for androgens and, most likely, interaction with appropriate genes. In addition, the androgen receptor seems to be upregulated in density by testosterone, amplifying its effects (38–40).

Growth hormone interacts critically with these activities of both cortisol and testosterone. With cortisol, the LPL expression is sensitively inhibited, not including gene transcription interactions, and lipolysis is now turned on to a high activity (Ottosson, unpublished). Growth hormone acts in synergism with testosterone in its LPL-inhibitory effect (Xu, unpublished) and is actually necessary for the full expression of the lipolytic stimulation of testosterone (Yang, Xu, Vikman, Edén, Björntorp, unpublished data).

In summary, this means that cortisol and insulin potentiate regulatory systems for lipid accumulation and inhibit lipolytic actions at the cellular level, whereas testosterone and growth hormone have opposite effects. From this it follows that one would expect the relative hypercortisolism and hyperinsulinemia in combination with low testosterone and growth hormone levels in visceral obesity to act efficiently to accumulate triglycerides in adipocytes. The reason why this is occurring mainly in visceral fat seems to be a specifically high density of steroid hormone receptors in this tissue in combination with a high density of adipocytes per unit weight. Furthermore, at least in rats, blood flow is higher and innervation denser in this than other depots (41, 42). These factors act in concert to create a fat depot with very high turnover. Perturbations of the secretion of hormones involved in the regulation of adipose tissue mass will be followed by more pronounced consequences in visceral fat than other adipose tissue regions for these reasons.

This synthesis of data from cellular and molecular studies agrees with clinical and physiological observations. As seen above, the balance between the lipid accumulating hormones (cortisol and insulin) on one side and the lipid mobilizing hormones (testosterone and growth hormone) on the other will be critical for the net effects on visceral adipose tissue mass. Conditions known to be followed by visceral accumulation are Cushing's syndrome (high cortisol and insulin, low growth hormone and testosterone), aging (normal cortisol and insulin, low growth hormone and testosterone), total growth hormone deficiency after hypophysectomy with substitution of other hormones (43), alcoholism (high cortisol) (20, 44), smoking (high cortisol) (19, 45), visceral obesity (high cortisol and insulin, low growth hormone and testosterone in men), and they all show a hormonal balance toward the lipid accumulating side. When Cushing patients are cured (Sjöström, personal communication), men with low testosterone are substituted with testosterone (46) and growth hormone–deficient patients with growth hormone (47), visceral depots decrease markedly, demonstrating that the suggested mechanisms probably are correct.

Female sex steroid hormones in women probably have similar effects as testosterone in the suggested chain of events. For example, with menopause and decreased levels of female sex steroid hormones, visceral fat increases, which can be prevented by hormone replacement therapy (48); and LPL in the characteristic adipose tissue of the gluteo-femoral regions of women is regulated by estrogen (49). The exploration of further detailed regulatory mechanisms of female sex steroid hormones has been severely hampered by the absence of specific receptors for these hormones in human adipose tissue (50, 51). However, evidence is now emerging suggesting that growth hormone secretion pattern may play a role in these regulations (52, and Yang *et al.*, un-published). It is therefore possible that the female sex steroid hormones act on adipose tissue triglyceride balance via regulation of the secretion pattern of growth hormone. Recent studies also suggest the possibility of modification of the androgen receptor by estrogen (unpublished data).

In summary, evidence has now emerged that strongly suggests that both cardinal symptoms of visceral obesity (insulin resistance and visceral fat accumulation) may in fact be due to the multiple endocrine abnormalities of that condition. It is also possible that visceral fat accumulation, secondarily via portal free fatty acids, amplifies insulin resistance in both the liver and muscles (7), as mentioned in a preceding section. The central endocrine abnormality seems to be located to the hypothalamo-adrenal axis, with a potential background in central serotonergic neurons, as reviewed above. It then becomes important to try to trace the background factors for this abnormality.

Pathogenetic Factors

Potential pathogenetic factors to the syndrome are most likely found in the central regulation of neuroendocrine secretions. When these become clearer, it will be easier to examine explanatory mechanisms, which now have to be speculative based mainly on circumstantial evidence.

As mentioned above, stress reactions might be involved as suggested by the aberrations in the hypothalamo-adrenal regulatory system. With submissive, depressive reactions to perceived stressful environmental factors, the hypothalamo-adrenal axis is reacting in this way, and the axis may be sensitized by repeated chronic challenges. The overwhelming part of the background literature in this area comes from animal studies, and the information is rather consistent. Because of the primitive lifesaving regulatory function of this part of the brain, it seems likely that the human should react similarly, though this is more difficult to observe because of overriding psychological mechanisms (53), and of course much more difficult to subject to conclusive experimental testing in humans. There are, however, observations in standardized test situations that suggest a reaction in humans similar to that in animals (54). Several studies (14, 15) have shown that such stress reactions might also be amplified in humans, as they are in rodents (17, 18). These observations strongly suggest that stress reactions of the cortisol-generating type are involved in the syndrome both at the physical level in terms of cold pressure test (14), use of alcohol, and smoking (19, 20), and at mental levels (14, 15).

Furthermore, other potential consequences of this type of stress re-action have been found, such as frequent sick leave in psychosomatic types of diseases (peptic ulcer, gastrointestinal bleeding), frequent use of free health facilities, and high scores in the generalized question of perceived stress. Use of alcohol and smoking is more frequent. Fur-thermore, infectious diseases seem to be more prevalent. This infor-mation is consistent in independent studies of both men and women in the population (55, 56). Additional information is available on women showing a high prevalence of mental disorders, including anx-iety and depression. Interestingly, the prevalence of using antidepres-sant drugs was apparently linearly related to the WHR, with a large difference between the first and fifth quintile of the WHR, suggesting that depressive equivalents may be of importance. Sleeplessness, use of sleeping pills, and nightmares were also prevalent (56). Recent stud-ies have also shown similar perturbations in men (Rosmond *et al.*, un-published). Several of these observations have now been confirmed (57, 58), providing a relatively suggestive base of information on the involvement of psychological, psychosomatic, and psychiatric fac-tors. Furthermore, the relationship between the WHR and smoking or the use of alcohol has been repeatedly described (44, 55, 56, 59), also including detailed CT-scan measurements (44). The latter is an important distinction because the WHR might be misleading in con-ditions in which muscle atrophy is involved, such as in excessive use of alcohol (44).

The impact of stressful situations varies with personality character-istics; stress is perceived differently among individuals (60). Personality variables, therefore, are of interest here, not least in relation to a poten-tial involvement of central serotonergic mechanisms. We have reported that women in the population with a high WHR have traits of "sen-sation seeking" behavior (56). This type of behavior is believed to be associated with low serotonergic drive (61) and would to some degree be consistent with the observations in CSF of low 5-HIAA levels in viscerally obese women (unpublished data). Clearly much work is needed in this sector.

Having observed signs of stress in endocrine, psychological, and psychosomatic variables, it becomes important to look for environmental factors that may be triggers for such reactions. We found (56) that men with a high WHR are afflicted by several socioeconomic and psychosocial handicaps. For example, they have a low level of education, perform a physical type of unskilled labor, have a low income, and belong to a low social class. Similar socioeconomic and psychosocial observations have subsequently been reported for other ethnic groups (62, 63). Recent studies also have demonstrated a clear correlation with divorce and living alone (unpublished data). It seems suggestive to lead this into a chain of events in which economical problems and a monotonous, dependent work situation may lead to perceived stress and reactions of the type described above. This is, however, less apparent in women (56), but the socioeconomic situation in Sweden is still very much dependent on the working conditions of the husband in a couple.

Hyperandrogenicity, a characteristic feature of women with this syndrome, has also potentially interesting connections with central regulatory mechanisms. As mentioned above there are apparent associations between hyperandrogenicity and low levels of 5-HIAA in the CSF (unpublished data). Furthermore, it has been found that women with a high level of education and an independent type of profession often have higher testosterone levels than other women. This might be considered to be a consequence of perceived stress, but it may also be looked upon in the reverse. Women might be assisted by aggressive behavior induced by testosterone to reach these kinds of professions against conventional resistance (64). Thus, there are suggestive connections between hyperandrogenicity and psychosocial factors in which neuroendocrine and serotonergic mechanisms might be involved. This area needs further exploration.

As mentioned above, women with the syndrome report more anxiety and depression, and there are clear relationships between antidepressant medication and the WHR (56). Depression is well known to be followed by increased activity along the CRF-hypothalamic axis (65) and by the involvement of serotonergic neurons centrally (66). This problem is also of further interest for studies.

As stated previously, this area is difficult to study conclusively in humans. However, valuable information can be obtained from animal experimentation. Of particular significance are studies in primates. In the cynomolgus monkey, Shively and Clarkson and their colleagues have recently performed experiments of significant relevance and interest to the human problem. These investigators submitted monkeys to standardized prolonged stressful events, which were followed by a submissive type of reaction, as well as the previously well-established endocrine reaction, including enlarged adrenals, presumably a consequence of stress and anovulation. This is an endocrine pattern similar to that seen in the human syndrome, though other hormonal abnormalities observed in humans have not yet been reported in the studies in monkeys. These primates further develop insulin resistance, accumulation of visceral adipose tissue, decreased glucose tolerance, elevated blood pressure, and coronary atherosclerosis (67, 70). This then is a picture that is very similar to that of the human syndrome with metabolic risk factors, hypertension, coronary atherosclerosis, diabetes, visceral accumulation of body fat, and insulin resistance with an endocrine background, detectable by standardized stress reactions. This close parallelism lends strong support to the suggestion we put forward several years ago, and have repeated (33, 71–76), that reaction to perceived stress with neuroendocrine reactions may provide the background for the syndrome.

Pathogenetic factors to the syndrome, then, seem to be found in stress reactions, use of alcohol, and smoking. In addition, a positive energy balance, based on increased energy intake and/or physical inactivity, is clearly the cause of the frequently accompanying obesity. Also, this factor probably has a central and neuroendocrine regulatory background. In addition to genetic factors (77), several undesirable lifestyle habits seem to be involved, and we have suggested that this condition should be labeled a "civilization syndrome" (33). It should be noted that the endocrine perturbations are similar to those found in aging. The syndrome discussed, therefore, has several features common with a condition of premature aging.

REFERENCES

1. Björntorp P. Abdominal fat distribution and disease: an overview of epidemiological data. *Ann Med.* 1992;24:15–18.
2. Bergstrom RW, Newell-Morris LL, Leonetti DL, Shuman WP, Wahl P, Fujimoto WY. Association of elevated fasting C-peptide level and increased intra-abdominal fat distribution with the development of NIDDM in Japanese-American men. *Diabetes.* 1990;39:104–111.
3. Marin P, Andersson B, Ottosson M, *et al.* The morphology and me-

tabolism of intraabdominal adipose tissue in men. *Metabolism*. 1992; 41:1242–1248.

4. Lapidus L, Bengtsson C, Larsson B, Pennert K, Rybo E, Sjöström L. Distribution of adipose tissue and risk of cardiovascular disease and death: 12-year follow-up of participants in the population study of women in Gothenburg, Sweden. *Br Med J*. 1984;289:1257–1261.

5. Larsson B, Svärdsudd K, Welin L, Wilhelmsen L, Björntorp P, Tibblin G. Abdominal adipose tissue distribution, obesity and risk of cardiovascular disease and death: 13-year follow-up of participants in the study of men born in 1913. *Br Med J*. 1984;288:1401–1404.

6. Lapidus L, Bengtsson C, Björntorp P, Lissner L. The quantitative relationship between "The Metabolic Syndrome" and abdominal obesity in women. *Obesity Res*. 1994;2:372–377.

7. Björntorp P. "Portal" adipose tissue as a generator of risk factors for cardiovascular disease and diabetes. *Arteriosclerosis*. 1990;10:493–496.

8. Enzi G, Gasparo M, Biondetti PR, Fiore S, Semosa M, Zurlo F. Subcutaneous and visceral fat distribution according to sex, age, and overweight, evaluated by computed tomography. *Am J Clin Nutr*. 1986;44:739–746.

9. Fujioka S, Matsuzawa Y, Tokunaga K, Tarui S. Contribution of intraabdominal fat accumulation to the impairment of glucose and lipid metabolism in human obesity. *Metabolism*. 1987;36:54–59.

10. Schteingart DE, Gregerman RI, Conn JW. A comparison of characteristics of increased adrenocortical function in obesity and in Cushing's syndrome. *Metabolism*. 1963;12:484–497.

11. Strain GW, Zumoff B, Strain JJ, *et al*. Cortisol production in obesity. *Metabolism*. 1980;29:980–985.

12. Glass AR, Burman KD, Dahms WT, *et al*. Endocrine function in human obesity. *Metabolism*. 1981;30:89–104.

13. Vague J, Vague P, Boyer J, Cloix MC. Anthropometry of obesity, diabetes, adrenal and beta-cell functions. In: Proceedings of the VII Congress of the International Diabetes Function. 1970;23:517–525. Excerpta Medica International Congress Series.

14. Mårin P, Darin N, Amemiya T, Andersson B, Jern S, Björntorp P. Cortisol secretion in relation to body fat distribution in obese premenopausal women. *Metabolism*. 1992;41:882–886.

15. Rebuffé-Scrive M. Neuroendocrine regulation of adipose tissue distribution and function. *Obesity Res.* 1993;1(suppl 2):1435. Abstract.
16. Pasquali R, Cantobelli S, Casimirri F, *et al.* The hypothalamo-pituitary-adrenal axis in obese women with different patterns of body fat distribution. *J Clin Endocrinol Metab.* 1993;77:341–346.
17. Sapolsky RM, Krey LC, McEwen BS. The neuroendocrinology of stress and aging: the glucocorticoid cascade hypothesis. *Endocr Rev.* 1986;7:284–301.
18. McEwen B. Adrenal steroid actions on brain: dissecting the fine line between protection and damage. In: Friedman MJ, Charney DS, Deutch AY, eds. *Neurobiological and Clinical Consequences of Stress: From Normal Adaptation to PTSD.* New York: Wiley; 1994.
19. Gossain VV, Sherma NK, Srivastava L, Michelakis AM, Rovner DR. Hormonal effects of smoking, II: effects on plasma, cortisol, growth hormone, and prolactin. *Am J Med Sci.* 1986;291:325–327.
20. Cicero TJ. Sex differences in the effects of alcohol and other psychoactive drugs on endocrine function. In: Israel Y, Kalant O, Kalant H, eds. *Research Advances in Alcohol and Drug Problems.* New York: Plenum;1980:544–593.
21. Starkman M, Gebarski S, Berent S, Schteingart D. Hippocampal formation volume, memory dysfunction and cortisol levels in patients with Cushing's syndrome. *Biol Psychiatry.* 1992;32:756–765.
22. Fuller RW. The involvement of serotonin in regulation of pituitary-adrenal function. *Front Neuroendocrinol.* 1992;13:250–270.
23. Conn PJ, Sanders-Bush E. Central serotonin receptors: effector systems, physiological roles and regulation. *Psychopharmacology.* 1987; 92:267–277.
24. Bray G, York D. Hypothalamic androgenetic obesity in experimental animals: an autonomic and endocrine hypothesis. *Physiol Rev.* 1979;59:719–809.
25. Seidell J, Björntorp P, Sjöström L, Kvist H, Sannerstedt R. Visceral fat accumulation in men is positively associated with insulin, glucose and C-peptide levels, but negatively with testosterone levels. *Metabolism.* 1990;39:897–901.
26. Haffner S, Valdez R, Stern M, Katz M. Obesity, body fat distribution and sex hormones in men. *Int J Obes.* 1993;17:643–649.
27. Khaw K, Chir B, Barrett-Connor E. Lower endogenous androgens predict central adiposity in men. *Am J Epidemiol.* 1992;2:675–682.
28. Simon D, Preziosi P, Barett-Connor E, *et al.* Interrelation between

plasma testosterone and plasma insulin in healthy adult men: the Telecom Study. *Diabetologia.* 1992;35:173–177.

29. Hartz A, Rupley D, Rimm A. The association of girth measurements with disease in 32 856 women. *Am J Epidemiol.* 1984;119: 71–80.

30. Mårin P, Kvist H, Lindstedt G, Sjöström L, Björntorp P. Low concentrations of insulin-like growth factor-I in abdominal obesity. *Int J Obes.* 1993;17:83–89.

31. Laatikainen T. Corticotropin-opioid peptides in reproduction and stress. *Ann Med.* 1991;23:489–496.

32. Eriksson E, Sundblad C, Lisjö P, Modigh K, Andersch B. Serum levels of androgens are higher in women with premenstrual irritability and dysphoria than in controls. *Psychoneuroendocrinology.* 1992;17:195–204.

33. Björntorp P. Visceral obesity: a "Civilization syndrome." *Obesity Res.* 1993;1:206–222.

34. Björntorp P. Androgens, the metabolic syndrome, and non–insulin-dependent diabetes mellitus. *Ann NY Acad Sci.* 1993;676:242–252.

35. Reaven GH. Role of insulin resistance in human disease. *Diabetes.* 1988;37:1595–1607.

36. Cigolini M, Smith U. Human adipose tissue in culture, VIII: studies on the insulin-antagonistic effect of glucocorticoids. *Metabolism.* 1979;28:502–510.

37. Ottosson M. The effects of cortisol on the regulation of lipoprotein lipase activity in human adipose tissue. *Int J Obes.* 1991;15(suppl 1):86.

38. Xu X, DePergola G, Björntorp P. Testosterone increases lipolysis and the number of beta-adrenoceptors in male rat adipocytes. *Endocrinology.* 1991;128:379–382.

39. Xu X, DePergola G, Eriksson P, *et al.* Postreceptor events involved in the up-regulation of β-adrenergic receptor mediated lipolysis by testosterone in rat white adipocytes. *Endocrinology.* 1993;132:1651–1657.

40. DePergola G, Xu X, Yang S, Giorgino R, Björntorp P. Up-regulation of androgen receptor binding in male rat fat pad adipose precursor cells exposed to testosterone: study in a whole cell assay system. *J Steroid Biochem Mol Biol.* 1990;37:553–558.

41. West DB, Prinz WA, Greenwood MRC. Regional changes in adipose

tissue, blood flow and metabolism in rats after a meal. *Am J Physiol.* 1989;257:R711–R716.

42. Rebuffé-Scrive M. Neuroregulation of adipose tissue: molecular and hormonal mechanisms. *Int J Obes.* 1991;15:83–86.

43. Brummer RJM, Lönn L, Grangård U, Bengtsson BÅ, Kvist H, Sjöström L. Adipose tissue and muscle volume determination by computed tomography in acromegaly, before and one year after adenectomy. *Eur J Clin Invest.* 1993;23:199–205.

44. Kvist H, Hallgren P, Jönsson L, *et al.* Distribution of adipose tissue and muscle mass in alcoholic men. *Metabolism.* 1993;42:569–573.

45. Shimokata H, Muller D, Andres R. Studies in the distribution of body fat, III: effects of cigarette smoking. *JAMA.* 1989;243:1828–1831.

46. Mårin P, Holmäng S, Gustafsson C, *et al.* Androgen treatment of abdominally obese men. *Obesity Res.* 1993;1:245–251.

47. Bengtsson BÅ, Edén S, Lönn L, *et al.* Treatment of adults with growth hormone deficiency with recombinant human growth hormone. *J Clin Endocrinol Metab.* 1992;76:309–317.

48. Haarbo J, Marslew U, Gottfredsen A, Christiansen C. Postmenopausal hormone replacement therapy prevents central distribution of body fat after menopause. *Metabolism.* 1991;40:323–326.

49. Rebuffé-Scrive M, Lönnroth P, Mårin P, Wesslau CH, Björntorp P, Smith U. Regional adipose tissue metabolism in men and postmenopausal women. *Int J Obes.* 1987;11:347–355.

50. Rebuffé-Scrive M, Brönnegård M, Nilsson A, Eldh J, Gustafsson JÅ, Björntorp P. Steroid hormone receptors in human adipose tissues. *J Clin Endocrinol Metab.* 1990;71:1215–1219.

51. Brönnegård M, Ottosson M, Böös J, Marcus C, Björntorp P. Lack of evidence for estrogen and progesterone receptors in human adipose tissue. *J Steroid Biochem Mol Biol.* 1994;51:275–281.

52. Vikman-Adolfsson K, Oscarsson J, Nilsson-Ehle P, Edén S. Growth hormone but not gonadal steroids influence lipoprotein lipase and hepatic lipase activity in hypophysectomized rats. *J Endocrinol.* 1994;140:203–209.

53. Folkow B. Stress, hypothalamic function and neuroendocrine consequences. In: Björntorp P, Smith U, Lönnroth P, eds. *Health Implications of Regional Obesity.* Acta Med Scand, Symp Ser 4, 1988;61–70.

54. Frankenhaeuser M. The sympathetic-adrenal and pituitary-adrenal response to challenge: comparisons between the sexes. In: Dom-

broski TM, Schmidt TH, Blümchen G, eds. *Biobehavioural Bases of Coronary Heart Disease. Human Psychophysiology.* Basel, Switz: Marc-Karger; 1983;2:91–105. Karger Biobehavioural Medicine Series.

55. Larsson B, Seidell J, Svärdsudd K, *et al.* Obesity, adipose tissue distribution and health in men: the study of men born in 1913. *Appetite.* 1989;13:37–44.

56. Lapidus L, Bengtsson C, Hällström T, Björntorp P. Obesity, adipose tissue distribution and health in women: results from a population study in Gothenburg, Sweden. *Appetite.* 1989;12:25–35.

57. Wing RR, Matthews KA, Kuller LH, Mellahn EN, Plantinga P. Waist to hip ratio in middle-aged women: associations with behavioural and psychosocial factors and with changes in cardiovascular risk factors. *Arterioscler Thromb.* 1991;11:1250–1257.

58. Leonetti DL, Bergstrom RW, Shuman WP, *et al.* Urinary catecholamines, plasma insulin and environmental factors in relation to body fat distribution. *Int J Obes.* 1991;15:345–357.

59. Pettersson P, Ellsinger B-M, Sjöberg C, Björntorp P. Fat distribution and steroid hormones in women with alcohol abuse. *J Intern Med.* 1990;228:311–316.

60. Karasek RA, Russel RS, Theorell T. Physiology of stress regeneration in job-related cardiovascular illness. *J Human Stress.* 1982;3:29–42.

61. Fowler CJ, von Knorring L, Oreland L. Platelet monoamine oxidase activity in sensation seekers. *Psychiatry Res.* 1980;3:273–279.

62. Georges E, Wear ML, Mueller WH. Body fat distribution and job stress in Mexican-American men of the Hispanic Health and Nutrition Exam Survey. *Am J Human Biol.* 1991;4:657–667.

63. Kaye SA, Folsom AR, Jacobs DR, Hughes GH, Flack JM. Psychosocial correlates of body fat distribution in black and white young adults. *Int J Obes.* 1993;17:271–277.

64. Purefoy FE, Koopmans LH. Androstenedione, testosterone, and free testosterone concentration in women of various occupations. *Soc Biol.* 1979;26:179–188.

65. Carrol BJ. The dexamethasone suppression test for melancholia. *Br J Psychiatry.* 1982;140:292–304.

66. Åsberg M, Thorn P, Träskman L, Bertilsson L, Ringberger V. Serotonin depression: a biochemical subgroup within the affective disorder. *Science.* 1976;191:478–480.

67. Kaplan J, Adams M, Clarkson R, Koritnik D. Psychosocial influ-

ences on female protection among cynomolgus macaques. *Atherosclerosis.* 1984;53:283–295.

68. Kaplan J, Adams M, Koritnik D, Rose J, Manuck S. Adrenal responsiveness and social status in intact and ovariectomized *Macaca fascicularis. Am J Primatol.* 1986;11:181–193.

69. Shively C, Clarkson TB, Miller CL, Weingard JW. Body fat as a risk factor for coronary artery atherosclerosis in female cynomolgus monkeys. *Arteriosclerosis.* 1987;7:226–231.

70. Jayo J, Shively C, Kaplan J, Manuck S. Effects of exercise and stress on body fat distribution in male cynomolgus monkeys. *Int J Obes.* 1993;17:597–604.

71. Björntorp P. Abdominal obesity and the development of non-insulin dependent diabetes mellitus. *Diabetes Metab Rev.* 1988;4:615–622.

72. Björntorp P. The associations between obesity, adipose tissue distribution and disease. *Acta Med Scand Suppl.* 1988;723:121–134.

73. Björntorp P. Possible mechanisms relating fat distribution and metabolism. In: Bouchard C, Johnston F, eds. *Fat Distribution During Growth and Later Health Outcomes.* New York: Alan R Liss; 1988;175–191.

74. Björntorp P. Visceral fat accumulation: the missing link between psycho-social factors and cardiovascular disease? *J Intern Med.* 1991;230:195–201.

75. Björntorp P. Metabolic abnormalities in visceral obesity. *Ann Med.* 1992;24:3–5.

76. Björntorp P. Psychosocial factors and fat distribution. In: Ailhuad G, Guy-Grand B, Lafontan M, Requier D, eds. *Obesity in Europe 91.* London: John Libbey & Co Ldt; 1992:377–387.

77. Bouchard C, Bray GA, Hubbard VS. Basic and clinical aspects of regional fat distribution. *Am J Clin Nutr.* 1990;52:946–950.

PHILIP BEALES, PETER KOPELMAN,
SHANTI VIJAYARAGHAVAN, and GRAHAM HITMAN

The Molecular Genetics of Obesity

ABSTRACT

Obesity is a multifactorial disease with a strong genetic component. The genetic component is suggested by adoption, twin, and
family studies. Segregation analysis of obesity suggests that the
disease predisposition is accounted for by a major gene (35%–
46%), polygenic loci (9%–42%), and environmental factors (25%–
48%). The best hope of identifying the major gene will be by linkage studies in obese sib-pairs by positional cloning; this type of
study is under way in several centers. The complementary approach is to study candidate genes in population association studies; this method has the power to detect both major and minor
gene effects, but is limited by the uncertainty of the primary biochemical defect and the chances of spurious results caused by poor
population stratification. So far, by this latter approach, we have
found associations between either obesity, body fat distribution,
or hyperinsulinemia, and the genes for insulin, apolipoprotein D,
and the glucocorticoid receptor. Interestingly, all these associations are also found with diabetes, suggesting an important genetic overlap between these two disorders.

Introduction

Obesity is an example of a multifactorial disease with a strong genetic
component. This is suggested by adoption, twin, and family studies
and further supported by examples of inherited monogenic disorders
(*e.g.*, Prader-Willi and Bardet-Biedl syndromes) and inherited animal
models of obesity. Sørensen *et al.* demonstrated among Danish adoptees
a significant correlation between their weight and that of their biological but not their adoptive parents or siblings (1). Stunkard went on to
study the body mass index (BMI) of identical and fraternal twins reared

534

apart and together (2). The intrapair correlation coefficients of identical twins reared apart were similar to those for twins reared together. In other words, sharing the same childhood environment did not contribute to the similarity of the BMI of twins later on in life. They concluded that genetic influences on BMI may account for as much as 70% of variance.

The situation is further complicated by the likely heterogeneity of obesity demonstrated by the topographical distribution of body fat, for example, central and gluteal obesity. Central obesity is characterized by hyperinsulinemia and insulin resistance, which are common to a number of other disorders, including diabetes, hypertension, and atherosclerosis (3). There is also evidence that the amount of intraabdominal visceral fat compared to subcutaneous fat is more affected by genetic than environmental factors. Bouchard and colleagues, in a study of twelve identical twins who were deliberately overfed, found a strong intrapair correlation for increases in the amount of intraabdominal visceral fat, with six times more variation between pairs than within pairs (4). The presence of a major gene in human obesity has been clearly demonstrated in family studies (5–8).

Genes Versus Environment

Many human diseases are inherited as simple Mendelian traits or are associated with chromosomal abnormalities. However, the majority of common diseases of adult life (diabetes mellitus, hypertension) and most congenital malformations (cleft lip and palate, neural tube defects) have complex etiologies (*i.e.,* genetic and environmental influences). The genetic predisposition to disease is thought to reflect the cumulative effect of genetic variation at several and possibly multiple loci, each with small effect on phenotype. Those diseases caused by the impact of many different genes are termed *polygenic,* and each gene has a small individual impact on phenotype. Multifactorial traits result from the interplay of multiple environmental factors with multiple genes. In practice, the terms *multifactorial* and *polygenic* are often used interchangeably.

Simple examples of genes interacting with environment are seen in phenylketonuria and celiac disease. Phenylketonuria is a single-gene disorder, inherited in an autosomal recessive fashion and occurring in northern European populations with a frequency of about one in twelve thousand births. It is caused by a deficiency of hepatic phenylalanine hydroxylase, which converts phenylalanine to tyrosine. When the child begins to eat a normal diet, phenylalanine accumulates to levels that if left will result in profound mental retardation. Strict restriction of dietary phenylalanine, if begun early in infancy, can lower plasma phenylalanine levels and prevent mental retardation. Celiac disease has a prevalence of one in two to three thousand in the United Kingdom and is characterized by gastrointestinal symptoms, loss of weight, and nutritional complications with failure-to-thrive in children. It is caused by gluten sensitivity, and this group of proteins must be eliminated from the diet to prevent further development or progression of the disease. Celiac disease has a clear-cut familial susceptibility and is likely to be polygenic. Genetic susceptibility is largely determined by multiple alleles of DQA1 and DQB1 genes located to the major histocompatibility complex on chromosome six (9). Since both the HLA-DQ alleles and the environmental factors are very common, it seems likely that other factors are also involved in the susceptibility to celiac disease.

In obesity, the majority of studies point to a major gene effect, disease predisposition accounted for by a combination of a major gene (35%–46% of total variance), polygenic loci (9%–42%), and environmental factors (25%–48%) (Fig. 1). It has been suggested that the major gene may define those patients with extreme obesity, whereas the polygenic effect may relate to the range from thin to fat.

A Strategy to Identify the Major Gene

With the advent of marker libraries covering the entire human genome, it is now possible to proceed to a random genomewide search. However, in order to implement such a stratagem, one must engage suitable clinical materials that might be drawn from: 1) very large single pedigrees; 2) nuclear families; 3) affected pedigree members (*e.g.*, sibling pairs, grandparent-grandchild pairs).

Linkage analysis follows segregation of a disease and DNA markers in affected families. When the marker and the disease are inherited together more often than would be expected by chance alone, they are said to be linked. In general terms, the closer the marker is to the gene, the less chance there is of a recombination event separating them, and the more chance there is of their segregating together.

Classical linkage analysis utilizes pedigrees to calculate log of the

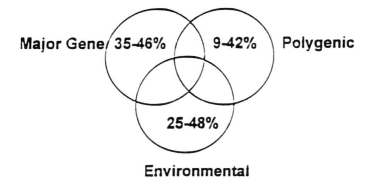

Figure 1. Gene-environment interaction.

odds (LOD) scores for linkage likelihood. The main limitations of this method are that the model of inheritance must be specified and that family collection is time consuming and costly. An alternative method of analysis is that of the affected pedigree member (sib-pair) linkage analysis. Two subtypes have been described: identity by state (IBS) and identity by descent (IBD). To perform sib-pair analysis one requires an unambiguous determination of the sib-IBD relations at the marker locus (10). Such information is usually available only if parents are available for study. In diseases such as non–insulin-dependent diabetes mellitus (NIDDM), the parents are more often not available and thus IBD relations are unknown. Weeks and Lange (11) have proposed the substitution of IBS relationships as a method of circumventing this problem and thus allowing sib-pair analysis to be performed in cases in which parents are unavailable. The IBD method, however, is likely to be the most powerful when, as is the case for obesity, both parents are alive and available for bleeding (12). In order to calculate the sample size needed for analysis one can use formulas devised by Feingold *et al.* (13) and Risch (14). To achieve 90% power using sib-pairs, we must make estimates of the risk ratio (λ_0) for an offspring of an affected individual compared with the general population prevalence. For obesity the relative risk is in the order of 2–4. Given that there may be a major gene contributing 40% of the total variance to the disorder, one can estimate that 200 to 400 sibling pairs and their parents will be required. In order to maximize the power of the analysis, sibling pairs should be sought in which it can be clearly demonstrated that one side of the family exhibits segregation of extreme obesity but the other side of the pedigree does not. Using this strategy, fewer sib-pairs would be needed; this has been confirmed by simulation experiments reported by Arlen Price (15).

A further drawback in utilizing linkage analysis is that we are looking for and assuming that a gene locus is the cause of the disease in question—in other words, a locus or allele that is "necessary" for disease expression. Greenberg (16) distinguishes two concepts: a necessary disease locus as described versus a "susceptibility locus." The latter refers to a locus that increases susceptibility or risk for the disease but that is not necessary for disease expression. In other words, an allele at some locus makes it more likely that a person will develop a disease, but the presence of that allele is not the determining factor in disease expression; it merely lowers the threshold for disease. The true determining factor could be environmental (*e.g.*, a virus) or genetic; for example, the susceptibility locus may alter the penetrance for the main locus. Referring to the example of celiac disease, gluten would be a necessary environmental determinant, whereas the disease-associated DQ alleles would be an example of a susceptibility locus. These two different models of a disease locus may lead to similar outcomes on association tests but to very different outcomes on linkage tests. If a necessary locus exists in linkage disequilibrium with a marker locus, then some allele of this locus will be found more frequently in the patient population than in the general population. The disease will be associated with an allele of the marker locus (*e.g.*, HLA region). The marker alleles will also segregate together with the disease within families, and linkage analysis will then show that genetic linkage exists between the disease and the marker locus. Thus, in the case of an associated necessary disease locus, not only is a marker allele associated with the disease, but the marker locus and the disease locus show positive results on linkage analysis. In contrast, if the locus involved is a susceptibility locus, then depending on how much additional risk is conferred by the susceptibility allele and how much risk there is without that allele, one may or may not observe a segregation of the disease with the marker. It may be that in the case of obesity we are seeing the cumulative actions of susceptibility loci at work, in which case the method of choice to investigate obesity-related genes will be the population association study.

A Strategy to Identify the Polygenic Component

POPULATION ASSOCIATION STUDIES

Population association studies have been used extensively in the past to study the genetic component of several diseases, and there have been some notable successes (Table 1).

In a population association study the distribution of a polymorphism of a candidate gene is compared between a group of subjects with disease and matched control subjects. The method relies on linkage disequilibrium between the disease-associated polymorphism and an etiological mutation in the candidate gene locus. If the disease is determined by multiple mutations in one gene (such as is the case for glucokinase and maturity onset diabetes of the young), then no association between the disease and the candidate gene will be found. The main problem of population association studies is their propensity to generate spurious results, leading to false positive or negative associations. It is likely that one of the main reasons for spurious results is hidden population stratifications between the test and control subjects, and great care should be taken to avoid this error.

MOLECULAR SCANNING OF CANDIDATE GENES

If there is a strong argument for choosing a particular candidate gene for obesity and if it is thought a mutant protein may be involved, the method of choice is molecular scanning of the candidate gene. The success of molecular scanning methodology relies on a point mutation in the candidate gene, leading to an amino acid substitution in the

Table 1. Population Association Studies

Disease	Genetic Marker
Alzheimer's disease	Apolipoprotein-E
Cardiovascular disease	Angiotensin
Insulin-dependent diabetes mellitus	HLA-DQ
Narcolepsy	HLA-DR2
Multiple sclerosis	HLA-DR2
Grave's disease	HLA-DR3
Psoriasis	HLA-Cw6, Cw7, Cw11

protein to distinguish mutant from wild type. The two most commonly used methods are the detection of single-stranded conformation polymorphisms (SSCP) and the detection of abnormal conformers by denaturing gel gradient electrophoresis (DGGE). These methods rely on mobility shifts caused by point mutations that can be detected electrophoretically. If an abnormal conformer is detected then the gene in question is sequenced.

REDUCTION OF THE COMPLEX PHENOTYPE

Obesity itself may be too complex as a phenotype to study, and perhaps the focus of attention should be on traits leading to the disease. Possible intermediate traits are listed in Table 2.

SELECTION OF A CANDIDATE GENE FOR OBESITY

The main problem with obesity is that the primary biochemical defect involved in the disease is unknown, though there are many clues to the abnormal biochemistry and physiology. The potential list of candidate genes and chromosomal regions is large, but a small selection is presented in Figure 2.

Preliminary Studies of Candidate Genes Selected Through Syndrome X

SYNDROME X

It has been suggested that resistance to insulin-stimulated glucose uptake is the abnormality underlying a number of common defects with polygenic inheritance—central obesity, NIDDM, glucose intolerance,

Table 2. Intermediate Traits and Obesity

Distribution of body fat
Insulin resistance
Other component of Syndrome X
Energy expenditure
Endocrine abnormality
Hypothalamic dysfunction

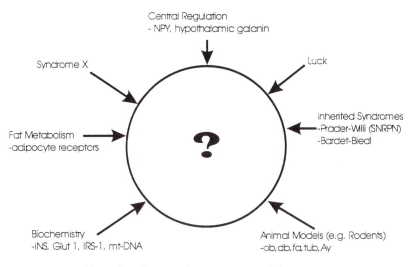

Central Regulation
- NPY, hypothalamic galanin

Syndrome X

Luck

inherited Syndromes
-Prader-Willi (SNRPN)
-Bardet-Biedl

Fat Metabolism
-adipocyte receptors

?

Biochemistry
-INS, Glut 1, IRS-1, mt-DNA

Animal Models (e.g. Rodents)
-ob, db, fa, tub, Ay

Figure 2. How to choose your candidate gene.

hyperinsulinemia, increased very low density lipoproteins triglyceride, decreased high density lipoproteins cholesterol, atherosclerosis, and hypertension. Reaven (17) has grouped together these variables into a possible single entity coined Syndrome X. This raises the possibility that all these associated diseases could have a common genetic origin. Our preliminary studies in obesity have concentrated on three genes that may be associated with Syndrome X, namely, the genes for insulin, the glucocorticoid receptor, and apolipoprotein D.

THE INSULIN GENE

The insulin (INS) gene has been cloned and localized to the short arm of chromosome 11 (11p15.5) (18). It is closely linked with a hypervariable region (HVR) of DNA, characterized by the variation in the number of tandem repeats 14 base pairs in length (19). There exist distinct size classes of alleles, depending on the number of repeats: class 1 alleles are 0–600 base pairs, class 2 are 600–1200 base pairs, and class 3 are greater than 1200 base pairs in length. Associations between NIDDM and the class 3 allele are controversial. Recent studies of the indigenous populations of southern India, in which the main determinant of diabetes is central obesity (20), have shown a positive association between the HVR and NIDDM (21). To investigate this further we studied a group of British Caucasoid severely obese women with normal glucose tolerance. A positive association between the class 3 allele and fasting hyperinsulinemia and with various indices of insulin secretion and resistance was demonstrated (22). As this region lies 5' to the INS gene we would postulate that the HVR is in linkage disequilibrium with mutations in the regulatory sequences important for transcriptional activity of the gene or, alternatively but less likely, that the HVR has a direct effect on gene regulation.

THE GLUCOCORTICOID RECEPTOR

Steroid hormone excess in man is associated with polycystic ovary syndrome, Cushing's syndrome, and steroid administration. In each of these, central obesity is a main feature often with accompanying hyperinsulinemia, glucose intolerance, and insulin resistance. Glucocorticoids when administered will result in increased glucose production, decreased glucose utilization, an effect on growth, and differentiation of adipose tissue. Diminution of steady-state levels of insulin mRNA by 80% is observed that can be reversed using a glucocorticoid receptor blocker. As glucocorticoids assume such a central role in the development of obesity, it would be reasonable to infer that an abnormality of the glucocorticoid receptor gene might likewise play a part. Similar to the insulin gene experiments, we therefore studied the same polymorphism in the population of southern India. An association was found between the glucocorticoid receptor gene polymorphism and diabetes (unpublished data).

APOLIPOPROTEIN D

We have previously described an association between the apolipoprotein D gene and NIDDM (23) and so have gone on to investigate a similar association with obesity. Using a Taq I restriction enzyme digestion, two alleles sized 2.2 kb and 2.7 kb were identified. Among the British Caucasoid group studied, we found a significant association of the 2.2 kb allele with obesity and hyperinsulinemia. This suggests an association between the apolipoprotein D polymorphism itself and obesity or linkage disequilibrium between the apolipoprotein D gene and another gene in close proximity (*e.g.,* the GLUT2 locus). Preliminary studies of GLUT2 polymorphism have failed to show any association with obesity. Hence the apolipoprotein D gene itself may be associated with obesity and hyperinsulinemia (24, 25).

Summary

Obesity is a multifactorial disease with a complex phenotype. The way to identify genes should be multifaceted in order to identify both the major and minor genes likely to be involved in the predisposition to obesity. We would suggest three main approaches to be adopted: positional cloning in affected sib-pairs, population association studies, and molecular scanning of candidate genes.

REFERENCES

1. Sørensen TIA, Price RA, Stunkard A, Shulsinger F. Genetics of obesity in adult adoptees and their biological siblings. *BMJ.* 1989;298: 87–90.
2. Stunkard AJ, Sørensen TIA, Hanis C, *et al.* An adoption study of human obesity. *N Engl J Med.* 1986;314:193–198.
3. Stunkard AJ, Harris JR, Rederson NL, McChearn GE. The body mass index of twins who have been reared apart. *N Engl J Med.* 1990;322:1483–1487.
4. Bouchard C, Tremblay A, Després J-P, *et al. N Engl J Med.* 1990;322: 1477–1482.
5. Moll PP, Burns TL, Lauer RM. The genetic and environmental sources of body mass index variability: the Muscatine ponderosity family study. *Am J Hum Genet.* 1991;49:1243–1255.
6. Hasstedt SJ, Ramirez ME, Kuida H, Williams RR. Recessive inheritance of a relative fat pattern. *Am J Hum Genet.* 1989;45:917–925.
7. Zonta LA, Jayakar SD, Bosiso M, Galante A, Pennetti V. Genetic analysis of human obesity in an Italian sample. *Hum Hered.* 1987; 37:129–139.
8. Paganini-Hill A, Martin AO, Spence MA. The S-leut anthropometric traits: genetic analysis. *Am J Phys Anthropol.* 1981;55:55–67.
9. Spurkland A, Sollid LM, Ronningen KS, *et al.* Susceptibility to develop celiac disease is primarily associated with HLA-DQ alleles. *Hum Immunol.* 1990;29(3):157–165.
10. Thomson G. Determining the mode of inheritance of RFLP-asso-

ciated diseases using the affected sib-pair method. *Am J Hum Genet.* 39:207–221.

11. Weeks DE, Lange K. The affected-pedigree-member method of linkage analysis. *Am J Hum Genet.* 1988;42:315–326.

12. Rich S. Mapping genes in diabetes: genetic epidemiological perspective. *Diabetes.* 1990;39:1315–1319.

13. Feingold E, Brown PO, Siegmund D. Gaussian models for genetic linkage analysis using complete high-resolution maps of identity-by-descent. *Am J Hum Genet.* 1993;53:234–251.

14. Risch N. Linkage strategies for genetically complex traits, II: the power of affected relative pairs. *Am J Hum Genet.* 1990;46:229–241.

15. Price RA. Obesity genes in human populations. In: Bray GA, Ryan DH, eds. *Molecular and Genetic Aspects of Obesity.* Pennington Center Nutrition Series, 5. Baton Rouge, LA: Louisiana State University Press; 1995:453–461.

16. Greenberg DA Linkage analysis of "necessary" disease loci versus "susceptibility" loci. *Am J Hum Genet.* 1993;52:135–143.

17. Reaven G. Role of insulin resistance in human disease. *Diabetes.* 1988;37:1595–1607.

18. Bell GI, Picket RL, Rutter WJ, *et al.* Sequence of human insulin gene. *Nature.* 1980;284:26–32.

19. Bell GI, Karam JH, Rutter WJ. Polymorphic cDNA region adjacent to 5′ end of the human insulin gene. *Proc Nat Acad Sci USA.* 1981; 78:5759–5763.

20. Ramachandran A, Snehalatha C, Dharmaraj D, *et al.* Preview of glucose intolerance in Asian Indians: urban-rural differences and significance of upper-body adiposity. *Diabetes Care.* 1991;15:1348–1355.

21. Kambo P, Hitman G, Mohan V, *et al.* The genetic predisposition to fibrocalculous pancreatic diabetes. *Diabetologia.* 1989;32:45–51.

22. Weaver JU, Kopelman PG, Hitman GA. Central obesity and hyperinsulinaemia in women are associated with polymorphism in the 5′ flanking region of the human insulin gene. *Eur J Clin Invest.* 1992; 22:265–270.

23. Weaver JU, Hitman GA, Kopelman PG. An association between a BclI restriction fragment length polymorphism of the glucocorticoid receptor locus and hyperinsulinaemia in obese women. *J Mol Endocrinol.* 1992;9:295–300.

24. Vijayaraghavan S, Hitman GA, Kopelman PG. Apolipoprotein D

polymorphism: a genetic marker for obesity and hyperinsulinae-mia. *J Clin Endocrinol Metab.* 1994;79:568–570.

25. Vijayaraghavan S, Hitman GA, Niven MJ, *et al.* Polymorphism of the apolipoprotein D gene: a genetic determinant of obesity, NIDDM, and hyperinsulinaemia. *Diabetologia.* 1993;36(suppl 1 A84):32. Abstract.

DAVID S. WEIGLE

Candidate Genes for Human Obesity
from Adipose Tissue

ABSTRACT

Efforts to identify genes associated with obesity are hampered by
the polygenic nature of this condition in humans. Although sib-
pair linkage studies using random markers may identify genes of
interest, the candidate gene approach offers a potential shortcut
to elucidate the genetics of obesity. There are several routes by
which candidate gene probes for linkage studies may be obtained:
1) The cDNA for known proteins playing key roles in fuel and
energy metabolism may be chosen on a plausibility basis. 2)
Probes for the human analogues of genes determined by positional
cloning to be responsible for the monogenic rodent obesity syndromes can be chosen. 3) The cDNA's for novel mRNA molecules
differentially expressed in obese and lean states can be obtained
by subtractive cloning techniques and used as candidate gene
probes. As an example of the latter approach, we obtained a partial
cDNA clone for a 5 kilobase mRNA expressed in macaque adipose
tissue at a higher level following the induction of dietary obesity.
Subsequent studies revealed that this mRNA was also expressed
at high levels in rapidly growing fibroblasts from various tissues.
Newer polymerase chain reaction–based techniques promise to
improve the specificity of subtractive cDNA cloning of state-specific mRNA species for use as probes in genetic linkage studies.

Introduction

Although a genetic contribution to obesity is widely accepted on the
basis of twin (1) and adoption (2) studies, it is clear that body-fat content does not follow a simple Mendelian inheritance pattern. Multiple
genes appear to interact to determine the total body energy store except, possibly, in extreme familial obesity (3) or the Prader-Willi syn-

546

drome (4), in which a smaller number of major genes may be involved. Cultural, environmental, and cognitive variables further obscure the heritable component of obesity and may account for as much as half of the transmission of body-fat content across generations (5). In the face of this complexity it is no surprise that the genetic basis of human obesity has not yet been clarified. Nevertheless, continued efforts to identify the genes involved in the regulation of body-fat content are justified by the likelihood that this knowledge will lead to new strategies to prevent or ameliorate this major health problem.

Positional cloning of obesity genes in extended families through the generation of log of the odds (LOD) scores using polymorphic markers will be extremely difficult in the absence of a defined inheritance pattern. A more promising approach might be to perform nonparametric sib-pair analysis, in which the square of the difference in body-fat content between pairs of siblings is regressed against the proportion of shared parental haplotypes at a particular gene locus (6). In theory, this latter technique could be undertaken using random chromosomal markers. Alternatively, markers for genes postulated a priori to contribute to obesity could be examined for linkage to body-fat content using sib-pair analysis. This candidate gene approach offers a potential shortcut to elucidate the genetics of obesity.

Candidate gene markers can be derived from several sources. One attractive approach would be to use probes for the human analogues of genes determined by positional cloning to be responsible for the monogenic rodent obesity syndromes. In this regard, the recent characterization of the gene associated with the mouse agouti locus is of great interest (7). Ectopic overexpression of this gene product is accompanied by pronounced obesity, diabetes, and the development of neoplasms. Another source of candidate gene probes could be the cDNA for known proteins playing key roles in energy intake, energy expenditure, or nutrient partitioning. Bouchard and coworkers have listed a number of these polypeptide molecules in a previous volume in this series (5). Finally, the cDNAs for novel mRNA molecules expressed differentially in obese and lean states could be obtained by subtractive or differential cloning techniques and used to identify candidate genes. Subtractive cloning was first used successfully by Davis and coworkers in 1984 to isolate the T cell antigen receptor (8). More recently, Reynet and Kahn used this method to identify a Ras-related protein overexpressed in the muscle of type II diabetics (9).

The principal advantage of subtractive cDNA cloning is that the function of the desired gene products need not be known in advance. The method typically yields a variety of cDNA molecules that are preferentially expressed in a certain tissue in a defined physiological state. The specificity of the cloned cDNA for the desired state is enhanced by multiple cycles of subtraction against excess cDNA from a source that differs minimally from the condition of the target tissue. For example, the subtraction of hepatoma cDNA against cDNA from normal liver has been used to clone sequences associated with neoplastic transformation in this tissue type (10). The specificity of sequences obtained by subtraction is generally verified by using the cloned cDNA as a probe to perform Northern analysis of the original tissues. Specific clones may then be used in genetic linkage studies or sequenced and studied further to assess the potential function of their protein products.

We have used subtractive cloning to isolate adipocyte cDNA molecules potentially involved in the regulation of body-fat mass and the pathogenesis of obesity (11). Our hypothesis is that as the triglyceride content of adipocytes increases, the cells produce one or more peptides that act either locally to inhibit further lipid deposition or systemically to reduce energy intake or increase energy expenditure. Thus, the adipocyte is postulated to participate actively in a negative feedback loop that prevents indefinite expansion of the total body-fat store. Defective synthesis or activity of one of these putative peptides could predispose to obesity. The animal data on which this hypothesis is based has been reviewed recently (12) and is briefly summarized below.

Evidence for Regulation of Total Adipose Mass

Perhaps the most direct evidence that body-fat mass is regulated comes from lipectomy and adipose tissue grafting studies in rodents. Under the correct experimental conditions, surgical removal of adipose tissue is followed by replacement of the lost adipose mass either locally or in areas remote from the surgical site (13–15). Similarly, adipose tissue grafts in rodents generally undergo atrophy unless the animal's fat mass is first reduced surgically (16). Human data are limited to a case report by Kral in which a woman who lost 55 kg through a combination of diet and lipectomy regained 37 kg of mass before she was lost to follow-up (17). A more recent study by Yost and coworkers found an increase in circumference of body regions remote from the surgical site in women undergoing suction lipoplasty procedures (18). The compensation observed following both lipectomy and fat grafting indicates that the total adipose mass is sensed, perhaps through a secretory product of adipocytes, and regulated by active adjustments in energy balance.

Several lines of evidence indicate that an inverse relationship between energy intake and deviations of adipose mass from base line may contribute to regulation of the total fat store. In rodents (11), nonhuman primates (11), and humans (19), an increase in fat mass produced by feeding a caloric excess is followed by a reduction in voluntary energy intake after termination of the overfeeding period. Conversely, a reduction in adipose mass produced by caloric restriction is followed by hyperphagia that abates only after the lost fat is restored (20). Perhaps most suggestive of a regulatory relationship between adipose mass and energy intake, the recovery of appetite following both induced weight gain and weight loss exactly parallels the return to base-line weight and body-fat content (Fig. 1). An increase in food consumption has been

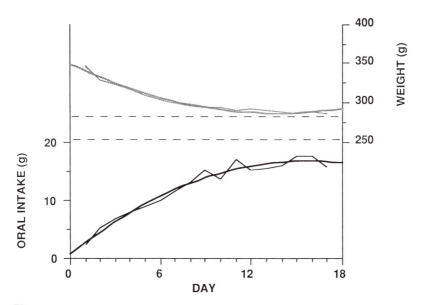

Figure 1.   Recovery of body weight and spontaneous daily consumption of chow blocks in a group of seven male Sprague-Dawley rats following cessation of gavage overfeeding on day 0. Dashed lines indicate base-line values of weight and oral intake after correcting for growth of control rats. Heavy lines represent best polynomial fits to data.

From reference 12 with permission.

demonstrated following surgical removal of white adipose tissue in weight-stable gold thioglucose obese mice (21) and, more recently, in mice that have undergone complete transgenic ablation of brown adipose tissue (22). All of these observations are consistent with the existence of a satiety signal, the strength of which is directly proportional to the total adipose mass. Such a signal has been demonstrated to be transmitted in the circulation both in serum transfer experiments and studies of parabiotic rodents (12).

Insulin has been postulated to be the adipose-related satiety signal, since the base-line circulating insulin level increases in proportion to fat mass (23). A recent report by Hulsey and Martin suggests that a satiety signal may be produced directly by adipose tissue, however. These workers demonstrated a reduction in chow intake of rats who received daily third cerebroventricular injections of an aqueous extract of adipose tissue collected from obese rats (24). Preliminary work in our laboratory suggested that this factor may actually be secreted by adipocytes (25). In view of these limited but provocative observations, the recognition that adipocytes secrete a variety of other polypeptides (26), and the plausibility of a role for adipocytes in the regulation of total body-fat stores, we decided to obtain cDNA clones for candidate adipocyte genes encoding a satiety factor or other molecules involved in energy homeostasis. Our experience illustrates both the strengths and weaknesses of using subtractive cloning to obtain candidate gene probes.

Subtractive Cloning of cDNA from the Adipose Tissue of an Obese Nonhuman Primate

The production of a satiety factor or any other adipocyte polypeptide acting as a negative regulator of total adipose tissue mass should be maximally induced in an animal that has been experimentally pushed above its normal body-fat content. Therefore, we developed a model of dietary obesity in the nonhuman primate *Macaca nemestrina* as a starting point for this work. Silastic gastrostomy tubes were surgically placed in three macaques and used to infuse excess calories in the form of a balanced liquid diet (11). A significant weight gain amounting to 20% of base-line body weight was induced after 40 to 50 days of this overfeeding protocol. Voluntary oral intake, which was measured daily, decreased dramatically as maximum weight gains were attained. Appetite returned to normal only after gastrostomy infusions were discontinued and the animals returned to their base-line weights. At the point of maximal weight gain, the omental adipose tissue of each animal was removed and flash frozen for later RNA preparation. A dramatic increase in intraabdominal and subcutaneous fat volume was noted in the animals at the time of laparotomy.

Poly (A)$^+$ RNA was isolated from the overfed macaque adipose tissue and used to prepare a cDNA library in lambda gt10 (11). The remaining poly (A)$^+$ RNA was used to prepare ^{32}P-labeled cDNA, which was hybridized to an excess of biotinylated poly (A)$^+$ RNA from the adipose tissue of an ad libitum–fed macaque. In this step, sequences present in both the induced-obese and nonobese states should have formed biotinylated RNA/DNA hybrids. These hybrids, as well as free biotinylated RNA, were then removed by addition of streptavidin and phenol/chloroform extraction according to the method of Sive and St. John (27). The remaining ^{32}P-cDNA, which should have been enriched in sequences specifically expressed in adipose tissue from the overfed animals, was then used as a probe to screen the cDNA library. Of 60 000 recombinants screened, 33 recombinants to which the subtracted probe mixture hybridized were isolated for secondary screening at a low plating density. In this second screening step, replica filters were probed with ^{32}P-labeled cDNA prepared from both overfed and ad libitum–fed macaque adipose tissue. Six phage clones demonstrated relatively greater hybridization to the overfed probe mixture. Of these, the one that exhibited the greatest differential hybridization signal was found to contain a 1.8 kilobase (kb) insert that was subcloned into pBluescript for further study.

Northern analysis using the radiolabeled 1.8 kb cDNA as a probe was performed on whole adipose tissue RNA from the three overfed macaques and two nonobese macaques. A native mRNA of approximately 5 kb detected in this analysis appeared to be expressed at a higher level in the overfed state as expected (11). The 5 kb mRNA was also detected in a pure fraction of adipocytes prepared by collagenase digestion of macaque omental adipose tissue. To better define the relationship of 5 kb mRNA levels to body-fat content, Northern analysis was performed on whole cell RNA prepared from retroperitoneal fat pads of fasted, ad libitum–fed, and gavage overfed rats. Densitometry of both the 5 kb mRNA and actin bands indicated a 50% induction of 5 kb relative to actin mRNA in the overfed obese state (Fig. 2). Inves-

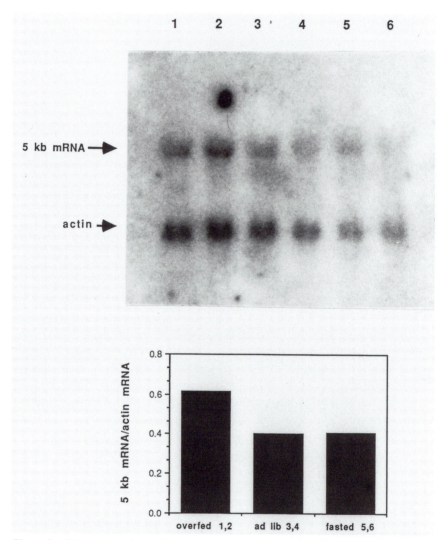

Figure 2. Upper panel: Northern analysis of whole-cell RNA prepared from retroperitoneal fat pads of gavage overfed (lanes 1 and 2), ad libitum–fed (lanes 3 and 4), and 48-hour fasted (lanes 5 and 6) rats. Each lane contains 10 μg of RNA from a separate animal. The blot was probe with radiolabeled 1.8 kb cDNA cloned from overfed macaque adipose tissue and a 2 kb beta-actin cDNA. Lower panel: Densitometric ratio of 5 kb mRNA to actin from this blot. Each bar represents the mean ratio computed from the indicated two lanes.

From reference 11 with permission.

tigation of other tissues revealed high levels of the 5 kb mRNA in the brain, lower levels in the liver, and no hybridization signal in the kidney, spleen, or skeletal muscle. Finally, the 5 kb mRNA was detected in subcutaneous adipose tissue biopsy specimens from human volunteers (11).

Given these results, we judged the 1.8 kb overfed macaque adipose tissue cDNA to be sufficiently interesting to justify an effort to obtain and sequence a full-length clone. Despite repeated efforts to this end, the longest clone obtainable from both oligo-dT and random-primed cDNA libraries using the 1.8 kb cDNA as a probe was 2.2 kb. It is likely that secondary mRNA structure prevented more complete 5' reverse transcription during library preparation. The 2.2 kb clone was sequenced and found to contain a 942 base pair (bp) open reading frame followed by 1243 bp of 3' untranslated sequence and a poly (A) tail. Searches of the 2.2 kb nucleic acid sequence and the predicted 314 amino acid sequence against all available DNA and protein data bases revealed no significant homology to characterized sequences. Similarly, a blocks search using the algorithm of Henikoff *et al.* (28) revealed no structural motifs that allowed the translation product to be placed into a known family of proteins.

At this point, Northern analyses using our available cDNA probes revealed the 5 kb mRNA to be present in fully differentiated postconfluent 3T3-F442A adipocytes. Surprisingly, the 5 kb message was also found at high levels in cells from this line in the preconfluent undifferentiated state. Further analysis demonstrated a strong 5 kb hybridization signal in RNA prepared from a variety of actively dividing fibroblast cell lines. These results suggested that the 5 kb message was not specific for adipocytes from animals in a state of markedly positive energy balance as originally thought. Rather, this message now appeared to be a potential marker for any tissue containing rapidly proliferating cellular elements, of which hyperplastic adipose tissue was only one example. The five remaining cDNA clones from the secondary screening of the macaque adipose tissue library were used as probes to perform additional Northern analyses of adipose tissue RNA from obese and lean rodent models. None of the mRNA species identified by these probes exhibited greater specificity for the obese state than we had already observed for the 5 kb mRNA. We therefore elected to defer further sequencing or linkage studies pending technical improvement of our subtraction cloning protocol.

Improved Techniques for Differential Cloning
of Candidate Gene cDNA Probes

Our experience illustrates that a single cycle of subtractive hybridization, which at best probably removes only 90% of shared sequences, is
not adequate to generate highly state-specific cDNA populations for
use as probes in genetic linkage studies. Ideally, Northern analysis performed with a differentially cloned cDNA probe should reveal at least
a tenfold increase in mRNA level relative to a noninduced gene transcript such as actin in the state of interest. Fortunately, creative new
applications of polymerase chain reaction (PCR) technology, two of
which are summarized below, promise to lead to improved results in
this area.

MULTIPLE CYCLE SUBTRACTION WITH PCR AMPLIFICATION

A disadvantage of all subtractive hybridization protocols is that both
specific and nonspecific losses of cDNA during processing can result
in an inadequate amount of material for direct cloning or probe generation. This is a particular problem if there is a limited amount of
starting tissue available, as may be the case for human biopsy specimens. Multiple cycles of subtraction dramatically improve the specificity of the selected cDNA but compound the problem of material loss.
Schweinfest and coworkers have suggested a way to circumvent this
problem, a modification of which is shown in Figure 3 (10). In this
scheme, starting tissue from both the desired and the alternative physiological states is first used to prepare poly (A)$^+$ RNA. Double-stranded
cDNA is then synthesized from each RNA preparation and used to
prepare two libraries in a high efficiency viral vector such as lambda
ZAP II that contains the F1 phage origin of replication. Using the
lambda ZAP II system, single-stranded DNA is next prepared from
each library with helper phage R408, and ssDNA from the alternative
state library is photobiotinylated. Hybridization between a ten- to
twentyfold excess of this biotinylated DNA and unmodified DNA from
the desired state library is performed, followed by removal of biotinylated hybrids and ssDNA with streptavidin. The resulting DNA,
which is now enriched in sequences specific to the desired state, is
subjected to further cycles of subtraction against excess biotinylated
DNA from the alternative state. With each round of subtraction the

MULTIPLE CYCLE cDNA SUBTRACTION WITH PCR AMPLIFICATION

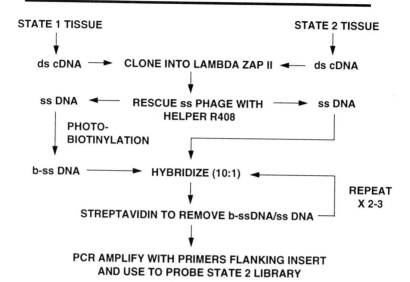

Figure 3. A protocol for state-specific cDNA cloning using multiple cycles of subtractive hybridization followed by PCR amplification of products.

Adapted with permission of the publisher, from reference 10. Copyright 1990 by Elsevier Science Inc.

specificity of the remaining DNA increases, but the overall recovery decreases. Ultimately, the subtracted DNA is amplified by PCR-using primers flanking the cloning casette and either sequenced directly or used as a probe to recover clones from the original desired state library.

DIFFERENTIAL mRNA DISPLAY USING PCR

Liang and Pardee have described an elegant technique to display limited cellular mRNA subpopulations in a manner that permits direct comparison of individual gene transcripts between alternative cell types (29). Their approach is similar in principle to using two-dimensional gel electrophoresis to compare the expression of specific cellular proteins following various experimental manipulations. Poly (A)$^+$ RNA from the two alternative states of the tissue or tissues to be compared is first reverse transcribed using oligo-dT plus two additional 3′ bases as a 3′ primer. An example of such a primer would be 5′-T_{11}CA-

3'. Since there are twelve different combinations of the last two 3' bases, omitting T as the penultimate base, each of these primers permits the synthesis of cDNA from only one-twelfth of the total mRNA population. The resulting cDNA is then subjected to PCR amplification using the same one of the twelve 3' primers and a 9 or 10 base pair 5' primer of arbitrary sequence. An arbitrary 5' primer of this length anneals to the cDNA strand at a position that is randomly distributed in distance from the poly (A) tail, but generally no farther than 500 bp away. The resulting PCR products are labeled with ^{35}S-dATP, run on a sequencing gel, and displayed by autoradiography. The fifty to one hundred amplified mRNA species resulting from each pair of primers are easily resolved on the gel, and differences in specific bands between alternative cell types or physiological states of the tissue of interest can be visualized easily. A differentially expressed band may be eluted from the gel, reamplified by PCR, and sequenced. If this partial sequence is judged to be of interest, the cDNA may be used as a marker in linkage studies or as a probe to obtain a full-length clone. The advantages of this technique over subtractive hybridization include greater speed, requirement for only tiny amounts of starting material, ability to detect both overexpressed and underexpressed mRNA species in the target tissues, and higher reproducibility.

Conclusions

The lack of a simple inheritance pattern reduces the likelihood that positional cloning efforts will identify genes critical for the development of human obesity in the near future. The alternative approach of sib-pair linkage studies is more feasible but requires the generation of markers for plausible candidate obesity genes. Based on the hypothesis that adipocytes participate in a negative feedback loop that contributes to the regulation of total body-fat mass, we employed subtractive cDNA cloning to identify adipocyte mRNA species expressed at a higher level following the induction of dietary obesity in a nonhuman primate. Due to the use of a single cycle subtraction protocol, the six cDNA clones that we obtained did not display sufficient selectivity for the obese state to justify further characterization or use as markers in linkage studies of obese kindreds. Subsequent improvements in PCR-based subtraction and differential mRNA display methods make it likely that future efforts along these lines will be more successful. The principal advantage of all of these techniques is that they require no knowledge of candidate gene function and, if the alternative states of starting materials are chosen wisely, could potentially provide a short-cut to the identification of obesity-related genes. The disadvantage of the candidate gene approach is that, unlike positional cloning, cumu-lative progress is not possible, since each marker is evaluated essen-tially in a hit-or-miss fashion. Ultimately, it appears likely that some combination of genetic and physiological approaches will be necessary to elucidate the complex pathogenesis of obesity.

REFERENCES

1. Stunkard AJ, Foch TT, Hrubec Z. A twin study of human obesity. *JAMA.* 1986;256:51–54.
2. Stunkard AJ, Sørensen TIA, Hanis C, *et al.* An adoption study of human obesity. *N Engl J Med.* 1986;314:193–198.
3. Price RA, Stunkard AJ. Commingling analysis of obesity in twins. *Hum Hered.* 1989;39:121–135.
4. Cassidy SB, Ledbetter DH. Prader-Willi syndrome. *Neurol Clin.* 1989;7:37–54.
5. Bouchard C, Tremblay A, Després J-P, Dériaz O, Dionne FT. The genetics of body energy content and energy balance: an overview. In: Bray GA, Ryan DH, eds. *The Science of Food Regulation: Food Intake, Taste, Nutrient Partitioning, and Energy Expenditure.* Penning-ton Center Nutrition Series, Baton Rouge, LA: Louisiana State Uni-versity Press; 1992:3–21.
6. Haseman JK, Elston RC. The investigation of linkage between a quantitative trait and a marker locus. *Behav Genet.* 1972;2:3–19.
7. Bultman SJ, Michaud EJ, Woychik RP. Molecular characterization of the mouse agouti locus. *Cell.* 1992;71:1195–1204.
8. Hedrick SM, Cohen DI, Nielsen EA, Davis MM. Isolation of cDNA clones encoding T cell-specific membrane-associated proteins. *Na-ture.* 1984;308:149–153.
9. Reynet C, Kahn CR. Rad: a member of the ras family overexpressed in muscle of type II diabetic humans. *Science.* 1993;262:1441–1444.
10. Schweinfest CW, Henderson KW, Gu J-R, *et al.* Subtraction hybrid-ization cDNA libraries from colon carcinoma and hepatic cancer. *Genet Anal Tech Appl.* 1990;7:64–70.
11. Wilson BE, Meyer GE, Cleveland JC Jr, Weigle DS. Identification of

candidate genes for a factor regulating body weight in primates. *Am J Physiol.* 1990;259:R1148–R1155.

12. Weigle DS. Appetite and the regulation of body composition. *FASEB J.* 1994;8:302–310.

13. Hamilton JM, Wade GN. Lipectomy does not impair fattening induced by short photoperiods or high-fat diets in female Syrian hamsters. *Physiol Behav.* 1988;43:85–92.

14. Larson KA, Anderson DB. The effects of lipectomy on remaining adipose tissue depots in the Sprague Dawley rat. *Growth.* 1978;42:469–477.

15. Faust IM, Johnson PR, Hirsch J. Adipose tissue regeneration following lipectomy. *Science.* 1977;197:391–393.

16. Liebelt RA, Vismara L, Liebelt AG. Autoregulation of adipose tissue mass in the mouse. *Proc Soc Exp Biol Med.* 1968;127:458–462.

17. Kral JG. Surgical reduction of adipose tissue hypercellularity in man. *Scand J Plast Reconstr Surg.* 1975;9:140–143.

18. Yost TJ, Rodgers CM, Eckel RH. Results of suction lipectomy relate to region-specific changes in adipose tissue lipoprotein lipase. *Clin Res.* 1992;40:104A.

19. Roberts SB, Young VR, Fuss P, et al. Energy expenditure and subsequent nutrient intakes in overfed young men. *Am J Physiol.* 1990;259:R461–R469.

20. Harris RBS, Kasser TR, Martin RJ. Dynamics of recovery of body composition after overfeeding, food restriction or starvation of mature female rats. *J Nutr.* 1986;116:2536–2546.

21. Liebelt RA, Ichinoe S, Nicholson N. Regulatory influences of adipose tissue on food intake and body weight. *Ann NY Acad Sci.* 1965;131:559–582.

22. Lowell BB, S-Susulic V, Hamann A, et al. Development of obesity in transgenic mice after genetic ablation of brown adipose tissue. *Nature.* 1993;366:740–742.

23. Porte D Jr, Woods SC. Regulation of food intake and body weight by insulin. *Diabetologia.* 1981;20:274–279.

24. Hulsey MG, Martin RJ. An anorectic agent from adipose tissue of overfed rats: effects on feeding behavior. *Physiol Behav.* 1992;52:1141–1149.

25. Hutson AM, Meyer GE, Weigle DS. Bioassay for a satiety factor produced by adipose tissue from overfed obese rats. *Clin Res.* 1992;40:60A.

26. Choy LN, Rosen BS, Spiegelman BM. Adipsin and an endogenous pathway of complement from adipose cells. *J Biol Chem.* 1992;267: 12736–12741.
27. Sive HL, St. John T. A simple subtractive hybridization technique employing photoactivatable biotin and phenol extraction. *Nucleic Acids Research.* 1988;16:10937.
28. Henikoff S, Henikoff JG. Automated assembly of protein blocks for data base searching. *Nucleic Acids Res.* 1991;19:6565–6572.
29. Liang P, Pardee AB. Differential display of eukaryotic messenger RNA by means of the polymerase chain reaction. *Science.* 1992;257: 967–971.

ROBERT D. NICHOLLS, CHRISTOPHER C. GLENN,
MICHELLE T. C. JONG, SHINJI SAITOH,
MARIA J. MASCARI, and DANIEL J. DRISCOLL

Molecular Pathogenesis of Prader-Willi Syndrome

ABSTRACT

Prader-Willi syndrome (PWS) is a complex genetic disorder associated with hyperphagia and consequent morbid obesity unless strict dietary control is maintained. Prader-Willi syndrome represents a valuable genetic model for obesity, since the chromosomal basis is known. Recent findings have clearly implicated the process of genomic imprinting in the pathogenesis of Prader-Willi syndrome, in which parental alleles of the etiological genes within the 15q11-q13 critical region are differentially marked and expressed during development.

Genetic data have suggested that at least two genes are needed in order to develop the classic Prader-Willi syndrome phenotype. To date, we have identified two imprinted genes that may be involved in the pathogenesis of the disorder. The *SNRPN* gene, encoding the SmN protein involved in mRNA splicing, and a novel zinc-finger protein encoding gene, *ZNF127*, both are expressed only from the paternal allele. The expression of each of these genes appears to correlate with DNA methylation imprints. Other workers have completed a yeast artificial chromosome contig of 15q11-q13 and are isolating other genes from the region of interest. Furthermore, imprinted genes are embedded within large differentially replicated chromosomal domains. Mutations in the imprinting process have also been found. In conclusion, the mechanism of imprinting appears to involve a complex interplay of events involving higher order chromatin structure of a large imprinted chromosomal region, with gene-specific events occurring at multiple genes within each imprinted domain. Further study of Prader-Willi syndrome patients, developmental gene expression, and animal models will be necessary to link each imprinted gene

560

in this region to each aspect of the Prader-Willi syndrome phenotype, particularly the hyperphagia responsible for obesity.

Obesity and the Clinical Phenotype of Prader-Willi Syndrome

Obesity, one of the major health problems in the modern world, has
important psychological and social consequences, yet almost nothing
is known about its molecular basis (1). There are a number of experimentally induced and genetic animal models of obesity, but these are
just beginning to yield to molecular analysis (1, 2) (see other papers in
this volume). Nevertheless, many insights are now being gained in an
understanding of the molecular pathogenesis of Prader-Willi syndrome
(PWS), a human genetic disorder associated with severe obesity that is
life threatening by the third decade without dietary and behavioral
intervention. The clinical phenotype of PWS (Fig. 1; Table 1), which
occurs in $\frac{1}{10\ 000}$ to $\frac{1}{20\ 000}$ births, is characterized by neonatal hypotonia
and developmental delay (Fig. 1a), followed by onset of hyperphagia
between one year and six years of age with subsequent severe obesity
(Fig. 1b, 1c), and other features including short stature, hypogonadism,
and mild to moderate mental retardation (Table 1) (2–5).

Hyperphagia in PWS appears to be driven by a failure to reach satiety, thought to be hypothalamic in origin (Table 2) (4, 5). This results
in a very high energy intake, which, coupled with low activity levels,
short stature, and a decreased caloric requirement, results in severe
obesity (Fig. 1c) that, without intervention, has potentially morbid consequences, most commonly caused by cardiopulmonary failure (Table
2). However, with modification of diet and behavior (6, 7), including
incorporation of an exercise program, significant weight losses can be
achieved (Fig. 1d) with medical, psychological, and social benefits to
the patient. Interestingly, even PWS individuals who have lost weight
and are near ideal weight for height still have 30% to 40% body fat,
and through skinfold measurements PWS infants have been found to
have obesity even before they are considered heavy by weight-for-
length criteria (8). Basal metabolic rate is considered normal, but
whether energy expenditure is low or normal when corrected for the
small fat-free mass typical of PWS is still controversial (9, 10). It is not
clear what significance, cause or effect, can be attributed to the tenfold
increased level of adipose tissue lipoprotein lipase, the enzyme that
regulates the uptake and storage of triglycerides, in PWS patients ver-

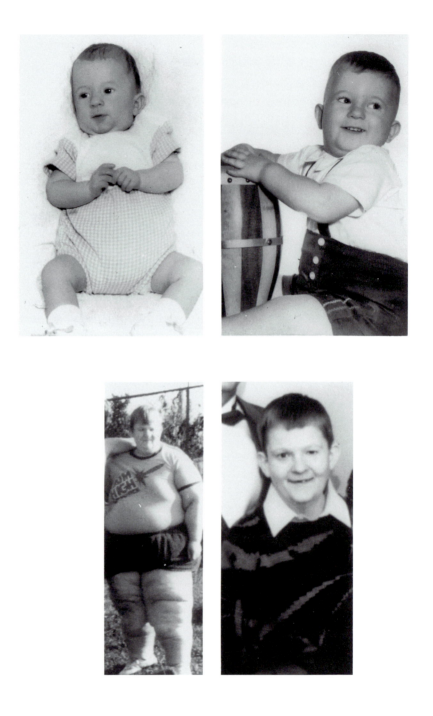

Table 1.   Clinical Phenotype of PWS.

Decreased fetal activity (perinatal)
Hypotonia (neonatal/infancy)
Feeding difficulties, failure to thrive (neonatal/infancy)
Developmental delay (neonatal/infancy)
Hyperphagia, obesity (onset between 1 and 6 years of age)
Hypogenitalism, hypogonadism
Cryptorchidism
Mild dysmorphism (narrow bifrontal diameter, almond-shaped eyes,
    downturned mouth, thin upper lip)
Mental retardation (mild to moderate)
Behavioral and emotional problems
Somnolence
Skin picking, decreased pain sensitivity
Short stature
Small hands and feet
Hypopigmentation of eyes, skin, hair (candidate gene identified)

Table 2.   Obesity and the PWS Patient

Hyperphagia—excess caloric intake
                    —inability to achieve satiety
Food-seeking behavior, obsession with food
Reduced caloric requirement (for fat-free mass)
Low activity levels
Thick, viscous saliva
Inability to vomit
Fat distribution predominantly truncal and proximal limb
30% to 40% body fat even when near ideal weight/height
Increased adipose tissue lipoprotein lipase
Diabetes mellitus in 10% to 20% patients
Cardiopulmonary compromise
Poor social acceptance, poor self-image

Figure 1.   Natural history of PWS clinical phenotype. The same individual is
shown (*A*) as an infant with neonatal hypotonia; (*B*) at 3 years of age; (*C*) at 21
years of age with severe obesity (reaching 400 lbs); and (*D*) at 30 years of age,
after significant weight loss. Note the small hands and characteristic facial features (narrow bifrontal diameter, almond-shaped eyes, thin upper lip, and
downturned corners of the mouth), particularly in (*A*) and (*B*), and the chub-
biness in (*B*) with progression to severe obesity in (*C*). Obesity in PWS is potentially life threatening in the third decade without intervention (3–5).

sus controls (11). Other biochemical, endocrine, and anatomical studies have not identified any consistent abnormality (2, 4, 5).

In this paper, we will discuss recent research toward identification of candidate genes in PWS, particularly the genes involved in obesity. Prader-Willi syndrome is of great interest for obesity research, since it is one of very few human obesities for which a specific genetic abnormality is known, and it is likely that a specific genetic determinant or determinants of this severe biological obesity can be identified in the next few years. This may have wider implications for understanding factors causing obesity in the general population.

Genomic Imprinting in PWS and Angelman Syndrome

Prader-Willi syndrome is associated with abnormalities in inheritance of chromosome 15q11-q13 (Fig. 2). Most commonly (75% of patients), large cytogenetic deletions of 15q11-q13 are found, and in all cases the deletion has been found to be paternal in origin (5, 12, 13). Interestingly, a second genetic disorder, Angelman syndrome (AS), is also associated with deletions of 15q11-q13, and these are indistinguishable in extent at the molecular level from the deletions found in PWS (12, 13, 16). Angelman syndrome is an entirely different clinical syndrome, associated with gait ataxia, tremulousness, seizures typically beginning after one to six years, an abnormal electroencephalogram, hyperactivity, severe mental retardation, absence of speech, microbrachycephaly, protruding tongue and drooling, and a happy disposition with inappropriate laughter (17). In contrast to the exclusively paternal deletion in PWS, these deletions are exclusively maternal in AS (12, 13).

Most of the remaining PWS patients have two normal copies of chromosome 15, but nondisjunction during parental gametogenesis and/or early embryonic development leads to the absence of a paternal chromosome 15 and the presence of two maternal chromosomes, termed maternal uniparental disomy (UPD) (12, 13, 18). A similar event leads to paternal UPD in AS, in a small proportion of cases (12, 13). Both deletion and UPD classes in either syndrome can be considered to be biologically equivalent, resulting in the loss of functional paternal genes for PWS or a functional maternal gene or genes for AS, respectively (Fig. 2). Conversely, it is likely that the corresponding maternal genes in PWS and paternal gene(s) in AS, respectively, are normally silent. Only with a genetic contribution from both male and female

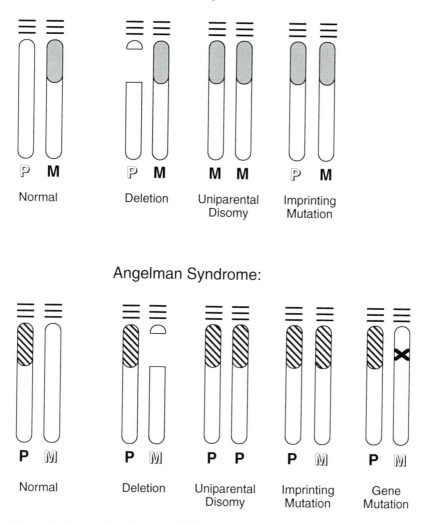

Figure 2. Molecular classes in PWS and AS. The paternal (P) and maternal (M) chromosome 15 is shown for normal individuals (left, top and lower) and for three classes of patients with PWS (top, right three panels) or four classes of patients with AS (lower, right four panels) (12, 13). The hatched regions indicate an inactive gene(s) in maternal (top) or paternal (lower) chromosome region 15q11q-13. The inactive locus is indicated by bold lettering (**M, P**) and the active locus by shadowed lettering (P, M). Note that the inactive locus has historically been defined as that imprinted, but recent studies indicate that sometimes the active genes may carry the imprinting mark (14, 15; C.C. Glenn, R.D. Nicholls, D.J. Driscoll, unpublished data). Deletion, uniparental disomy, and the rare imprinting mutation class occur for both PWS and AS, but a putative class of patients with a gene mutation in a single imprinted gene (cross) occurs in AS but not PWS (12, 13).

parents does normal development occur (Fig. 2). A third class of PWS
and AS patients is considered below. However, the parent-of-origin
inheritance patterns strongly implicate the phenomenon of genomic
imprinting in the etiology of PWS and AS. Sporadic or familial PWS
patients with biparental inheritance are very rare (see below), suggesting that PWS results from abnormal expression of at least two imprinted genes, in contrast to AS, in which this fourth class occurs and
in which mutations probably occur in a single imprinted gene (12, 13,
19–21) (Fig. 2).

Nearly all the phenotypic features of PWS and AS appear to be man-
ifested by imprinted genes, since deletion and UPD patients have almost identical phenotypes (5, 12, 13). The exception is for hypopigmentation (Table 1), commonly associated with 15q11-q13 deletions in
PWS and AS patients, in which a candidate gene has been cloned and
is not imprinted (22, 23). Inactivating mutations in this pigment gene
are the most common cause of tyrosinase-positive (type II) oculocutaneous albinism (22, 23). This is the only component of the PWS and AS
phenotype for which a likely candidate gene is known at this time.

Genomic imprinting refers to the process whereby specific genes are
differentially marked during parental gametogenesis, resulting in the
differential expression of these genes in the embryo and adult. Pronu-
clear transplantation and breeding studies in the mouse during the
early 1980s first demonstrated that paternal and maternal inheritance
was unequal in mammals, followed by mouse transgene studies that
implicated a role for DNA methylation in the imprinting process (24).
More recently, several functionally imprinted endogenous genes have
been identified in the mouse, including *Igf2, H19, Igf2r* (13–15, 25),
Snrpn (26, 27), and *U2afbp-rs* (28, 29). In the last few years, a role for
genomic imprinting has also been recognized in human genetic disease
(12, 13, 18, 30, 31) and tumorigenesis (32), but one of the best models
for imprinting in the human is PWS and AS. Imprinting has been evolutionarily conserved for the human *IGF2, H19,* and *SNRPN* genes
(32–35), but apparently not for *IGF2R* (37).

Molecular Diagnosis of PWS and a
Model to Identify Imprinted Genes

Molecular diagnosis of PWS (and AS) (12, 13) is based on molecular
cytogenetic deletion analysis by fluorescent in situ hybridization (FISH)

and on DNA studies that determine the parental inheritance based on dinucleotide repeat analysis in patients and parents, or on differential DNA methylation between parentally inherited alleles (12, 13, 19, 33, 38). The advantage of the latter technique is that it is alone in identifying affected PWS and AS individuals from all three classes of patients that have been proven to exist (Fig. 2), it does not require parental DNA, and it is the only one of these techniques that can be used for research purposes as an assay to identify and study imprinted gene regions (12, 13, 19, 33, 38–40). Since cultured cells from PWS patients with a deletion or UPD have only a maternal chromosome present, and similar cells from AS patients with a deletion or UPD have only the paternal chromosome present, it is theoretically possible to identify differentially imprinted DNA sequences, mRNA transcripts, or proteins using such a model system (Fig. 3). We and others have used this system for mRNA expression studies (13, 33, 35, 36) (Fig. 4a), DNA methylation (12, 13, 19, 33, 38–40) (Fig. 4b, 4c), and DNA replication studies (12, 13, 41, 42) (Fig. 5).

Cloning of the PWS Chromosomal Region and Identification of Candidate Genes

Four approaches have been taken to identify candidate genes for PWS and for AS: 1) A search for DNA methylation imprints at loci throughout 15q11-q13 (12, 13, 19, 33, 38–40) (Fig. 4b, 4c); 2) cloning of a yeast artificial chromosome (YAC) contig (16, 43) and exon trapping (45); 3) random mapping of clones to the region (see 12); 4) identification of smaller deletions in rare AS and PWS patients that has identified small AS and PWS critical regions (16, 43, 46). We (Fig. 4a) (33) and others (34, 35) have shown that the small nuclear ribonucleoprotein polypeptide N (*SNRPN*) gene is the first gene in the PWS region to be functionally imprinted, since it is expressed only from the paternal chromosome, as previously found in the mouse (26, 27). This feature makes this gene a candidate to have a role in at least some aspect of the PWS phenotype, and for a mouse model (27) that shows maternal UPD spanning genes syntenic to those located in the PWS/AS region (22, 44) and an imprinted phenotype (Fig. 5b).

Following the identification of the first DNA methylation imprint in a mammalian gene (19), DNA methylation imprints have been found in a total of three loci in 15q11-q13, *ZNF127* (DN34), PW71, and *SNRPN*

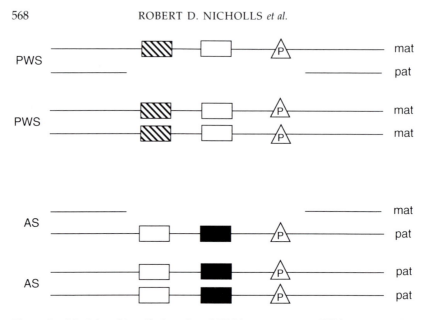

Figure 3. Model to identify imprinted DNA sequences, mRNAs, or proteins in PWS and AS. The maternal (mat) and paternal (pat) chromosome region 15q11-q13 is shown for PWS patients (upper) with a deletion (broken line) or uniparental disomy, and for AS patients (lower) with a deletion or uniparental disomy. Active (open boxes) or inactive (hatched and filled boxes) genes are indicated, as are genes not subject to genomic imprinting and thus in which both alleles are expressed (triangles; shown here is the one known example in 15q11-q13, the *P* gene that is involved in pigment biosynthesis [22, 23]). Clearly, PWS patients of either molecular class have only a maternal chromosome region 15q11-q13 present, and similarly AS patients in these two classes have only a paternal 15q11-q13 region, allowing maternally and paternally imprinted genes, their mRNA transcripts, or translated proteins, to be identified in cells derived from the patients (12, 13, 19).

(Fig. 4b, 4c) (12, 13, 19, 33, 36, 39, 40). Such imprints are recognized as epigenetic differences in DNA methylation between the two parental alleles (Fig. 4b, 4c), and this type of modification satisfies all requirements necessary for specifically marking parental alleles in the germ line and for subsequent maintenance during embryonic and adult development (12, 13, 25, 47). Thus, PWS patients with a deletion or UPD have only a maternal DNA methylation imprint, whereas AS patients in these two molecular classes have only a paternal methylation imprint (see Figs. 3, 4b, 4c). Biparental AS patients do not typically have the characteristic AS DNA methylation imprint (12, 19), perhaps expected from hypothetical mutations that may affect an encoded protein. The *SNRPN* (Figs. 4a, 5a, 5b) (33–35) and the *ZNF127* mouse homolog (36) (Fig. 5b) have been shown to be functionally imprinted, and this correlates with DNA methylation (Figs. 4c, 5), as found for other mouse imprinted genes (13–15, 25). If *ZNF127* is also imprinted in humans, it would also be a candidate to have a role(s) in the PWS clinical phenotype.

An Imprinted Genetic Domain in PWS

PW71 and *SNRPN* map to the PWS critical region (13, 38, 43), but chromosome rearrangements in 15q11-q13 alter DNA methylation imprints at distant loci, including the *ZNF127* gene (39), suggesting that the regulation of imprinted genes may involve a domain structure and that genes outside the small critical regions cannot be ruled out from having an effect on the phenotype.

Interestingly, we (Fig. 4b) (39) and others (40) have identified a third class of AS patients (see above), commonly occurring in sibships, in which the patients have biparental inheritance of an apparently intact chromosome but in which DNA methylation imprints at *ZNF127* and PW71 show only a paternal methylation imprint. A similar class of affected PWS sibs has also been found (40), with biparental inheritance and maternal only DNA methylation imprints. Therefore, the paternal chromosome in these PWS patients carries a maternal methylation imprint, and the maternal chromosome in the AS patients carries a paternal methylation imprint. In both the PWS and AS families, it is likely that the normally active parental allele has been silenced by an imprinting mutation. Since the two loci studied are about 1.5 megabases (Mb) apart (16), the data are consistent with a *cis*-acting mutation (13, 39, 40). A mutation in the germ line of one grandparent might result in a failure to reset the imprinting signal in the parental germ line, which results in the disease phenotype and familial occurrence (40). In one of the PWS familial cases, a small deletion overlapping the *SNRPN* gene was identified (40), which may indicate the location of a *cis*-acting sequence controlling the 15q11-q13 imprinted gene region. Multiple imprinted genes might be affected by this imprinting control element, or ICE (13), and recent data are consistent with the likelihood that multiple imprinted loci may be found in 15q11-q13 (33–36, 45).

The effect of translocations and imprinting mutations on DNA meth-

(a)

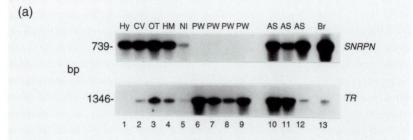

```
       Hy CV OT HM  NI  PW PW PW PW    AS AS AS   Br
739-                                                      SNRPN
bp
1346-                                                      TR
       1  2  3  4   5   6  7  8  9     10 11 12   13
```

(b)

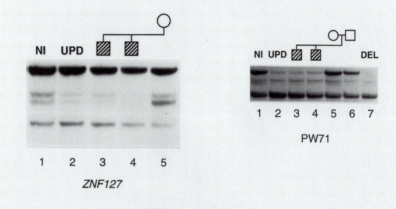

```
    NI  UPD  [hatched] [hatched]           NI UPD [hatched][hatched]    DEL

    1   2    3    4    5                    1  2   3   4   5  6   7

         ZNF127                                    PW71
```

(c)

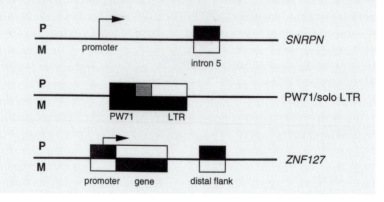

```
P  ─────────┬──────────────■──────────────  SNRPN
M            promoter       □
                         intron 5

P  ─────────■■■▨□□──────────────────────  PW71/solo LTR
M           ■■■  □□
            PW71   LTR

P  ──────■□─■■□──────────■─────────────  ZNF127
M        □■  ■■□          □
         promoter gene   distal flank
```

ylation imprints, as discussed above, suggests that 15q11-q13 represents an imprinted chromosome region. More direct evidence for this
hypothesis has come from an analysis of the timing of DNA replication
of imprinted genes and flanking loci (12, 41, 42, 47). Most genes replicate synchronously during S phase in the cell cycle; however, all known

---

Figure 4.   Identification of candidate genes and imprinting mutations in PWS
and AS. (a) Functional imprinting of *SNRPN* expression is identified by analysis
of mRNA from cultured cells of PWS and AS patients (33). cDNA was made
from mRNA of various cell types by reverse transcription followed by polymerase chain reaction (PCR) amplification with gene-specific primers, and hybridization of a Southern blot with a *SNRPN* probe (top) or a transferrin receptor (TR; lower) control probe. Note the absence of *SNRPN* product in PWS
patients (PW, lanes 6–9, fibroblasts or lymphoblasts) but its presence in normal
(Nl, lane 5) and AS fibroblasts (lanes 10–12), normal human brain (Br), hyda-
tidiform mole (HM), ovarian teratoma (OT), chorionic villus (CV), and a chromosome 15–specific somatic cell hybrid (Hy).
Reproduced from reference 33, by permission of Oxford University Press.

(b) Identification of an AS family with an apparent imprinting mutation affecting DNA methylation imprints at the *ZNF127* (left) and PW71 (right) loci
(39). DNA from peripheral blood leukocytes is digested with a methyl-sensitive
(*Hpa*II) and a non–methyl-sensitive restriction enzyme, Southern blotted, and
probed. For both loci, a normal (Nl) control (lane 1) shows an identical pattern
to the parents (lanes 5, 6), whereas the two affected AS siblings (lanes 3, 4) have
a significant reduction in intensity of the middle two bands (left) or upper band
(right), which is an identical methylation pattern to the unrelated AS patients
with uniparental disomy (UPD, lane 2) or a deletion (DEL, lane 7). Although
not shown here, PWS patients have a reduction of the lower band for *ZNF127*
(19) and for PW71 (38), indicating parent-of-origin specific DNA methylation
at these loci (see Fig. 4c). These loci are about 1.5 Mb apart in chromosome
15q11-q13, and families with affected PWS siblings and methylation imprint
alterations at these two loci also have been found recently (40).
Adapted and reproduced with permission from reference 39.

(c) DNA methylation imprints at three loci (*SNRPN*, top [33]; PW71, center [38];
ZNF127, lower [19, 36]) in the PWS and AS chromosomal region. The paternal
(P) and maternal (M) alleles are shown, along with parental allele-specific methylation (filled box), lack of methylation (open boxes, when at least 50% of cells
are unmethylated at this site), or a partially methylated state (hatched box; 80%
of cells are methylated). Transcription initiation sites are indicated by the arrow,
and LTR represents an endogenous retroviral-like long terminal repeat.
Adapted from data in references 19, 33, 36, 38.

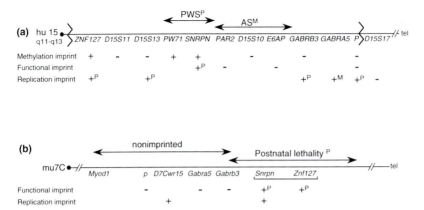

Figure 5. Features of imprinted loci in the PWS and AS chromosomal region in humans and the syntenic region in mouse. (a) Human (hu) chromosome 15q11-q13, illustrating PWS and AS critical regions (arrows), which involve the absence of paternal (P) or maternal (M) genetic contributions, respectively. Known genetic loci are listed from the centromere (filled circle) toward the telomere (tel), and the common deletion end points are demarcated by vertical zigzag lines (12, 13, 16, 43). Underneath are shown the presence (+) or absence (−) of a DNA methylation imprint, functional imprint, or replication imprint, at each locus tested. For functional imprints, P or M represents the expressed allele, and for the replication imprint, P or M represents the allele that replicates early in the cell cycle. (b) Mouse (mu) chromosome 7C region, syntenic to the PWS/AS region in humans. Symbols are as above. The relative order of *Snrpn* and *Znf127* is not yet known (bracket). The developmental phenotypes of radiation-induced deletions spanning from *Myod1* through *Gabrb3* are not imprinted, showing that no functionally imprinted loci causing a phenotype lie in this segment (22, 44). However, maternal UPD for the central region of mouse chromosome 7 causes a postnatal lethality phenotype that is imprinted (27).

Adapted and reproduced with permission from reference 13. Copyright © 1994 University of Chicago.

imprinted genes in humans and mice replicate asynchronously, with the paternal allele usually replicating before the maternal allele (Fig. 5a, 5b) (41). Relatively large, 1–3 Mb, chromosomal regions showed differential DNA replication (41). In the distal region of 15q11-q13, the *GABRA5* locus shows maternal early replication (Fig. 5a) (42), but since this region maps distal of the AS critical region, the significance of this finding is not known. Likewise, it is not known how differential DNA replication of a chromosomal domain and differential DNA methylation at individual loci are coordinated. In addition, it is likely that specific proteins expressed during male or female gametogenesis are involved in specification of the epigenetic imprint (12, 47), in addition to DNA methylation (14, 15, 25, 47).

Concluding Remarks

It has been suggested that the mechanism of imprinting involves a complex interplay of events involving large imprinted chromosomal regions, with gene-specific events occurring at multiple genes within each imprinted domain. We have identified two candidate genes, *SNRPN* and *ZNF127*, for PWS, and it is likely that additional candidate imprinted genes will also be found (45) (R.D. Nicholls *et al.*, unpublished data). Further study of individual imprinted genes, including analysis of expression during the different developmental phases that occur in PWS, a search for mutations in each imprinted gene in PWS-like patients, and animal models are necessary to link imprinted DNA sequences in this region to each aspect of the PWS phenotype.

One interesting possibility for imprinted disorders, such as PWS and AS, is that they may be amenable to therapeutic intervention based on pharmacological or other modification of the imprinted state. Since the phenotype in at least the majority of patients results from the "unmasking" of normally silent gene(s), rather than mutant alleles, an understanding of the molecular mechanisms of imprinting may make it possible to turn the silenced allele back on. Since imprinting mutations affect either PWS or AS specifically, and no patient has been observed to have a collection of imprinted disorders, it is possible that distinct regulation can be found for each imprinted locus, meaning that they may each be correctable independently. Therapy would be particularly valuable for PWS patients, in whom prevention of the failure to reach satiety would remove the biological drive to morbid obesity.

Recently, other imprinted genes (*ZNF127* [36]; *IPW* [48]) or anonymous transcripts (*PAR-1, PAR-5* [49]) have been identified in the human. In addition, the molecular basis of PSW and AS imprinting mutations has been discovered, identifying an imprinting center (IC) controlling resetting of imprinting throughout chromosome 15q11-q13 (50).

ACKNOWLEDGMENTS

This paper is dedicated to all the supportive families of individuals with PWS. Thanks to Jim Amos-Landgraf for preparation of figures and to Bernhard Horsthemke for a preprint of his work. This work was supported by a grant from the March of Dimes Birth Defects Foundation to Robert D. Nicholls, and grants from the American Cancer Society and National Institutes of Health to Robert D. Nicholls and Daniel J. Driscoll. Robert D. Nicholls is a Pew Scholar in Biomedical Sciences.

REFERENCES

1. Friedman JM, Leibel RL. Tackling a weighty problem. *Cell.* 1992;69: 217–220.
2. Bray GA, Dahms WT, Swerdloff RS, Fiser RH, Atkinson RL, Carrel RE. The Prader-Willi syndrome: a study of 40 patients and a review of the literature. *Medicine (Baltimore).* 1983;62:59–80.
3. Holm VA, Cassidy SB, Butler MG, *et al.* Prader-Willi syndrome: consensus diagnostic criteria. *Pediatrics.* 1993;91:398–402.
4. Cassidy SB. Prader-Willi syndrome. *Curr Probl Pediatr.* 1984;14:1–55.
5. Butler MG. Prader-Willi syndrome: current understanding of cause and diagnosis. *Am J Med Genet.* 1989;35:319–332.
6. Altman K, Bondy A, Hirsch A. Behavioral treatment of obesity in patients with Prader-Willi syndrome. *J Behav Med.* 1978;1:403–412.
7. Holm VA, Pipes PL. Food and children with Prader-Willi syndrome. *Am J Dis Child.* 1976;130:1063–1067.
8. Butler MG, Butler RI, Meaney FJ. The use of skinfold measurements to judge obesity during the early phase of Prader-Labhart-Willi syndrome. *Int J Obes.* 1988;12:417–422.
9. Schoeller DA, Levitsky LL, Bandini LG, Dietz WW, Walczak A. Energy expenditure and body composition in Prader-Willi syndrome. *Metabolism.* 1988;37:115–120.
10. Davies P, Joughin C, Livingstone MBE, Barnes ND. Energy expenditure in the Prader-Willi syndrome. In: Cassidy SB, ed. *Prader-Willi Syndrome.* Berlin: Springer-Verlag; 1992;H61;181–187. NATO ASI Series.
11. Schwartz RS, Brunzell JD, Birman EL. Elevated adipose tissue lipoprotein lipase in the pathogenesis of obesity in Prader-Willi syndrome. In: Holm VA, Sulzbacher S, Pipes PL, eds. *Prader-Willi Syndrome.* Baltimore: University Park Press; 1981;137–143.
12. Nicholls RD. Genomic imprinting and candidate genes in the Prader-Willi and Angelman syndromes. *Curr Opin Genet Dev.* 1993; 3:445–456.

13. Nicholls RD. Invited editorial: new insights reveal complex mechanisms involved in genomic imprinting. *Am J Hum Genet.* 1994;54: 733–740.

14. Stöger R, Kubicka P, Liu C-A, *et al.* Maternal-specific methylation of the imprinted mouse *Igf2r* locus identifies the expressed locus as carrying the imprinting signal. *Cell.* 1993;73:61–71.

15. Brandeis M, Kafri T, Ariel M, *et al.* The ontogeny of allele-specific methylation associated with imprinted genes in the mouse. *EMBO J.* 1993;12:3669–3677.

16. Mutirangura A, Jayakumar A, Sutcliffe JS, *et al.* A complete YAC contig of the Prader-Willi/Angelman chromosome region (15q11-q13) and refined localization of the *SNRPN* gene. *Genomics.* 1993; 18:546–552.

17. Clayton-Smith J, Pembrey ME. Angelman syndrome. *J Med Genet.* 1992;29:412–415.

18. Nicholls RD, Knoll JHM, Butler MG, Karam S, Lalande M. Genetic imprinting suggested by maternal heterodisomy in non-deletion Prader-Willi syndrome. *Nature.* 1989;342:281–285.

19. Driscoll DJ, Waters MF, Williams CA, *et al.* A DNA methylation imprint, determined by the sex of the parent, distinguishes the Angelman and Prader-Willi syndromes. *Genomics.* 1992;13:917–924.

20. Meijers-Heijboer EJ, Sandkuijl LA, Brunner HG, *et al.* Linkage analysis with chromosome 15q11-q13 markers shows genomic imprinting in familial Angelman syndrome. *J Med Genet.* 1992;29:853–857.

21. Wagstaff J, Knoll JHM, Glatt KA, Shugart YY, Sommer A, Lalande M. Maternal but not paternal transmission of 15q11-q13–linked nondeletion Angelman syndrome leads to phenotypic expression. *Nature Genet.* 1992;1:291–294.

22. Rinchik EM, Bultman SJ, Horsthemke B, *et al.* A gene for the mouse pink-eyed dilution locus and for human type II oculocutaneous albinism. *Nature.* 1993;361:72–76.

23. Lee S-T, Nicholls RD, Bundey S, Laxova R, Musarella M, Spritz RA. Mutations of the *P* gene in type II oculocutaneous albinism, Prader-Willi syndrome plus albinism, and "autosomal recessive albinism." *N Engl J Med.* 1994;330:529–534.

24. Stewart CL. Genomic imprinting in the regulation of mammalian development. *Adv Dev Biol.* 1993;2:73–118.

25. Surani MA. Silence of the genes. *Nature.* 1993;366:302–304.

26. Leff SE, Brannan CI, Reed ML, *et al.* Maternal imprinting of the

mouse *Snrpn* gene and conserved linkage homology with the Prader-Willi syndrome region. *Nature Genet.* 1992;2:259–264.

27. Cattanach BM, Barr JA, Evans EP, *et al.* A candidate mouse model for Prader-Willi syndrome which shows an absence of *SNRPN* expression. *Nature Genet.* 1992;2:270–274.

28. Hatada I, Sugama T, Mukai T. A new imprinted gene cloned by a methylation-sensitive genome scanning method. *Nucleic Acids Res.* 1993;21:5577–5582.

29. Hayashizaki Y, Shibata H, Hirotsune S, *et al.* Identification of an imprinted U2af binding protein related sequence on mouse chromosome 11 using RLGS method. *Nature Genet.* 1994;6:33–40.

30. Hall JG. Genomic imprinting: review and relevance to human diseases. *Am J Hum Genet.* 1990;46:857–873.

31. Junien C. Beckwith-Wiedemann syndrome, tumourigenesis and imprinting. *Curr Opin Genet Devel.* 1992;2:431–438.

32. Feinberg AP. Genomic imprinting and gene activation in cancer. *Nature Genet.* 1993;4:110–113.

33. Glenn CC, Porter KA, Jong MTC, Nicholls RD, Driscoll DJ. Functional imprinting and epigenetic modification of the human *SNRPN* gene. *Hum Mol Genet.* 1993;2:2001–2005.

34. Reed M, Leff SE. Maternal imprinting of human *SNRPN*, a gene deleted in Prader-Willi syndrome. *Nature Genet.* 1994;6:163–167.

35. Nakao M, Sutcliffe JS, Durtschi B, Mutirangura A, Ledbetter DH, Beaudet AL. Imprinting analysis of three genes in the Prader-Willi/Angelman region: *SNRPN*, E6-associated protein, and *PAR-2* (*D15S225E*). *Hum Mol Genet.* 1994;3:309–315.

36. Jong MTC, Glenn CC, Saitoh S, *et al.* A novel imprinted RING zinc-finger gene and overlapping antisense transcript within the Prader-Willi syndrome and syntenic mouse genetic regions. Submitted 1995.

37. Kalscheuer VM, Mariman EC, Schepans MT, Rehder H, Ropers H-H. The insulin-like growth factor type-2 receptor gene is imprinted in the mouse but not in humans. *Nature Genet.* 1993;5:74–78.

38. Dittrich B, Buiting K, Groß S, Horsthemke B. Characterization of a methylation imprint in the Prader-Willi syndrome chromosome region. *Hum Mol Genet.* 1993;2:1995–1999.

39. Glenn CC, Nicholls RD, Robinson WP, *et al.* Modification of 15q11-q13 DNA methylation imprints in unique Angelman and Prader-Willi patients. *Hum Mol Genet.* 1993;2:1377–1382.

40. Reis A, Dittrich B, Greger V, *et al.* Imprinting mutations suggested by abnormal DNA methylation patterns in familial Angelman and Prader-Willi syndromes. *Am J Hum Genet.* 1994;54:741–747.

41. Kitsberg D, Selig S, Brandeis M, *et al.* Allele specific replication timing of imprinted gene regions. *Nature.* 1993;364:459–463.

42. Knoll JHM, Cheng S-D, Lalande M. Allele specificity of DNA replication timing in the Angelman/Prader-Willi syndrome imprinted chromosomal region. *Nature Genet.* 1994;6:41–46.

43. Buiting K, Dittrich B, Groß S, *et al.* Molecular definition of the Prader-Willi syndrome chromosome region and orientation of the *SNRPN* gene. *Hum Mol Genet.* 1993;2:1991–1994.

44. Nicholls RD, Gottlieb W, Russell LB, Davda M, Horsthemke B, Rinchik EM. Evaluation of potential models for imprinted and non-imprinted components of human 15q11-q13 syndromes by fine structure homology mapping in the mouse. *Proc Natl Acad Sci USA.* 1993;90:2050–2054.

45. Beaudet AL, Nakao M, Durtschi BA, Mutirangura A, Ledbetter DH, Sutcliffe JS. Molecular analysis of the Prader-Willi/Angelman critical region identifies a cluster of imprinted genes. *J Cell Biochem Suppl.* 1994;18A:205.

46. Saitoh S, Kubota T, Ohta T, *et al.* Familial Angelman syndrome caused by imprinted submicroscopic deletion encompassing $GABA_A$ receptor β3-subunit gene. *Lancet.* 1992;339:366–367.

47. Razin A, Cedar H. DNA methylation and genomic imprinting. *Cell.* 1994;77:473–476.

48. Wevrick R, Kerns JA, Francke U. Identification of a novel paternally expressed gene in the Prader-Willi syndrome region. *Hum Mol Genet.* 1994;3:1877–1882.

49. Sutcliffe JS *et al.* Deletions of a differentially methylated CpG-island at the *SNRPN* gene define a putative imprinting control region. *Nature Genet.* 1994;8:52–58.

50. Buiting K, Saitoh S, Groß S, Dittrich B, Schwartz S, Nicholls RD, Horsthemke B. Inherited microdeletions in the Angelman and Prader-Willi syndromes define an imprinting center on human chromosome 15. *Nature Genet.* 1995;9:395–400.

PART VII

Transgenic Models of Obesity

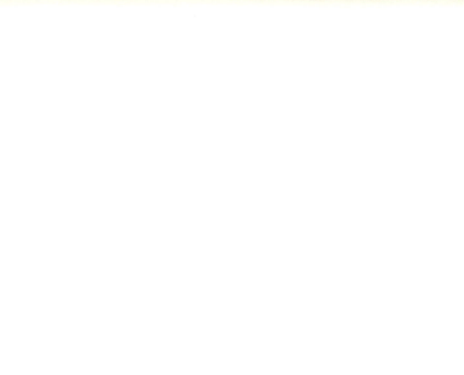

ANNE-MARIE CASSARD-DOULCIER, BRUNO MIROUX,
SUSANNE KLAUS, MARIANNE LAROSE,
ODETTE CHAMPIGNY, CORINNE LEVI-MEYRUEIS,
CHANTAL GELLY, SERGE RAIMBAULT,
FRÉDÉRIC BOUILLAUD, and DANIEL RICQUIER

Molecular Studies of the Uncoupling Protein in Animals and Humans

ABSTRACT

Brown adipose tissue is a tissue specialized in the production of heat, which is important for the maintenance of body temperature during cold exposure and awakening from hibernation in small and newborn mammals, including the human baby. This tissue may also buffer an excess of ingested calories. Heat production in brown adipose tissue is due to a controlled uncoupling of the mitochondrial respiratory chain. This is achieved by the uncoupling protein (UCP), a proton carrier in the inner mitochondrial membrane, unique to mitochondria of brown adipocytes. We are studying the mechanisms that restrict UCP gene transcription to brown adipocytes, the expression of UCP in primary cultures and its control by β_3-adrenoreceptors, the expression of UCP in human adipocytes, and the functional organization of UCP in the membrane.

Using cell transfection and transgenic mice, we obtained evidence that a region encompassing 3 kb of DNA upstream of the transcription start site contains positive and negative elements controlling UCP gene transcription. Trans-factors related to NF1, Ets 1, and Sp1 proteins bind UCP gene promoter. Evidence for expression of β_3-adrenoreceptor in brown adipocytes in primary culture was obtained. This expression precedes UCP emergence. Using immunodetection or Northern analysis, we demonstrated UCP expression in fat biopsies obtained from newborn or adult humans; however, such a study cannot be taken as a measurement of brown fat activity in humans. To study UCP structure, we generated a library of bacterial clones randomly expressing short subsequences of UCP fused to the MalE periplasmic protein of *Escherichia coli*. Then, we selected antibodies directed against certain subsequences and used them to study the topological organization of UCP. The orientation of five out of six predicted α-helices was determined and allowed us to propose a membranous folding.

Introduction

Small and newborn mammals, including humans, possess brown adipose tissue, the function of which is thermogenesis. Such heat production is essential at birth, during arousal from hibernation, and during exposure to a cold environment (1). Thermogenesis in brown adipocytes results from controlled uncoupling of respiration. This unique mechanism is due to the uncoupling protein (UCP), a proton carrier specifically expressed in brown adipocytes and located in the inner membrane of brown adipocyte mitochondria (2, 3). Contrary to white adipose tissue, the function of which is energy storage, brown adipose tissue functions are fat oxidation and energy dissipation. Morphologically, brown adipocytes are characterized by numerous mitochondria and multilocular lipid droplets. However, in terms of gene expression, the only true qualitative difference known so far between brown and white adipocytes is the expression of UCP in brown adipocytes. Several in vivo studies have demonstrated that UCP synthesis in brown adipocytes is strongly activated by norepinephrine released by sympathetic fibers at the surface of brown adipocytes (1, 4). The β-adrenoreceptor, now termed β$_3$-adrenoreceptor, involved in brown adipocyte activation and UCP synthesis has been cloned and shown to be present in both brown and white adipocytes (5). In this paper we present an analysis of regulatory elements in the UCP gene promoter and a study of the contribution of β$_3$-adrenoreceptor to UCP expression. The occurrence of UCP in human brown fat is also discussed. Finally, an analysis of the functional organization of UCP is presented.

Analysis of UCP Gene Promoter

Besides the question of molecular mechanisms responsible for the norepinephrine activation of UCP gene transcription, the main question is that of mechanisms that restrict UCP gene expression to brown adipocytes. These mechanisms have recently been advanced by the isolation and sequencing of genomic clones for mouse (6), rat (7), and human (8) UCP. The start site of transcription of mouse and rat UCP gene has been localized as well as several DNase I-hypersensitive sites (7, 9). Using transgenic mice bearing either a UCP minigene (9) or a chloramphenicol acetyltransferase (CAT) construct (10), evidence was obtained that the main *cis*-elements regulating UCP gene transcription are located in 3 kb or 4.5 kb of DNA upstream of the transcriptional start site of mouse and rat UCP gene, respectively. In order to identify these *cis*-elements, different deletions were made in the 4.5 kb long rat UCP gene promoter fused to CAT DNA and analyzed by transfection into in vitro differentiated brown adipocytes or into CHO cells (Fig. 1). A large deletion that removed the sequence from bp -4551 to bp -896 strongly reduced the CAT activity in transfected brown adipocytes but had no effect in Chinese hamster ovary (CHO) cells. To dissect the 5'-regulatory region further, several other deleted CAT constructs were generated. These constructs allowed us to identify a strong positive element of 211 base pairs (bp) at -2.5 kb. To analyze this element, it was placed upstream of the heterologous TK gene promoter of herpes simplex virus. The 211-bp AatII-ApaI element stimulated expression of this herologous promoter 15-fold in brown adipocytes and 6-fold in CHO cells. When the 211-bp element was placed upstream of the minimal promoter of UCP, a 32-fold activation was recorded both in brown adipocytes and in CHO cells. Similar activations were measured, whatever the orientation of the 211-bp element. These experiments confirmed that the AatII-ApaI element alone does not determine the cellular specificity of UCP gene transcription (10). In order to approach other regulatory elements, more 3' deletions were created in the promoter. Interestingly, such deletions preferentially activated CAT expression in CHO cells, suggesting that a silencer was involved in the inhibition of UCP gene expression in cells that do not transcribe this gene (Fig. 1).

Further analysis of the enhancer and silencer elements was achieved using DNase I and band-shift experiments. Data are given in Figure 2. In the enhancer element, two footprints (FP1 and FP2) were observed at positions bp $-2444/-2423$ and bp $-2352/-2319$. In the silencer domain adjacent to the transcriptional start site, five boxes A–E, able to bind nuclear extracts, were delineated at the positions indicated in Figure 2. In addition, two C/EBP binding sites were also identified in this region of the promoter. Another study (11), dealing with the or-

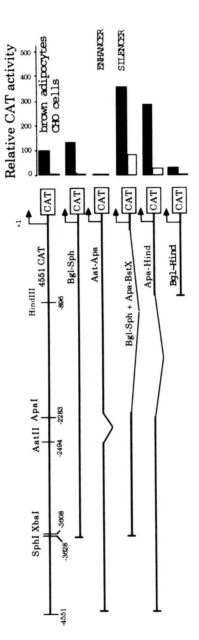

Figure 1. Delineation of *cis*-elements in the UCP promoter. Different CAT-DNA constructs were transfected either in cultured brown adipocytes or in CHO cells. A 211-bp AatII-ApaI enhancer was identified. A 3' deletion induced CAT activity especially in CHO cells, suggesting the presence of a silencer element.

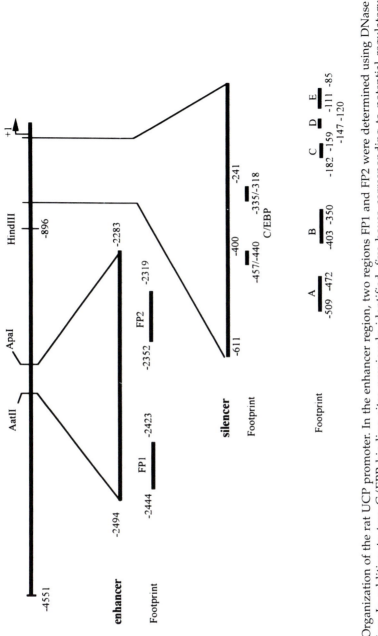

Figure 2. Organization of the rat UCP promoter. In the enhancer region, two regions FP1 and FP2 were determined using DNase I footprinting. In addition to two C/EBP binding sites previously identified, five boxes corresponding to potential regulatory elements were detected in the region containing silencer elements.

ganization of the murine UCP promoter, also identified enhancer and silencer regions and described in the enhancer regulatory elements homologous to rat FP1 and FP2. The regulation of UCP gene transcription is thought to result from an interaction between an enhancer region and a silencer region (10, 11).

Control of UCP Expression by β_3-Adrenoreceptors

Over the past few years the involvement of β_3-adrenoreceptor in UCP expression in brown adipose tissue (BAT) was demonstrated (1). Such a conclusion was obtained either from in vivo studies (12) or from treatment of in vitro differentiated brown adipocytes (13, 14, 15). Other studies were made with immortalized cell lines (16, 17, 18, 19). An immortalized cell line expressing UCP was obtained from a hibernoma of a transgenic mouse (16). This mouse contained a transgene with the adipocyte-specific regulatory region from adipocyte P2 (aP2) gene fused to SV40 transforming genes. This mouse developed hibernomas (brown fat tumors) from which cell lines were derived. One of these cell lines, HIB 1B, was found to express UCP when stimulated by cyclic adenosine monophosphate (cAMP) or catecholamines. Investigation of adrenergic receptors regulating the stimulation of UCP synthesis demonstrated that β_3-adrenergic agonists were much less effective than nonspecific β_3-adrenergic agonists (Fig. 3), and that the expression of β_3-adrenoreceptors was weak in HIB 1B cells. In fact, other cell lines were derived from hibernomas of aP2-SV40 transgenic mice. Figure 3 shows UCP mRNA expression in such a cell line termed 1B/8 (Champigny, Ross, Spiegelman, and Ricquier, unpublished data). In comparison with HIB 1B cells, stimulated 1B/8 cells expressed higher UCP mRNA level; in addition they better responded to BRL 37344 compound, which is a specific agonist of β_3-adrenergic receptors.

The β_3-adrenoreceptor mRNA was easily detected in Siberian hamster brown adipocytes in culture (19). Such an mRNA was also detected in cultured brown preadipocytes. The onset of UCP mRNA expression in differentiating brown adipocytes is delayed with respect to that of β_3-adrenoreceptor expression. Whereas UCP expression requires full differentiation of brown adipocytes, expression of β_3-adrenoreceptor in brown preadipocytes suggests that β_3-adrenoreceptor expression is a prerequisite to UCP synthesis. In comparison with immortalized cell

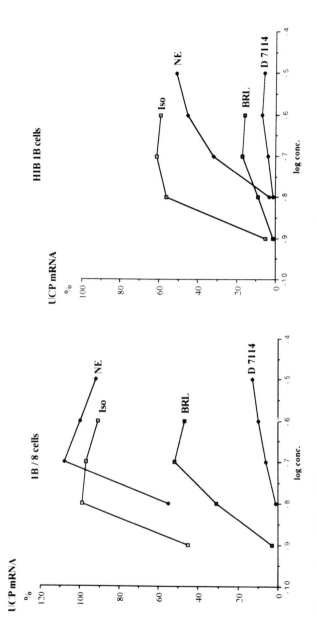

Figure 3. Stimulation of UCP mRNA in two immortalized cell lines derived from aP2-SV40 transgenic mice. Cells were treated for 4 hours with norepinephrine (NE), isoproterenol (Iso), BRL 37344 (Smith Kline Beecham pharmaceuticals), or D7114 (ICI-Zeneca pharmaceuticals). UCP mRNA is expressed as % of the value corresponding to 1B/8 cells treated by 10^{-8} M isoproterenol. 1B/8 cells treated by BRL 37344 β_3-adrenoreceptor agonist express higher UCP mRNA level than HIB 1B cells.

lines, it was generally observed that β_3-adrenoreceptor agonists in primary cultures are as potent as noradrenaline with respect to UCP mRNA induction (20, 21, 22).

UCP Expression in Human Adipose Tissue

Although it is generally said that BAT is not an important tissue in large mammals, the predicted low contribution of this tissue to human thermogenesis is only based on the impossibility of directly measuring BAT activity. In fact, BAT in infants accounts for about 1% of body weight (23), about the same proportion as BAT in rodents. Although typical BAT has been described in human adults (24) and especially in individuals who have spent a lot of time outdoors (25), or in alcoholic patients (26), quantification of BAT in adults is much more difficult. Analysis of UCP or its mRNA can be used to identify brown adipocytes. The uncoupling protein was easily detected in perirenal, retroperitoneal, subscapular adipose tissue of several infants (23, 27, 28). In agreement with previous reports, high UCP and UCP mRNA levels were measured in perinephric fat obtained from patients undergoing surgery for a pheochromocytoma (23). Since UCP gene transcription is known to be very sensitive to norepinephrine stimulation, it is assumed that UCP induction in patients with pheochromocytoma is the consequence of elevated catecholamine secretion. Actually, we detected UCP and/ or UCP mRNA in perirenal fat from eleven patients out of a group of nineteen individuals without pheochromocytoma (27). These patients had primary aldosteronism, pelviureteric syndrome, kidney adenocarcinoma, or kidney infarction. Kortelainen *et al.* (28) have also reported the immunodetection of UCP in fat excised from around the common carotid arteries and from around the thoracic aorta of several human adults. These data suggest that BAT is likely to be present in a larger number of adults than expected. The question of BAT thermogenesis in adult humans and of its contribution to body weight regulation is still open. Recently, two allelic forms of human UCP gene were discovered and a correlation between one allele and a high-fat gain over a period of ten years was observed (29). It does not mean that UCP gene is directly involved in fat gain, but it can be concluded that UCP gene polymorphism may be taken as an index to predict the ability of humans to gain fat.

The Functional Organization of UCP

Although it is a proton transporter, UCP belongs to the family of mitochondrial anion transporters such as the ADP/ATP carrier, the phosphate carrier, the oxoglutarate carrier, and the citrate carrier (30). These proteins share extensive sequence homologies and seem to result from triplication and divergence of an ancestral sequence. It is believed that all these carriers share the same organization in the membrane. The complete understanding of catalytic activity of UCP requires the identification of its catalytic center. In order to approach this question, a study of the topological organization of UCP was undertaken (31). We constructed a library of fusion proteins made of various fragments of UCP fused to *Escherichia coli* MalE protein (32). The screening of this library by an antiserum against UCP allowed cloning of several DNA short fragments identifying epitopes. Antibodies specific for these different epitopes were then purified and assayed either with mitoplasts or with inverted mitochondrial vesicles. This strategy allowed us to distinguish between epitopes facing the mitochondrial matrix and epitopes orientated toward the intermembrane space and led to the identification of the folding of UCP into the mitochondrial membrane (32). More recently several mutants of UCP were constructed and studied in collaboration with Eduardo Rial in Madrid. It was shown that no cysteine residue is essential for UCP activity (33); three amino acids essential for the nucleotide inhibition of UCP were also identified (34). A mutant of UCP deleted of phenylalanine 267, lysine 268, and glycine 269 was still able to transport protons but was insensitive to guanosine diphosphate. Analysis of other mutants could lead to the identification of residues participating to proton transport and residues mediating free fatty acid activation of this transport.

REFERENCES

1. Himms-Hagen J. Brown adipose tissue thermogenesis: interdisciplinary studies. *FASEB J*. 1990;11:2890–2898.
2. Klaus S, Casteilla L, Bouillaud F, Ricquier D. The uncoupling protein UCP: a membranous mitochondrial ion carrier exclusively expressed in brown adipose tissue. *Int J Biochem*. 1991;23:791–801.
3. Cannon B, Nedergaard J. The biochemistry of an inefficient tissue: brown adipose tissue. *Essays Biochem*. 1985;20:111–164.

4. Ricquier D, Mory G. Factors affecting brown adipose tissue in animals and man. *Clin Endocrinol Metab.* 1984;13:501–520.

5. Arch JRS, Kaumann AJ. β and atypical β-adrenoreceptors. *Med Res Rev.* 1993;13:663–729.

6. Kozak LP, Britton JH, Kozak UC, Wells JM. The mitochondrial uncoupling protein gene: correlation of exon structure to transmembrane domains. *J Biol Chem.* 1988;263:12274–12277.

7. Bouillaud F, Raimbault S, Ricquier D. The gene for rat uncoupling protein: complete sequence, structure of primary transcript and evolutionary relationship between exons. *Biochem Biophys Res Commun.* 1988;157:783–792.

8. Cassard AM, Bouillaud F, Mattei MG, *et al.* Human uncoupling protein gene: structure, comparison with rat gene and assignment to the long arm of chromosome 4. *J Cell Biochem.* 1990;43:255–264.

9. Boyer BB, Kozak LP. The mitochondrial uncoupling protein gene in brown fat: correlation between DNase-I hypersensitivity and expression in transgenic mice. *Mol Cell Biol.* 1991;11:4747–4756.

10. Cassard-Doulcier AM, Gelly C, Fox N, *et al.* Tissue-specific and β-adrenergic regulation of the mitochondrial uncoupling protein gene: control by cis-acting elements in the 5′-flanking region. *Mol Endocrinol.* 1993;7:497–506.

11. Kozak UC, Kopecky J, Teisenger J, Enerbäck S, Boyer B, Kozak LP. An upstream enhancer regulating brown-fat-specific expression of the mitochondrial uncoupling protein gene. *Mol Cell Biol.* 1994;14:59–67.

12. Champigny O, Ricquier D, Blondel O, Mayers RM, Briscoe MG, Holloway BR. β_3-Adrenoceptor stimulation restores message and expression of brown fat mitochondrial uncoupling protein (UCP) in adult dogs. *Proc Natl Acad Sci USA.* 1991;88:10774–10778.

13. Rehnmark S, Néchad M, Herron D, Cannon B, Nedergaard J. Alpha-adrenergic and beta-adrenergic induction of the expression of the uncoupling protein thermogenin in brown adipocytes differentiated in culture. *J Biol Chem.* 1990;265:16464–16471.

14. Kopecky J, Baudysova M, Zanolti F, Janikova D, Pavelka S, Houstek J. Synthesis of mitochondrial uncoupling protein in brown adipocytes differentiated in cell culture. *J Biol Chem.* 1990;165:22204–22209.

15. Klaus S, Cassard-Doulcier AM, Ricquier D. Development of Phodopus sungorus brown adipocytes in primary culture: effect of an

atypical β-adrenergic agonist, insulin and triiodothyronine on differentiation, mitochondrial development and expression of the uncoupling protein UCP. *J Cell Biol.* 1991;115:1783–1790.

16. Ross SR, Choy L, Graves RA, *et al.* Hibernoma formation in transgenic mice and isolation of a brown adipocyte cell line expressing the uncoupling protein gene. *Proc Natl Acad Sci USA.* 1992;89:7561–7565.

17. Kozak UC, Held W, Kreutter D, Kozak LP. Adrenergic regulation of the mitochondrial uncoupling protein gene in brown fat tumor cells. *Mol Endocrinol.* 1991;6:763–772.

18. Benito M, Porras A, Santos E. Establishment of permanent brown adipocyte cell lines achieved by transfection with SV40 large T antigen and ras genes. *Exp Cell Res.* 1993;209:248–254.

19. Klaus S, Choy L, Champigny O, *et al.* Characterization of the novel brown adipocyte cell line HIB 1B: adrenergic pathways involved in regulation of uncoupling protein gene expression. *J Cell Sci.* 1994;107:313–319.

20. Klaus S, Muzzin P, Revelli JP, *et al.* Control of B₃-adrenergic receptors in Siberian hamster brown adipocyte in culture. *Mol Cell Endocrinol.* 1995;109:189–195.

21. Champigny O, Holloway BR, Ricquier D. Regulation of UCP gene expression in brown adipocytes differentiated in primary culture: effects of the acid metabolite of a new β-adrenoreceptor agonist, ICI D 7114. *Mol Cell Endocrinol.* 1992;86:73–82.

22. Bronnikov G, Houstek J, Nedergaard J. β-Adrenergic, cAMP-mediated stimulation of proliferation of brown fat cells in primary culture. *J Biol Chem.* 1992;267:2006–2013.

23. Lean MJ. Brown adipose tissue and obesity. In: Belfiore F, Jeanrenaud B, Papalia D, eds. *Obesity: Basic Concepts and Clinical Aspects.* Basel, Switzerland: Karger;1992:37–49.

24. Hassi J. The brown adipose tissue in man. *Acta Univ Ouluensis Anat Path Microbiol.* 1977;1:1–93.

25. Huttunen P, Hirvonen J, Kinnula V. The occurrence of brown adipose tissue in outdoor workers. *Eur J Appl Physiol.* 1981;46:339–45.

26. Huttunen P, Kortelainen ML. Long-term alcohol consumption and brown adipose tissue in man. *Eur J Appl Physiol.* 1989;60:418–424.

27. Garruti G, Ricquier D. Analysis of uncoupling protein and its mRNA in adipose tissue of adipose deposits of adult humans. *Int J Obes.* 1992;16:383–390.

28. Kortelainen ML, Pelletier G, Ricquier D, Bukowiecki LJ. Immuno-histochemical detection of human brown adipose tissue uncoupling protein in an autopsy series. *J Histochem Cytochem.* 1993;41:759–764.

29. Oppert JM, Vohl MC, Chagnon M, *et al.* DNA variation in the uncoupling protein (UCP) gene and human body fat. *Int J Obes.* 1994; 18:526–531.

30. Walker JE, Runswick MJ. The mitochondrial transport protein superfamily. *J Bioenerg Biomembr.* 1993;25:435–446.

31. Miroux B, Casteilla L, Klaus S, *et al.* Antibodies selected from whole antiserum by fusion proteins as tools for the study of mitochondrial membranous protein topology: evidence that the N-terminal extremity of the sixth alpha helix of the uncoupling protein is facing the matrix. *J Biol Chem.* 1992;267:13603–13609.

32. Miroux B, Frossard V, Raimbault S, Ricquier D, Bouillaud F. The topology of the brown adipose tissue mitochondrial uncoupling protein determined with antibodies against its antigenic sites revealed by a library of fusion proteins. *EMBO J.* 1993;12:2739–2745.

33. Arechaga I, Raimbault S, Prieto S, *et al.* Cysteine residues are not essential for uncoupling protein function. *Biochem J.* 1993;296:693–700.

34. Bouillaud F, Arechaga I, Petit PX, *et al.* A sequence related to a DNA recognition element is essential for the inhibition by nucleotides of the proton transport through the mitochondrial uncoupling protein. *EMBO J.* 1994;13:1990–1997.

BRADFORD B. LOWELL, VEDRANA S. SUSULIC,
ANDREAS HAMANN, JOEL A. LAWITTS,
JEAN HIMMS-HAGEN, BERT B. BOYER,
LESLIE KOZAK, and JEFFREY S. FLIER

Transgenic Ablation of Brown Adipose Tissue

ABSTRACT

Brown fat is an important site of regulated energy expenditure. This observation has led to the suggestion that brown fat functions to maintain energy balance and prevent obesity. To directly test this hypothesis, we have produced transgenic mice that have a deficiency of brown fat due to the directed expression of diphtheria toxin A-chain. These animals are characterized by efficient metabolism and obesity. As the mice age, they also become hyperphagic, suggesting the possibility of a direct link between brown fat function and appetite regulation. In addition, obese animals develop severe insulin resistance. This study demonstrates that brown adipose tissue plays a critical role in the nutritional homeostasis of mice.

Brown adipose tissue (BAT), by virtue of its capacity for uncoupled mitochondrial respiration, has been implicated as an important site of regulated, adaptive energy expenditure (1, 2, 3). In tissues other than BAT, fuel oxidation is linked to the energy needs of the cell (*i.e.*, calories are expended only if work has been performed). The mitochondria of BAT are unique, however, in that they possess uncoupling protein (UCP), a 32 kd mitochondrial proton transporter that functions to uncouple respiration by dissipating the mitochondrial proton electrochemical gradient (4, 5). This capacity permits BAT to expend calories unrelated to the performance of work with the net result of heat generation. Two key roles have been proposed for this tissue: generation of heat during cold exposure (nonshivering thermogenesis) (6), and protection from obesity during the ingestion of excess calories (diet-induced thermogenesis) (1). The role of BAT in mediating diet-induced thermogenesis has led to the suggestion that BAT activity contributes to metabolic inefficiency and, as such, might provide a cellular and molecular explanation for protection against obesity.

Obesity results when caloric intake chronically exceeds energy expenditure. In genetic models of obesity, such as *ob/ob*, *db/db*, and A^y mice and *fa/fa* rats, it is well established that there are two abnormalities: increased food intake and decreased energy expenditure (7). Many studies have attempted to determine whether dysfunction of BAT contributes to decreased energy expenditure and obesity in these animals. Genetic forms of rodent obesity are characterized by decreased sympathetic nervous system activity in BAT (3, 8, 9). This appears to result in a variety of secondary disturbances in BAT function, such as reduced thyroxine 5′-deiodinase activity, decreased UCP mRNA, and mitochondrial UCP concentration, and reduced mitochondrial guanosine diphosphate (GDP) binding (thought to reflect UCP activity) (2, 3). However, some workers have found normal UCP mRNA in obese rodents (10, 11). Since the causative mutations in genetically obese rodents are unknown or uncharacterized, and the animals possess numerous abnormalities likely to be unrelated to abnormal function of BAT, it has not been possible to use these models to determine the quantitative importance of brown fat dysfunction in the development of obesity. Attempts to define the function of BAT through surgical ablation or denervation have not been successful, since BAT exists in many diffuse depots and has substantial capacity for regeneration and hypertrophy (12). Therefore, the role of BAT in the regulation of body weight has remained unclear.

In the present study, recently reported in *Nature* (13), we have utilized an alternative, transgenic approach. The goal was to create lines of mice with genetically ablated BAT through the use of a suicide DNA vector in which regulatory elements in the UCP gene drive BAT specific expression of diphtheria toxin A-chain (DTA). Native diphtheria toxin is composed of A- and B-chains which are linked by disulfide bonds. The B-chain recognizes a cell surface receptor and promotes endocytosis. Once inside the cell, the A-chain catalyzes the ribosylation of elongation factor-2 resulting in cell death. Through selective genetic expression of the A-chain, programmed cell death is targeted to a specified cell lineage. A-chain protein released during cell death is nontoxic to neighboring cells, since the B-chain is lacking. Previous studies have used similar or related technology to create mice that lack various tissues (14). In the present study, we have succeeded in producing two lines of mice that have decreased BAT and marked obesity. In one line, BAT regenerates later in life and obesity resolves. In the other line, BAT deficiency persists and the transgenic mice develop massive obesity complicated by severe insulin resistance. Initially, the obesity develops in the absence of hyperphagia, demonstrating that BAT-deficient mice have decreased energy expenditure. Interestingly, the transgenic animals later develop increased food intake in addition to decreased overall thermogenesis, suggesting the possibility that control of food intake may be influenced by brown fat function.

Characterization of 16-Day-Old Mice

UCP-1 is a UCP minigene that has previously been shown in transgenic mice to be expressed exclusively in BAT (15). The genetic ablation vectors (Fig. 1) were constructed to include all of UCP-1 plus an additional 850 base pairs (bp) of 5′ distal UCP sequence. Full-strength DTA (16) or a slightly less toxic version termed 176 (17) was inserted into the first exon of the UCP minigene at position +120, preceding the UCP start codon located at position +232 to create UCP-DTA and UCP-176, respectively.

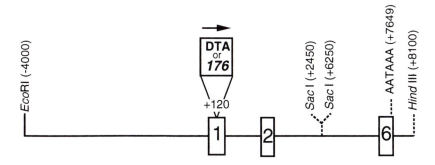

Figure 1. UCP-DTA and UCP-176 transgenes. DTA and 176 were cloned into the UCP minigene as previously described (13). The vector was injected into the pronuclei of fertilized FVB/N mouse embryos. Numbers shown are relative to the UCP transcription start site, and the arrow represents the orientation of DTA and 176 coding sequence. Methods for all data shown in Figures 1–6 are described in reference 13.

Figure from reference 13.

Two lines of mice were created (UCP-DTA and UCP-176), each of which has ablated BAT and extreme obesity. Upon gross visual inspection of 16-day-old transgenic heterozygous offspring from both lines, it was apparent that the interscapular BAT depot had been nearly completely (UCP-176) or partially (UCP-DTA) replaced by white adipose tissue. Although it was difficult to visualize any remaining brown adipose tissue in the UCP-176 line, a BAT remnant was always observed in the UCP-DTA line. The remnant from the UCP-DTA line at age 16 days weighed about one-half of control BAT interscapular depots (data not shown). In order to quantitate the degree of BAT ablation, immunoblotting with UCP antisera was used to assess the interscapular BAT depot content of UCP, a brown adipocyte lineage specific marker (5, 10), whose expression reflects the functional status of the tissue. The interscapular BAT depot was chosen for UCP quantitation, since it is well circumscribed and represents a major depot of BAT in mice. As seen in Figure 2A, UCP-DTA mice had a modest decrease in interscapular UCP content. In the case of UCP-176 mice, UCP per depot was markedly decreased with the signal being visible only when the lanes were overloaded 25-fold. To more accurately estimate UCP content we utilized phosphor-imaging of immunoblots and compared signals from unknown BAT homogenates and purified mouse UCP standards. In 16-day-old UCP-DTA transgenic mice, UCP content was decreased by 68%, and in UCP-176 transgenic mice, UCP content was reduced by 96% (Fig. 2B).

Obesity in 16-day-old mice was assessed by quantitating total body lipid stores. Total body lipid was increased by 31% in UCP-DTA mice and by 68% in UCP-176 mice (Fig. 2C), thus correlating with their relative deficiency of BAT. This degree of obesity at 16 days is comparable to that found in other murine models of genetic- (*ob/ob, db/db*) or hypothalamic lesion– (monosodium glutamate) induced obesity.

Development of Obesity and Its Metabolic Complications

A longitudinal study was conducted in which heterozygous offspring of the UCP-DTA founder were weaned at age 2.7 weeks and housed separately in plastic cages at 24°C with free access to chow (Purina Formulab Chow 5008, 6.5% fat by weight) and water. Body weight and food intake were monitored until 8.4 weeks, when the majority of animals were sacrificed and further analyzed. Linear growth (nasal-anal

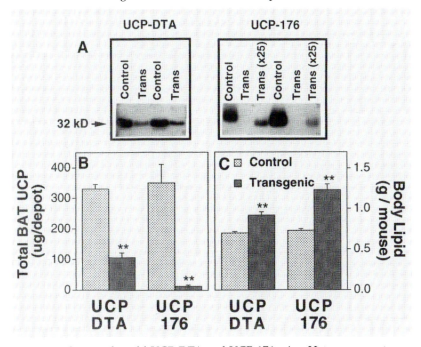

Figure 2. Sixteen-day-old UCP-DTA and UCP-176 mice. Heterozygous trans-genic mice and their nontransgenic littermates were analyzed at age 16 days, prior to weaning [UCP-DTA: control = 12 (7 female, 5 male), transgenic = 13 (7 female, 6 male); UCP-176: control = 8 (5 female, 3 male), transgenic = 7 (4 female, 3 male)]. (*A*) Immunoblotting of BAT homogenates for UCP. Each lane contains 1/2000 of the total depot protein content except for lanes labeled "(×25)," in which 25 times that amount was loaded. (*B*) Quantitation of UCP. Immunoblots of BAT interscapular homogenates were prepared with 5 µg of homogenate protein per lane and purified mouse UCP standards (25 µg to 1000 ng) and analyzed with a phosphor-imager. Total interscapular BAT depot UCP was determined by adjusting for total interscapular depot protein content. (*C*) Total body lipid content. Lipid content was assessed using the alcoholic KOH digestion method. All values are shown as mean +/- SE (** = $P < 0.01$).
Figure from reference 13.

length) and body composition were assessed and serum was assayed for various metabolites and hormones. A small subset of female control and transgenic mice were maintained until age 19 weeks, when similar analyses were performed. Linear growth was normal in 8.4-week-old male and female transgenic animals (data not shown), which is in con-trast to most other forms of genetic rodent obesity in which growth is usually stunted (7). Body weight became noticeably greater at age 5.5 weeks and then increased steadily (Fig. 3). When examined at similar ages, males had a greater degree of weight gain, but with advancing age (19 weeks) females also became massively overweight.

Interscapular BAT UCP content was decreased by 87% in 8.4-week-old transgenic males, 60% in 8.4-week-old transgenic females, and 71% in 19-week-old transgenic females (Fig. 4A). Total body lipid (Fig. 4B) was increased by 4-fold and 2.5-fold in 8.4-week-old male and female transgenic mice, respectively, and by 6-fold in 19-week-old transgenic females. Lean body mass, as reflected by body protein content, was increased by 28% in transgenic 8.4-week-old males ($P < 0.01$), 12% in 8.4-week-old females (not significant), and by 17% in 19-week-old females (not significant). This tendency toward increased lean body mass is in contrast to other rodent models of obesity in which lean body mass is decreased (7), but it is similar to human obesity in which lean body mass is usually increased (18).

The serum glucose level (Fig. 4C) was increased in all transgenic groups and was maximally increased by twofold in 19-week-old fe-

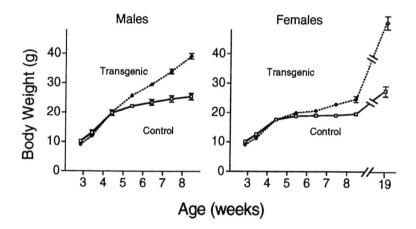

Figure 3. Body weight of heterozygous UCP-DTA mice and their nontransgenic littermates. Study design is as described in the text. Numbers of mice used in the study as shown in Figures 3, 4, and 5 are as follows: 8.4-week-old UCP-DTA (male = 5, female = 4), controls (male = 5, female = 13); 19-week-old UCP-DTA (female = 3), controls (female = 3). Values are shown as mean $+/-$ SE.

Figure from reference 13.

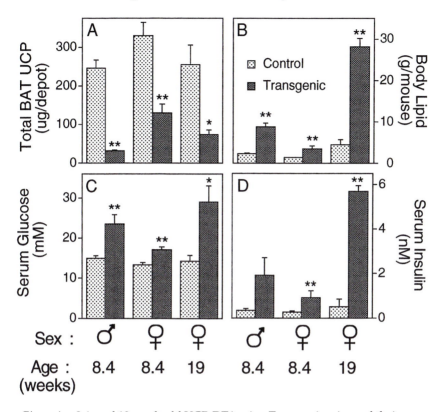

Figure 4. 8.4- and 19-week-old UCP-DTA mice. Transgenic mice and their non-transgenic littermates were analyzed as indicated below. Following euthanasia with carbon dioxide in the fed state, interscapular BAT and serum were obtained. Values are shown as mean $+/-$ SE (* $= P < 0.05$ and ** $= P < 0.01$). (*A*) Total interscapular BAT UCP and (*B*) total body lipid content were determined as described in Figure 2. (*C*) Serum glucose and (*D*) serum insulin were determined as described in reference 13.

males. The serum insulin level (Fig. 4D) was also increased in all transgenic groups and was maximally increased by 12-fold in 19-week-old females. A modest increase in serum glucose concurrent with a marked increase in serum insulin demonstrates the presence of severe insulin resistance. Insulin and glucose levels were normal in 16-day-old transgenic UCP-DTA mice, suggesting that glucose intolerance, hyperinsulinemia, and insulin resistance develop as obesity progresses and is not a direct or immediate consequence of BAT ablation.

The UCP-176 line differs dramatically from the UCP-DTA line with respect to the status of BAT ablation over time. Despite a more complete ablation of BAT at 16 days (96% reduction in UCP, Fig. 2A, B), UCP content was only minimally reduced in 8-week-old UCP-176 transgenic mice (data not shown). Since all 16-day-old UCP-176 transgenic animals had massive ablation, the minimal ablation in older UCP-176 transgenic animals implies regeneration of BAT. Tissue regeneration has been noted in another genetic ablation study (14). Although the mechanism responsible for regeneration is not understood at present, it is important to note that although UCP-176 mice are extremely obese at age 16 days (Fig. 2C), total body lipid stores are normal at age 8 weeks (data not shown). Reversal of obesity following regeneration of BAT provides compelling evidence that obesity in these mice is a consequence of BAT deficiency.

UCP-DTA Mice Develop Hyperphagia

Both male and female controls maintained nearly constant levels of food intake from week 5 to week 8 (Fig. 5). In contrast, male transgenic

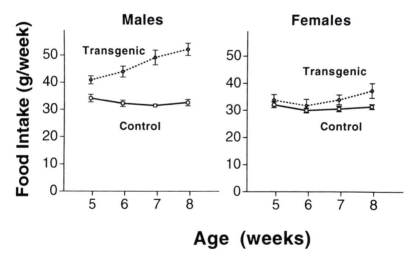

Figure 5. Food intake in UCP-DTA mice. Food was weighed at the beginning and end of each week. The difference was assumed to represent grams of chow eaten per week. No evidence of spillage was noted. Values are shown as mean +/− SE.

mice ingested 20% more than controls at week 5 and this increased steadily to 58% above controls by week 8. Female transgenic mice ingested the same as controls at weeks 5 and 6, but this also increased steadily to 19% above control food intake by week 8. In additional studies, hyperphagia has been uniformly observed in UCP-DTA transgenic mice over the age of 7 weeks. However, the age at which hyperphagia begins varies between week 5 and week 7.

It is conceivable that hyperphagia in UCP-DTA mice is the consequence of an unexpected lesion in some location other than BAT. One such possibility would be expression of the transgene in the hypothalamus, where it is known that ablative lesions can produce hyperphagia and obesity (7). This would be unexpected, however, since the endogenous UCP gene is not known to be expressed in any tissue other than BAT (5, 10). Using polymerase chain reaction, we and others (Daniel Ricquier, personal communication) have been unable to detect endogenous UCP mRNA in the hypothalamus. In order to directly address the possibility of a hypothalamic lesion in UCP-DTA mice, we have histologically examined the brains of UCP-DTA transgenic mice. The volume of all nuclei was normal. Additional functional evidence against a hypothalamic lesion is the fact that UCP-DTA male and female mice can reproduce and grow normally, processes that are sensitive to hypothalamic disturbance. Although the evidence against a hypothalamic lesion is strong, we cannot definitively rule out the existence of a lesion that specifically affects appetite and not fertility or growth, and is unable to be detected on histological analysis.

In addition to the two lines described above, we have generated three nontransmitting UCP-DTA founders that were analyzed at age 26 weeks (13). Two founders were mosaic for the transgene and one was infertile. These founders had diminished BAT, were significantly overweight, and had a large increase in total body lipid. In addition, these founders were markedly hyperphagic. The presence of brown fat deficiency, obesity, and hyperphagia in these additional founder animals essentially rules out the possibility that these phenotypic features of the UCP-DTA mice could be due to positional integration effects.

Energy Expenditure Is Decreased in UCP-DTA Mice

Given the function of BAT as a site of thermogenesis, it would be predicted that mice with a deficiency of BAT and living at a temperature below thermoneutrality would have a reduction in energy expenditure. However, the presence of hyperphagia in the UCP-DTA line complicates the demonstration of this defect. In order to address this point, an additional group of UCP-DTA transgenic and control male littermates were analyzed at age 6 weeks, prior to the development of hyperphagia (Fig. 6A). Although food intake was not increased, total body lipid content was increased by 2.4-fold. Increased fat mass in the absence of hyperphagia demonstrates that UCP-DTA mice have decreased energy expenditure.

Brown and white adipose tissue possesses an "atypical" β-adrenergic receptor subtype termed β_3 (19–22). It possesses unique pharmacological properties, and specific agonists have been synthesized. Administration of such agonists to rodents increases oxygen consumption by more than two-fold, demonstrating the remarkable potential of this signaling pathway to augment energy expenditure. Since the β_3-adrenergic receptor (β_3AR) is expressed predominantly in brown and white adipose tissue (20–22), it has been suspected that the marked increase in oxygen consumption caused by these agents is due to the activation of BAT. A highly selective β_3AR agonist, CL 316,243 (23), was administered to control and transgenic male and female littermates, and the increase in oxygen consumption was assessed (Fig. 6B). The measurements were performed at an ambient temperature of 28°C to ensure that BAT would be quiescent prior to drug administration. Accordingly, the pretest metabolic rate was equal in control and transgenic animals. The response to CL 316,243 was reduced in transgenic mice by 50%. This finding demonstrates that UCP-DTA mice have a functional deficiency of BAT.

Cold exposure increases oxygen consumption of rodents by at least twofold. In acutely exposed animals, it is estimated that about 60% of this response is the result of shivering (24), and the rest is mediated by "nonshivering" thermogenesis primarily in BAT (6). Thermoregulation represents the balance between heat generation (shivering and nonshivering thermogenesis) and heat conservation (piloerection and redistribution of blood flow) and is regulated by the hypothalamus (25). Genetically obese mice (ob/ob and db/db), which are thought to have BAT dysfunction, become profoundly hypothermic and die following brief cold exposure (26). This behavior has led many to conclude that the role of BAT in thermoregulation following acute cold exposure is vital. However, these animals have additional defects in hypothalamic

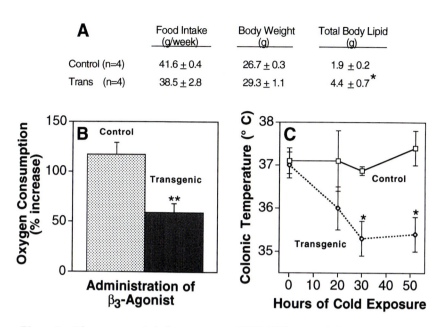

A	Food Intake (g/week)	Body Weight (g)	Total Body Lipid (g)
Control (n=4)	41.6 ± 0.4	26.7 ± 0.3	1.9 ± 0.2
Trans (n=4)	38.5 ± 2.8	29.3 ± 1.1	4.4 ± 0.7*

Figure 6. Thermogenesis in heterozygous UCP-DTA mice. (*A*) Total body lipid content of UCP-DTA mice prior to the development of hyperphagia. Male UCP-DTA mice and their control littermates were weaned at 2.7 weeks and group housed, 2 control and 2 transgenic mice per cage (4 total/cage). At 5.5 weeks of age, they were separated and housed individually. Food intake was monitored over the following week after which the mice were euthanized and analyzed for total body lipid content. (*B*) Thermogenic response to CL (CL 316,243), a β_3-adrenoceptor selective agonist. UCP-DTA (2 male and 8 female) and control (3 male and 4 female) littermates were weaned at age 2.7 weeks, then separated and housed individually at age 4.5 weeks. Mice were 62–69 days old at the time of CL administration. Male and female control mice responded similarly to the CL compound. (*C*) Colonic temperature during cold exposure. Female UCP-DTA (n = 6) and control (n = 3) littermates were weaned at age 2.7 weeks, individually housed at age 4.5 weeks (at 24°C), and acutely cold exposed to 4°C at age 8 weeks with food available ad libidum. Colonic temperature was measured using a YSI model 43 tele-thermometer equipped with a series 500 probe (Yellow Springs Instrument Co., Inc, Yellow Springs, Ohio). All values are shown as mean +/− SE (* = $P < 0.05$, ** = $P < 0.01$). Methods are as described in reference 13.

Figure from reference 13.

function (7) that probably contribute to their defective thermoregulation. Indeed, at room temperature (24°C) genetically obese mice maintain their body temperature at about two degrees below normal (26). To address the effect of isolated BAT dysfunction on thermoregulation, control and UCP-DTA littermates were exposed to 4°C for 52 hours. At 24°C, both control and transgenic mice had a rectal temperature of 37°C. During cold exposure, the control mice maintained their temperature at 37°C, but the transgenic mice gradually decreased to 35.3°C by 30 hours and maintained that temperature at 52 hours. Unlike *ob/ob* mice, UCP-DTA animals have only a minor decrease in body temperature in response to cold exposure. Thus, BAT dysfunction sufficient to produce massive obesity causes only a minor disturbance in thermoregulation following cold exposure.

Discussion

A thorough understanding of the physiologic function of BAT has remained uncertain, given the unavailability of a pure model of chronic BAT deficiency. We have addressed this issue by creating lines of transgenic mice with primary BAT deficiency caused by BAT-specific expression of a toxigene. The resulting animals have brown fat deficiency, decreased energy expenditure, obesity, and hyperphagia. Some have taken the view that the dominant function of BAT is to maintain body temperature during cold stress, and that its role, if any, in the regulation of energy balance is minor. In contrast, the present study suggests that the role of BAT in the regulation of energy balance is substantially greater than many workers would have anticipated.

Obesity and non–insulin-dependent diabetes mellitus (NIDDM) are prevalent diseases and relevant animal models of these conditions are needed. The UCP-DTA mouse has many features in common with obesity as it appears in most humans, and lacks many of the features found in other rodent models that are atypical of human disease. For instance, most other rodent genetic- and hypothalamic lesion–induced models of obesity are characterized by reduced fertility or infertility, stunted linear growth, and decreased lean body mass (7). Exceptions include the *A^y* mouse and the gold thioglucose (GTG) hypothalamic lesioned mouse, both of which have accelerated linear growth and increased lean body mass. The UCP-DTA mice, similar to humans with obesity, have normal fertility, normal linear growth, and increased lean body mass. Finally, one confounding aspect of rodent models of obesity is the nearly universal finding of elevated corticosterone (the circulating mouse glucocorticoid) (7). With the exception of patients with Cushing's disease, glucocorticoid levels are normal in human obesity. Since glucocorticoids are widely known to have anti-insulin and obesity inducing actions, the relevance of these obese rodent models for human obesity and NIDDM could be limited. In UCP-DTA mice, corticosterone levels were not elevated (data not shown). For these reasons, the UCP-DTA mouse should be a valuable tool in efforts to better understand the pathogenesis and pathophysiology of obesity and NIDDM in humans.

This study provides compelling evidence that BAT plays a critical role in the regulation of energy balance in mice. Although previous correlative studies suggested that BAT could influence systematic energy balance, the extent of obesity and metabolic derangement seen in these BAT-deficient mice is consistent with the most liberal estimates regarding the metabolic importance of this tissue. Brown adipose tissue is present in humans (27, 28) and can hypertrophy in response to stimuli as in patients with pheochromocytomas (29), a catecholamine-secreting tumor. However, the functional significance and quantitation of BAT in humans with and without obesity are at present unknown and should be the focus of future investigations.

ACKNOWLEDGMENTS

We wish to thank Anna-Lisa Kates for providing us with UCP Western blotting reagents and methodology, Ian Maxwell for providing pIBI130-DT-A and pIBI-176, Ronald Lechan for performing hypothalamic histology, Jean-Pierre Flatt for assisting us with carcass analysis methodology, Tom Claus of American Cyanamid Co., Pearl River, NY for providing CL 316,243, the National Research Council of Canada for providing the computerized equipment for the measurement of oxygen uptake, and Kemp Herzberg of the Beth Israel Transgenic Facility for assisting with the generation of transgenic mice. This work was supported by grants from the National Institutes of Health to Bradford B. Lowell, Jeffrey S. Flier, and Leslie P. Kozak, from Miles Inc. to Bradford B. Lowell and Jeffrey S. Flier, and from the Medical Research Council of Canada to Jean Himms-Hagen.

REFERENCES

1. Nicholls DG, Locke RM. Thermogenic mechanisms in brown fat. *Physiol Rev.* 1984;64:1–64.

2. Klaus S, Casteilla L, Bouillaud F, Ricquier D. The uncoupling protein UCP: a membraneous mitochondrial ion carrier exclusively expressed in brown adipose tissue. *Int J Biochem.* 1991;23:791–801.

3. Rothwell NJ, Stock MJ. A role for brown adipose tissue in diet-induced thermogenesis. *Nature.* 1979;281:31–35.

4. Trayhurn P, Mercer SW. Brown adipose tissue thermogenesis in obese animals. *Biochem Soc Trans.* 1986;14:236–239.

5. Himms-Hagen J. Brown adipose tissue thermogenesis and obesity. *Prog Lipid Res.* 1989;28:67–115.

6. Foster DO, Frydman ML. Tissue distribution of cold-induced thermogenesis in conscious warm- or cold-acclimated rats reevaluated from changes in tissue blood flow: the dominant role of brown adipose tissue in the replacement of shivering by nonshivering thermogenesis. *Can J Physiol Pharmacol.* 1979;57:257–270.

7. Bray GA, York DA. Hypothalamic and genetic obesity in experimental animals: an autonomic and endocrine hypothesis. *Physiol Rev.* 1979;59:719–809.

8. Knehans AW, Romsos DR. Reduced norepinephrine turnover in brown adipose tissue of *ob/ob* mice. *Am J Physiol.* 1982;242:E253–E261.

9. Young JB, Landsberg L. Diminished sympathetic nervous system activity in the genetically obese (*ob/ob*) mouse. *Am J Physiol.* 1983;245:E148–E154.

10. Jacobsson A, Stadler U, Glotzer MA, Kozak LP. Mitochondrial uncoupling protein from mouse brown fat: molecular cloning, genetic mapping and mRNA expression. *J Biol Chem.* 1985;260:16250–16254.

11. Ricquier D, Bouillaud F, Toumelin P, *et al.* Expression of uncoupling mRNA in thermogenic or weakly thermogenic brown adipose tissue. *J Biol Chem.* 1986;261:13905–13910.

12. Rothwell NJ, Stock MJ. Surgical removal of brown fat results in rapid and complete compensation by other depots. *Am J Physiol.* 1989;257:R253–R258.

13. Lowell BB, S-Susulic V, Hamman A, *et al.* Development of obesity in transgenic mice after genetic ablation of brown adipose tissue. *Nature.* 1993;366:740–742.

14. Breitman ML, Bernstein A. Engineering cellular deficits in transgenic mice by genetic ablation. In: Grosveld F, Kollias G, eds. *Transgenic Animals*. Boston: Academic Press; 1992:129–145.

15. Boyer BB, Kozak LP. The mitochondrial uncoupling protein gene in brown fat: correlation between DNase I hypersensitivity and expression in transgenic mice. *Mol Cell Biol*. 1991;11:4147–4156.

16. Maxwell IH, Maxwell F, Glode LM. Regulated expression of a diphtheria toxin A-chain gene transfected into human cells: a possible strategy for inducing cancer cell suicide. *Cancer Res*. 1986;46:4660–4664.

17. Maxwell F, Maxwell IH, Glode LM. Cloning, sequence determination and expression in transfected cells of the coding sequence for the tox 176 attenuated diphtheria toxin A chain. *Mol Cell Biol*. 1987; 7:1576–1579.

18. Forbes GB, Welle SL. Lean body mass in obesity. *Int J Obes*. 1983;7: 99–107.

19. Emorine LJ, Marullo S, Briend-Sutren M-M, *et al*. Molecular characterization of the human β_3-adrenergic receptor. *Science*. 1989;245: 1118–1121.

20. Granneman JG, Lahners KN, Chaudhry A. Molecular cloning and expression of the rat β_3-adrenergic receptor. *Mol Pharmacol*. 1991;40: 895–899.

21. Muzzin P, Revelli J-P, Kuhne F, *et al*. An adipose tissue-specific β-adrenergic receptor. *J Biol Chem*. 1991;266:24053–24058.

22. Nahmias C, Blin N, Elalouf J-M, Mattei MG, Strosberg AD, Emorine LJ. Molecular characterization of the mouse β_3-adrenergic receptor: relationship with the atypical receptor of adipocytes. *EMBO J*. 1991; 10:3721–3727.

23. Bloom JD, Dutia MD, Johnson BD, *et al*. Disodium (R,R)-5-[2-[[2-(3-Chlorophenyl)-2-hydroxyethyl]-amino]propyl]-1,3-benzodioxole-2,2-dicarboxylate (CL 316,243): a potent β-adrenergic receptor agonist virtually specific for β_3 receptors: a promising antidiabetic and antiobesity agent. *J Med Chem*. 1992;35:3081–3084.

24. Davis TRA, Johnston DR, Bell FC, Cremer BJ. Regulation of shivering and nonshivering heat production during acclimation of rats. *Am J Physiol*. 1960;198:471–475.

25. Gordon CJ, Heath JE. Integration and central processing in temperature regulation. *Annu Rev Physiol*. 1986;48:595–612.

26. Davis TRA, Mayer J. Imperfect homeothermia in the hereditary

obese-hyperglycemic syndrome of mice. *Am J Physiol.* 1954;177: 222–226.

27. Garruti G, Ricquier D. Analysis of uncoupling protein and its mRNA in adipose tissue deposits of adult humans. *Int J Obes.* 1992; 16:383–390.

28. Krief S, Lonnqvist F, Raimbault S, *et al.* Tissue distribution of β₃-adrenergic receptor mRNA in man. *J Clin Invest.* 1993;91:344–349.

29. Ricquier D, Nechad M, Mory G. Ultrastructural and biochemical characterization of human brown adipose tissue in pheochromo-cytoma. *J Clin Endocrinol Metab.* 1982;54:803–807.

LESLIE P. KOZAK, ULRIKE KOZAK, GEORGE CLARKE,
SVEN ENERBÄCK, and JAN KOPECKY

Genes of Energy Balance:
Modulation in Transgenic Mice

ABSTRACT

An efficient metabolism, essential for survival in a foraging, physically active primitive culture, has been postulated to lead to obesity and diabetes in modern man. We seek to understand the genetic basis of energy efficiency with transgenic mouse models.
Two genetic models have been developed: 1) Overexpression of
the cytoplasmic NAD-linked glycerol-3-phosphate dehydrogenase generates a futile ATP cycle that burns off energy and results
in a depression of nonshivering thermogenesis and a reduction in
white fat lipid stores. These effects are observed in normal transgenic mice and in transgenic mice also homozygous for the diabetes (db) gene. The results indicate that modulations in the basic
pathways of carbohydrate and lipid metabolism can have profound effects on energy efficiency. 2) The second model alters energy efficiency by modulating expression of the mitochondrial uncoupling protein, a key step in the pathway of nonshivering
thermogenesis. A transgene of the Ucp coding sequence under
control of the fat-specific aP2 gene promoter has been produced
in order to evaluate the consequences of constitutive Ucp expression in brown fat and ectopic expression in white fat. On the
C57BL/6J background, no change in body weight is observed, but
a striking redistribution of regional fat occurs. In addition to the
regional redistribution, when the transgene is combined with the
A^{vy} gene, a 20% reduction in total body weight occurs because of
the reduction in fat depots.

In a paper published in 1962, James Neel (1) postulated that the high
frequency of non–insulin-dependent diabetes among primitive peoples

recently exposed to modern Western culture was caused by the presence of a thrifty genotype. This genotype was viewed as providing an individual with the efficient metabolism necessary for survival in primitive cultures characterized by regular episodes of fasting, intense physical activity, and a low-fat diet. In contrast, in modern cultures characterized by overeating, a sedentary life-style, and a high-fat diet, the efficient metabolism of the thrifty genotype causes obesity. Viewed from this perspective, obesity in humans is an evolutionary disease whose etiology is found in the failure of biological evolution to keep pace with cultural evolution.

We are interested in evaluating that part of the evolutionary problem in obesity that is determined by genetically based differences in the efficiency of energy metabolism. Investigations have shown that alterations in the hormonal state of the animal can cause major changes in the course of obesity (2) and that the genetic background of an animal can alter the characteristics and progression of the obese condition (3, 4); nevertheless, these studies have not led to the identification of genes that are critical in the control of energy efficiency. At present we do not know the biochemical function of any of the genetic mutations that cause obesity in mice. An alternative approach is to use transgenic methods and homologous recombination to alter the expression of genes that might be expected to be important in the control of energy balance. Some of these transgenic studies that encode genes for GLUT4 (5) and the glucocorticoid receptor (6) are described in other conference papers. When these studies are conducted in mice, in which several genetically determined models of obesity are available, it is possible to recombine transgenes with an obese model such as the *db/db* mouse and determine the effects of the transgene on the obese phenotype. In this paper we wish to describe the consequence of alterations in the expression of the *Gdc-1* and the *Ucp* genes on obesity in mice.

Glycerol-3-Phosphate Dehydrogenase

The NAD-linked glycerol-3-phosphate dehydrogenase (EC-1.1.1.8; GPDH) is a cytoplasmic enzyme that catalyzes the reduction of dihydroxyacetone phosphate, a substrate of glycolysis, to form glycerol-3-phosphate. Although it is present in virtually all cells and tissues of the animal, the fact that the highest levels of activity are found in adipocytes (7) and that its appearance during the differentiation of the adipocyte is coincident with the accumulation of triglycerides (8, 9) suggested that the primary function of the enzyme was to provide the substrate for triglyceride and phospholipid synthesis (10). White has also postulated that the function of GPDH in muscle was to remove the reduced NAD that is formed during anaerobic glycolysis (11). The first clue that this view of the function of GPDH was too limited and possibly secondary to its real function came with the discovery of the null mutant for the Gdc-1 gene (12, 13). This null allele, Gdc-1^0, was found as the common allele in the BALB/cHeA strain of mouse. BALB/cHeA mice were normal in their morphological, physiological, and reproductive functions. Most surprising was the lack of any reduction in the weight of fat depots on the animal (Table 1). Furthermore, even though the highest levels of GPDH are normally found in the brown fat in which expression is also induced during exposure to cold, these mice can thermoregulate normally when placed in the cold.

The absence of a phenotype in the Gdc-1 null mouse was very perplexing, given the pivotal location of the enzyme at the interface of carbohydrate and lipid metabolism. In addition, expression of the Gdc-1 gene is controlled by a variety of tissue specific mechanisms that suggested some unique tissue specific functions. Experiments analyzing the regulatory mechanisms controlling the expression of Gdc-1 in

Table 1. Body Weight, Liver Weight, and White Fat Pad Weights in BALB/cByJ and BALB/cHeA Mice

	BALB/cByJ		BALB/cHeA	
	Male n = 8	Female n = 12	Male n = 14	Female n = 12
Body weight (grams)	33.74 ± 0.61	28.19 ± 0.53	32.79 ± 0.58	28.20 ± 0.67
Liver weight (grams)	1.58 ± 0.08	1.20 ± 0.03	1.65 ± 0.08	1.37 ± 0.12
Omental fat pad weight (grams)	0.12 ± 0.01	0.26 ± 0.02	0.09 ± 0.02	0.22 ± 0.04
Retroperitoneal fat pad weight (grams)	0.52 ± 0.06	0.83 ± 0.08	0.39 ± 0.05	0.71 ± 0.09

Data are presented as mean and standard error. Body weight, liver weight, and fat pad weights were not significantly different between strains.

transgenic mice provided our next clues into the function of GPDH (14). We produced transgenic mice with a DNA fragment carrying the complete *Gdc-1* coding sequence. Three separate transgenic lines were produced, each of which carried approximately twenty gene copies. The control of the expression of the transgene in these lines appeared normal in that cell- and tissue-specific expression was essentially indistinguishable from that of nontransgenic mice, as determined by immunohistology. Yet despite this similarity in the pattern of the *Gdc-1* transgene expression, the absolute level of GPDH produced in tissues of the transgenic mice was greatly elevated. Each line produced an exceptionally high level of GPDH protein, with the highest expression found in the brown fat of the A1 line, in which GPDH constituted approximately 60% of the soluble protein of the tissue (Table 2). Very high levels of GPDH were also present in the Bergman glial cells of the cerebellum and the proximal tubule cells of the kidney (Fig. 1). Considering this high level of expression, it was surprising that initially no abnormal phenotype could be detected. As the mice aged to a point at which they should have been accumulating depots of white fat, we noticed a striking lack of white fat in the interscapular region and a clear hypertrophy of the brown fat (Fig. 2A). Further inspection of the mice revealed a generalized reduction in white fat accumulation in both subcutaneous and the peritoneal depots (Fig. 2B). Determinations of the developmental profile of fat depots showed that the increase in

Table 2. GDPH Enzyme Activities in Transgenic Lines

	+ / +	A1	A2	A3
	(μ/mg protein)			
BAT	4.5 ± 1.4	218 ± 33 (48)	76 ± 27	74 ± 28
Liver	0.34 ± 0.16	60 ± 14 (176)	21 ± 8	21 ± 7
Kidney	0.77 ± 0.28	52 ± 12 (67)	26 ± 12	17 ± 2
WAT	0.94 ± 0.28	61 ± 27 (65)	38 ± 22	35 ± 16
Spleen	0.05 ± 0.02	15 ± 4 (300)	4.9 ± 1.1	4.2 ± 0.3
Cerebellum	0.71 ± 0.40	94 ± 20 (134)	34 ± 19	34 ± 5

Data are presented as the mean ± SD of determinations in five animals for each genotype. Data from males and females at ≈7 weeks of age were pooled. Transgenic mice were heterozygous for the transgene complex and homozygous for the *Gdc-1* null allele at the endogenous gene. The control (+/+) mice were the BALB/cByJ inbred strain. Numbers in parentheses refer to the ratio of activity in A1 to +/+ animals.
Reprinted with permission from reference 14.

KIDNEY   CEREBELLUM   TESTIS

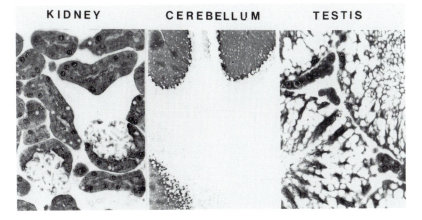

Figure 1.   Immunoperoxidase localization of GPDH in kidney, cerebellum, and testis of the A_1 transgenic. Magnification, 400×. (For the staining procedure and a comparison to normal mouse tissues, see reference 7.) Immunostaining for the GPDH was not detected in tissues from *Gdc-1* null BALB/cHeA mice (data not shown).

brown fat and decrease in white fat were evident during early postnatal development and continued until approximately one year of age when the study was terminated (Table 3). No other abnormality has been detected; the mice breed normally and live up to 30 months of age.

The first insights into the mechanism determining this loss of white fat came from the histological analysis of the hypertrophied brown fat. The brown fat from a transgenic mouse shows a striking resemblance to that of denervated mice or mice maintained at thermoneutrality at which the adipocytes are laden with fat droplets (15), suggesting that the brown fat was thermogenically dormant (Fig. 3). If this interpretation is correct then the level of *Ucp* should also be reduced in the transgenic mice, and this was indeed the case (Fig. 4).

These data suggested that overexpression of GPDH had established a mechanism for burning off excess calories that are normally stored in white fat depots. To further test this idea we crossed the *Gdc-1* transgenic mice to genetically obese *dbm/dbm* mice to produce mice homozygous for the *db* gene and carrying at least one complex of the transgene. The homozygous *db* transgenic mice had a reduction in body weight to levels indistinguishable from the +/+ control mice. This

A   B

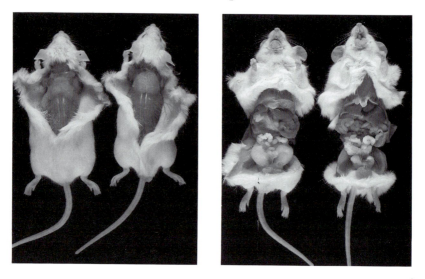

Figure 2. (*A*) Dorsal view of A_1 transgenic mice (*right*) and littermate controls (*left*) illustrating the increase in brown fat size in A_1 transgenic mice. Note also the reduction of subcutaneous fat in A_1 transgenic mice. (*B*) Ventral view shows the reduction in omental and epididymal fat in the peritoneal cavity of A_1 transgenic mice (*right*). (*Left*) Control.

Reprinted with permission from reference 14, copyright 1991 Macmillan Magazines Limited.

occurred even though the transgenic *db/db* mice were as hyperphagic as nontransgenic *db/db* mice. Homozygous *db* mice cannot tolerate cold; however, transgenic *db/db* mice are resistant to cold even though the expression of *Ucp* in the brown fat is barely detectable. These results indicate that the *Gdc-1* transgene is able to establish a mechanism for burning off calories that produces sufficient heat to inactivate the brown fat and yet still protect the animal during exposure to cold.

This physiological effect of the *Gdc-1* gene provides evidence for a thermogenic mechanism that has not heretofore been realized. The major function of GPDH is generally considered to be in lipid metabolism in which it provides the glycerol backbone of triglycerides and phospholipids. The first clue that GPDH may have a different or additional function came from the discovery of the *Gdc-1* null mutant mouse, which shows no deficit in its ability to synthesize and accumulate fat stores. An alternative pathway for the synthesis of glycerol-3-phos-

Table 3. Weights of Interscapular Brown Fat and Parietal (Female) or Epididymal (Male) White Fat in Aging Transgenic Mice and Littermate Controls

Transgenic Line	Age	BAT		WAT	
		Tg/+	+/+	Tg/+	+/+
A1	10[a]	0.076 ± 0.020 (10)	0.044 ± 0.012 (9)*	0.04 ± 0.02 (5)	0.05 ± 0.03 (7)
A1	1.0	0.14 ± 0.03 (5)	0.08 ± 0.02 (7)*	not detected (5)	0.24 ± 0.10 (3)
A1	1.5	0.20 ± 0.03 (5)	0.13 ± 0.02 (3)*	0.13 ± 0.10 (3)	0.26 ± 0.10 (3)*
A3	2.0	0.27 ± 0.03 (3)	0.12 ± 0.04 (3)*	0.07 ± 0.08 (3)	0.48 ± 0.26 (3)*
A1	5.0	0.28 ± 0.03 (3)	0.10 ± 0.02 (3)*	0.18 ± 0.04 (5)	0.30 ± 0.06 (4)*
A2	5.0	0.16 ± 0.03 (5)	0.11 ± 0.01 (4)*	0.10 ± 0.09 (3)	3.00 ± 1.53 (2)*
A1	8.5	0.43 ± 0.17 (3)	0.26 ± 0.13 (2)	0.19 ± 0.09 (4)	1.15 ± 0.94 (4)*
A3	8.5	0.40 ± 0.13 (4)	0.09 ± 0.03 (4)*	0.13 ± 0.16 (4)	2.08 ± 0.54 (5)*
A1	10.5	0.58 ± 0.09 (4)	0.14 ± 0.04 (5)*		

The data are presented as the mean ± of the wet weights in grams. The number of animals of each genotype in a litter is indicated in parentheses.
*Statistically significant differences between genotypes ($P < 0.05$), determined by Student's t test.
[a] Comparisons at each age (months) were made with transgenic (Tg/+) and nontransgenic (+/+) animals within a litter except for the 10-day mice, which came from two separate litters.

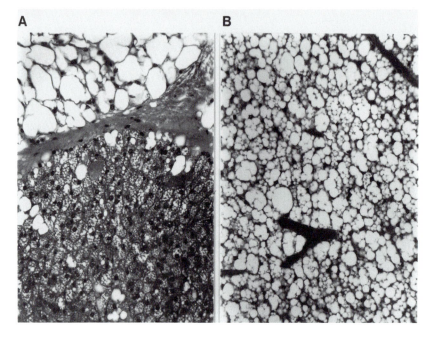

Figure 3. Comparison of the morphology of brown fat from a normal mouse (*A*) with that from a transgenic mouse (*B*). Tissues were fixed in Bouin's fixative and embedded in paraffin, and sections were stained with hematoxylin and eosin. Magnification, 150×.

Reprinted with permission from reference 14, copyright 1991 Macmillan Magazines Limited.

phate from dihyroxyacetone phosphate by the direct acylation of the latter by glycerol phosphate acyltransferase is capable of providing the substrate for lipid synthesis (16). The effects of overexpression of *Gdc-1* on energy balance and thermogenesis suggest that an important function for *Gdc-1* is in regulating energy balance. Glycerol-3-phosphate dehydrogenase is located at the interface of carbohydrate and lipid metabolism, where it converts dihydroxyacetone phosphate to glycerol-3-phosphate. It is also at the interface of cytoplasm and the mitochondria, where it can function to shuttle reducing equivalents generated by active glycolysis into the mitochondria, since glycerol-3-phosphate is permeable to the mitochondria but NADH is not. The subsequent transfer of electrons to the respiratory chain by the mitochondrial glycerol-3-phosphate oxidase completes the shuttle mechanism (17). Lardy has previously postulated that this shuttle mechanism

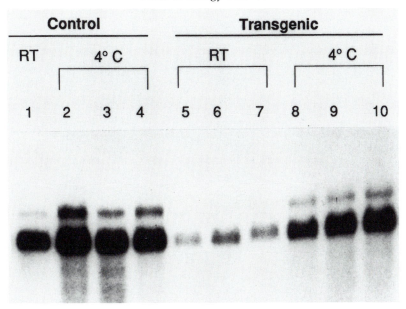

| Control | | | | | Transgenic | | | | |

Figure 4. Northern blot illustrating reduced levels of *Ucp* mRNA in the brown fat of A_1 transgenic mice maintained at room temperature and induction of *Ucp* mRNA when mice are placed in the cold (4°C). Each lane contained 5μg of total RNA.

Reprinted with permission from reference 14, copyright 1991 Macmillan Magazines Limited.

could provide a thermogenic mechanism that could be important in the control of obesity (18). It may also contribute to the increased thermogenesis of the *Gdc-1* transgenic mice; however, since the mitochondrial glycerol-3-phosphate oxidase would be rate limiting, additional mechanisms of thermogenesis are required.

Figure 5 provides a view of the known pathways associated with the synthesis and degradation of glycerol phosphate. Note that a fourth pathway in which glycerol-3-phosphate can be hydrolyzed to glycerol and inorganic phosphate has been described in yeast under nutrient conditions that lead to the accumulation of triose phosphate and NADH (19). The function of the phosphatase would be to limit the accumulation of glycerol phosphate, a tendency that would be extremely strong in the *Gdc-1* transgenic mice as a result of the high levels of GPDH. If a glycerol-3-phosphatase was active in some tissues of the mouse, it would establish a futile cycle in which high energy phosphate

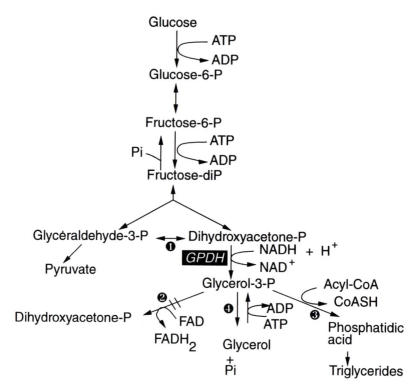

Figure 5. Metabolic pathways associated with the synthesis and degradation of glycerol phosphate.

from adenosine triphosphate (ATP) was transferred to glycerol phosphate via hexokinase and phosphofructokinase steps of glycolysis and GPDH and dephosphorylation by the phosphatase completed the cycle. Additional futile ATP cycles involving the turnover of triglycerides has also been postulated (20). Given the pivotal location of GPDH in energy metabolism, several thermogenic mechanisms could participate in the thermogenic phenotype generated by its overexpression.

The *Gdc-1* transgenic mouse provides compelling evidence for the importance of thermogenic mechanisms based on simple enzymes of carbohydrate metabolism to control obesity in animals, even in animal models such as the *db/db* mouse in which the primary defect may lie in a feeding disorder controlled by the central nervous system (21). To further establish the importance of metabolic thermogenic mechanisms to control obesity, we are attempting to manipulate energy efficiency and obesity through the altered genetic expression of the mitochondrial uncoupling protein. Since the only known function of the uncoupling protein is to produce heat, interpretation of the results may be more direct than that of GPDH overexpression, in which alterations of metabolite levels may have additional effects.

The Mitochondrial Uncoupling Protein

The function of the mitochondrial uncoupling protein (UCP) as the critical component in brown fat nonshivering thermogenesis (22) suggested that the manipulation of *Ucp* expression could alter the overall energy balance in an animal and, correspondingly, the degree of obesity. Reductions in *Ucp*-derived thermogenesis would contribute to the obese state of the animal, whereas increases in *Ucp* expression would reduce the amount of body fat in an animal. To reduce the amount of brown fat–derived thermogenesis we constructed a transgenic mouse carrying the diphtheria toxin gene under control of the *Ucp* gene regulatory region (23). Since any cell in which diphtheria toxin is produced should be killed, a transgene in which the expression of the diphtheria toxin gene is regulated by the *Ucp* promoter should destroy the brown fat. As predicted, these animal are obese (24).

In a second experiment to use the *Ucp* gene to alter energy balance, we constructed a transgene in which the *Ucp* coding sequence was regulated by the *aP2* promoter (25). Since this promoter is specific for both white fat and brown fat, it is possible to express the *Ucp* gene in white fat as well as brown fat. In addition, the *aP2* gene is constitutively expressed in fat so that the *Ucp* transgene will be expressed independent of the need for nonshivering thermogenesis. The initial analysis of the *aP2-Ucp* transgenic mouse showed that on a normal C57BL/6J background the total body weights of the mice were indistinguishable from nontransgenic littermate controls (manuscript in preparation). By immunoblot analysis UCP was expressed in both subcutaneous and peritoneal white fat depots of transgenic mice at about 10% the level that is found in brown fat. No UCP was found in the white fat depots of the nontransgenic mice. Surprisingly, there was no difference in the amount of UCP detected in the brown fat of transgenic and nontransgenic mice.

In order to increase our ability to detect an effect of the *aP2-Ucp* transgene on energy balance, it was recombined with the A^{vy} gene, a gene which among its several pleiotropic effects in the mouse also causes obesity (26). This genetic combination resulted in approximately a 25% reduction of body weight at six months of age (Table 4). Examination of the mice also showed that a redistribution of fat depots occurred with a depletion of subcutaneous fat depots and an increase in gonadal fat depots. This finding of fat redistribution in the A^{vy} transgenic mice led us to reexamine the *aP2-Ucp* transgenic mice on the normal C57BL/6J background. Similar to the A^{vy} mice, a major redistribution of fat occurred whereby subcutaneous depots were drastically reduced and gonadal fat increased; however, on the normal C57BL/6J background, the *aP2-Ucp* transgenic and nontransgenic mice did not differ in their total body weight. These changes in fat deposition in the transgenic mice were strong in female mice but weak in the males. No reductions in the amount of interscapular brown fat could be detected.

Conclusion

Two novel mechanisms for increasing thermogenesis have been introduced into mice by transgenic techniques. The first mechanism based on the overexpression of the *Gdc-1* gene was an unexpected finding and will be discussed below. The second mechanism, based upon the ectopic expression of *Ucp* in white fat, was achieved by design. At present we have not quantified the degree of heat that each system generates. If, however, the reduction in fat content of an A^{vy} mouse is used as an estimator, the GPDH system is burning off many more calories than the UCP system. The strength of the GPDH could be due to the higher number of transgene copies and the broad expression of the

Table 4. Effects of Transgenes on Body Weight of A^{vy} Mice

Group	Count	Mean	Std. Dev.
A^{vy}-Ucp	9	40.0	5.1
A^{vy} control	10	48.5	6.1
A^{vy}-Gdc	4	33.6	3.4
A^{vy} control	5	49.7	4.0

A^{vy}-Ucp mice carry the A^{vy} gene at the agouti locus and the *aP2-Ucp* transgene; the A^{vy} control mice are nontransgenic littermates. A^{vy}-Gdc mice carry the A^{vy} gene and the *Gdc* transgene. The groups of mice carried both males and females approximately six months of age. The A^{vy}-Ucp and A^{vy}-Gdc-1 mice were significantly different from their controls.

Gdc-1 gene to all tissues of the animal. The GPDH system seems to reduce white fat stores in a uniform manner; that is, it acts on both subcutaneous and peritoneal fat depots. In contrast, ectopic expression of *Ucp* in nonobese animals seems to redistribute the fat depots without reductions in total lipid stores; in genetically obese mice reductions in total fat depots were detected. Since the type of regional distribution of fat in human obesity is important with regard to human susceptibility to heart disease and diabetes, the *aP2-Ucp* transgenic mouse could provide a model system to investigate mechanisms that cause differences in regional fat distribution.

ACKNOWLEDGMENTS

The research described in this paper was supported by grants from the National Institutes of Health and the Pfizer Corporation. The Jackson Laboratory is fully accredited by the American Association of Laboratory Animal Care.

REFERENCES

1. Neel JV. Diabetes mellitus: a "thrifty" genotype rendered detrimental by "progress." *Am J Hum Genet.* 1962;14:353–362.
2. Shimomura Y, Bray GA, Lee M. Adrenalectomy and steroid treat in obese (*ob/ob*) and diabetic (*db/db*) mice. *Horm Metab Res.* 1987;19:295–299.
3. Coleman DL, Hummel KP. The influence of genetic background on the expression of the obese (*ob*) gene in the mouse. *Diabetologia.* 1973;9:287–293.
4. Hummel K, Coleman DL, Lane PW. The influence of genetic background on the expression of mutations at the diabetes locus in the mouse: C57B1/KsJ and C57B1/6J strains. *Biochem Genet.* 1972;7:1–13.
5. Shepherd PR, Gnudi L, Tozzo E, Yang H, Leach F, Kahn BB. Adipose cell hyperplasia and enhanced glucose disposal in transgenic mice overexpressing GLUT4 selectively in adipose tissue. *J Biol Chem.* 1993;268:22243–22246.
6. Pepin M-C, Pothier F, Barden N. Impaired type II glucocorticoid receptor function in mice bearing antisense RNA transgene. *Nature.* 1992;355:725–728.

7. Ratner PL, Fisher M, Burkart D, Cook JR, Kozak LP. The role of mRNA levels and cellular localization in control of sn-glycerol-3-phosphate dehydrogenase expression in tissues of the mouse. *J Biol Chem.* 1981;256:3576–3579.

8. Cook JR, Kozak LP. sn-Glycerol-3-phosphate dehydrogenase gene expression during mouse adipocyte development in vivo. *Dev Biol.* 1982;92:440–448.

9. Wise LS, Greene H. Participation of one isozyme of cytosolic glycerophosphate dehydrogenase in adipose conversion of 3T3 cells. *J Biol Chem.* 1979;254:273–275.

10. Kornberg A, Pricer WE. Enzymatic esterification of ∂-Glycerophosphate by long chain fatty acids. *J Biol Chem.* 1953;204:345–357.

11. White HB, Kaplan NO. Separate physiological roles for two isozymes of pyridine nucleotide-linked glycerol-3-phosphate dehydrogenase in chicken. *J Mol Evol.* 1972;1:158–172.

12. Hilgers J, van Nie R, Ivanyi D, *et al.* Genetic differences in BALB/c sublines. *Current Topics in Microbiology.*

13. Prochazka M, Kozak UC, Kozak LP. A glycerol-3-phosphate dehydrogenase null mutant in BALB/cHeA mice. *J Biol Chem.* 1989;264:4679–4683.

14. Kozak LP, Kozak UC, Clarke GT. Abnormal brown and white fat development in transgenic mice overexpressing glycerol 3-phosphate dehydrogenase. *Genes Dev.* 1991;5:2256–2264.

15. Sidman RL, Fawcett DW. The effect of peripheral nerve sections on some metabolic responses of brown adipose tissue in mice. *Anat Rec.* 1954;118:487–507.

16. Hajra AK, Agrnaoff B. Reduction of palmitoyl dihydroxyacetone phosphate by mitochondria. *J Biol Chem.* 1968;243:3542–3543.

17. Estabrook RW, Sacktor B. Alpha-glycerophosphate oxidase of flight muscle mitochondria. *J Biol Chem.* 1958;233:1014–1019.

18. Lardy H, Su CY, Kneer N, Wielgus S. Dehydroepiandosterone induces enzymes that permit thermogenesis and decrease metabolic efficiency. In: Lardy H, Stratman, eds. *Hormones, Thermogenesis, and Obesity.* New York: Elsevier, 1989.

19. Gancedo C, Gancedo JM, Sols A. Glycerol metabolism in yeasts. *Eur J Biochem.* 1968;5:165–172.

20. Newsholme EA, Stanley JC. Substrate cycles: their role in control of metabolism with specific references to liver. *Diabetes Metab Rev.* 1987;3:295–305.

21. Coleman DL. Effects of parabiosis of obese with diabetes and normal mice. *Diabetologia.* 1973;9:294–298.
22. Nicholls DG, Locke RM. Thermogenic mechanisms in brown fat. *Physiol Rev.* 1984;64:1–64.
23. Boyer BB, Kozak LP. The mitochondrial uncoupling protein gene in brown fat: correlation between DNAse hypersensitivity and expression in transgenic mice. *Mol Cell Biol.* 1991;11:4747–4756.
24. Lowell BB, S-Susulic V, Hamann A, *et al.* Development of morbid obesity in transgenic mice following the genetic ablation of brown adipose tissue. *Nature.* 1993;366:740–742.
25. Ross SR, Graves RA, Greenstein A, *et al.* A fat-specific enhancer is the primary determinant of gene expression for adipocyte P2 *in vivo. Proc Natl Acad Sci USA.* 1990;87:9590–9594.
26. Wolff GL, Roberts DW, Galbraith DB. Prenatal determination of obesity, tumor susceptibility, and coat color pattern in viable yellow (*Avy/a*) mice: the yellow mouse syndrome. *J Hered.* 1986;77:151–158.

LUIGI GNUDI, PETER R. SHEPHERD,
EFFIE TOZZO, and BARBARA B. KAHN

Selective Overexpression in Adipose Cells in Transgenic Mice of GLUT4: The Major Insulin Regulatable Glucose Transporter

ABSTRACT

To investigate the potential role of the GLUT4 glucose transporter in the pathogenesis of obesity and in in vivo glucose homeostasis, we developed a transgenic model in which we overexpressed the major insulin-regulatable glucose transporter specifically in white and brown adipose tissue. The adipose specific transgene was generated by ligating the human GLUT4 genomic sequence with the promoter-enhancer element of the fatty acid binding protein gene, *aP2*. Two lines of transgenic mice were created that overexpress GLUT4 six- to ninefold in white adipose tissue and three- to fivefold in brown adipose tissue.

Transgenic mice showed increased glucose tolerance and lower fed insulin levels. In isolated adipocytes of transgenic mice from different fat depots (perigonadal, subcutaneous, and perirenal), basal glucose transport was twenty to thirty times greater and insulin-stimulated transport was two to four times greater than in cells from nontransgenic mice. Body lipid content was increased approximately threefold in transgenic mice versus nontransgenic mice of both sexes, and at different ages. Cell size was unaltered, but fat cell number was increased about twofold in transgenic versus nontransgenic mice. The adipose cell hyperplasia and enhanced glucose disposal with lower plasma insulin levels in transgenic mice is a unique model that dissociates obesity from insulin resistance.

Glucose transport in mammalian tissues occurs by facilitated diffusion mediated by specific glucose transporter proteins (1–3). Six genes have been cloned that encode for distinct transporter proteins, which facilitate diffusion of sugars (glucose or fructose) across the cell membrane. GLUT4 is the major insulin-regulated glucose transporter and has a unique tissue distribution with expression almost exclusively in muscle and fat (1).

Insulin-resistant states such as obesity and diabetes are characterized by a reduction in glucose uptake in muscle and fat (4). In both humans and rodents these states are associated with markedly altered expression of GLUT4 in adipocytes (1, 5–7) but not in skeletal muscle (8–10). Instead, the insulin resistance in muscle appears to result from impaired function of GLUT4 (1, 8).

Muscle is responsible for 80% of the insulin-mediated glucose disposal in vivo, and relatively little glucose is taken up by adipose tissue (11). Thus, the physiological impact of GLUT4 regulation in fat in insulin-resistant states needs to be elucidated. Specifically, the concept that increased partitioning of nutrients to fat may play a role in the development of obesity deserves investigation.

Evidence for this pathogenic phenomenon comes from longitudinal studies in the genetically obese Zucker rat (12). Obesity in Zucker rats is associated with early overexpression of GLUT4 in adipose tissue of rats at 5 to 10 weeks age. As obesity and hyperinsulinemia progress, expression of GLUT4 in adipocytes is suppressed, so that at 20 weeks of age GLUT4 levels in adipose cells of obese rats are 50% lower than in lean littermates (Fig. 1). Thus, increased glucose uptake into fat as a result of overexpression of GLUT4 may contribute to the development of obesity in these rats and in other obese models (13). After obesity has been present for a period of time, down-regulation of GLUT4 expression may represent an adaptation to limit further progression of the obese state.

In these obese Zucker rats GLUT4 expression in skeletal muscle (14) is not subject to regulation during the development of obesity (Fig. 2). This suggests that in the obesity found in the Zucker rat, tissue-specific regulation of GLUT4 may alter nutrient partitioning, favoring the development of the obese state.

To see whether increased expression of GLUT4 selectively in fat can modulate glucose disposal in vivo, and whether increased glucose transport into adipose cells can alter nutrient partitioning so as to cause obesity, we developed transgenic mice that overexpress GLUT4 selectively in adipose cells. Transgenic mice were generated by ligating the

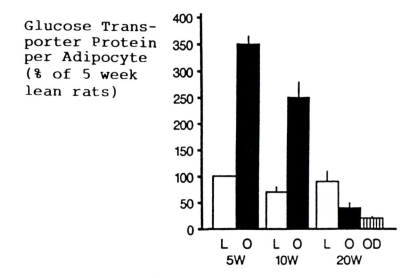

Figure 1. GLUT4 protein levels in epididymal adipose cells of lean (L) and obese (O) Zucker rats at 5, 10, and 20 weeks of age. Values represent densitometry performed on Western blots and are expressed as percent of values in 5-week-old lean Zucker rats. Also shown are GLUT4 levels in acutely streptozotocin-induced diabetic/obese (OD) Zucker rats at 20 weeks of age.

fat-specific promoter enhancer from the fatty acid binding protein gene *aP2* (15), to 6.3 kb of the genomic sequence of the human GLUT4 gene (16) containing all 11 exons and 10 introns and the consensus polyadenylation signal. The construct maintains the consensus transcription initiation site in the promoter/enhancer, and the ATG translation initiation codon in the GLUT4 gene (Fig. 3).

This DNA construct was injected into the pronucleus of fertilized mouse ova followed by reimplantation into pseudopregnant female mice (17, 18). Forty-two offspring were analyzed, and seven of these had the transgene incorporated in their genomic DNA. Two of these overexpressed the GLUT4 protein at high levels selectively in fat.

Northern blotting of total RNA from adipose tissue revealed two distinct transcripts in transgenic mice: the endogenous GLUT4 mRNA at 2.7 kb and the human GLUT4 transcript (transgene) at 3.5 kb. The human GLUT4 message was not detectable in nontransgenic mice. Western blotting for the GLUT4 protein revealed that GLUT4 was overexpressed six- to ninefold in white fat and three- to fivefold in brown

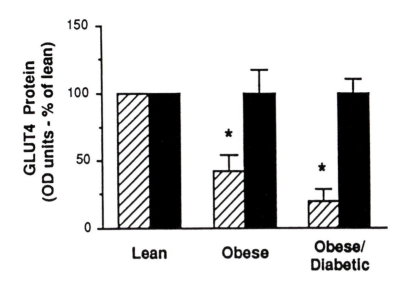

Figure 2. GLUT4 protein levels in skeletal muscle (■) and adipose cells (▨) in 20-week-old lean, obese, and acutely streptozotocin-induced diabetic/obese (OD) Zucker rats. GLUT4 was determined by Western blotting.

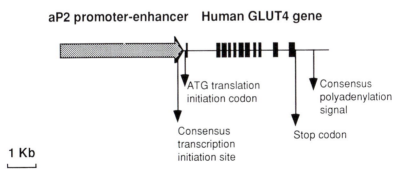

Figure 3. Schematic representation of the transgene construct. 5.4 kb of mouse genomic DNA containing the mouse aP2 fatty acid binding protein promoter and enhancer elements (15) was fused to 6.3 kb of human genomic DNA (16) containing all 11 exons of the human GLUT4 gene.

fat with no overexpression in skeletal muscle, heart, liver, brain, or kidney (19) (Fig. 4).

To determine the effect of GLUT4 overexpression in adipose cells on in vivo glucose disposal we performed intraperitoneal glucose tolerance tests. All mice were matched for sex and age; in fact, all studies

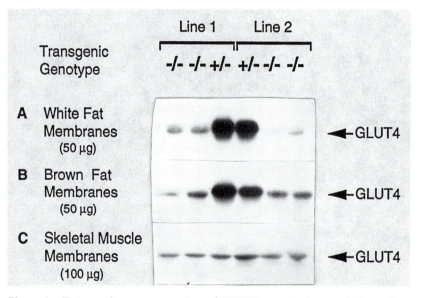

Figure 4. Fat-specific overexpression of GLUT4 protein in two independent lines (#1 and #2) of transgenic FVB mice. Fat and muscle membranes from mice heterozygous for the transgene ($+/-$) or nontransgenic littermates ($-/-$) were prepared, and SDS-PAGE and immunoblotting for GLUT4 were performed. Micrograms of protein loaded in each lane are indicated on the figure.

Figure 5. Glucose tolerance test in transgenic mice heterozygous for the transgene and in nontransgenic littermates. After an overnight fast, D-glucose (1 mg/g body weight) was injected intraperitoneally in awake mice, and blood glucose was determined on samples from the tail vein. Data shown in each panel represent 2 to 3 mice per group and are representative of results in a total of 17 nontransgenic and 20 transgenic mice, comprising seven sets of littermates ranging in age from 7 to 11 weeks. Values are expressed as $\bar{x} \pm$ SEM.

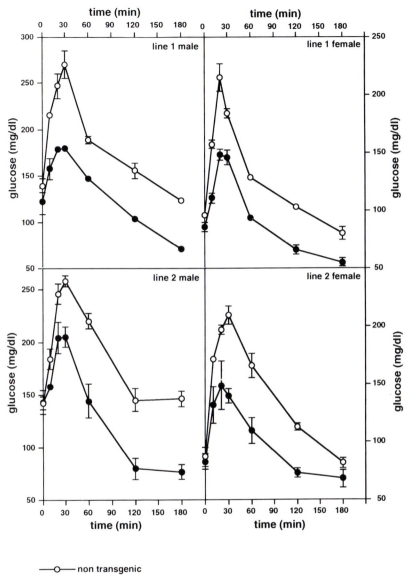

line 1 male

line 1 female

line 2 male

line 2 female

—○— non transgenic
—●— transgenic

values are expressed as $\bar{x} \pm$ SEM

were carried out in littermates for both transgenic lines. D-glucose (20%, 1 mg/g body weight) (20) was injected intraperitoneally in awake mice that had been fasted overnight. Blood glucose was measured at time 0 and 10, 20, 30, 60, 120, and 180 minutes after glucose injection (Fig. 5). In one transgenic line, fasting glucose was lower than in controls. Transgenic mice from both lines had a markedly blunted response curve to glucose administration compared with nontransgenic littermates, indicating increased glucose tolerance. At 30 minutes after intraperitoneal glucose injection the blood glucose levels were significantly lower in transgenic mice. The plasma insulin levels at the same time also showed a tendency to be reduced in transgenic animals. Confirming this tendency, insulin levels in fed animals were significantly reduced by 40% in both male and female transgenic mice versus nontransgenic mice. The increased insulin-mediated glucose disposal observed in transgenic mice (with similar or lower insulin concentrations) indicates that these mice are more sensitive to insulin.

To better understand the phenotype obtained with the overexpression of GLUT4 in fat, we then studied the fat cell itself in in vitro studies. Glucose transport into fat cells was performed at a glucose concentration of 3 µmol, a concentration low enough that transport is rate limiting for glucose metabolism. In cells from GLUT4 overexpressing mice, basal glucose transport was 20- to 30-fold greater than the basal transport in cells of nontransgenic mice, and approximately 1.5-fold greater than the maximal insulin effect obtained with the nontransgenic cells (Fig. 6). At 80 nmol insulin concentration, glucose transport into the transgenic fat cell was 4-fold greater than into fat cells from nontransgenic mice.

To analyze whether the massive flux of glucose into the fat cell would preferentially direct nutrients into fat and result in obesity, growth rate and body composition were evaluated. Growth curves showed no difference in weight between nontransgenic and transgenic mice until 5 to 6 weeks of age. Then the transgenics gained weight more rapidly. This difference in weight (3–4 grams, about a 10% increase of body weight) between nontransgenic and transgenic mice was evident in both sexes and both transgenic lines.

The increase in body weight observed in the transgenic mice is entirely due to an increase in body lipid. Transgenic mice were 15% lipid, versus 5% lipid in nontransgenic mice. This obese phenotype (Fig. 7) was confirmed in both transgenic lines and in both males and females.

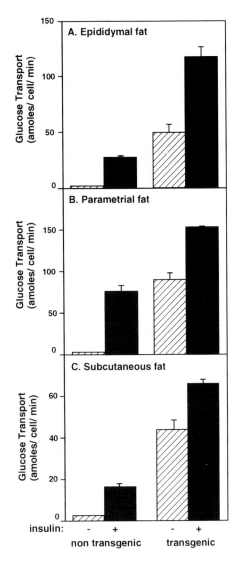

Figure 6. Glucose transport in isolated adipocytes from mice heterozygous for the transgene and nontransgenic littermates. *A*) Epididymal adipose cells from 19.5-week-old line #1 male mice. *B*) Parametrial adipose cells from 10-week-old line #2 female mice. *C*) Subcutaneous adipose cells from 12-week-old line #2 male mice. Each experiment was carried out on pooled cells from 2 to 3 littermates per group. Results are means ±SEM and are representative of 6 separate glucose transport experiments.

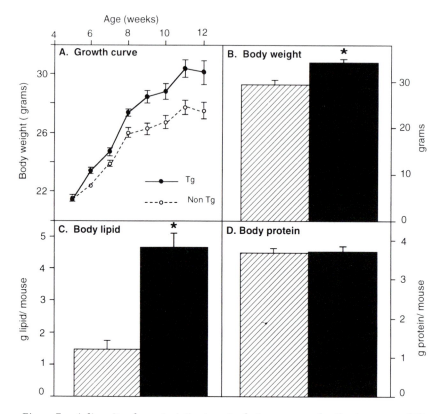

Figure 7. Adiposity characteristics in mice heterozygous for the transgene (■) and nontransgenic (▨) littermates. *A*) Representative growth curves in line #1 male mice from 5 to 12 weeks of age. Weights are the same in transgenic and nontransgenic littermates up to 5 weeks of age. *B*) Body weight in male mice from 18 to 21 weeks of age. *C*) Total body lipid in male mice 18 to 21 weeks of age. *D*) Total body protein in male mice 18 to 21 weeks of age. Results shown in panels *B, C,* and *D* are for combined lines #1 and #2 male mice (n = 6–8 in each group). Similar results were obtained for female mice from both lines #1 and #2 ranging in age from 9 to 26 weeks. Results are mean ± SEM. *$P < 0.02$.

Reproduced, with permission, from reference 19. Copyright © The American Society for Biochemistry and Molecular Biology.

To determine if the increase in fat percentage was due to an increase in cell size, cell number, or a combination of the two, we measured cell size in different fat depots. There was no difference in fat cell size expressed as micrograms of lipid per cell between nontransgenic and transgenic mice in perigonadal (epididymal and perimetrial), perirenal,

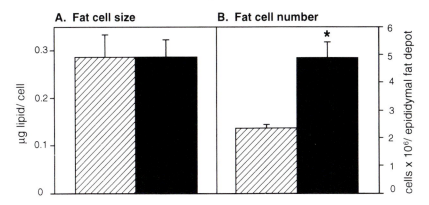

Figure 8. Adipocyte size and number for mice heterozygous for the transgene (■) and nontransgenic (▨) littermates. Adipocyte number was determined by osmic acid fixation and counting in a Coulter Counter. Adipocyte size was calculated by dividing the milligram of lipid in an aliquot of isolated cells by the number of cells in the same aliquot. Adipocyte number per fat depot was calculated by dividing the milligram of lipid per depot by the microgram of lipid per cell. Results are means ±SEM for 6 to 10 mice per group. *A)* Epididymal fat cell size. *B)* Number of fat cells per epididymal fat depot. *$P < 0.005$.

omental, or subcutaneus fat depots. The estimated number of fat cells was increased approximately twofold in the epididymal depot (Fig. 8).

In summary, overexpression of GLUT4 selectively in fat results in increased whole-body glucose disposal and increased adiposity that results primarily from increased fat cell number with no change in fat cell size. Thus, the GLUT4 glucose transporter is a major determinant of glucose homeostasis in vivo. Overexpression of GLUT4 in fat without any other manipulation of insulin signaling or cellular metabolism enhances glucose tolerance. Furthermore, overexpression of GLUT4 in fat alters nutrient partitioning so as to cause obesity. The increased flux of glucose into the fat cell appears to foster the replication of immature adipocytes and/or their differentiation into mature adipocytes.

REFERENCES

1. Kahn BB. Facilitative glucose transporters: regulatory mechanisms and dysregulation in diabetes. *J Clin Invest.* 1992;89:1367–1374.

2. Pessin J, Bell G. Mammalian facilitative glucose transporter family: structure and molecular regulation. *Annu Rev Physiol.* 1992;54:911–930.

3. Burant C, Sivitz W, Fukumoto H, *et al.* Mammalian glucose transporters: structure and molecular regulation. *Recent Prog Horm Res.* 1991;47:349–388.

4. Olefsky JM, Kolterman OG, Scarlett JA. Insulin action and resistance in obesity and non insulin dependent type II diabetes mellitus. *Am J Physiol.* 1982;243:E15–E30.

5. Garvey WT, Maianu L, Huecksteadt TP, Birnbaum MJ, Molina JM, Ciaraldi TP. Pretranslational suppression of a glucose transporter protein causes insulin resistance in adipocytes from patient with non-insulin-dependent diabetes mellitus and obesity. *J Clin Invest.* 1991;87:1072–1081.

6. Garvey WT, Huecksteadt TP, Birnbaum MJ. Pretranslational suppression of an insulin-responsive glucose transporter in rats with diabetes mellitus. *Science.* 1989;245:60–63.

7. Kahn BB, Charron MJ, Lodish HF, Cushman SW, Flier JS. Differential regulation of two glucose transporters in adipose cells from diabetic and insulin-treated diabetic rats. *J Clin Invest.* 1989;84:404–411.

8. Kahn BB, Rossetti L, Lodish HF, Charron MJ. Decreased in vivo glucose uptake but normal expression of GLUT1 and GLUT4 in skeletal muscle of diabetic rats. *J Clin Invest.* 1991;87:2197–2206.

9. Pedersen O, Bak JF, Andersen PH, *et al.* Evidence against altered expression of GLUT1 or GLUT4 in skeletal muscle of patients with obesity or NIDDM. *Diabetes.* 1990;39:865–870.

10. Kahn BB, Rosen AS, Bak JS, *et al.* Expression of GLUT1 and GLUT4 glucose transporters in skeletal muscle of humans with insulin dependent diabetes mellitus: regulatory effects of metabolic factors. *J Clin Endocrin Metabol.* 1992;74:1101–1109.

11. DeFronzo RA. The triumvirate: beta cell, muscle, liver. *Diabetes.* 1988;37:667–687.

12. Pedersen O, Kahn CR, Kahn BB. Divergent regulation of the GLUT1 and GLUT4 glucose transporters in isolated adipocytes from Zucker rats. *J Clin Invest.* 1992;89:1964–1973.

13. Cousin B, Agou K, Leturque A, Ferre P, Girard J, Penicaud L. Molecular and metabolic changes in white adipose tissue of the rat

during development of ventromedial hypothalamic obesity. *Eur J Biochem.* 1992;207:377–382.

14. Kahn BB, Pedersen O. Suppression of GLUT4 expression in skeletal muscle of rats that are obese from high-fat feeding but not from high-carbohydrate feeding or genetic obesity. *Endocrinology.* 1992; 132:13–22.

15. Ross SR, Graves RA, Greenstein A, *et al.* A fat-specific enhancer is the primary determinant of a gene expression for adipocyte P2 in vivo. *Proc Natl Acad Sci USA.* 1990;87:9590–9594.

16. Buse JB, Yasuda K, Lay TP, *et al.* Human GLUT4 muscle/fat glucose transporter gene: sequence, promoter characterization and genetic variations. *Diabetes.* 1992;41:1436–1446.

17. Merlino GT. Transgenic animals in biomedical research. *FASEB J.* 1991;5:2996–3001.

18. Koretsky AP. Investigation of cell physiology in the animal using transgenic technology. *Am J Physiol.* 1992;262 (2P + 1):C261–C275.

19. Shepherd PR, Gnudi L, Tozzo E, Yang H, Leach F, Kahn BB. Adipose cell hyperplasia and enhanced glucose disposal in transgenic mice overexpressing GLUT4 selectively in adipose tissue. *J Biol Chem.* 1993;268:22243–22246.

20. Kaku K, Fiedorek FT, Province M, Permutt MA. Genetic analysis of glucose tolerance in inbred mouse strains. *Diabetes.* 1988;37:707–713.

NICOLAS BARDEN

Transgenic Mice Expressing Glucocorticoid Receptor Antisense RNA: A Model for Exploring the Role of Glucocorticoids in Obesity

ABSTRACT

The introduction of genes into the germ line of mice offers the possibility to generate precise animal models for human genetic disease. By use of an appropriate promoter, this approach can have the advantage of affecting the expression of a specific gene in a single tissue and at a certain time in development. Through interaction with a cellular receptor, corticosteroid hormones govern a large range of metabolic processes affecting development, physiological homeostasis, and behavioral patterns. Using a fragment of type II glucocorticoid receptor cDNA coupled, in a reverse orientation to produce antisense RNA, to a human neurofilament gene promoter element, we have been able to produce transgenic mice that have a reduced glucocorticoid binding capacity in the brain. Hyperactivity of the hypothalamic-pituitary-adrenal axis, demonstrated by elevated early morning plasma corticosterone and adrenocorticotrophic hormone levels, a flattening of the circadian rhythm of corticosteroid secretion, and a resistance to suppression of corticotrope activity by exogenous corticosteroids are consequences of this reduction in glucocorticoid receptors. Although at birth these transgenic mice do not differ in weight from normal controls, they become markedly obese in late life. This weight gain can be reversed by administration of drugs that increase glucocorticoid receptor gene expression and subsequently normalize components of the hypothalamic-pituitary-adrenal axis. Since a reduction in glucocorticoid receptors precedes elevation of hormone levels in these animals, they may be useful in elucidating the role that glucocorticoid hormones play in the etiology of obesity.

636

Introduction

Glucocorticoid hormones govern a large range of metabolic processes that can affect both development and physiological homeostasis. They regulate cell growth and differentiation, modify neuronal and peripheral metabolism, and may influence feeding and behavioral patterns (1). A role for glucocorticoids in the development of obesity caused by different etiologies also has often been noted (2–4). Their mechanism of action in this process remains unclear but may be related to modulation of both feeding behavior (5, 6) and metabolism (7).

In order to exert their biological actions, corticosteroids must first bind to a cellular receptor. Corticosterone, the major adrenal corticosteroid found in rodents, can bind to two different types of receptors. Although the type II, or glucocorticoid receptor, is widespread throughout the brain, pituitary gland, and peripheral tissues, the type I, or mineralocorticoid receptor, has a much more restricted distribution and, in the central nervous system, is localized to the hippocampus, septum, amygdala, and brain stem nuclei. Both types of receptor have been purified (8, 9), the cDNAs for rat, mouse, and human receptors have been cloned (10–13), and their functional domains have been characterized (14). Although adrenal steroids have a well-known negative feedback effect on the hypothalamic-pituitary-adrenal (HPA) axis that leads to suppression of glucocorticoid secretion, their precise site of action remains controversial (15). One means of studying the physiological role of corticosteroid receptors and, subsequently, glucocorticoids in obesity would be the reduction of glucocorticoid receptor concentrations provoked by formation of glucocorticoid receptor antisense RNA in brain tissues.

Antisense RNA can prevent the normal expression of several different gene products in both cell cultures and intact mice (16–19). When expressed in the nucleus, antisense RNA is believed to form a double-stranded complex with the endogenous mRNA precursor, and once this hybrid molecule is formed it is rapidly degraded by nucleases-specific for double-stranded regions. By use of an appropriate promoter, antisense RNA formation can be directed to specific cell types, and this approach can affect the expression of a specific gene in a single tissue and at a certain time in development. Introduction into the germ line of mice of transgenes that generate antisense RNA molecules thus offers the possibility to generate precise animal models for investigation of the normal physiological role of defined proteins as well as for human disease states.

We have previously constructed an antisense RNA, complementary to the 3' noncoding region of the glucocorticoid receptor mRNA and have shown its efficacy in decreasing functional glucocorticoid receptor levels in cells maintained in culture (20). Incorporation of this antisense RNA–generating construct in transgenic animals offers possibilities for elucidating the role of the glucocorticoid receptor in HPA axis regulation.

Antisense RNA Generation

Glucocorticoid receptor antisense RNA was transcribed from 1815 base pairs (bp) of the 3' noncoding region of the rat glucocorticoid receptor cDNA inverted downstream from a human neurofilament (NF-L) gene promoter element (Fig. 1). The 3' noncoding region of the glucocorticoid receptor mRNA, which contains the least degree of homology with other members of the steroid hormone superfamily of genes, was used to avoid cross-inhibition of other receptor activity.

Specificity of Corticosteroid Receptor Antisense RNA Action

When cotransfected with a glucocorticoid responsive reporter plasmid (MMTV-CAT) into leukocyte tyrosine kinase (LTK)–cells, the glucocorticoid receptor antisense RNA construct (pNFLAsGR) efficiently reduced functional glucocorticoid receptor levels (Fig. 2). Stable transfectants bearing the same glucocorticoid receptor antisense gene fragment construction had a 50% to 70% decrease in glucocorticoid receptors as evidenced by a ligand binding assay with the type II glucocorticoid receptor-specific ligand ^{3}[H]-RU 28362 (20). The specificity of antisense RNA action can be seen by the failure of the glucocorticoid antisense RNA (pNFLAsGR) to inhibit mineralocorticoid receptor–mediated activation of MMTV-CAT in the presence of aldosterone (Fig. 2). The corticosteroid receptor antisense RNA used here specifically and effectively diminishes its cognate receptor production when transfected into cell lines. Its mechanism of action is not known with certainty, but the very low level of transgene transcripts in tissue extracts (20) together with the markedly reduced glucocorticoid receptor mRNA level sug-

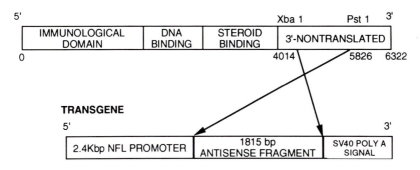

GR cDNA

Figure 1. Schematic representation of the structure and construction of the NFL-AsGR constructs used to direct the transcription of antisense RNA with a sequence complementary to that of regions of the mouse glucocorticoid recep- tor mRNA molecule. Plasmid NFL-AsGR was constructed by cloning a 1815 bp fragment of the 3' noncoding region of the rat glucocorticoid receptor cDNA in the reverse orientation downstream from the human neurofilament gene promoter. The plasmid containing the human neurofilament L gene promoter (pNF-L, gift of Dr. J. P. Julien) was linearized by digestion with Hind III, which cleaves at a sequence at the 3' end of the promoter. Extruding sequences were filled in with the Klenow fragment of DNA polymerase and a blunted Xba 1- Pst 1 fragment of the pSG-1 plasmid (gift of Dr. R. Miesfeld; this cDNA clone is a derivative of pRM16 [10]) was inserted into pNF-L in a reverse orientation. Finally, we added a Pst 1-Bam H1 fragment of the VP1 gene of SV40 that con- tains a polyadenylation signal. The glucocorticoid receptor cDNA sequence containing the least degree of homology with other steroid receptors (3' non- translated region) was used to generate antisense RNA and thus avoid cross inhibition of other steroid receptor activity.

gests that double-stranded sense:antisense RNA hybrids are formed and are rapidly degraded by nucleases.

Glucocorticoid Receptor Antisense RNA Transgenic Mouse

We have obtained transgenic mice following microinjection of the glu- cocorticoid receptor antisense gene into the pronucleus of fertilized oo- cytes obtained from superovulated prepubertal females (Fig. 3). The presence of the antisense construct in founder mice and their offspring was established by Southern blot analysis of DNA purified from the tail. Mice that were positive for integration of the chimæric NFL-AsGR served as founder animals for the development of individual transgenic

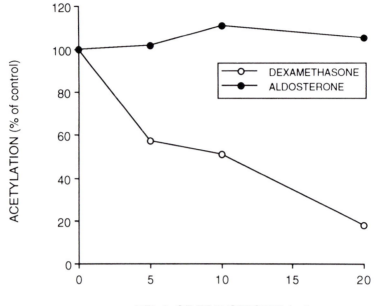

Figure 2. Specificity of inhibition of glucocorticoid receptor activity by anti-sense RNA. The promoter activity of the reporter plasmid (pMTVCAT) when transiently cotransfected with NFL-AsGR in LTK⁻ cells in the presence of dex-amethasone (0.1 µmol) or in CV1 cells in the presence of aldosterone (1 µmol) was determined. The recombinant DNA construct (NFL-AsGR, 0–20 µg) was precipitated with pRSV Lac Z (2.5 µg) and the reporter plasmid pMTVCAT (10 µg) and introduced for 5 hours into 2×10^6 LTK⁻ cells or for 14–16 hours into 1×10^6 CV1 cells. The mineralocorticoid receptor expression vector pRShMR (1µg) was also introduced into CV1 cells. Dexamethasone (LTK⁻ cells) or al-dosterone (CV1 cells) was added 24–48 hours after transfection, and the cells were harvested 24 hours later and assayed for CAT activity (at constant β-galactosidase activity for each CAT assay).

lines. Of the five founder mice that initially screened positive for the presence of the transgene (21), three have now been bred to homozy-gosity.

All three permanent transgenic lines established display a charac-teristic phenotype, the most remarkable aspect of which is a late onset development of marked obesity (Fig. 4). Transgenic animals have a greatly increased fat deposition and, at around 6 months of age, are as much as twice the weight of normal mice. This accumulation of fat in different adipose tissue regions is observed even though transgenic mice eat 15% less chow than do normal mice (22). Marked metabolic changes, which precede the development of overt obesity, are apparent in young transgenic animals. These include a significant increase in serum triglyceride concentrations and a decrease in energy expenditure, suggested by a decreased oxygen consumption, during the first hours of the dark phase of the diurnal cycle. The percentage of body fat is increased by 5%, with no change in body protein, and although lipoprotein lipase activity was significantly decreased in the heart and muscle of young animals, no decrease was seen in white adipose tissue. A tendency toward hyperinsulinemia was also noted as well as decreased noradrenergic activity of both heart and brown adipose tissue (22).

HPA Axis Regulation in Transgenic Mice

Effects of the antisense RNA on the level of glucocorticoid receptor mRNA in various tissues was measured by Northern blot analysis. Endogenous glucocorticoid receptor mRNA strands were detected in all tissue analyzed in transgenic mice. In different brain regions of the three different transgenic lines analyzed (hypothalamus, frontal cortex, hippocampus), we observed a maximal 50% to 70% decrease of the glucocorticoid receptor mRNA compared to controls. Although the transgene is not expressed in all tissues, some expression can be detected outside the central nervous system including the pituitary gland and, to a much lesser degree, in the liver (21). The 2.4 kb neurofilament promoter region used in these animals is thus not sufficient to generate complete tissue-specific expression, as has been noted in other transgenic mice incorporating this element (23).

The decreased glucocorticoid receptor mRNA concentrations were reflected by decreases in functional glucocorticoid binding activity. Scatchard analysis of glucocorticoid binding to hippocampal extracts showed fewer glucocorticoid receptor binding sites when compared to control mice (Fig. 4). The transgene incorporated into the genome was designed to disrupt normal HPA axis function, and this was found to be the case as evidenced by both elevated early morning adrenocorticotrophic hormone (ACTH) and corticosterone levels (Table 1). When measured in the afternoon or early evening, however, corticosterone and ACTH concentrations did not differ between control and trans-

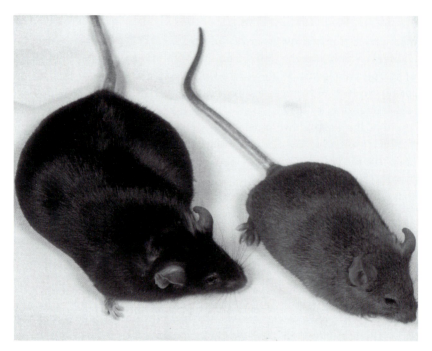

Figure 3. Transgenic mice expressing glucocorticoid receptor antisense RNA. Glucocorticoid receptor antisense transgenic mice (transgenic mouse, line 1.3, *left;* normal mouse, *right*) were produced by microinjection of a ≈4.9 kb Nde1-Ase1 fragment excised from pNFL-AsGR plasmid (see Fig. 1) into the male pronucleus of fertilized mouse oocytes obtained from superovulated prepubertal females (C3H X c57BL/6F2) 20 hours after treatment with human chorionic gonadotropin (45). The DNA fragment had been previously gel purified by filtration through an Elutip-D column (Schleicher and Schuel, Inc.) and its concentration adjusted to 3 µg/mL in 10 mmol Tris and 0.1 mmol EDTA. Injected embryos were reimplanted into pseudopregnant outbred CD1 females, and offspring were screened for transgene integration by tail blotting with ^{32}P-labeled probe. DNA was extracted from 1–2 cm tail pieces by incubating in 0.7 mL of 50 mmol tris hydrochloride-100 mmol EDTA, pH 8.0, 0.5% sodium dodecyl sulfate and 350 µg of proteinase K for 16 hours at 55° with agitation. DNA was phenol-chloroform extracted, ethanol precipitated, and resuspended in 10 mmol tris hydrochloride-1 mmol EDTA, pH 8.0. For Southern blot analysis (46), 15 µg of total genomic DNA of each mouse was digested with Bam H1, electrophoresed on 1.0% agarose gels, and transferred to nylon filters (Hybond N$^+$, Amersham). Filters were prehybridized for 2 hours at 42°C (in 50% formamide, 5X SSPE [1X SSPE is 0.15M NaCl, 0.01M NaH$_2$PO$_4$, 0.001M EDTA], 6X Denhardt's, 0.5% SDS, and 200µg/mL denatured salmon sperm DNA) and

(continued)

genic animals, and the typical pattern of diurnal secretion of these hormones was flattened in the transgenic mice. Characteristics similar to what we see in the transgenic animals (lower B_{max} for glucocorticoid binding with elevated serum corticosterone and ACTH concentrations) also have been reported (24), though not universally acclaimed (25), in the obese *fa/fa* Zucker rat. Besides causing alterations in the base-line levels of ACTH and corticosterone secretion patterns, the presence of the antisense RNA also rendered the transgenic mouse HPA axis less sensitive to glucocorticoid feedback inhibition (26). Although in normal mice injection of 1 μg/100g body weight of dexamethasone six hours prior to blood sampling was sufficient to completely suppress corticosterone levels, in transgenic mice a tenfold higher concentration was required to achieve the same effect (26).

Several antidepressant drugs have been shown to increase glucocorticoid receptor mRNA concentrations (27, 28), and we tested their effects on glucocorticoid receptor function by monitoring type II glucocorticoid receptor mRNA levels, type II glucocorticoid receptor binding activity, and HPA axis modification in the transgenic mice. Type II glucocorticoid receptor mRNA concentration, measured in the brain of normal or transgenic mice, was increased following antidepressant treatment. This increase in type II glucocorticoid receptor mRNA was translated into functional glucocorticoid receptors as shown by elevated type II glucocorticoid receptor binding activity in the brain of antidepressant-treated normal or transgenic mice (29). The correlation between glucocorticoid receptor mRNA levels and functional glucocorticoid binding activity in brain regions strongly suggests that antidepressants increase type II glucocorticoid receptor gene expression in vivo, as they have been shown to do in vitro (30). No significant change in the type II glucocorticoid receptor mRNA concentration and gluco-

---

hybridized overnight at 42°C to a ^{32}P-labeled Bam H1-Bam H1 fragment containing a part of both the NF-L promoter and the antisense glucocorticoid receptor cDNA fragment. After hybridization, filters were washed twice for 15 minutes each in 2XSSC with 0.5% SDS (sodium dodecyl sulfate) at room temperature, once for 30 minutes in 2X SSC (1X SSC is 0.15M NaCl, 0.015M sodium citrate), 0.5% SDS at 42°C, and once for 30 minutes in 0.1X SSC, 0.5% SDS at 65°C. Founder animals positive for transgene integration were bred as lines by mating first with (C3H X c57BL/6)F1 wild-type mice and subsequently as homozygotes. Homozygotic lines have been derived from three of the founder transgenic mice.

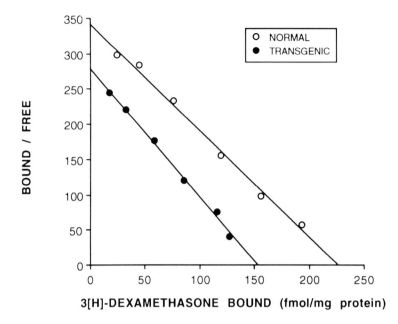

Figure 4. [³H]-dexamethasone binding activity of hippocampus in normal and transgenic mice. Scatchard plots of saturation binding data of normal (open symbols) and transgenic line 1.3 (full symbols) were performed with [³H]-dexamethasone binding data. Tissue was homogenized in 30 mmol Tris, 1 mmol EDTA, 10 mmol molybdate, 10% (v/v) glycerol, and 1 mmol dithiothreitol (TEDGM, pH 7.4). After centrifugation at 105 000g for 45 minutes at 0°C, an aliquot of the cytosol was incubated with [³H]-dexamethasone (Spec. act. 44.7 Ci/mmol, Amersham). Concentration range 1–25 nmol for Scatchard analysis (47) for 20–24 hours at 4°C. The amount of nonspecific binding was determined in parallel incubations of the labeled steroid in the presence of a 500-fold excess of unlabeled RU 28362. Sephadex LH20 (Pharmacia) columns equilibrated with TEDGM buffer were used to separate bound from unbound steroid. Following incubation, 100 µL aliquots of the incubates were loaded into the columns, washed with 100 µL of TEDGM, and eluted with 400 µL of TEDGM into minivials. The vials were then filled with 5 mL of aqueous counting cocktail Formula A-963 (New England Nuclear, Boston, MA) and counted in a LKB scintillation counter at 40% efficiency. Protein content was determined by the method of Bradford (48).

corticoid binding capacity of the liver of antidepressant-treated transgenic mice was observed (30). Finally, presumably as a result of increased glucocorticoid receptor binding activity in the brain, and more efficient glucocorticoid negative feedback action, a reduction in the

Table 1. Effects of Antidepressant Treatment on ACTH and Corticosterone Concentrations in Normal and Transgenic Mice

Animals	ACTH (pg/mL plasma)	Corticosterone (ng/mL plasma)
Normal mice	109 ± 14 (28)	42 ± 6 (28)
Normal mice/amitriptyline	129 ± 19 (29)	46 ± 7 (29)
Transgenic mice	198 ± 21 (29)	55 ± 13 (29)
Transgenic mice/amitriptyline	130 ± 16 (28)*	27 ± 3 (28)*

Hormone content of blood plasma from individual animals (n is shown in parentheses) was measured by specific radioimmunoassay using commercially available kits (ICN Biomedical Inc., USA). Where indicated, animals were treated with amitryptiline (10 mg/kg body weight) for three weeks prior to sacrifice. Results shown are the mean ± SEM. Differences between means were tested by the Duncan-Kramer (44) test after analysis of variance.
*$P < 0.05$ vs untreated transgenic mice.

HPA axis activity of transgenic mice, shown by decreased ACTH and corticosterone concentrations, was produced (Table 1). Longer-term treatment of transgenic animals with these same antidepressant drugs resulted in significant decreases in body weight (Fig. 5).

Discussion

Although introduction into eukaryotic cells of either antisense RNA or vectors expressing antisense RNA has been widely used to decrease the level of the final product of the complementary sense mRNA, only a limited success has been achieved with these same approaches in transgenic animals (16, 31). Although the reasons for this discrepancy are not clear, antisense RNA technology has been successfully used here to decrease the glucocorticoid receptor level in mouse tissues and to cause marked disturbance in HPA axis regulation. One consequence of this disturbance is an increased plasma ACTH concentration in transgenic animals that could reflect a failure of glucocorticoids to inhibit HPA axis activity at either or both central and pituitary sites. Disruption of the normal diurnal rhythm of ACTH and corticosterone secretion argues in favor of at least one site of action in the central nervous system. However, since glucocorticoid receptor concentrations are also decreased in the pituitary gland (21), it is possible that this represents an additional site at which glucocorticoid feedback inhibition of ACTH secretion could be affected. In these transgenic mice, morning ACTH

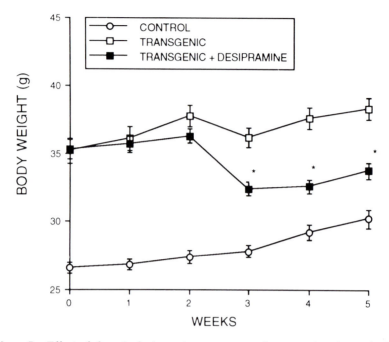

Figure 5.   Effect of chronic desipramine treatment of transgenic mice on body weight. Mice were injected intraperitoneally with desipramine (20 mg/kg body weight) once per day for up to five weeks. Results shown are the mean ± SEM (n = 8). Differences between means were tested by the Duncan-Kramer (44) test after analysis of variance.
$P < 0.01$ vs untreated transgenic mice.

concentrations are elevated to a greater degree than are morning corticosterone levels, suggesting that the adrenal gland may become refractory to continuous stimulation from ACTH. Glucocorticoids are known to decrease the number of their cognate receptors in both the hippocampus and the pituitary gland (32, 33). Thus the elevated corticosterone levels of the transgenic mice, which are secondary to decreased glucocorticoid receptor levels, could contribute to even further glucocorticoid receptor down-regulation. The development of obesity in these animals is of interest concerning the elevated corticosteroid concentrations. Although a role for glucocorticoids in the development of obesity and modification of glucocorticoid receptor concentrations in obese animals has been implied by numerous studies (25, 34–40) it has never been clear which of these two factors was initiative. In the present studies, animals were designed to have decreased glucocorticoid receptor concentrations, and changes in corticosteroid levels are secondary to this modification. Hyperinsulinemia is usually seen in obese animals and the transgenic mice also have an inclination toward this disposition. In this respect it is of interest that similar changes to what we see in the transgenic mice, including decreased levels of brain glucocorticoid receptors, are reported in the genetically diabetic (*mdb/mdb*) mouse (41).

Hypothalamus-pituitary-adrenal axis dysfunction is frequently seen in patients with major depression (42), and defective glucocorticoid feedback inhibition is the principal event that could explain this pathophysiology. Antidepressant drugs have been shown to increase corticosteroid receptor concentrations (27, 28), and chronic treatment of transgenic animals with desipramine can normalize not only the HPA axis of these animals but also weight gain. At the present time the mechanism of action of antidepressant drugs is not clear. However, it is of interest that fenfluramine, frequently used as an anorexic agent in the treatment of obesity, has certain characteristics in common with antidepressant agents including blockade of serotonin reuptake (43). It is thus possible that the action of this drug on the HPA axis also stems from a decrease in glucocorticoid receptor concentrations.

In conclusion, the animals we have developed with defective glucocorticoid receptor regulation have important changes in the HPA axis. These endocrine modifications lead to secondary changes in behavior and several other systems including the immune system, energy balance, and lipid metabolism. These animals may be important, not only for the investigation of the role of corticosteroid receptors in the regulation of HPA axis activity, but also for studies on the role of corticosteroids in the etiology of obesity.

ACKNOWLEDGMENTS

This work was supported in part by grants from the Medical Research Council of Canada and the Stanley Foundation.

REFERENCES

1. Funder JW, Sheppard K. Adrenocortical steroids and the brain. *Annu Rev Physiol.* 1987;49:397–411.

2. Yukimura Y, Bray GA, Wolfsen AR. Some effects of adrenalectomy in the fatty rat. *Endocrinology.* 1978;103:1924–1928.

3. Fletcher JM. Effects of adrenalectomy before weaning in the genetically obese Zucker rat *(fa/fa). Br J Nutr.* 1986;56:141–151.

4. Freedman MR, Horwitz BA, Stern JS. Effects of adrenalectomy and glucocorticoid replacement on development of obesity. *Am J Physiol.* 1986;250:R595–R607.

5. Debons AF, Zurek LD, Tse CS, Abrahamsem S. Central nervous system control of hyperphagia in hypothalamic obesity: dependence on adrenal glucocorticoids. *Endocrinology.* 1986;118:1678–1681.

6. Castonguay TW. Glucocorticoids as modulators in the control of feeding. *Brain Res Bull.* 1991;27:423–428.

7. Dubuc PU. Interactions between insulin and glucocorticoids in the maintenance of genetic obesity. *Am J Physiol.* 1992;263:E550–E555.

8. Wrange O, Okret S, Radojéiè M, Carlstedt-Duke C, Gustafsson J-Å. Characterization of the purified activated glucocorticoid receptor from rat liver cytosol. *J Biol Chem.* 1984;259:4534–4541.

9. Wrange O, Carlstedt-Duke C, Gustafsson J-Å. Purification of the glucocorticoid receptor from rat liver cytosol. *J Biol Chem.* 1979;254:9284–9290.

10. Miesfeld R, Okret S, Wikström A-C, Wrange O, Gustafsson J-Å, Yamamoto KR. Characterization of a steroid hormone receptor gene and mRNA in wild-type and mutant cells. *Nature.* 1984;312:779–781.

11. Miesfeld R, Rusconi S, Godowski PJ, *et al.* Genetic complementation of a glucocorticoid receptor deficiency by expression of cloned receptor cDNA. *Cell.* 1986;46:389–399.

12. Hollenberg SM, Weinberger C, Ong ES, *et al.* Primary structure and expression of a functional human glucocorticoid receptor cDNA. *Nature.* 1985;318:635–641.

13. Arriza JL, Simerly RB, Swanson LW, Evans RM. The neuronal mineralocorticoid receptor as a mediator of glucocorticoid response. *Neuron.* 1988;1:887–900.

14. Gustafsson J-Å, Carlstedt-Duke J, Poellinger L, *et al.* Biochemistry, molecular biology, and physiology of the glucocorticoid receptor. *Endocr Rev.* 1987;8:185–234.

15. Bradbury MJ, Strack AM, Dallman MF. Lesions of the hippocampal efferent pathway (fimbria-fornix) do not alter sensitivity of adre-

nocorticotropin to feedback inhibition by corticosterone in rats. *Neuroendocrinology.* 1993;58:396–407.

16. Katsuki M, Sato M, Kimura M, Yofohama M, Kobayashi K, Nomura T. Conversion of normal behavior to shiverer by myelin basic protein antisense cDNA in transgenic mice. *Science.* 1988;241:593–595.

17. Izant JG, Weintraub H. Constitutive and conditional suppression of exogenous genes by anti-sense RNA. *Science.* 1985;229:345–351.

18. Kim SK, Wold BJ. Stable reduction of thymidine kinase activity in cells expressing high levels of anti-sense RNA. *Cell.* 1985;42:129–138.

19. McGarry TJ, Lindquist S. Inhibition of heat shock protein synthesis by heat-inductible antisense RNA. *Proc Natl Acad Sci USA.* 1986;83:399–403.

20. Pepin M-C, Barden N. Decreased glucocorticoid receptor activity following glucocorticoid receptor antisense RNA gene fragment transfection. *Mol Cell Biol.* 1991;11:1647–1653.

21. Pepin M-C, Pothier F, Barden N. Impaired type II glucocorticoid receptor function in transgenic mice expressing antisense RNA. *Nature.* 1992;355:725–728.

22. Richard D, Chapdelaine S, Deshaies Y, Pepin M-C, Barden N. Energy balance and lipid metabolism in transgenic mice bearing an antisense glucocorticoid receptor gene construct. *Am J Physiol.* 1993;265:R146–R150.

23. Julien J-P, Beaudet L, Tretjakoff I, Peterson A. Neurofilament gene expression in transgenic mice. *J Physiol (Paris).* 1990;84:50–52.

24. Douglas White B, Martin RJ. Alterations in the binding characteristics of glucocorticoid receptors from obese Zucker rats. *J Steroid Biochem.* 1990;36:681–686.

25. Langley SC, York DA. Increased type II glucocorticoid-receptor numbers and glucocorticoid-sensitive enzyme activities in the brain of the obese Zucker rat. *Brain Res.* 1990;533:268–274.

26. Stec I, Barden N, Reul JMHM, Holsboer F. Dexamethasone non-suppression in transgenic mice expressing antisense RNA to the glucocorticoid receptor. *J Psychiatr Res.* 1994;28:1–5.

27. Pepin M-C, Beaulieu S, Barden N. Antidepressants regulate glucocorticoid receptor messenger RNA concentrations in primary neural cultures. *Mol Brain Res.* 1989;6:77–83.

28. Peiffer A, Veilleux S, Barden N. Antidepressant and other centrally-

acting drugs regulate glucocorticoid receptor messenger RNA levels in rat brain. *Psychoneuroendocrinology.* 1991;16:505–515.

29. Pepin M-C, Pothier F, Barden N. Antidepressant drug action in a transgenic mouse model of the endocrine changes seen in depression. *Mol Pharmacol.* 1992;42:991–995.

30. Pepin M-C, Govindan MV, Barden N. Increased glucocorticoid receptor gene promoter activity following antidepressant treatment. *Mol Pharmacol.* 1992;41:1016–1022.

31. Munir MI, Rossiter BJF, Caskey CT. Antisense RNA production in transgenic mice. *Somatic Cell Mol Genet.* 1990;16:383–394.

32. Svec F, Rudis M. Glucocorticoids regulate the glucocorticoid receptors in the AtT-20 cell. *J Biol Chem.* 1981;256:5984–5987.

33. Tornello S, Orti E, DeNicola AF, Rainbow TC, McEwen BS. Regulation of glucocorticoid receptor in brain by corticosterone treatment of adrenalectomized rats. *Neuroendocrinology.* 1982;35:411–417.

34. Langley SC, York DA. Glucocorticoid receptor numbers in the brain and liver of the obese Zucker rat. *Int J Obes.* 1992;16:135–143.

35. Langley SC, York DA. Effects of antiglucocorticoid RU 486 on development of obesity in obese *fa/fa* Zucker rats. *Am J Physiol.* 1990; 259:R539–R544.

36. Guillaume-Gentil C, Rohner-Jeanrenaud F, Abramo F, Bestetti GE, Rossi GL, Jeanrenaud B. Abnormal regulation of the hypothalamo-pituitary-adrenal axis in the genetically obese *fa/fa* rat. *Endocrinology.* 1990;126:1873–1888.

37. King BM. Glucocorticoids and hypothalamic obesity. *Neurosci Biobehav Rev.* 1988;12:29–37.

38. McGinnis R, Walker J, Margules D. Genetically obese (*ob/ob*) mice are hypersensitive to glucocorticoid stimulation of feeding but dramatically resist glucocorticoid-induced weight loss. *Life Sci.* 1987; 40:1561–1570.

39. Plotsky PM, Thrivikraman KV, Watts AG, Hauger RL. Hypothalamic-pituitary-adrenal axis function in the Zucker obese rat. *Endocrinology.* 1992;130:1931–1941.

40. Tsai HJ, Romsos DR. Glucocorticoid and mineralocorticoid receptor-binding characteristics in obese (*ob/ob*) mice. *Am J Physiol Endocrinol Metab.* 1991;261:E495–E499.

41. Webb ML, Flynn JJ, Schmidt TJ, Margules DL, Litwack G. Decreased glucocorticoid binding and receptor activation in brain of

gentically diabetic (*mdb/mdb*) mice. *J Steroid Biochem.* 1986;25:649–657.

42. Holsboer F, Spengler D, Heuser I. The role of corticotropin-releasing hormone in the pathogenesis of Cushing's disease, anorexia nervosa, alcoholism, affective disorders and dementia. *Prog Brain Res.* 1992;93:385–417.

43. Brindley DN. Neuroendocrine regulation and obesity. *Int J Obes.* 1992;16:S73–S79.

44. Kramer CY. Extension of multiple range tests to group means with unequal number of replications. *Biometrics.* 1956;12:307–310.

45. Hogan B, Costantini F, Lacy E. *Manipulating the Mouse Embryo: A Laboratory Manual.* Cold Spring Harbor, NY: Cold Spring Harbor Laboratory Press; 1986:153–186.

46. Southern EM. Detection of specific sequences among DNA fragments separated by gel electrophoresis. *J Mol Biol.* 1975;98:503–517.

47. Scatchard G. The attractions of proteins for small molecules and ions. *Ann NY Acad Sci.* 1949;51:660.

48. Bradford MM. A rapid method for quantification of microgram quantities of protein utilizing the principle of protein-dye binding. *Anal Biochem.* 1976;72:248–254.

Contributors to Volume 5

GÉRARD AILHAUD
Centre de Biochimie UMR 134 CNRS
Université de Nice-Sophia Antipolis
Faculté des Sciences
Parc Valrose
06108 Nice cédex 2
France

AKIRA AKABAYASHI
Rockefeller University
1230 York Avenue
New York, NY 10021

PETER ARNER
Karolinska Institute
Department of Medicine
Huddinge University Hospital
S-141 86 Huddinge (Stockholm)
Sweden

MELISSA A. AUSTIN
University of Washington
Department of Epidemiology
Box 357236
Seattle, WA 98195

NICOLAS BARDEN
Molecular Psychogenetics
CHUL
2705 Blvd. Laurier
Ste-Foy, Quebec GIV 4G2
Canada

RAYMOND BAZIN
INSERM U 177
15 rue de l'Ecole de Medecine
75270 Paris Cedex 06
France

PHILIP BEALES
Medical Unit
Royal London Hospital
Whitechapel
London, E1 1BB
United Kingdom

NICOLE BÉGIN-HEICK
Department of Biochemistry
University of Ottawa
Ottawa, Ontario KIH M5
Canada

HANS-RUDOLF BERTHOUD
Pennington Biomedical Research
    Center
6400 Perkins Road
Baton Rouge, LA 70808

PER BJÖRNTORP
Department of Heart and Lung
    Diseases
Sahlgren's Hospital
University of Göteborg
S-413 45 Göteborg
Sweden

JUAN J. BONAVERA
Department of Physiology
College of Medicine
University of Florida
Gainesville, FL 32610

CLAUDE BOUCHARD
Physical Activity Sciences
    Laboratory
Laval University
Ste-Foy, Québec
G1K 7P4
Canada

FRÉDÉRIC BOUILLAUD
CNRS/CEREMOD
9 rue Jules Hetzel
92190 Meudon
France

ANNE BOULOUMIÉ
Unité INSERM 317
Institut Louis Bugnard
CHU Rangueil
Bât. L3
31054 Toulouse Cedex
France

BERT B. BOYER
Jackson Laboratory
600 Main Street
Bar Harbor, Maine 04609

GEORGE A. BRAY
Pennington Biomedical Research
    Center
6400 Perkins Road
Baton Rouge, LA 70808

H. DOUGLAS BRAYMER
Pennington Biomedical Research
    Center
6400 Perkins Road
Baton Rouge, LA 70808

DAVID N. BRINDLEY
328 Heritage Medical Research
    Centre
Lipid and Lipoprotein Research
    Group
University of Alberta
Edmonton, Alberta
T6G 2S2 Canada

JOHN D. BRUNZELL
University of Washington School of
    Medicine
Department of Medicine, Box 356426
Division of Metabolism,
    Endocrinology, and Nutrition
Seattle, WA 98195

TRUDY L. BURNS
Department of Preventive Medicine
    and Environmental Health
College of Medicine
2800 Steindler Building
University of Iowa
Iowa City, IA 52242

CHRISTIAN CARPÉNÉ
Unité INSERM 317
Institut Louis Bugnard
CHU Rangueil
Bât. L3
31054 Toulouse Cedex
France

ANNE-MARIE CASSARD-
    DOULCIER
CNRS/CEREMOD
9 rue Jules Hetzel
92190 Meudon
France

ISABELLE CASTAN
Unité INSERM 317
Institut Louis Bugnard
CHU Rangueil
Bât. L3
31054 Toulouse Cedex
France

ODETTE CHAMPIGNY
CNRS/CEREMOD
9 rue Jules Hetzel
92190 Meudon
France

GEORGE CLARKE
Jackson Laboratory
600 Main Street
Bar Harbor, ME 04609

JOHN D. DAVIS
Department of Psychiatry
Cornell University Medical College
  and Bourne Behavioral Research
  Laboratory
New York Hospital—Cornell
  Medical Center
Westchester Division
21 Bloomingdale Road
White Plains, NY 10605

DANIEL J. DRISCOLL
Division of Genetics
Department of Pediatrics, College of
  Medicine
University of Florida
Gainesville, FL 32610

MICHAEL G. DUBE
Department of Neuroscience
College of Medicine
University of Florida
Gainesville, FL 32610

ISABELLE DUGAIL
INSERM U 177
15 rue de l'Ecole de Medecine
75270 Paris Cedex 06
France

SVEN ENERBÄCK
University of Göteborg
Department of Molecular Biology
Medicinareg
S-431 69 Göteborg
Sweden

JANIS S. FISLER
Division of Cardiology, 47-123 CHS
UCLA Medical Center
10833 Le Conte Avenue
Los Angeles, CA 90095-1679

JEFFREY S. FLIER
Charles A. Dana Research Institute
  and the Harvard-Thorndike
  Laboratory of Beth Israel Hospital
Department of Medicine
Beth Israel Hospital and Harvard
  Medical School
Boston, MA 02215

JEFFREY M. FRIEDMAN
Howard Hughes Medical Institute
The Rockefeller University
1230 York Avenue
New York, NY 10021

MARK I. FRIEDMAN
Monell Chemical Senses Center
3500 Market Street
Philadelphia, PA 19104

WILFRED Y. FUJIMOTO
University of Washington School of
  Medicine
Department of Medicine, Box 356426
Division of Metabolism,
  Endocrinology, and Nutrition
Seattle, WA 98195

CHANTAL GELLY
CNRS/CEREMOD
9 rue Jules Hetzel
92190 Meudon
France

CHRISTOPHER C. GLENN
Division of Genetics
Department of Pediatrics, College of
  Medicine
University of Florida
Gainesville, FL 32610

LUIGI GNUDI
Department of Medicine
Beth Israel Hospital and Harvard
  Medical School
Boston, MA 02215

JO GOUDEY-LEFEVRE
Pennington Biomedical Research
  Center
6400 Perkins Road
Baton Rouge, LA 70808

DANIELLE GREENBERG
Department of Psychiatry
Cornell University Medical College
  and Bourne Behavioral Research
  Laboratory
New York Hospital-Cornell Medical
  Center
Westchester Division
21 Bloomingdale Road
White Plains, NY 10605

PAUL GRIMALDI
Centre de Biochimie UMR 134 CNRS
Université de Nice-Sophia Antipolis
Faculté des Sciences
Parc Valrose
06108 Nice cédex 2
France

MICHÈLE GUERRE-MILLO
INSERM U 177
15 rue de l'Ecole de Medecine
75270 Paris Cedex 06
France

ISABELLE HAINAULT
INSERM U 177
15 rue de l'Ecole de Medecine
75270 Paris Cedex 06
France

ERIC HAJDUCH
INSERM U 177
15 rue de l'Ecole de Medecine
75270 Paris Cedex 06
France

ANDREAS HAMANN
Charles A. Dana Research Institute
  and the Harvard-Thorndike
  Laboratory of Beth Israel Hospital
Department of Medicine
Beth Israel Hospital and Harvard
  Medical School
Boston, MA 02215

LUIS HERNANDEZ
University of Los Andes
Merida, Venezuela

JEAN HIMMS-HAGEN
Department of Biochemistry
Faculty of Medicine
University of Ottawa
Ottawa, Ontario K1H 8M5
Canada

GRAHAM HITMAN
Medical Unit
Royal London Hospital
Whitechapel
London, E1 1BB
United Kingdom

BARTLEY G. HOEBEL
Department of Psychology
Green Hall
Princeton University
Princeton, NJ 08544-1010

GÖKHAN S. HOTAMISLIGIL
Harvard School of Public Health
Department of Nutrition
665 Huntington Ave.
Boston, MA 02115

MICHELLE T. C. JONG
Division of Genetics
Department of Pediatrics, College of
  Medicine
University of Florida
Gainesville, FL 32610

BARBARA B. KAHN
Diabetes Unit
Beth Israel Hospital
330 Brookline Ave.
Boston, MA 02215

PUSHPA S. KALRA
Department of Physiology
College of Medicine
University of Florida
Gainesville, FL 32610

SATYA P. KALRA
Department of Neuroscience
College of Medicine
University of Florida
P.O. Box 100244
Gainesville, FL 32610-0244

SUSANNE KLAUS
CNRS/CEREMOD
9 rue Jules Hetzel
92190 Meudon
France

MITCHELL L. KLEBIG
University of Tennessee Medical
    Center
Human Immunology and Cancer
    Program
Box 2, Room 231
1924 Alcoa Highway
Knoxville, TN 37920-6999

JAN KOPECKY
Institute of Physiology
Czech Academy of Sciences
Prague, Czech Republic

PETER KOPELMAN
Medical Unit
Royal London Hospital
Whitechapel
London, E1 1BB
United Kingdom

LESLIE KOZAK
Jackson Laboratory
600 Main Street
Bar Harbor, ME 04609

ULRIKE KOZAK
Jackson Laboratory
600 Main Street
Bar Harbor, ME 04609

MAX LAFONTAN
Unité INSERM 317
Institut Louis Bugnard
CHU Rangueil
Bât. L3
31054 Toulouse Cedex
France

MARIANNE LAROSE
CNRS/CEREMOD
9 rue Jules Hetzel
92190 Meudon
France

DOMINIQUE LARROUY
Unité INSERM 317
Institut Louis Bugnard
CHU Rangueil
Bât. L3
31054 Toulouse Cedex
France

RONALD M. LAUER
Departments of Pediatrics,
    Preventive Medicine, and
    Environmental Health
College of Medicine
University of Iowa
Iowa City, IA 52242

MARCELLE LAVAU
INSERM U 177
15 rue de l'Ecole de Medecine
75270 Paris Cedex 06
France

JOEL A. LAWITTS
Department of Pathology
Beth Israel Hospital and Harvard
    Medical School
Boston, MA 02215

SARAH FRYER LEIBOWITZ
Rockefeller University
1230 York Avenue
New York, NY 10021

CORINNE LEVI-MEYRUEIS
CNRS/CEREMOD
9 rue Jules Hetzel
92190 Meudon
France

LING LIN
Pennington Biomedical Research
    Center
6400 Perkins Road
Baton Rouge, LA 70808

BRADFORD B. LOWELL
Charles A. Dana Research Institute
    and the Harvard-Thorndike
    Laboratory of Beth Israel Hospital
Department of Medicine
Beth Israel Hospital and Harvard
    Medical School
Boston, MA 02215

GREGORY P. MARK
Princeton University
Princeton, NJ 08544-1010

MARIA J. MASCARI
Medical Genetics Resources, Inc.
5400 Chambershill Road
Harrisburg, PA 17111

BRUNO MIROUX
CNRS/CEREMOD
9 rue Jules Hetzel
92190 Meudon
France

LAURA E. MITCHELL
St. Louis University
School of Public Health
3663 Lindell Blvd.
St. Louis, MO 63108

PATRICIA PEYSER MOLL
Department of Epidemiology
School of Public Health
University of Michigan
Ann Arbor, MI 48109

RAYMOND NEGREL
Centre de Biochimie UMR 134 CNRS
Université de Nice-Sophia Antipolis
Faculté des Sciences
Parc Valrose
06108 Nice cédex 2
France

DAVID N. NEVIN
University of Washington School of
    Medicine
Department of Medicine, Box 356426
Division of Metabolism,
    Endocrinology, and Nutrition
Seattle, WA 98195

ROBERT D. NICHOLLS
Department of Genetics
Case Western Reserve University
10900 Euclid Ave.
Cleveland, OH 44106-4955

MARCO PARADA
University of Los Andes
Merida, Venezuela

MARINA PUIG DE PARADA
University of Los Andes
Merida, Venezuela

EMMANUEL POTHOS
Princeton University
Princeton, NJ 08544-1010

R. ARLEN PRICE
Department of Psychiatry
University of Pennsylvania
415 Curie Blvd. CRB-145B
Philadelphia, PA 19104-6140

ANNIE QUIGNARD-BOULANGÉ
INSERM U 177
15 rue de l'Ecole de Medecine
75270 Paris Cedex 06
France

PEDRO RADA
University of Los Andes
Merida, Venezuela

SERGE RAIMBAULT
CNRS/CEREMOD
9 rue Jules Hetzel
92190 Meudon
France

TIMOTHY G. RAMSAY
Pennington Biomedical Research
    Center
6400 Perkins Road
Baton Rouge, LA 70808

D. C. RAO
Washington University School of
    Medicine
Division of Biostatistics
Box 8067
660 South Euclid Avenue
St. Louis, MO 63110

NANCY E. RAWSON
Monell Chemical Senses Center
3500 Market Street
Philadelphia, PA 19104

DANIEL RICQUIER
CNRS/CEREMOD
9 rue Jules Hetzel
92190 Meudon
France

VIOLAINE ROLLAND
INSERM U 177
15 rue de l'Ecole de Medecine
75270 Paris Cedex 06
France

ABHIRAM SAHU
Department of Neuroscience
College of Medicine
University of Florida
Gainesville, FL 32610

SHINJI SAITOH
Department of Pediatrics
Hokkaido University School of
    Medicine
Kita 15
Nishi 17
Kita-Ku Sapporo 060
Japan

JEAN-SEBASTIEN SAULNIER-
    BLACHE
Unité INSERM 317
Institut Louis Bugnard
CHU Rangueil
Bât. L3
31054 Toulouse Cedex
France

ROBERT S. SCHWARTZ
University of Washington School of
    Medicine
Department of Medicine
Harborview Medical Center
Gerontology and Geriatric Medicine
Seattle, WA 98104

PETER L. SHEPHERD
Department of Medicine
Beth Israel Hospital and Harvard
    Medical School
Boston, MA 02215

GERARD P. SMITH
Department of Psychiatry
Cornell University Medical College
    and Bourne Behavioral Research
    Laboratory
New York Hospital-Cornell Medical
    Center
Westchester Division
21 Bloomingdale Road
White Plains, NY 10605

THORKILD IA SØRENSEN
Institute of Preventive Medicine
Copenhagen Hospital Corporation
Kommunehospitalet
DK-1399 Copenhagen
Denmark

BRUCE M. SPIEGELMAN
Dana Farber Cancer Institute and
    Department of Cell Biology
Harvard Medical School
Boston, MA 02115

A. DONNY STROSBERG
Laboratoire
    d'ImmunoPharmacologie
    Moléculaire
Institut Cochin de Génétique
    Moléculaire
75014 Paris
France

VEDRANA S. SUSULIC
Charles A. Dana Research Institute
    and the Harvard-Thorndike
    Laboratory of Beth Israel Hospital
Department of Medicine
Beth Israel Hospital and Harvard
    Medical School
Boston, MA 02215

MICHAEL G. TORDOFF
Monell Chemical Senses Center
3500 Market Street
Philadelphia, PA 19104

EFFIE TOZZO
Department of Medicine
Beth Israel Hospital and Harvard
   Medical School
Boston, MA 02215

GARY E. TRUETT
Pennington Biomedical Research
   Center
6400 Perkins Road
Baton Rouge, LA 70808

PHILIPPE VALET
Unité INSERM 317
Institut Louis Bugnard
CHU Rangueil
Bât. L3
31054 Toulouse Cedex
France

SHANTI VIJAYARAGHAVAN
Medical Unit
Royal London Hospital
Whitechapel
London, E1 1BB
United Kingdom

CHEUN-NEU WANG
328 Heritage Medical Research
   Centre
Lipid and Lipoprotein Research
   Group
University of Alberta
Edmonton, Alberta
T6G 2S2 Canada

YIBING WANG
Pennington Biomedical Research
   Center
6400 Perkins Road
Baton Rouge, LA 70808

CRAIG H. WARDEN
Division of Cardiology, 47-123 CHS
UCLA Medical Center
10833 Le Conte Avenue
Los Angeles, CA 90024-1679

DAVID S. WEIGLE
Endocrinology, Box 359757
Harborview Medical Center
325 Ninth Ave.
Seattle, WA 98104

DAVID B. WEST
Pennington Biomedical Research
   Center
6400 Perkins Road
Baton Rouge, LA 70808

J. E. WILKINSON
Department of Pathobiology
College of Veterinary Medicine
University of Tennessee
Knoxville, TN 37916

HUIJUN WONG
Pennington Biomedical Research
   Center
6400 Perkins Road
Baton Rouge, LA 70808

R. P. WOYCHIK
Biology Division
Oak Ridge National Laboratory
P.O. Box 2009
Oak Ridge, TN 37831-8077

BARBARA YORK
Pennington Biomedical Research
   Center
6400 Perkins Road
Baton Rouge, LA 70808

DAVID A. YORK
Pennington Biomedical Research
   Center
6400 Perkins Road
Baton Rouge, LA 70808

Index

Accumbens
  dopamine release in, 263–76
Adenosine, 421, 422, 423, 438
  and adenylyl cyclase, 425, 426
  antilipolytic effects of, 442, 444–45
  and antilipolysis, 420, 426, 428
  and fattening, 429
  and lipolysis, 416, 418–19
Adenosine A1-receptor(s), 423, 430
  and antilipolysis, 416, 418, 421
Adenosine A2-receptor, 421–22
Adenosine deaminase, 418, 419, 425, 478
Adenosine triphosphate (ATP), 318, 327–30, 331, 618
Adenylyl cyclase
  and adrenalectomy, 193, 194
  and β-adrenergic agonists, 189–90
  and β-adrenergic receptors, 404, 405, 407, 410
  effect of guanosine triphosphate (GTP) on, 191–92
  fat cell, 431–32
  in fat deposits, 427–28
  and G proteins, 419–20, 424–25, 426
  inhibition of, 416, 419, 421, 425
  and lipolysis, 418, 419, 424
  in *ob/ob* mice, 186, 187, 194
  and sex steroids, 428
Adipocytes, 177, 550, 581
  and regulation of body-fat mass, 548, 556
  See also Fat cell(s)
Adipose tissue
  abdominal, 344
  and α_2-adrenoceptors, 427–31
  and β-adrenergic receptors, 411, 412
  candidate genes for human obesity from, 546–57

distribution phenotypes in the Québec Family Study, 477
and fat depots, 417
fatty acids from, 340
function of, 582
G-protein levels in the *db/db* mouse, 188–89
heterogeneity of obesity and metabolism of, 443–44
and insulin-like growth factors, 373–97
and lipid and lipoprotein metabolism, 342
and lipolysis, 438, 444–45
lipoprotein lipase, 561, 563
mouse, 189–91, 193
of obese rats, 177–80
and obesity, 206
of the *ob/ob* mouse, 186, 187
overexpression of GLUT4 in, 624–33
site-specific properties of, 417
and stress, 527
in the study of fat cell function, 417
from subcutaneous depots, 432
TNF-α from, 206–208, 212
triglyceride(s) in, 439, 523, 524
and uncoupling protein (UCP) expression, 588
visceral, 516–17, 522, 523
of Zucker rats, 180–81
See also Body fat; Brown adipose tissue (BAT); Fat(s)
Adrenal steroids, 35, 37, 39
  and β-adrenoreceptor function in obesity, 192–93
  and neuropeptides, 11, 238–39

661